TEXTBOOK OF DERMATOLOGY

VOLUME 3

NEOPLASTIC, OCCUPATIONAL, AESTHETIC, AND EMERGENCY DERMATOLOGIC DISORDERS

Dr. Mariya Kharodawala

ALLIED HEALTH PRESS

Textbook of Dermatology

Volume 3: Neoplastic, Occupational, Aesthetic, and Emergency Dermatologic Disorders

Author: **Dr. Mariya Kharodawala**

Allied Health Press
4164 Lakeshore Road
Burlington ON L7L 1A4
Canada
www.alliedhealthpress.com
Email: orders@arclereducation.com

ISBN: 978-1-77956-827-4

Allied Health Press publishes wide variety of books and eBooks. For more information about Allied Health Press and its products, visit our website at www.alliedhealthpress.com

ABOUT THE AUTHOR

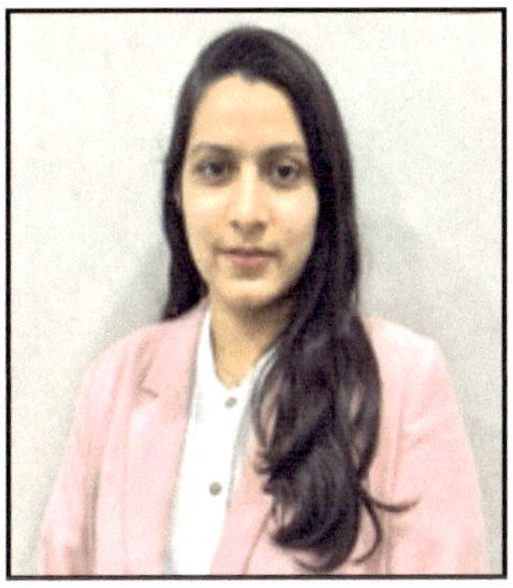

Dr. Mariya Kharodawala holds an MBBS degree with a gold medal from The Maharaja Sayajirao University of Baroda and an MD in Dermatology, Venereology, and Leprosy from B. J. Medical College, Pune, both of which are among the premier medical institutes in India. She is currently working as a Senior Resident in Dermatology. Her areas of interest include clinical dermatology, dermatopathology, and academic writing. Over the years, she has contributed to peer-reviewed journals and actively participated in national and international conferences. Her professional journey is driven by a passion for continuous learning, research, and teaching. Alongside her academic pursuits, she is committed to bridging the gap between medical knowledge and public awareness through digital platforms. Reviewing this comprehensive dermatology textbook has been an intellectually rewarding experience, and she is delighted to contribute to the academic growth of future dermatologists.

Brief Table of Contents

Chapter Openers

A list of Chapter Outline is presented providing a brief Introduction to what will be covered in the chapter.

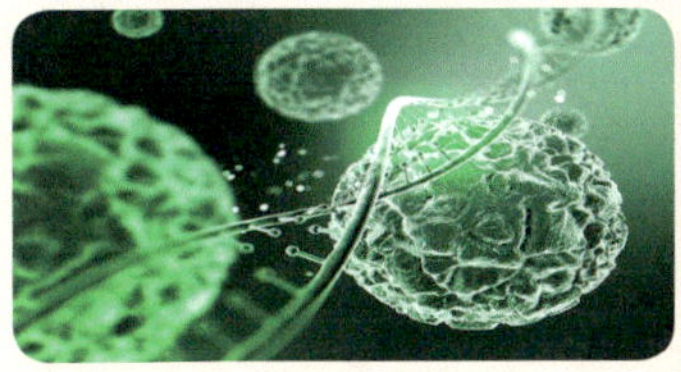

LEARNING OBJECTIVES

After studying this chapter, you will be able to:

1. Discuss the scientific method in biology;
2. Explain the cell theory;
3. Discuss the genetics and heredity;
4. Evolution and natural selection;
5. Focus on ecology and ecosystems;
6. Learn about human biology;
7. Evaluate the plant biology;
8. Explain the microbiology;
9. Focus on current trends in biology.

Introduction

Often referred to as the science of life, biology is a broad field of study aimed at comprehending the several kinds of life on Earth, from tiny creatures to sophisticated multicellular entities. Comprising several subfields, including molecular biology, ecology, and evolutionary biology, each of which advances our knowledge of living systems, this field clarifies the mechanisms controlling life events, including development, reproduction, and interaction with the surroundings, which is the central goal of biology. Moreover, biology fills in the void between the natural sciences and medicine by offering a necessary understanding of health, illness, and the interactions between organisms and their environments. Dealing with urgent global issues such as climate change, biodiversity loss, and new diseases depends on an awareness of these complex biological interactions, therefore highlighting the critical part biology plays in modern civilization. Fundamentally, biology explores and tests ideas about the living world using the scientific method. Through methodical observation and experimentation,

1.1. The Scientific Method in Biology

Learning Outcome

1. Describe the steps of the scientific method;
2. Focus on hypothesis formation;
3. Learn about experimental design.

Learning Outcomes

The beginning of each section of every chapter contains a set of Learning Outcomes that inform students of concepts they should understand. These outcomes help students understand what they should be able to do if they have mastered the material in that section.

Test Your Knowledge

Throughout each chapter, Test Your Knowledge cues you to note which topics have been covered and to self-test your understanding of the material presented.

Test Your Knowledge

1. Explain why correlation does not imply causation in scientific experiments.
2. How does the scientific method help reduce the influence of personal opinions in research?

Chapter Summary

The Summary Section appear at the end of each chapter and summarize main concepts covered throughout the chapter. These points provide key concepts in an engaging and meaningful way.

Summary

The investigation of biological principles highlights the importance of a comprehensive view of life by reflecting the intricate interactions that occur within living systems. The complexity of biology goes beyond individual species or systems, as this essay highlights; it also includes the interactions that mold ecosystems and affect biodiversity. Researchers can conduct in-depth analyses of metabolomic data using sophisticated technologies like MetaboAnalyst, which offer insights into the molecular mechanisms underlying these interactions. As demonstrated by the developments in MetaboAnalyst, for example, the integration of diverse omics data promotes a thorough understanding of metabolic pathways and helps identify important biological markers necessary for research on development and disease (Chong et al., 2018). Additionally, the phenomenon of ecological invasions is a key component of biological research and a vital field of study. The introduction of non-native species into unfamiliar habitats has significant ramifications and calls for multidisciplinary management strategies. Examining the origins and effects of these biological incursions, invasion science has become a crucial field that highlights the need to comprehend ecological dynamics and community interactions. As interest in biological invasions increases, new findings are emerging that put conventional ecological theories and practices to the test. The importance of incorporating various scientific viewpoints is shown by this developing discipline, which also highlights how invasive species shape ecosystems and advances our knowledge of ecological resilience (David et al., 2013). When taken as a whole, these discoveries from invasion science and metabolomics highlight the value of multidisciplinary biology research. Fostering cross-disciplinary collaboration and utilizing technological breakthroughs to improve our comprehension of intricate biological interactions are crucial as we look to the future of biological research. In addition to deepening our understanding of the complexities of life, this method lays the groundwork for tackling urgent environmental issues. Future studies can ensure the continued relevance of biology in a world that is constantly changing by acknowledging the interconnection of biological systems and opening the door to creative solutions that support sustainability and biodiversity conservation. We might imagine a thorough comprehension of life that serves both academia and society at large through ongoing investigation and integration of scientific knowledge.

Knowledge Assessment

The chapter includes material designed to review and reinforce each content. It includes Critical Thinking Questions to help test of your understanding of information presented in the chapter and Short answer Questions to review your understanding of the key concepts presented in the chapter.

Critical Thinking Questions

1. **Who is known as the "Father of Modern Biology"?**
    a. Aristotle
    b. Charles Darwin
    c. Gregor Mendel
    d. Louis Pasteur
2. **What is the basic unit of life?**
    a. Atom
    b. Molecule
    c. Cell
    d. Organism
3. **Which branch of biology studies the interaction of organisms with their environment?**
    a. Genetics
    b. Ecology
    c. Physiology
    d. Botany
4. **Which macromolecule is the main source of energy for living organisms?**
    a. Proteins
    b. Lipids
    c. Carbohydrates
    d. Nucleic acids
5. **DNA is primarily responsible for which function in living organisms?**
    a. Energy production
    b. Protein synthesis
    c. Storing genetic information
    d. Regulating body temperature

Short Answer Questions

1. What is biology, and why is it important to study biology?
2. What are the three main domains of life, and how are they different from one another?
3. Define homeostasis and give an example of how it works in living organisms.
4. What is the cell theory, and why is it fundamental to biology?
5. How do autotrophs and heterotrophs differ in the way they obtain energy?
6. What is the scientific method, and how is it applied in biological research?
7. Discuss how biology helps address global challenges such as climate change, disease, and food security.
8. Explain the levels of biological organization from the smallest unit to the largest. Provide examples at each level.
9. Describe the relationship between structure and function in biology, giving specific examples from cells or organs.
10. How has the discovery of genetics shaped our understanding of inheritance and variation among organisms?

Supplementary Materials

Key Terms: A list of key terms is given for quick reference

KEY TERMS FROM THIS CHAPTER

Annotation enrichment analysis	Biological structure	Cell
Cell theory	Cellular structure	Ecology
Ecosystems	Genetics	Human biology
Microbiology	Natural selection	Organism
Plant biology		

Further Resources: Recommendations for additional readings, websites, and multimedia resources.

References

1. Argelaguet, R., Velten, B., Arnol, D., Dietrich, S., Zenz, T., Marioni, J. C., Buettner, F., et al. (2018). Multi-omics factor analysis—A framework for unsupervised integration of multi-omics data sets. *Molecular Systems Biology, 14*. https://doi.org/10.15252/msb.20178124.
2. Bacher, S., Blackburn, T. M., Essl, F., & Genovesi, P. (2017). *Socio-Economic Impact Classification of Alien Taxa (SEICAT)*. https://core.ac.uk/download/286567949.pdf (accessed on 8th March 2025).
3. Barnett, R., Brace, S., Cucchi, T., & Dobney, K. (2013). *Divergent Evolutionary Processes Associated with Colonization of Offshore Islands*. https://core.ac.uk/download/20664364.pdf (accessed on 8th March 2025).

Detailed Table of Contents

CHAPTER 5

Occupational Skin Diseases 139

CHAPTER 6

Drug Reactions and Adverse Cutaneous Drug Eruptions 173

CHAPTER 12

Dermatologic Emergencies and Treatment 379

Index 413

LIST OF FIGURES

LIST OF TABLES

PREFACE

The skin, as the largest of all the organs in the body, is not only a physical covering but also a reflection of internal health. It can manifest signs of systemic disease, environmental exposure, emotional status, and drug hypersensitivity. Cutaneous diseases in the clinical context are very diverse in presentation and severity, ranging from benign lesions and cosmetic complaints to potentially fatal malignancies and complex systemic diseases. Understanding the structure, function, and response mechanisms of the skin is the basis for identifying and treating many disorders.

Dermatology has undergone significant change in the last few decades due to advances in medical imaging, molecular diagnostics, immunotherapy, and cosmetic technology. Traditional diagnostic acumen is now supported by computer aids and non-invasive techniques, expanding the horizons of care and accuracy. Once considered incurable, diseases are now managed using targeted therapies. Moreover, growing demand for cosmetic treatments and heightened awareness of skin health have expanded the clinician's scope in clinical dermatology beyond treatment, making it a dynamic practice in which patient-centered innovation intersects with clinical medicine.

Textbook of Dermatology: Volume 3 has been designed to address advanced and specialized areas of dermatological science, with emphasis on oncologic, occupational, psychocutaneous, and aesthetic fields. It is part of a comprehensive series of books designed to provide students of dermatology, residents, and practicing clinicians with precise, well-organized information that is valuable and evidence-based. The volume has been founded on recent research, clinical guidelines, and the opinions of experts to provide a well-concerted and current reference to aid learning and professional practice.

Chapter 1 describes an overview of cysts and benign skin tumors, discussing frequent lesions such as epidermoid cysts, dermatofibromas, and seborrheic keratoses. Clinical presentation, diagnostic difficulty, and treatment with excision and conservative treatment are discussed in the chapter.

Chapter 2 is dedicated to premalignant and malignant skin tumors such as basal cell carcinoma, squamous cell carcinoma, and melanoma. Chapter 2 provides diagnostic criteria, risk factors, histologic types, staging systems, and new treatment modalities, including Mohs micrographic surgery and immunotherapy.

Chapter 3 covers cutaneous lymphomas and metastases to the skin. It explains cutaneous T-cell and B-cell lymphoma classification, staging techniques, cutaneous manifestations of internal neoplasms, and the application of biopsy and imaging in diagnosis and treatment planning.

Chapter 4 covers photodermatoses and ultraviolet-induced dermatoses. They consist of polymorphous light eruption, chronic actinic dermatitis, and photoallergic reactions, and prevention, photoprotection, and patient counseling measures.

Chapter 5 examines occupational skin diseases and their conditions , such as irritant and allergic contact dermatitis, occupational acne, and phototoxic reactions. It examines risk factors by industry, prevention, and medico-legal aspects in occupational dermatology.

Chapter 6 examines drug reactions and adverse cutaneous drug eruptions. Its subject matters are exanthematous eruptions, Stevens-Johnson syndrome, toxic epidermal necrolysis, and drug-induced hypersensitivity syndromes. The chapter focuses on early recognition and appropriate intervention.

Chapter 7 presents aesthetic treatments and cosmetic dermatology. It covers the applications of botulinum toxin, dermal fillers, microdermabrasion, and rejuvenation skin treatments , such as selection of patients, safety of procedures, and ethical considerations in aesthetic practice.

Chapter 8 addresses lasers and light therapy in dermatology, emphasizing their use in the management of vascular lesions, pigmentary disorders, scars, and tattoos. It covers the types of lasers, treatment parameters, post-treatment care, and potential complications.

Chapter 9 deals with cryotherapy, electrosurgery, and chemical peeling. The treatments are addressed in terms of technique, indications, contraindications, and management of complications, providing practical information for the clinic setting.

Chapter 10 discusses hair and nail diseases, including alopecia areata, telogen effluvium, onychomycosis, and nail dystrophies. The diagnostic approach and preferred therapy are investigated with visual aids and case examples.

Chapter 11 addresses psychodermatology and psychocutaneous disorders. It discusses skin disorders influenced by the psychological domain, such as trichotillomania, delusional parasitosis, and neurotic excoriations, with a focus on diagnostic nuances and the value of interdisciplinary consultation.

Chapter 12 introduces the reader to acute presentations such as Stevens-Johnson syndrome, toxic epidermal necrolysis, and angioedema. Triage principles, supportive care measures, and coordination with critical care are addressed. Emergency interventions for immediate action are centered on reducing morbidity and mortality in such emergent presentations.

This book is intended for dermatology residents, practicing dermatologists, general practitioners with an interest in skin disorders, and allied health professionals involved in dermatologic care. It is also suitable for postgraduate students seeking an advanced understanding of skin disease management. With a blend of clinical insight, procedural techniques, and technology integration, this volume supports both academic learning and real-world application in a field where science and patient care continue to progress together.

1

BENIGN SKIN TUMORS AND CYSTS

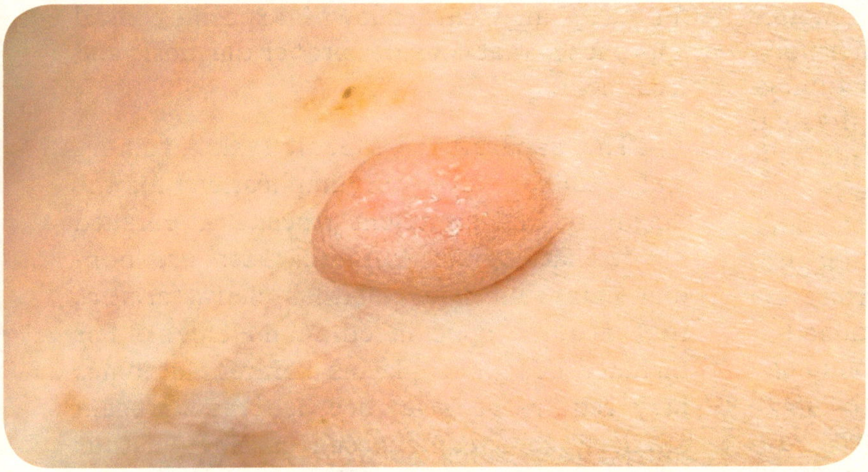

Introduction

The dermatologic specialty encompasses a wide range of conditions, among which skin tumors and cysts are of particular significance due to their frequency and comparatively low danger to patient health. These tumors, even if generally asymptomatic and benign, can lead to emotional distress and physical issues in affected individuals. Information on tumor biological pathways is crucial not only for accurate diagnosis but also for treatment planning. Furthermore, the etiology of benign skin tumors often stems from genetic and environmental factors and therefore warrants a more thorough study of how these forces interact to shape skin health. This initial examination lays the foundation for a more in-depth examination of the types, characteristics, and implications of benign skin tumors and cysts in clinical practice. One fascinating line of inquiry in benign skin tumor research is the relationship between many genetic diseases and the development of particular tumor types. For example, Cowden syndrome (CS), which predisposes to multiple hamartomas, is focused on genetic

LEARNING OBJECTIVES

After studying this chapter, you will be able to:

1. Understand the types of benign skin tumors and skin cysts
2. Explain how to diagnose benign skin tumors and cysts
3. Describe treatment options for managing benign skin tumors and cysts
4. Define the complications and risks associated with benign skin tumors and cysts
5. Discuss effective prevention and management strategies for benign skin tumors and cysts

predisposition for some benign tumors , such as trichilemmomas, which at times are equivocal with other skin malformations. The role of human papillomavirus (HPV) in the development of such tumors complicates the clinical picture because it can be detected in the majority of CS-related benign growths, making it challenging for medical professionals to distinguish benign from malignant tumors. These findings are significant for improving diagnosis reliability and proper patient management, implying a relevant dermatology presentation-genetics interface (Schaller et al., 2003). Furthermore, the importance of benign cutaneous tumors extends beyond reductionistic physical complaints to affect patients' quality of life, self-esteem, and social interactions. Where lesions evolve into cosmetically disfiguring lesions, the psychological impact can be pathological and result in many patients presenting for treatment not only for medical indications but also for cosmetic alleviation. The dermatology specialty is thus forced to balance the need for comprehensive medical management with the need to address patients' concerns about appearance. This interdisciplinary approach to benign skin tumors and cysts illustrates the need for continued research and education in dermatology, preparing practitioners to deliver well-informed and empathetic care to those afflicted by these disorders. In so doing, stakeholders can better treat both the medical and psychosocial concerns surrounding skin tumors, setting an example for interdisciplinary treatment models in dermatology (Abbasi et al., 2015).

Definition of Benign Skin Tumors and Cysts

Dermatology is the field of skin diseases, and among them, benign skin tumors and cysts stand out as especially notable because they are so prevalent and usually benign. Benign skin tumors are abnormal growths that arise from skin structures and cells and are characterized by their non-cancerous nature. These tumors may present as actinic keratoses, seborrheic keratoses, or dermatofibromas, all typically appearing as benign lesions on the skin surface. Cysts, which are fluid or semi-solid content pouch-like structures, tend to arise from hair follicles, glands, or connective tissues, and hence become a common occurrence in dermatology. Both benign tumors and cysts are of great significance in patient management because of their recognizable nature and low potential for malignancy, which allows for specific clinical approaches that consider proper diagnosis and treatment.

The separation of benign skin tumors and cysts can have great implications for the diagnostic and treatment procedures pursued by dermatologists. Both diseases are non-malignant but have distinct characteristics that require specialized management. For instance, benign neoplasms keratoacanthomas may require removal because they present similarly to squamous cell carcinoma, thus necessitating proper differentiation. On the other hand, cysts , such as epidermoid cysts will only require drainage or observation unless symptomatic. Such nuances help dermatologists correctly address the patient's concerns, thus ensuring physical and psychological well-being. Furthermore, with the development of medical technology, the pressure on diagnostic tools increases, and the importance of proper assessment and accurate classification of such skin lesions in daily practice comes to the fore (Bas et al., 2022). Furthermore, the effects of benign skin tumors and cysts extend beyond mere definitions, affecting research, clinical guidelines, and patient education. Detailed guidelines, provided by the National Comprehensive Cancer Network (NCCN) for skin check-ups, inform practitioners on best practices, diagnostic evaluation, and appropriate treatment regimen for patients presenting with skin conditions (Heller, 2020). This way, patients receive evidence-based care for their respective conditions. Since patients tend to require explanation and direction about their skin condition, the work of dermatologists is not just curing but also educating patients about the benign condition of such tumors and cysts. This combined attention strengthens the therapeutic relationship between patient and physician, where skin conditions can be well managed and followed up (Figure 1.1).

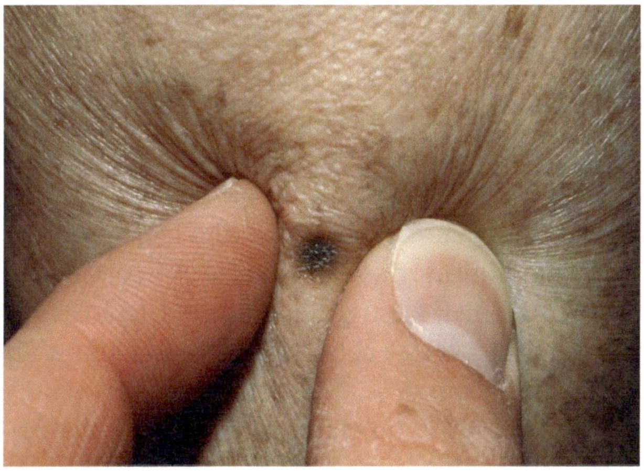

Figure 1.1. Benign skin tumor.

Source: https://media-us.amboss.com/media/thumbs/big_58a6ce12a3b39.jpg.

Importance of Studying Dermatological Conditions

Dermatologic illnesses are relevant not only to develop effective modes of treatment but also to understand the broader significance that skin health confers on overall well-being. The skin is a vital barrier and plays a significant role in immune protection, temperature control, and sensory function. Thus, benign skin neoplasms and cysts, as harmless as they may be, can significantly impact a patient's quality of life. By studying common dermatologic conditions, clinicians are better positioned to establish diagnostic criteria and treatment algorithms that serve the diverse patient population. In addition, more information and research on benign tumors can prevent unnecessary concern with regard to potential malignant transformation, hence enhancing a better-informed conversation between clinicians and patients about cutaneous health (Abbasi et al., 2015). Understanding of benign skin tumors and cysts will also assist in shaping dermatological research and clinical practice. The emergence of innovative techniques of treatment, such as the cryogenic technology that Dr. V.I. Kochenov has developed, has altered the approaches to addressing various dermatological issues. The technology assists in the successful treatment of conditions , such as epithelial cysts and skin hemangiomas with minimal side effects. The benefit of cryogenic procedures is not only the removal of lesions with success but also highly cosmetic improvements with minimal scarring (Kochenov et al., 2017).

The study of these procedures allows dermatologists to refine their skills and use the latest scientific advancements, thereby enhancing patient satisfaction and results. Furthermore, the study of dermatological disease forms the basis of interdisciplinary research that can progress the field further. The intersection of dermatology and technology, such as data mining to predict patient outcome, is a growing field of study. For instance, recent studies have demonstrated the capacity of machine learning algorithms to predict survival rates of patients with different forms of cancer, and it has been suggested that these same techniques can be utilized to assess the prognosis of benign skin tumors (Abbasi et al., 2015). By encouraging coordination between dermatologists, oncologists, and data scientists, scientists are able to develop holistic perspectives of skin health, which will assist in making better treatment guidelines. Eventually, the improved understanding of benign skin tumors and cysts equips health professionals with what they require to treat the nuances of skin conditions in a better manner.

1.1. Types of Benign Skin Tumors

Learning Outcome

1. Describe common types of benign skin tumors.
2. Explain characteristics and appearance of each type.
3. Understand prevalence of benign skin tumors and cysts.

Among the many benign skin lesions, seborrheic keratosis is one of the most prevalent. It has its waxy, raised nature and the color can vary from light tan to black and tends to appear in groups on the trunk, face, and extremities. Seborrheic keratosis arises from squamous cells in the epidermis and is a non-malignant growth that typically becomes more prevalent with age. Even though they are not usually harmful, such tumors sometimes inflame or itchy, and some individuals will want them removed. Seborrheic keratosis must be distinguished from other skin lesions because some forms of melanoma can appear somewhat alike. This highlights the importance of accurate diagnosis and the potential role of dermoscopy in improving detection and skin lesion analysis, like distinguishing benign from malignant tumors (Menzies et al., 2008).

Another fascinating group of benign skin tumors is dermatofibromas, which occur as hard, raised nodules on the skin, typically on the lower extremities. These fibrotic neoplasms typically represent localized reactive hyperplasia of fibroblasts and are normally asymptomatic but may, on occasion, be tender if irritated. Dermatofibromas typically present as brown or tan-colored lesions with a classic dimpling on compression. Although benign and normally self-limiting, dermatofibromas may occasionally be mistaken for more serious disease, such as dermatologic malignancy. Thus, appropriate histological examination is mandatory to provide the appropriate management and determine the nature of the tumors. Additionally, they depict the complexity and variety of benign skin neoplasms that can be encountered in clinical dermatology and the necessity of appropriate patient assessment in differential diagnoses (Menzies et al., 2008). Lastly, trichilemmomas represent benign follicular hair neoplasms that can be seen in humans, particularly in the context of diseases , such as Cowden syndrome. These neoplasms typically present as small, flesh-colored papules on the face, preferring the periorbital and perioral areas. Trichilemmomas are generally considered benign lesions, but of interest is their association with the human papillomavirus (HPV), complicating their pathological basis and treatment. HPV DNA has been detected in a high percentage of the lesions, suggesting a potential viral cause in their development. The overlapping clinical presentation of benign skin tumors and HPV-related skin lesions calls for increased vigilance and precise evaluation by physicians, especially in patients with an extensive clinical history like Cowden syndrome (Burgdorf, Schaller et al., 2003). This illustrates the intricate interrelationship between viral infection and benign skin tumors and proves the utility of precise dermatologic examinations.

1.1.1. Common Types: Seborrheic Keratosis, Lipomas, and Dermatofibromas

Among all benign neoplasms of the skin, seborrheic keratosis ranks among the most frequently seen in dermatology. Lesions occur in a classic scaly, waxy manner and range from light tan to dark brown color. Seborrheic keratoses are usually seen on sun-damaged areas of the skin and are benign tumors that most frequently present in middle-aged to older patients. They are thought to arise as a consequence of both environmental exposure and genetic predisposition, including ultraviolet light. Studies report that a significant number of elderly patients present with this condition during dermatological visits (Irene et al., 2023). Treatment of seborrheic keratoses is rarely indicated, with patients only opting for removal if the lesions become problematic or cosmetically undesirable (Figures 1.2, 1.3).

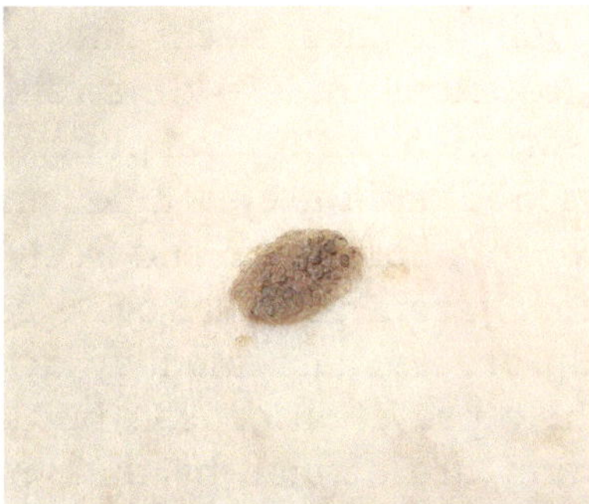

Figure 1.2. Seborrheic keratosis close-up.

Source: https://upload.wikimedia.org/wikipedia/commons/thumb/a/a3/Seborrheic_keratosis_closup.jpg/800px-Seborrheic_keratosis_closup.jpg.

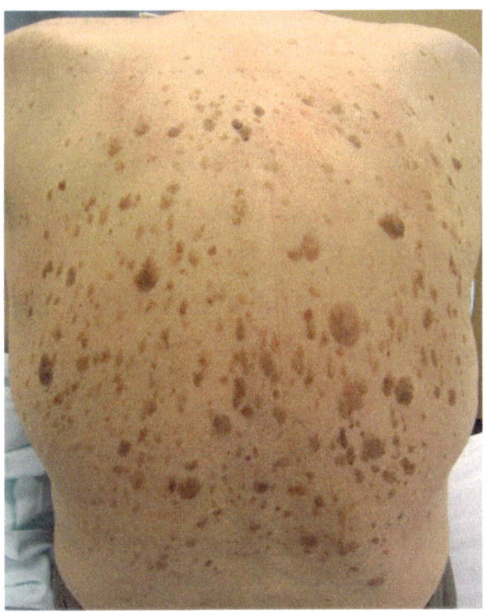

Figure 1.3. Many seborrheic keratoses on the back of a person with Leser–Trélat sign due to colon cancer.

Source: https://upload.wikimedia.org/wikipedia/commons/thumb/8/84/Seborrheic_keratosis_on_human_back.jpg/800px-Seborrheic_keratosis_on_human_back.jpg.

Lipomas, which are the second most common type of benign skin tumor, are fatty, soft tumors that arise just beneath the surface of the skin. The lesions are benign and are usually painless, feeling like rubbery nodules that are movable. Unlike seborrheic keratosis, lipomas are composed of adipose tissue and may occur anywhere on the human body, although they most commonly occur on the trunk, shoulders, and arms. Although lipomas are generally benign, multiple lipomas (lipomatosis) may require further testing. Lipomas are expected to persist uneventfully, though in some patients, cosmetic or pain concerns may require removal by surgery (Cocuz et al., 2021). The majority of lipomas exist in a static growth pattern, highlighting the benign quality of lipomas in dermatologic assessment (Figure 1.4).

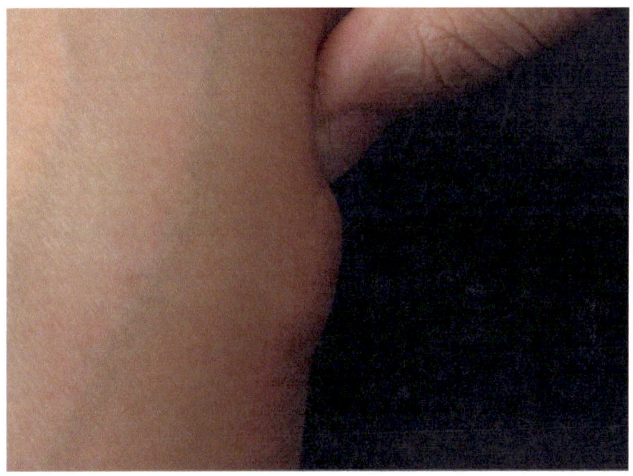

Figure 1.4. Lipoma on forearm.

Source: https://upload.wikimedia.org/wikipedia/commons/3/37/Lipoma_02.jpg.

Dermatofibromas are another type of benign skin tumor, and they are recognized by their hard, papular nodules, often with a prodigious dimpling effect when pinched. They are most frequently seen on the extremities and are brown to reddish-brown, and they are often mistaken for other lesions, such as skin tags or warts. Although dermatofibromas are benign and usually do not require treatment, they are a concern due to their resemblance to other serious skin conditions. Clinically, the lesions are usually found in middle-aged to young adults, and diagnosis is often made on the basis of clinical presentation and, if necessary, histopathologic examination (Irene et al., 2023). The patients typically present them as asymptomatic, but like seborrheic keratoses and lipomas, dermatofibromas are sometimes removed for cosmetic reasons or if they become pesky (Figure 1.5).

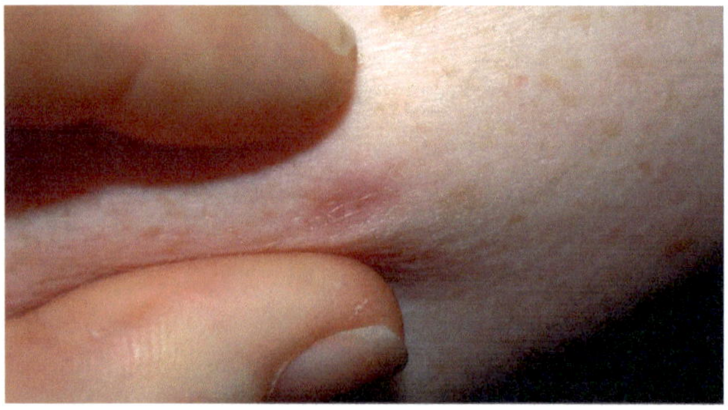

Figure 1.5. A dermatofibroma is a nodule made of fibrous tissue.

Source: https://www.medicalnewstoday.com/articles/318870#what-is-it.

1.1.2. Characteristics and Appearance of Each Type

The characteristics of benign skin tumors vary significantly by type and affect their appearance and clinical picture. Seborrheic keratosis is domed, brown papules that are warty-looking or have a "stuck-on" appearance, and sometimes barnacle-like when growing on the skin. The tumors are usually asymptomatic, but if they are scratched, itching can occur. On the other hand, dermatofibromas, which are firm nodules that commonly appear on the extremities, are brown or tan in color with a center depression, thus easy to recognize. They normally form after skin trauma and are most often mistaken for other life-threatening illnesses, clinical evaluation for proper diagnosis is critical. Understanding these characteristics is valuable for dermatologists because it aids in distinguishing benign tumors from malignant tumors and identifying appropriate treatment, as well as reassuring patients. Understanding the appearance of various cysts is also valuable in dermatology because of their wide variation in clinical presentation. Epidermoid cysts are commonly on the face, neck, and trunk and are small, rounded, under-skin swellings with a smooth surface and a central punctum, which is the open mouth of the cyst. Epidermoid cysts are commonly full of keratin and freely movable on palpation. In contrast, pilar cysts, commonly on the scalp, are less hard and may lack an open mouth. Their presentation can be deceptive; however, they are defined by their pattern of growth and absence of inflammation.

An accurate understanding of such presentations helps dermatologists make appropriate diagnoses, which is important to choose appropriate treatment strategies. The categorization of benign skin tumors and cysts also requires knowledge of their growth patterns and the likelihood of evolution over time. For instance, while most nevi (moles) remain stationary and only enlarge with age, atypical nevi also change in color and size, which would qualify them for monitoring due to their risk. Tuberous sclerosis complex, characterized by the presence of more than one benign growth named hamartomas, also includes cutaneous manifestations angiofibromas and shagreen patches that appear distinctively on the skin. They are harmless in nature but do present a diagnostic challenge with their unpredictable nature and overlapping characteristics with other skin diseases. Continuous professional education and understanding of these diverse benign tumors and cysts enhance clinical knowledge in dermatology clinics and ultimately benefit patient care by enabling early and accurate intervention (Northrup et al., 2013; Heller, 2020) (Figure 1.6).

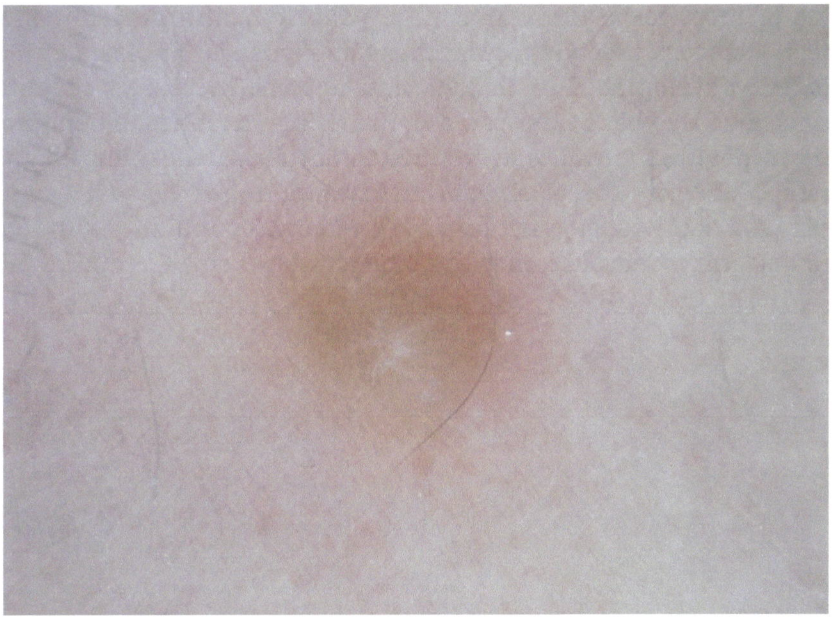

Figure 1.6. Dermoscopic features of the patient's dermatofibroma. Central white scar-like patch with delicate pigment network in dermatofibroma of the leg.

Source: https://www.researchgate.net/profile/Evelin-Paterno/publication/261748909/figure/fig2/AS:213910205538305@1428011575645/Dermoscopic-feature-of-dermatofibroma-of-the-patient-Central-white-scar-like-patch-with.png.

1.1.3. Prevalence and Demographics Affected

The prevalence of benign skin tumors and cysts varies greatly among different populations, based on a multifactorial combination of environmental, lifestyle, and genetic factors. Studies have established that the most frequent type of benign skin tumor, seborrheic keratoses, is seen most frequently in individuals older than 50 years, with higher frequencies among patients with light complexion types. On the other hand, dermatofibromas are seen more in European and African American populations suggesting that genetic predispositions might be involved in developing these cutaneous lesions. The rise in the prevalence of benign neoplasms can be credited to an increase in exposure to UV radiation, especially in regions with higher sunlight exposure, which indicates environmental causes for the formation of such tumors. Understanding these trends is essential for tailoring public health interventions to early detection and control of benign skin lesions. Age and ethnicity are significant factors influencing the types of benign skin tumors and cysts that individuals develop. Lipomas, for instance, are most likely to arise in middle-aged adults, whereas epidermoid cysts are most likely to be found in teenagers and young adults. This suggests that age-dependent biological functions may predispose individuals to certain skin lesions. Gender difference is also evident, as some tumors, including pilomatrixomas, are more common in females, while others, including lipomas, present in a more even gender distribution. The interplay between demographic variables and disease prevalence underscores the need for dermatologists to consider the individual patient's sociocultural background and risk factors in the design of diagnostic and treatment protocols. In addition, the situation of benign skin cysts and tumors is being redefined due to the influence of lifestyle patterns and more generic health determinants. With a shift in demographics, especially urban, lifestyle factors like sun exposure, smoking, and diet are becoming key risk factors for the development of benign skin lesions. Increased sedentary behavior and reduced skin shielding have also been implicated in the rising incidence of benign tumors. Moreover, disparities in access to healthcare can lead to differential prevalence and diagnostic rates across socioeconomic strata. Managing these aspects is paramount for dermatology professionals, as increased awareness and knowledge can empower affected populations, potentially leading to earlier intervention and improved outcomes for benign skin diseases (Figure 1.7).

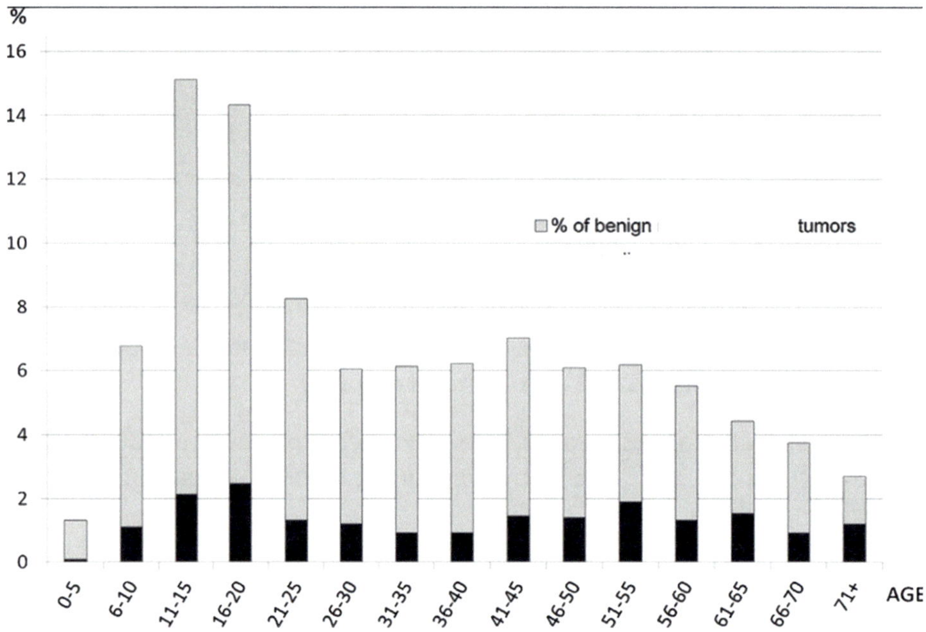

Figure 1.7. Depiction of the age distribution of the total percentage of benign tumors shown in the form of a bar graph. The results are sorted in five-year intervals.

Source: https://www.researchgate.net/profile/Orlic-Dubravko/publication/272523058/figure/fig1/AS:558758984404997@1510229931844/Depiction-of-the-age-distribution-of-total-percentage-of-benign-and-malignant-tumors.png

Test Your Knowledge

1. What is the typical appearance of seborrheic keratosis on the skin?
2. Which type of benign skin tumor commonly appears in older adults and is not usually found in children?
3. How does a dermatofibroma typically feel when palpated?

1.2. Types of Skin Cysts

Learning Outcome

1. Describe epidermoid cysts, pilar cysts, and steatocystomas.
2. Discuss the formation and underlying causes of skin cysts.
3. Differentiate between cysts and tumors.

Skin cysts are a heterogeneous group of benign cutaneous lesions that vary widely in composition, frequency, and presentation. Epidermoid cysts are perhaps the most common among them, occurring from the proliferation of epidermal cells in a confined space in the skin. These cysts can present as firm, rounded masses and occur anywhere on the body. Sebaceous cysts, often confused with epidermoid cysts, come from sebaceous glands and contain a central punctum that can expel a fatty substance. Whereas infections are true infections, these cysts are typically asymptomatic; inflammation or infection can be painful and require treatment. Understanding the differences among these cysts is essential for accurate dermatologic diagnosis and treatment.

Pilar cysts or trichilemmal cysts are also a prevalent variety and occur most frequently on the scalp. They are of hair follicle cell origin histologically and may be filled with keratinous material that is typically denser than the material within epidermoid cysts. While they are generally not symptomatic, pilar cysts may be bothersome due to the growth pattern, which can cause concern in patients due to their appearance. In addition, the existence of family patterns has also been described, suggesting an underlying genetic component to such cysts. Elucidation of the familial patterns and genetic background of pilar cysts underscores the need for meticulous patient history-taking during dermatological consultation to inform a tailored management strategy and reassure the patient. In dermatology, the clinical relevance of such cystic formations, particularly in relation to diagnostic imaging modalities, can enhance the quality of patient care. Recent advances in techniques , such as photoacoustic imaging (PAI), enable dermatologists to visualize cyst structures better, and hopefully discriminate cyst types from related skin lesions. PAI's capability to provide structural and functional data may enhance diagnostic and surveillance methods by combining the advantages of optical resolution with acoustic depth penetration. By using advanced imaging techniques in routine dermatological practice, clinicians can provide more accurate patient assessment and customized treatment advice, thereby optimizing care for benign cysts and skin tumors (Attia et al., 2019; Northrup et al., 2021).

1.2.1. Epidermoid Cysts, Pilar Cysts, and Steatocystomas

Epidermoid cysts, also known as epidermal inclusion cysts, are the most common type of skin cyst encountered in dermatology. Epidermoid cysts arise in the infundibular portion of hair follicles and are characterized by a sac of keratin that can create a dome-shaped protrusion beneath the skin.

They are typically slow-growing and can occur on any site of the body, but most often on the face, neck, and trunk. While presentation is often benign clinically, clinicians must rule out other cystic lesions that warrant alternative management, including lipomas or abscesses. Treatment is observation of asymptomatic lesions or surgical excision if the cyst becomes painful, infected, or cosmetically disfiguring. Information regarding the etiology and pathology of epidermoid cysts is critical to the effective management of patients in the practice of dermatology (Figure 1.8).

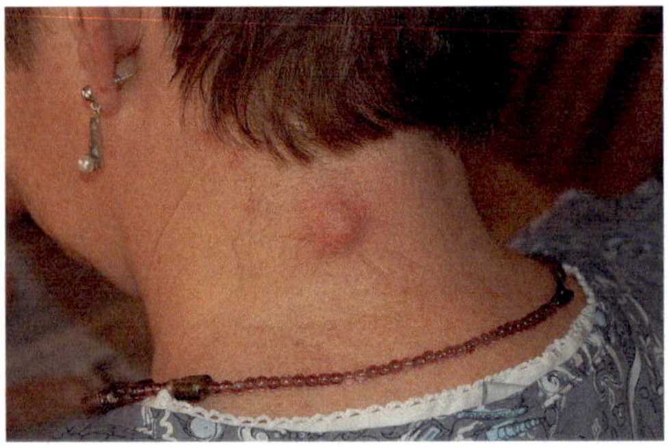

Figure 1.8. An inflamed epidermoid cyst (aka epidermal inclusion cyst or sebaceous cyst) on the neck.

Source: https://upload.wikimedia.org/wikipedia/commons/thumb/d/da/Inflamed_epidermal_inclusion_cyst.jpg/1024px-Inflamed_epidermal_inclusion_cyst.jpg.

Pilar cysts, or trichilemmal cysts, are a common variant of skin cysts that most commonly occur on the scalp. They arise from the hair follicle's outer root sheath and are typically characterized by a hard, smooth, and possibly mobile nodule. Unlike epidermoid cysts, pilar cysts are typically not filled with keratin within a sac but by a lined stratified squamous epithelium.

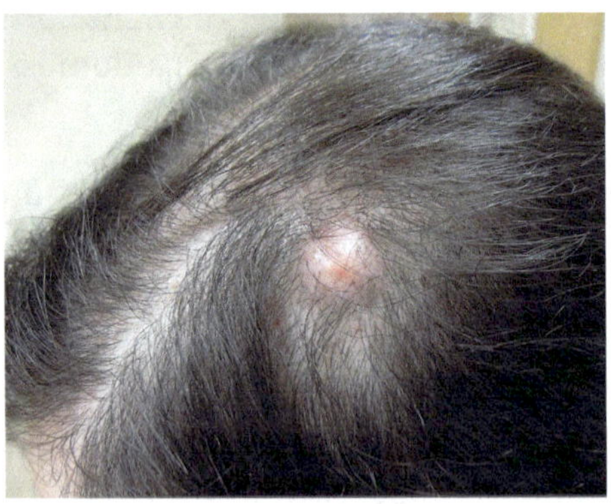

Figure 1.9. Pilar (trichilemmal) cysts are common fluid-filled growths (cysts) that form from hair follicles.

Source: https://my.clevelandclinic.org/-/scassets/images/org/health/articles/23092-pilar-cyst.

They usually present as a solitary lesion, but multiple lesions can occur, particularly in familial cases with a genetic predisposition. Pilar cysts are generally asymptomatic and require little treatment unless they are infected or inflamed. Surgical excision remains the preferred treatment, and due to its tendency to recur if not entirely removed, clinicians must be careful to excise the entire cyst and also the lining. Pilar cyst information positions the dermatologists in a better position to provide specific and proper care (Oakley, 2017) (Figure 1.9).

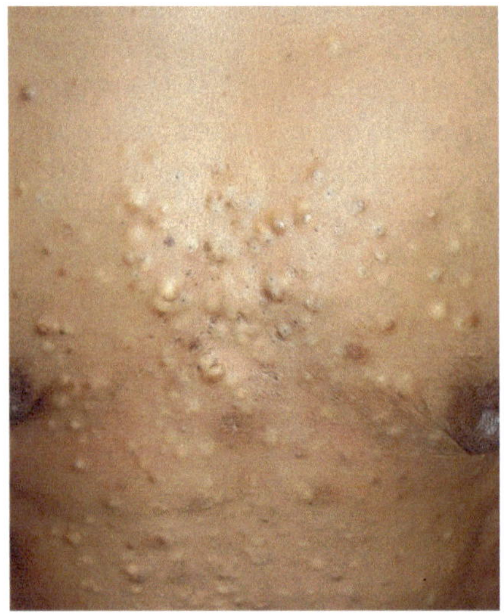

Figure 1.10. Steatocystoma multiplex.

Source: https://www.pcds.org.uk/imager/gallery/clinical/steatocytoma-multiplex/10249/steatocystoma-multiplex1_fee391183f15cb4d62773032fe0be92d.jpg.

Steatocystomas are another group of benign cystic lesions that are generally underestimated during dermatological evaluation. Steatocystomas develop from sebaceous glands and are characterized by having sebaceous material present in their cavities. Steatocystomas in clinically evident form are smooth, round nodules that may be of variable size and occur most frequently on the trunk, upper extremities, and chest. They may become troublesome with respect to the odor associated with them or secondary infection. Remarkably, steatocystomas are heritable, particularly in conditions such as steatocystoma multiplex, in which multiple cysts exist. Incision and drainage for symptomatic lesions are often adequate, but complete excision is the ideal method to affirmatively treat. Greater information regarding steatocystomas and their differing features is extremely significant to dermatologists in order to avoid misdiagnosis and in order to assure patients and counsel them appropriately (Oakley, 2017) (Figure 1.10).

1.2.2. Formation and Underlying Causes of Skin Cysts

Skin cysts, so prevalent in dermatology, are caused predominantly by the obstruction of sebaceous glands or hair follicles. Keratinization, inflammation, and trauma are the most frequent culprits behind such obstructions and lead to the formation of a fluid-filled or semisolid sac-like structure. Epidermoid cysts, for example, arise when epidermal cells proliferate into the dermis layer of skin and form an encapsulated cyst of varied size. It should be remembered that cysts may also be linked with inherited disorders, such as Gardner syndrome, which emphasizes the role of genes in impacting cyst formation. Understanding such etiologic mechanisms is crucial for effective treatment and control, as it enables dermatologists to tailor interventions to the clinical presentation and risk factors. Inflammation is also the key determinant of skin cyst formation. Conditions , such as acne and hidradenitis suppurativa not only block ducts physically but also induce inflammatory responses that may hasten the formation of cysts. In this case, the body reacts to infected hair follicles or acne lesions by forming tender cysts that require attention. In addition, pilar cyst formation, typically in the scalp, is likely to be caused by keratin deposition and variants in association with hormonal change. Such a multifaceted interaction between inflammation and cyst formation underscores the need for a comprehensive understanding within dermatology practice to optimize therapies and prophylactic measures. The underlying disease may predispose to cyst formation; however, the necessity of a complete patient assessment remains. For instance, sebaceous cysts can be more frequent with oily skin types or a history of trauma to the skin. Cysts can also serve as markers for underlying disease states; disease processes , such as steatocystoma multiplex illustrate the need for additional diagnostic testing to rule out other potential medical conditions. Where cysts are recurrent or present alongside other symptoms , such as pain or disfigurement, further investigation into other relevant benign tumors is indicated. This prudence ensures that experts maintain excellent standards of care and consider broader implications of cutaneous presentation, thereby fostering improved patient outcomes in diagnosis and treatment (Guirguis et al., 2024; Heck et al., 2024) (Figure 1.11).

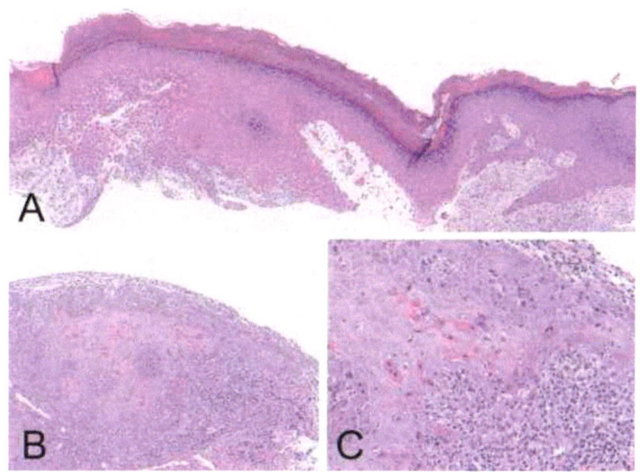

Figure 1.11. The cystic lesion shows an epidermal cyst with keratinized epithelium (A). Atypical keratinized cells are also seen, suggesting squamous cell carcinoma (B and C).

Source: https://www.researchgate.net/profile/Masanori-Hisaoka/publication/275058382/figure/fig1/AS:269642480484367@1441299185280/The-cystic-lesion-shows-an-epidermal-cyst-with-keratinized-epithelium-A-Atypical.png.

1.2.3. Differences Between Cysts and Tumors

In dermatology, particularly in the diagnosis of benign dermatological diseases, it is essential to distinguish cysts from tumors. Cysts are typically fluid-filled sacs that form within tissues, typically as a result of infection, blockage, or damage to tissue. They vary in size and may occur on any region of the body, appearing as soft, mobile swellings beneath the skin. On the other hand, tumors are abnormal tissue growths that may be fluid-filled or solid and can result from various cellular abnormalities. While benign tumors (lipomas) are non-cancerous, they may still require treatment depending on size and site. The two are distinguished in clinical practice when surgical treatment is available: cysts must be drained or removed, whereas tumors may require removal to prevent further complications or malignancy, depending on the situation. Cysts and tumors may present similar postoperative challenges, but their treatment approaches may differ substantially. Both are often the subject of surgical removal, especially in situations in which they are symptomatic or causing cosmetic problems. In benign tumors, complete excision may be warranted to ensure removal of all diseased tissue and to reduce the risk of recurrence. In cysts, simple drainage may be sufficient if complications like infection arise, as cysts can recur if the causative condition is not addressed. Moreover, histopathological analysis of both conditions following excision supports the differential diagnosis, confirms the nature of the lesion, and guides further therapeutic action. Identification of these nuances is important for optimal patient management in dermatologic practice, enabling proper diagnosis and effective treatment of skin conditions. Evolving methods of patient evaluation, such as teledermatology, improved availability and quality of skin lesion diagnosis, including tumors and cysts. Teledermatology facilitates efficient remote consultation and examination, permitting primary care physicians to treat a vast array of skin diseases in the elderly based on the diversity of lesions observed in this population. While assessing skin diseases in patients 60 years old and above patients, there were numerous cases, including benign lesions like epidermoid cysts and benign neoplasms that were successfully treated through teledermatology (Mara et al., 2020). This new approach not only enhances diagnostic accuracy but also streamlines follow-ups and referrals, hence optimizing dermatology healthcare resources. Understanding how to differentiate cysts from tumors, coupled with incorporating technology in therapeutic interventions, portends improved patient outcomes and satisfaction in dermatologic management (Figure 1.12).

CHARACTERISTIC	CYST	TUMOR
FAST-GROWING		✓
RED AND SWOLLEN	✓	
BLACKHEAD IN CENTER	✓	
WHITE, YELLOW, OF GREEN DISCHARGE	✓	
FIRM		✓
TENDER	✓	
ABLE TO MOVE AROUND UNDER SKIN	✓	

Figure 1.12. Cysts versus tumors.

Source: https://encrypted-tbn0.gstatic.com/images?q=tbn:ANd9GcRmYm0PCZchFX_1X3yZ05d_wZg9SytFj91LKQ&s.

Test Your Knowledge

1. What is the main cause of an epidermoid cyst?
2. What distinguishes steatocystomas from other cysts in terms of content?
3. How do cysts differ from tumors in terms of structure?

1.3. Diagnosis of Benign Skin Tumors and Cysts

Learning Outcome

1. Explain clinical examination techniques for the diagnosis of benign skin tumors and cysts.
2. Understand the role of imaging and biopsy in diagnosis.
3. Focus on differential diagnosis considerations for skin tumors and cysts.

Diagnosing benign skin tumors and cysts requires an intimate familiarity with the morphological characteristics and clinical manifestations of such lesions. Practitioners usually rely on a combination of patient history, physical examination, and imaging tests to sort out benign from malignant conditions. Physical examinations typically include features such as color, texture, and size, which can be used to distinguish among common types such as seborrheic keratosis, lipomas, and epidermoid cysts. Secondly, dermatoscopy has become a dermatologist's treasure, providing an extended view of the skin surface. It aids in clearer visualization of lesion structures, facilitating easier diagnosis and informed management decisions. A correct diagnosis is important, as it not only influences treatment options but also alleviates patient anxiety regarding malignancy. Histopathological examination is the most important diagnostic feature of benign cysts and skin tumors. Although many lesions are correctly diagnosed on clinical presentation, biopsy remains a gold standard tool for differentiation of benign processes from more malevolent neoplasms. Biopsies, such as excisional or incisional biopsies, provide useful information about the cellular architecture and characteristics of the lesions. The histology can reveal significant features, such as the cells involved or the pattern, which are typical of various benign skin tumors. For instance, in trichodiscomas, some follicular lesions observed under microscopic examination can determine diagnoses that would be hard to establish using visual criteria alone. Histopathology thus forms a vital component of dermatology's diagnostic process, complementing clinical assessments. Teledermatology is becoming a valuable adjunct to the diagnosis and treatment of benign skin tumors and cysts, especially for the elderly seeking convenient care. The ability to conduct consultations remotely enables the dermatologist to evaluate many skin diseases without seeing the patient, leading to early treatment of common lesions such as seborrheic keratosis and epidermoid cysts. Studies demonstrate that a high proportion of benign dermatoses are effectively managed through teledermatology, underscoring its value in enhancing patient access to specialist services. With high patient satisfaction, teledermatology not only facilitates accurate diagnosis but also conserves healthcare resources by reserving face-to-face appointments for complex cases. With the integration of teledermatology into practice, dermatologists are able to address the growing need for dermatological treatment while ensuring patients receive adequate and timely management of benign cysts and tumors (Giavina et al., 2020).

1.3.1. Clinical Examination Techniques

Clinical examination techniques are integral to the evaluation and diagnosis of benign skin tumors and cysts in dermatology. This typically begins with a thorough patient history that may inform potential risk factors and symptomatology. Clinicians must be able to recognize specific characteristics of benign lesions size, shape, color, and texture, to differentiate them appropriately from their malignant counterparts. Methods typically include clinical inspection under adequate lighting and dermatoscopy, which enhances visualization of underlying structures. This is more so in the examination of lesions related to hereditary syndromes like Cowden syndrome, whose early identification can dramatically influence patient prognosis, as explained in (Hildenbrand et al., 2001). Because these benign growths can also exhibit morphological features typical of malignancies, integration of clinical examination is necessary for appropriate and safe patient management.

Palpation of the lesions to assess consistency and mobility is another essential element of the clinical examination. It will be able to differentiate the type of cyst or tumor; benign lesions are firm and mobile, whereas malignant tumors are fixed to deep structures. During palpation, dermatologists can also assess tenderness, fluctuance, or other signs of infection or complications, which may alter management protocols. Furthermore, a complete assessment includes evaluation of the regional lymph nodes, particularly when systemic conditions may be involved. This multimodal assessment approach ensures a more precise diagnosis and underscores the importance of diligent clinical techniques in distinguishing benign skin tumors from potential malignancies. By paying close attention to detail, practitioners can best serve patients. Clinical examination techniques are also being advanced by technological innovations, including teledermatology and artificial intelligence diagnostic tools. These technologies can assist clinical examination by incorporating ancillary information from imaging studies or algorithmic assessment, thereby facilitating the identification of benign skin tumors and cysts. For instance, machine learning software has been shown to predict patient outcomes for various skin diseases with high accuracy, underscoring the need for accurate diagnosis in practice, as evidenced by studies cited in Abbasi et al. (2015). Not only does this multidisciplinary approach strengthen the clinician's toolkit, but it also empowers patients to make decisions about their dermatologic management. Finally, a robust clinical examination technique is inevitable in the management of benign cysts and tumors, yielding proper intervention and improved patient health outcomes (Figure 1.13).

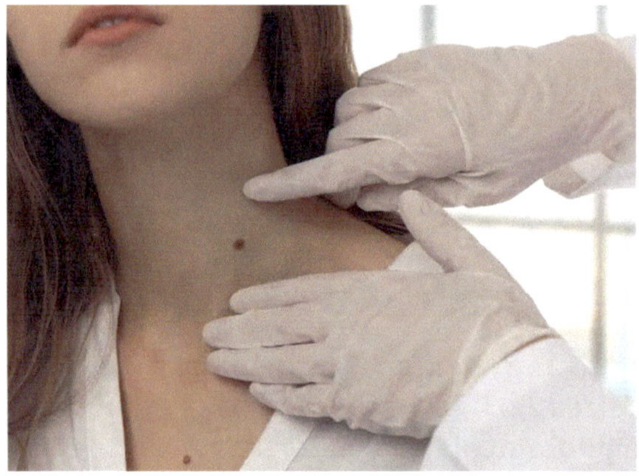

Figure 1.13. Clinical examination techniques are fundamental in the evaluation and diagnosis of benign skin tumors and cysts.

Source: https://media.post.rvohealth.io/wp-content/uploads/2020/08/Benign_Tumors-732x549-thumbnail-1-732x549.jpg.

1.3.2. Role of Imaging and Biopsy in Diagnosis

Imaging plays a significant role in the diagnosis of benign cysts and skin tumors and provides useful information for clinical decision-making. Techniques, such as CT scans, MRI, and ultrasound can help delineate the characteristics of the suspicious lesions. The use of ultrasound, in particular, is widely used because it is non-invasive and can differentiate solid from cystic masses. This differentiation is essential because it allows clinicians to decide if further diagnostic tests, such as biopsy, are needed. While imaging is highly informative about tumor size, location, and shape, it is the correlation of these imaging observations with clinical correlation that leads to an accurate diagnosis. Biopsy remains the gold standard for the exact diagnosis of benign skin neoplasms and cysts. By taking a tissue sample, dermatologists are able to analyze the histological characteristics of the lesion, which are most important for its nature assessment. Shave biopsies, punch biopsies, and excisional biopsies are the most common methods, each of which is chosen according to the size and location of the lesion. Histopathology analysis after biopsy may demonstrate significant characteristics, including cellular makeup and the status of any atypical cells, which can potentially have implications for therapeutics. Furthermore, histopathological examination can distinguish between skin tumor subtypes, confirming benign conditions like seborrheic keratosis or lipomas and ruling out malignant processes that mimic benign lesions on clinical or imaging studies. The integration of imaging and biopsy results makes overall diagnostic planning achievable to provide proper treatment for patients with benign skin tumors and cysts. As demonstrated in Cowden syndrome, where the early recognition of mucocutaneous manifestations during the course can detect underlying malignancies, the use of a combination of these modalities enhances clinical outcomes. If imaging finds an uncharacteristic lesion, biopsy is not only required for diagnosis but also to plan treatment and establish patient prognosis. Lastly, the roles of imaging and biopsy are non-substitutable in an integrated diagnostic procedure, both for identifying benign lesions and for safeguarding against potential malignancies, thereby maximizing patient care (Hildenbrand et al., 2001; Abbasi et al., 2015).

1.3.3. Differential Diagnosis Considerations

In the diagnosis of benign skin tumors and cysts, differential diagnosis is most important to prevent inappropriate therapy and management. Dermatologists must distinguish among a number of skin lesions, including seborrheic keratoses, dermatofibromas, and lipomas, because each of them has distinct features. For instance, seborrheic keratoses are most commonly seen as waxy, elevated lesions with a stuck-on appearance, while dermatofibromas present with firm, elevated nodularity and may demonstrate the “dimple sign” with lateral compression. The insidious onset of such lesions necessitates careful clinical assessment, in which a complete patient history and physical examination support accurate diagnosis. The discussion of the clinical presentation and typical presentations of benign neoplasms is very important; however, one must remain aware of those characteristics that may raise suspicion of malignant change so as to avoid misdiagnosis and inappropriate management of the patient.

With differential diagnosis, Cowden syndrome is among the syndromes to be taken into consideration, particularly in cases when patients come in with multiple skin tumors. Cowden syndrome is a rare epithelium and connective tissue tumor condition that features benign skin lesions, which can mimic common dermatologic presentations. Health professionals should exercise caution when evaluating a patient with multiple skin lesions, as these manifestations may indicate underlying syndromic associations. Premature diagnosis of Cowden syndrome is crucial, since its associated malignancies, for example, breast and thyroid carcinoma, have severe medical implications. Furthermore, familiarity with the genetic basis of such an illness is valuable for guiding familial screening guidelines. The fact that the development of some mucocutaneous lesions of Cowden syndrome can be utilized as markers of diagnosis guides the clinician’s management of the patient’s overall medical care, including both dermatological and oncologic considerations. In diagnosing benign skin tumors, it is critical to incorporate an extensive differential diagnostic strategy into the diagnostic workup that encompasses both prevalent and rare conditions. The evaluation should not be limited to benign tumors but should also include cysts that may mimic malignant lesions. A well-balanced approach can involve imaging techniques, such as ultrasound or dermatoscopy, to further define a lesion's character. These instruments enable clinicians to distinguish shallow cysts from more complex lesions that may require biopsy or surgical resection for definitive diagnosis. An in-depth investigation of patient symptomatology and demographics narrows the differential diagnosis, reducing the risk of overlooking significant conditions. Lastly, ongoing education and familiarity with evolving dermatologic literature, such as the syndromic presentations that have been described, for instance, in Cowden syndrome, significantly enhance diagnostic accuracy and patient outcomes in dermatology (Hildenbrand et al., 2001).

Test Your Knowledge

1. What is the first step in diagnosing a benign skin tumor or cyst?
2. When is a biopsy typically recommended for a skin lesion?
3. Why is it important to consider a differential diagnosis when examining a skin nodule or cyst?

1.4. Treatment Options

Learning Outcome

1. Discuss monitoring strategies in the management of benign skin tumors and cysts.
2. Understand surgical removal and other intervention methods for skin tumors and cysts.
3. Describe non-invasive treatments and their effectiveness.

In the management of benign skin tumors and cysts, the therapy is diverse and needs to be tailored in the individual case based on the nature of the tumors and the patient's overall condition. Most benign lesions , such as seborrheic keratosis or epidermoid cysts, are optimally treated with a policy of watchful waiting if the lesions are asymptomatic. This conservative strategy allows careful observation, and as experience in teledermatology indicates, a large majority of cases could probably be treated successfully without requiring in-clinic consultations. For instance, studies prove that it is possible for teledermatology to treat a significant proportion of dermatoses, making diagnoses and providing recommendations for treatment in collaboration with primary care physicians, thus promoting accessibility while minimizing waiting times (Mara et al., 2020). Where treatment is required, the modalities vary with the specific skin tumor or cyst involved. Surgical excision remains the norm for complete resection of most benign lesions, offering definitive treatment with no risk of recurrence. Modalities , such as cryotherapy and laser therapy are also being employed for some benign tumors, offering minimally invasive techniques without extensive scarring and recovery time. Particularly, patients with conditions like Gardner Syndrome, where there are epidermoid cysts, can be especially challenging. Conservative management, that is, observation using imaging techniques like MRI, has been found to benefit them particularly where complications are not developing (Heller, 2020).

Further, medical interventions may well supplement physical interventions. In cases of inflammation or discomfort, topical corticosteroids or emollients may provide symptomatic relief. The option of treatment also must include patient choice and potential impact on quality of life. Collaboration through teledermatology enhances communication between patients and providers, facilitating shared decision-making that considers patients' values. In summary, as knowledge of benign skin tumors advances, the range of therapeutic modalities continues to shift, driven by both clinical developments and patient-centered practices that expand access to dermatologic care (Mara et al., 2020).

1.4.1. Observation and Monitoring Strategies

Proper observation and monitoring strategies are important components of the treatment of benign skin tumors and cysts, enabling early detection of changes that may require further action. Regular follow-up clinics allow dermatologists to monitor changes in size, shape, and color of a tumor or cyst, such that any changes can be addressed in time. The use of standardized observation protocols, including photographic documentation of lesions, can enable more accurate comparisons over time. Such rigorous monitoring practices not only facilitate differentiation between benign and potentially malignant lesions but also provide patients with reassurance. By establishing a robust baseline through early evaluations, healthcare workers can detect atypical growth patterns that may indicate the need for biopsy or surgical intervention. With visual observation, advances in technology in imaging and diagnosis supplement the observational techniques used in dermatology. Dermostudies and high-frequency ultrasonography allow skin lesions to be analyzed non-destructively with specified detail regarding their morphology without excisional biopsies. These imaging methods can significantly increase diagnostic precision, particularly in differentiating malignant from benign tumors, thereby preventing unnecessary surgery. As well as this, the integration of genetic and molecular testing has become more important, especially in challenging-to-assess situations where there are unusual features. Using resources such as FISH and RT-PCR, specifically for diseases such as DFSP, dermatologists are in a position to make informed decisions regarding the necessity and timing of procedures based on genetic markers indicating disease progression (Cassalia et al., 2025).

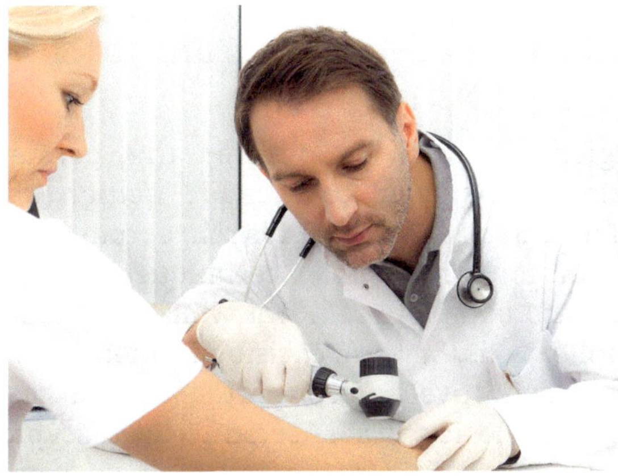

Figure 1.14. Effective observation and monitoring strategies are essential components in the management of benign skin tumors and cysts.

Source: https://static.wixstatic.com/media/08367c_0039b0e88b2b4301ae05c904bf20da64~mv2.jpg/v1/fill/w_980,h_743,al_c,q_85,usm_0.66_1.00_0.01,enc_avif,quality_auto/08367c_0039b0e88b2b4301ae05c904bf20da64~mv2.jpg.

Cooperation between the patient and dermatologist is crucial in monitoring and observation of benign skin cysts and tumors. Educating patients regarding the warning signs for potential change, such as rate increase or color alteration, allows them to take a more active role in their medical care. Regular communication and follow-up consultations are employed to foster understanding and surveillance, and to remind patients about their skin health. Moreover, such collaborative plans can enhance the therapeutic relationship, thereby improving treatment adherence and patient outcomes. Teledermatology for follow-ups also provides a new avenue to enhance monitoring, especially for those patients residing at distant locations. Through technology, healthcare providers are able to stay in contact with patients, ensuring timely evaluation while ensuring monitoring plans adapt based on unique situations and requirements (Abbasi et al., 2015) (Figure 1.14).

1.4.2. Surgical Removal and Other Intervention Methods

Surgical removal is one of the primary interventions used to manage benign skin tumors and cysts. Procedures range from simple excision to more complex techniques designed to ensure complete removal while minimizing complications. Surgical excision is often favored for its definitive nature, particularly in cases where the lesion is suspected to have atypical features or potential for recurrence. Furthermore, techniques such as Mohs micrographic surgery are used for tumors located in cosmetically sensitive areas, thereby maximizing tissue preservation and optimal aesthetic outcomes. The choice of surgical technique often depends on factors , such as tumor size, location, and the patient's overall health. Ultimately, successful excision can lead to a significant reduction in the likelihood of recurrence and can alleviate any associated symptoms, as well as provide psychological relief for patients concerned about the appearance of their skin. In addition to surgical options, other intervention methods are increasingly used to manage benign skin tumors and cysts. These approaches may include laser therapy, cryotherapy, and chemical peels, which can effectively treat specific types of lesions with minimal invasiveness. Laser therapy is particularly advantageous for superficial lesions, offering precise tissue targeting while minimizing damage to surrounding tissues. Cryotherapy, which uses extreme cold to destroy abnormal tissue, has also gained popularity due to its efficiency and relatively rapid recovery. Chemical peels can be effective for superficial skin lesions and help improve skin texture, although they may not be suitable for deeper tumors. While these non-surgical methods are promising, they often come with limitations regarding depth of penetration and complete removal, necessitating careful consideration when selecting the appropriate intervention for each specific case. Emerging techniques and technologies are enhancing the landscape of intervention methods for benign skin tumors and cysts.

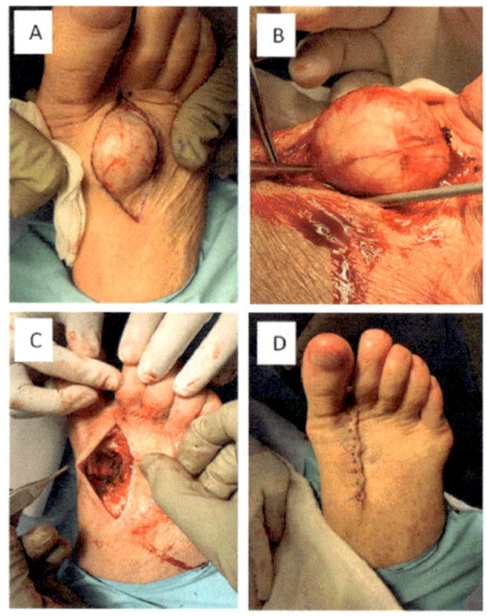

Figure 1.15. Surgical approach for excision of the mass. Intraoperative visualization of the well-encapsulated large benign tumor.

Source: https://www.researchgate.net/profile/Paul-Armanasco/publication/350931078/figure/fig2/AS:1016738581856259@1619420776643/Surgical-approach-for-excision-of-the-mass-Intraoperative-visualisation-of-the.png.

For instance, the integration of molecular diagnostic techniques and novel therapeutic agents is enabling a more personalized treatment approach. The identification of specific genetic markers associated with certain benign tumors prompts consideration of targeted therapies that could complement traditional surgical methods. Moreover, advances in imaging technologies have improved diagnostic accuracy, facilitating the distinction between benign and malignant lesions. As highlighted in recent literature, surgical excision remains the standard treatment for many benign tumors, particularly when malignancy is a concern, as seen with dermatofibrosarcoma protuberans (DFSP) (Cassalia et al., 2025). By embracing an integrated approach that combines surgical and non-surgical methods, clinicians can better tailor treatment strategies to individual patient needs, optimizing outcomes while minimizing risks associated with benign skin tumors and cysts (Fang et al., 2022) (Figure 1.15).

1.4.3. Non-Invasive Treatments and Their Effectiveness

Minimally invasive therapy is becoming the preferred treatment of benign skin tumors and cysts, primarily due to their reduced risk of complications and shorter recovery time. Modalities , such as laser therapy, cryotherapy, and topical agents have been found to perform differently as therapies for these conditions. Laser therapy, for instance, has been shown to be highly effective in treating vascular lesions, enabling cosmetic improvement with minimal tissue damage. This therapy illustrates advances in dermatologic treatments, in which patient care encompasses the effectiveness and psychological benefits of maintaining skin integrity. Moreover, with growing awareness of skin cancer, non-surgical therapy can be applied as a first-line treatment to allow dermatologists to observe and treat benign lesions to the best possible extent without subjecting patients to excessive invasive therapy. When evaluating the cost-effectiveness of non-invasive treatments, current studies have shown significant advantages over the conventional method. Teledermoscopy allows for rapid referrals in a way that dermatologists can triage and assess potential skin cancers more quickly. Studies contrasting teledermoscopy with traditional written referrals revealed that patients attained clinical resolution approximately 26 days earlier with the non-invasive method, which may be a game-changer in dermatology (Snoswell et al., 2018). Whereas the starting costs are slightly higher with teledermoscopy, the attendant benefits of earlier diagnosis and patient satisfaction underscore its growing relevance in contemporary dermatology practice. Emphasizing this efficiency in an age when healthcare resources are limited and earlier interventions directly improve patient outcomes is of utmost significance. Furthermore, the range of non-surgical therapies available for cysts and benign skin tumors necessitates ongoing research to inform clinical best practice. Dermatologists must continually weigh the effectiveness of such therapy against potential risks as well as patient-specific considerations , such as age, health status, and preference. Patient education and involvement cannot be overstressed, as educated patients are more likely to participate in their treatment programs, thereby ensuring greater adherence and satisfaction. By integrating advances in non-invasive therapies and robust patient-centered practices, dermatologists can establish an inclusive model that considers both clinical effectiveness and patients' overall health (Katsina et al., 2014). This integration strategy not only enhances treatment outcomes but sets a precedent for future advances in dermatology.

Test Your Knowledge

1. When is observation and monitoring an appropriate strategy for a benign skin tumor or cyst?
2. What is the most definitive treatment for a symptomatic or cosmetically concerning lipoma or cyst?

1.5. Complications and Risks

Learning Outcome

1. Understand the potential for misdiagnosis and its implications.
2. Describe risks associated with surgical procedures.
3. Focus on the psychological impact of benign skin tumors and cysts.

Treatment of benign skin tumors and cysts in dermatology is routinely associated with various risks and complications that clinicians are prepared to manage. Although such lesions are not malignant, treatment can have adverse effects. Scarring is possible secondary to incisions, particularly if excision of larger cysts or tumors is included, which may pose significant cosmetic problems for patients. Also, it has a possibility of site infection, an avoidable complication that needs close post-operative monitoring and rigorous preventative control, such as antibiotic prophylaxis. In children, where benign tumors occur more frequently, the physical and psychological aspects of surgery must be approached with sensitivity because children may respond differently both to the procedure and the process of recovery, emphasizing the importance of a practice that balances the need for surgery against potential complications (Lucas et al., 2007).

Misdiagnosis is another grave risk that lies in the treatment of benign skin tumors. Skin lesions, although generally benign, can in some cases present with features that could be mimetic of malignant tumors. Such mimicry can lead to unwarranted interventions if a tumor is mistaken for another one, exposing patients to avoidable surgical complications and increased psychological suffering. Additionally, in certain benign tumors, particularly those occurring in children, there exists clinical behavior heterogeneity, which complicates the planning of treatment (Maniaci et al., 2024). Histopathologic evaluation resulting in correct diagnosis is necessary but relies on familiarity with the range of benign entities, as incorrect identification can delay appropriate therapy and lead to complications from untreated lesions. Further, while benign skin tumors and cysts have good prognoses, complications in treating them can impact long-term outcomes. For instance, the recurrence of the tumor can occur due to incomplete resection in surgical procedures, necessitating further procedures with their respective risks. Dermatologists must examine the resection margins when removing the tumor to minimize recurrence rates. Furthermore, some benign lesions, such as pilomatrixomas, are by nature recurrent, and therefore constant vigilance is needed even after resection (Lucas et al., 2007). This underlines the importance of follow-up post-surgery and patient education for the detection of recurrence. Therefore, while benign in nature, the management of skin tumors and cysts has a complex combination of risks that have to be addressed by practitioners in order to have the optimal benefit to patients.

1.5.1. Potential for Misdiagnosis and Its Implications

In dermatology, accurate diagnosis of benign cysts and cutaneous tumors is critical, as misdiagnosis can lead to patient anxiety as well as inappropriate therapy. A case such as nodular melanoma, for which prompt identification is essential, illustrates the potential consequences of misdiagnosis. Inability to diagnose a malignant tumor when it is still in its initial stages not only puts patient outcomes at risk but also complicates follow-up treatments. For instance, misdiagnosis of a virulently growing cancer like nodular melanoma (NM) as a benign lesion can result in long delays, allowing the malignancy to develop uncontrollably and eventually impacting survival rates. Accuracy in the diagnosis of benign skin cysts and tumors is therefore important, and healthcare providers need to be more vigilant about the risk of misdiagnosis. Misdiagnosis of supposedly benign conditions , such as dermatofibrosarcoma protuberans (DFSP), is particularly challenging due to its clinical appearance, which may be similar to that of less malignant tumors or vascular lesions. Treatment has frequently been delayed in such patients, which may lead to increased morbidity concerning the advancement of the disease. DFSP, despite being a low-grade soft tissue sarcoma, can be misinterpreted as a benign lesion, leading to unwarranted delay in surgical intervention. Therefore, the subtleties of DFSP's distinction from other benign types demonstrate the need for thorough diagnostic protocols. Techniques such as the detection of the COL1A1-PDGFB fusion gene are important for ensuring accurate diagnoses and avoiding misdiagnosis. Such molecular approaches, tertiary in function, impart a level of specificity necessary to maximize patient management. The implications of misdiagnosis extend beyond clinical outcomes; they also affect patient relationships and overall healthcare costs. When benign tumors or cysts are inappropriately characterized, patients are unnecessarily subjected to treatment or procedures, with attendant ethical issues regarding patient autonomy and informed consent. Furthermore, misdiagnosis-related adverse effects, including psychological distress as a result of unwarranted fears regarding malignancy, can adversely affect the quality of life for patients. By making differential diagnostic techniques more robust, for example by integrating histopathology with advanced imaging modalities, clinicians can minimize such risks. Interdisciplinary collaboration within the health system must take priority to enhance awareness and education about the pitfalls of diagnosing benign tumors, thereby enabling optimal management with evidence-based treatment and reducing the risk of misdiagnosis and its consequences.

1.5.2. Risks Associated with Surgical Procedures

Surgical removal of benign skin tumors and cysts, although in most cases regarded as run-of-the-mill, naturally carries risks that must be well considered. Complications following dermatologic surgery can be minor or major, ranging from infection and scarring to anesthesia-related complications. The occurrence of postoperative infection is a severe complication because it can cause prolonged healing time, and thereby additional procedures or antibiotic treatment. Moreover, the possibility of scarring remains a primary concern, particularly in areas that are exposed, like the face and neck, where patients can develop psychological trauma due to cosmetic outcomes. Practitioners and patients must be well-informed of such risks since informed consent not only includes stating the benefits of surgery but also the possible complications that can arise during the healing process. In children, the choice to have surgical treatment of benign tumors is particularly sensitive due to the unique physiological and psychological considerations involved. Evidence reveals a variety of benign neoplasms of the skin that are frequent in children and need adequate investigation before surgery (Fang et al., 2022). Additionally, the type of anesthesia used—local or general—can present special risks, particularly for younger patients who may respond differently from adults. The challenge is finding the balance between the need for the surgery and the emotional and psychological impact on the child. Thus, the dermatologist must carefully evaluate the tumor's size, location, and impact on the child's quality of life, while keeping parents adequately informed about the potential risks and consequences of the operation (Fang et al., 2022). In addition, the postoperative period is also fraught with a set of risks that can influence the outcome of the operation. Aside from the short-term physical complications, the patients may be exposed to psychological consequences, such as anxiety regarding recovery and apprehension related to the visibility of scars. For instance, the possibility of requiring repeat surgeries due to complications or less-than-desirable cosmetic results is particularly daunting for individuals. A judicious preoperative consultation on risks and alternatives can also dispel some of these anxieties by setting realistic expectations for outcomes and recovery. Lastly, effective communication between the surgeon and patient is crucial for reinforcing agreement on treatment goals and dispelling any fear the patient may have about the risks of surgical treatment for benign skin cysts and tumors (Fang et al., 2022) (Figure 1.16).

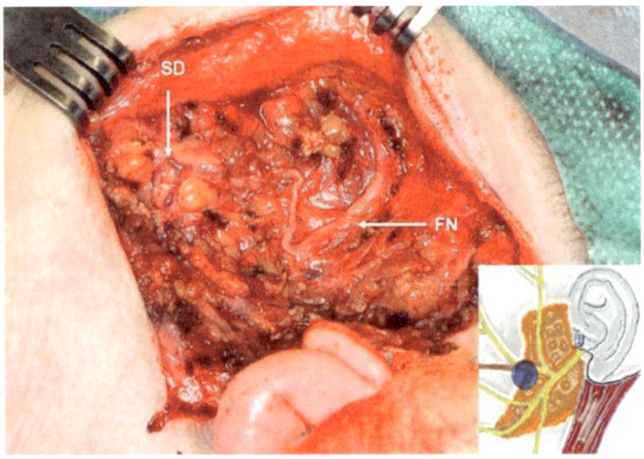

Figure 1.16. Surgical site after removal of a benign tumor of the anterior part of the left PG. Preserved Stensen's duct (SD) and branches of the FN can be seen.

Source: https://www.researchgate.net/publication/343440054/figure/fig8/AS:960116824223747@1605921097540/Surgical-site-after-removal-of-benign-tumor-of-the-anterior-part-of-the-left-PG.jpg.

1.5.3. Psychological Impact of Benign Skin Tumors and Cysts

The presence of benign cysts and skin tumors has a significant effect on the psychological well-being of patients. Though medically harmless, these conditions leave patients unnecessarily distressed. Appearance fears are often associated with low self-esteem and a negative self-image. Anxiety is developed by patients due to potential stigma and social judgment over their skin ailment. The psychological effect can be particularly dramatic in adolescents and young adults, who are probably already under intense social stress.

Moreover, the prolonged duration of benign skin conditions can lead to frustration and helplessness, which in turn exacerbate their psychological effects. Awareness of these emotional effects is important in dermatology in order to provide comprehensive patient care encompassing both physical and mental health issues. Besides the self-esteem problems in the case of benign skin cysts and tumors, patients also present with high anxiety regarding carcinoma fears. Even if the lesions are diagnosed as benign, patients tend to harbor a persistent fear of malignancy. The anxiety takes root because of a lack of knowledge about the nature of the condition, as well as the medical technology utilized in the management of the same. The psychic burden is intensified when the patient believes that their skin condition detracts from their professional or social status. The psychological implications of benign skin tumors, therefore, extend beyond simple appearance and represent deep-seated fears of inadequacy and rejection.

Addressing these fears in a therapeutic environment may enhance patient outcomes and demonstrates the need for an integrated model of practice in dermatology. Moreover, the role of healthcare professionals in managing the psychological impact of benign skin tumors and cysts cannot be replaced. Education and effective communication can empower patients by demystifying their disease and establishing a good patient-doctor relationship. It can reduce anxiety and improve satisfaction with care by assuring patients that the tumors are not malignant and responding appropriately to patients' concerns. Furthermore, psychiatric therapy, for example, counseling or support groups, can help resolve the emotional distress of these conditions. Greater coordination between dermatologists and mental health providers could maximize this process so that patients are provided with comprehensive care that addresses both their physical and emotional needs. With the creation of the science of dermatology, the detection and management of the psychological impact of benign skin tumors become central in enhancing overall patient well-being.

Test Your Knowledge

1. What is a major risk of misdiagnosing a malignant lesion as a benign tumor or cyst?
2. What are common risks associated with the surgical removal of skin cysts or tumors?
3. What psychological effects might patients experience due to visible benign skin tumors or cysts?

1.6. Prevention and Management

Learning Outcome

1. Describe lifestyle factors influencing skin health.
2. Focus on regular skin checks and self-examinations for maintaining skin health.

Effective prevention and treatment of benign skin tumors and cysts are essential in dermatology to reduce the risk of malignant transformation, particularly in high-risk individuals. One such strategy is protection measures against the sun for reducing ultraviolet (UV) radiation, the major risk factor for skin ailments, such as basal cell carcinomas (BCCs). The increasing incidence of skin cancer, particularly in areas of high UV exposure, underscores the importance of public education campaigns that emphasize the use of sunscreen, protective clothing, and seeking shade during peak sun hours. Strong educational programs can empower individuals to take personal responsibility for their skin health, thereby helping prevent the onset of benign lesions and reducing the health burden associated with the treatment of skin tumors and cysts, ultimately supporting broader public health objectives. Along with preventive therapy, treatment of benign skin tumors and cysts depends on a broad-based approach suitable to the individual case requirements and specific features of the tumor. Treatment measures vary significantly based on the size, location, and nature of the tumor or cyst, in addition to the patient's age and overall well-being. Traditional removal by surgery remains a usual procedure, especially in lesions with cosmetic concerns or a higher risk of complications if not treated. Alternatively, superficial lesions with minimal recurrence risk can be managed with therapies cryosurgery, curettage, and cautery. All management strategies will require a full assessment and consultation with the patient for potential outcomes, risks, and the importance of follow-up for any change over time, with a focus on responsible skin care practices. The role of vaccination in the prevention of certain benign skin tumors and their malignancies is gaining prominence, particularly for beta human papillomavirus (HPV) types that may have a causative role in cutaneous squamous cell carcinoma (cSCC). HPV-related skin pathology involves a diversity of lesions and necessitates universal immunization programs of high-risk individuals, including immunocompromised patients who may already harbor HPV infection. Evidence from research shows that vaccination against beta HPV at an early stage will likely decrease the formation of skin tumors in the long term. As technology advances in this research, it becomes clear that including vaccination in current treatment procedures in dermatology is more important. Health professionals must remain current with recent vaccination options, thereby promoting an active approach to the prevention and treatment of skin cancers and ultimately enhancing patient care and quality of life, according to recent evidence on HPV's role in dermato-oncology (Meyer, T., & Stockfleth, E., 2024). Moreover, ongoing monitoring of treatment response is necessary, particularly given the varying efficacy of marketed skin cancer treatments, as reported in the literature on BCC treatment options (Carrillo et al. & Carranza, 2024).

1.6.1. Lifestyle Influences on Skin Health

The complex interplay between lifestyle factors and skin well-being is of primary importance, particularly in the context of benign skin tumors and cysts in dermatology. Environmental factors UV radiation exposure, significantly impact skin integrity. UV exposure not only precedes malignant changes but also leads to the development of benign lesions, that is, seborrheic keratosis and actinic keratosis. Healthy habits , such as regular application of sunscreens, protective clothing, and shade-seeking during the peak sun, can help to reverse the impact. Surprisingly, research has found that implementing these preventive measures substantially reduces the incidence of various skin growths, thereby making the case for greater public education and awareness regarding skin health and healthy lifestyle practices more compelling. Nutrition and proper hydration are equally important factors determining skin health. High-antioxidant, high-vitamin, high-healthy-fat diets have been shown to increase skin elasticity and repair. Omega-3 fatty acids, for instance, can reduce inflammation, which is an important component in preventing some benign skin irregularities. Hydration also helps the skin maintain homeostasis, promoting a healthy-looking glow and aiding cell regeneration. In contrast, diets heavy in processed foods and carbohydrates can exacerbate such conditions as acne and are indirectly likely to be involved in benign tumor or cyst formation. Thus, a nutritious diet, combined with regular hydration, can promote better skin outcomes and reduce the risk of dermatological disorders. Stress management is also a significant aspect of skin well-being to consider. Chronic stress has been linked with numerous dermatoses, including psoriasis and atopic dermatitis, which are likely to give rise to benign skin lesions. The endocrine stress response, characterized by hypercortisolism, can disrupt skin barrier function and its associated healing process. Integrating stress-reduction techniques, such as mindfulness, yoga, and exercise, can enhance skin resilience. Better mental health leads to better overall health, and that is converted to skin health. Accordingly, the prevention and management of benign skin tumors and cysts are contingent on addressing lifestyle factors, including stress, diet, and sun protection. This results in maximum dermatological function and wellness.

1.6.2. Regular Skin Checks and Self-Examinations

Regular self-examination and periodic skin examination are essential components of skin maintenance and early detection of potential issues, particularly benign skin tumors and cysts. Through the practice, people develop a sense of awareness of any changes in their skin, and early detection of abnormality , such as new moles, change in size or color of pre-existing moles, or unusual changes in the skin can be achieved. By performing monthly self-examinations, individuals can establish a personal baseline for their skin's characteristics, thereby making it easier to identify deviations that require professional evaluation. Dermatologists promote regular skin checks as part of a comprehensive health plan, emphasizing the role of proactive measures in preventing more severe issues in the future. In the era of increasing skin cancer cases and increased awareness of the skin, the need to know the role of self-examination is essential. Research indicates that early identification of changes in the skin will lead to an early diagnosis and better prognosis for curing various skin conditions , such as benign tumors. (Mahajan et al., 2023) emphasizes the importance of incorporating periodic skin examinations as a component of preventive healthcare and suggests that the healthcare system place great emphasis on educating about skin health.

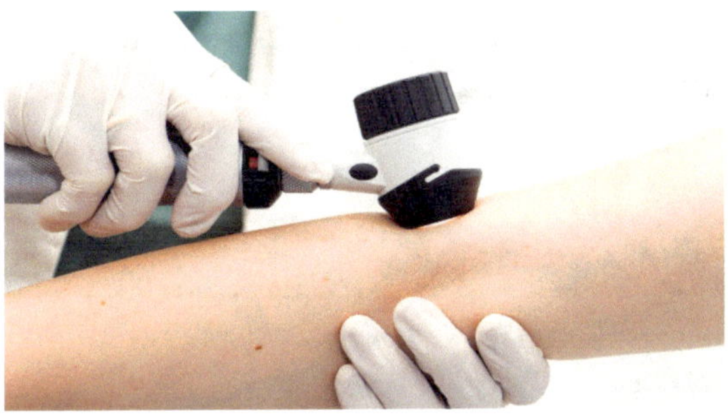

Figure 1.17. Regular skin checks and self-examinations are critical for maintaining skin health and detecting potential issues early, particularly for benign skin tumors and cysts.

Source: https://sundoctors.com.au/wp-content/uploads/2024/08/melanoma-1.jpg.

Regular screening by healthcare workers, combined with self-monitoring, can do wonders in increasing the likelihood of early detection so that benign tumors and cysts, which at times disguise more sinister issues, are detected early on. Moreover, the discourse on skin health is evolving in light of technological advances, including artificial intelligence, which is reshaping dermatological treatment. The application of AI to detect skin lesions has the potential to enhance the accuracy of benign tumor diagnosis and thereby reduce the workload of healthcare personnel while improving patient outcomes. (Karalis, 2024) documents the rapid adoption of AI in clinical specialties, noting its potential benefits in dermatology. As individuals go in for regular skin checks and capitalize on the technological innovations available, it creates opportunities for a more effective and educated trajectory towards skin health, thereby establishing an active partnership between patients and providers in the care of benign skin tumors and cysts (Figure 1.17).

1.6.3. Importance of Patient Education and Awareness

Patient education and awareness regarding benign cysts and skin tumors cannot be overstated in dermatology. An educated patient is in a better position to identify early signs and symptoms of cutaneous disease, which is particularly crucial in distinguishing between benign and potentially malignant lesions. For example, seborrheic keratosis (SK), the most prevalent benign skin tumor of adults, can resemble more harmful varieties of skin cancer and pose potential misdiagnosis in the event of a lack of patient awareness regarding the conditions' features. Awareness can better prepare patients to seek early medical consultation, which in turn turns into better treatment results and reduced psychological distress following ambiguous diagnoses. Therefore, robust educational programs to demystify the nature, presentation, and management of illnesses such as SK can go a long way toward ensuring patient compliance and satisfaction, as well as increased agency in dermatological management (Sutedja et al., 2022). Awareness programs on benign skin tumors and cysts also assist in the promotion of general dermatological health literacy among the population. Greater awareness about the types, risk factors, and treatment options enables individuals to practice preventive action

, such as routine dermatological check-ups and sun protective strategies. Because the majority of benign lesions like keratoacanthomas (KAs) are on sun-damaged skin, educating patients concerning the impact of the sun is two-fold: not only does it educate them regarding benign neoplasms, but also promotes habits that could potentially reduce the risk of future skin malignancies. Comprehensive community outreach activities that emphasize the importance of skin patient education can be the deciding factor in eliminating the fear and stigma around skin diseases and thus encouraging individuals to seek care without any fear (Patnode, 2012).

Finally, the psychological and emotional impacts of benign skin tumors underscore the importance of effective patient education and awareness. Conditions , such as SKs and KAs, self-limited though they may be, are not life-threatening but can drastically impact a patient's self-esteem and quality of life because they are visible to others. Knowledge that self-limited and benign tumors can, in most cases, be helpful in dispelling concern about unexpected skin lesions. Secondly, by educating patients on the available treatment choices, health care providers can enable individuals to make their own decisions regarding their care, thereby creating an equal patient-physician relationship. Through comprehensive education courses, patients can learn to have realistic expectations while also understanding the value of regular follow-ups. This empowerment entails active participation in their dermatological care, thereby advancing the overall purpose of patient-centered care in the management of benign skin tumors and cysts (Patnode, 2012; Gradia et al., 2022).

Test Your Knowledge

1. How can regular skin self-examinations help in managing benign skin tumors and cysts?
2. What lifestyle factors can help maintain healthy skin and potentially reduce the formation of cysts?
3. Why is patient education important in the management of benign skin lesions?

SUMMARY

The diagnosis of benign skin tumors and cysts is a valuable aspect of dermatologic practice. Not only are they difficult to diagnose and treat, but they also affect patient appearance and overall well-being. The knowledge that primary care physicians (PCPs) have regarding dermatologic surgery is significant because their beliefs will ultimately determine whether patients are referred for surgical treatment. Statistics show that the majority of PCPs recognize dermatologic surgeons as the most qualified experts to carry out many cutaneous procedures, including the removal of benign tumors and cysts. This observation underscores the value of ongoing education and communication among PCPs and dermatologists to ensure the optimal outcome of patients with dermatologic conditions, thereby reiterating the crucial role played by specialized training and expertise in the successful management of these benign lesions (Nuha et al., 2024).

Early diagnosis and management of benign skin tumors and cysts cannot be overstressed. Cutaneous disorders , such as epidermal cysts, which occur not infrequently but are rarely documented, may lead to cosmetic concerns or, in severe cases, complications if left untreated. Histopathologic confirmation remains essential in order to establish an accurate diagnosis since clinical presentations may vary widely among patients and generally lead to misdiagnosis. Familiarity with the histological characteristics and the risk of complications, namely cyst rupture or secondary infection, also informs treatment. An understanding of these factors challenges healthcare professionals to employ proactive strategies in their diagnosis and treatment of benign skin tumors, thereby minimizing potential morbidity from these otherwise benign lesions (Li et al., 2021).

Finally, treatment of benign skin tumors and cysts needs to address a holistic approach to treatment through both clinical acumen and patient education. Discussing with patients the nature of their diseases, the potential for treatment, and potential complications fosters an alliance that can result in greater treatment adherence and patient satisfaction. As dermatology continues to evolve, clinical practice guidelines and training programs need to align with the realities of these conditions, enabling practitioners to address the nuances of each case. This holistic approach not only supports clinical practice but also gives more insight into benign skin lesions in the context of the general dermatologic health (Li et al., 2021; Nuha et al., 2024).

Among the new diagnostic techniques of benign skin tumors and cysts is the application of reflectance confocal microscopy (RCM). This new, non-surgical imaging technology provides real-time images of the epidermis and superficial dermis, offering near-histological precision and high contrast for assessing skin lesions. The use of RCM in clinical dermatology practice is a significant shift from conventional histopathology, which will enable clinicians to accurately diagnose benign and malignant tumors without exposing patients to invasive methods. Uses of RCM go beyond a few dermatological diseases, enhancing diagnostic accuracy and patient management and ultimately the overall clinical outcomes. Continued study and use of this technology promise greater insight into skin neoplasms as well as providing a more patient-centered practice of dermatology, particularly for cases involving benign tumors and cystoid lesions. (Fang et al., 2022)

Another key area of interest discussed in the research on benign skin tumors and cysts is the psychological component associated with these diseases, particularly in stressed populations.

A pertinent investigation of women prisoners highlighted the prevalence of skin disorders, with benign conditions of eczema and acne being significantly mentioned amongst the female prisoners. The investigation revealed that 34% of the participants had acne, with other prevalent diseases being hair loss and dry skin. Secondly, the financial repercussions of such skin diseases cannot be underestimated; a considerable proportion of the respondents indicated financial loss and the need to spend money to be treated. This also proves the need for an inclusive dermatology that treats not only the physiological presentation of skin tumors and cysts but also their very severe psychological effect on patients, exemplifying the intricate relationship between mental and dermatological health. (Kocat Aürk et al., 2014) Finally, the controversies regarding benign skin tumors and cysts emphasize the importance of early detection and treatment. Having an understanding of the common characteristics of the various benign conditions is crucial for dermatologists since early treatment can prevent complications and enhance patients' quality of life. Further, continued development of diagnostic tools , such as RCM and the incorporation of psychological aspects are a reflection of the growing acknowledgment of the multifaceted nature of dermatological practice. By addressing both the clinical and emotional components of skin health, dermatologists can develop balanced treatment approaches. As ongoing research continues to unveil the numerous facets of benign skin tumors and their treatment, their integration into practice will ultimately yield improved patient outcomes and a more advanced understanding of dermatological disease.

KEY TERMS FROM THIS CHAPTER

- Adipose tissue
- Benign skin tumors
- Clinical examination techniques
- Cryotherapy
- Cystic lesions
- Dermatologic specialty
- Environmental factors
- Epidermoid cysts
- Hair follicles
- Benign processes
- Biopsies
- Cowden syndrome (CS)
- CS-related benign growths
- Dermatologic assessment
- Dermatology
- Epidermis
- Gardner syndrome
- HPV-related skin lesions calls

CRITICAL THINKING QUESTIONS

1. **Which of the following is the most common type of benign skin tumor?**
   a. Squamous cell carcinoma
   b. Basal cell carcinoma
   c. Seborrheic keratosis
   d. Melanoma
2. **A 25-year-old patient presents with a slow-growing, mobile, subcutaneous nodule on the back. It is not painful but has a central punctum. What is the most likely diagnosis?**
   a. Lipoma
   b. Epidermoid cyst
   c. Dermatofibroma
   d. Keloid
3. **Which of the following is an appropriate treatment for a symptomatic lipoma?**
   a. Surgical excision
   b. Radiation therapy
   c. Oral antibiotics
   d. Cryotherapy
4. **What is a potential complication of an untreated epidermoid cyst?**
   a. Metastasis
   b. Malignant transformation
   c. Rupture and secondary infection
   d. Autoimmune reaction
5. **Which of the following strategies can help prevent recurrence of benign skin cysts after removal?**
   a. Avoiding all dairy products
   b. Regular use of topical steroids
   c. Daily skin brushing
   d. Complete surgical excision of the cyst wall

Short Answer Questions

1. What are the distinguishing characteristics of seborrheic keratosis, lipomas, and dermatofibromas?
2. What are the main differences between epidermoid cysts, pilar cysts, and steatocystomas?
3. Why is a biopsy sometimes necessary in evaluating skin lesions?
4. What are the main treatment approaches for benign skin tumors and cysts?
5. What are potential complications associated with the surgical removal of skin tumors or cysts?
6. How can lifestyle choices influence the development or management of skin cysts and tumors?
7. Why is patient education important in the prevention and early management of benign skin conditions?

Answer to Critical Thinking Questions

1. (c); 2. (b); 3. (a); 4. (c); 5. (d)

REFERENCES

1. Abbasi, R., Amiri Gharghani, M., Montazeri, M., et al. (2015). A rule-based classification model to predict colon cancer survival. *Basic Dermatology*. https://core.ac.uk/download/33492544.pdf (accessed on 21st July 2025).
2. Mahajan, A., Chakrabarty, N., Majithia, J., Ahuja, A., Agarwal, U., Suryavanshi, S., Biradar, M., Sharma, P., Raghavan, B., Arafath, R., & Shukla, S. (2023). Multisystem Imaging Recommendations/Guidelines: In the pursuit of Precision Oncology. *Indian Journal of Medical and Paediatric Oncology*, *44*(01), 002–025. https://doi.org/10.1055/s-0043-1761266M. A. Katsina, I. V. Tsikhanouskaya, V. P. Adaskevich. (2014). *Basic Dermatology*. https://core.ac.uk/download/80151520.pdf (accessed on 21st July 2025).
3. Alfurayh, N. A., Almishary, M., & Alghamdi, K. M. (2024). Perceptions and attitudes of primary care physicians toward dermatologic surgery. *Clinical, Cosmetic and Investigational Dermatology, 17*, 41–49. https://www.semanticscholar.org/paper/ae9b6db4415d2d5b507d076fef409dff2200d518 (accessed on 21st July 2025).
4. Amalina Binte Ebrahim Attia, Balasundaram, G., Moothanchery, M., Dinish, U. S., Bi, R., Ntziachristos, V., & Olivo, M. (2019). A review of clinical photoacoustic imaging: Current and future trends. *Photoacoustics, 16*, 100144. https://doi.org/10.1016/j.pacs.2019.100144 (accessed on 21st July 2025).
5. Menzies, S. W., Moloney, F. J., Byth, K., Avramidis, M., Argenziano, G., Zalaudek, I., Braun, R. P., Malvehy, J., Puig, S., Rabinovitz, H. S., Oliviero, M., Cabo, H., Bono, R., Pizzichetta, M. A., Claeson, M., Gaffney, D. C., Soyer, H. P., Stanganelli, I., Scolyer, R. A., Guitera, P., ... Kreusch, J. (2013). Dermoscopic evaluation of nodular melanoma. *JAMA dermatology*, *149*(6), 699–709. https://doi.org/10.1001/jamadermatol.2013.2466(accessed on 21st July 2025).
6. Snoswell, C. L., Caffery, L. J., Whitty, J. A., Soyer, H. P., & Gordon, L. G. (2018). Cost-effectiveness of Skin Cancer Referral and Consultation Using Teledermoscopy in Australia. *JAMA dermatology*, *154*(6), 694–700. https://doi.org/10.1001/jamadermatol.2018.0855(accessed on 21st July 2025).
7. Balsamo, F., Cardoso, P. A. S., do Amaral, S. A., Theodoro, T. R., Gehrke, F. de S., da Silva Pinhal, M. A., Bianco, B., et al. (2020). Birt-Hogg-Dubé syndrome with simultaneous hyperplastic polyposis of the gastrointestinal tract: Case report and review of the literature. *BMC Medical Genetics, 21*. https://doi.org/10.1186/s12881-020-0991-8 (accessed on 21st July 2025).
8. Lucas, A., Betlloch, I., Planelles, M., Martínez, T., Pérez-Crespo, M., Mataix, J., & Belinchón, I. (2007). Non-melanocytic benign skin tumors in children. *American journal of clinical dermatology*, *8*(6), 365–369. https://doi.org/10.2165/00128071-200708060-00006(accessed on 21st July 2025).
9. Cassalia, F., Danese, A., Cocchi, E., Vaienti, S., Bolzon, A., Franceschin, L., Mazzetto, R., Caroppo, F., Melandri, D., & Belloni Fortina, A. (2025). Congenital Dermatofibrosarcoma Protuberans-An Update on the Ongoing Diagnostic Challenges. *Cancers*, *17*(1), 158. https://doi.org/10.3390/cancers17010158(accessed on 21st July 2025).
10. Bevers, T. B., Helvie, M. A., Bonaccio, E., Calhoun, K. E., Daly, M. B., Farrar, W. B., Garber, J. E., et al. (2018). Breast cancer screening and diagnosis, version 3.2018, NCCN clinical practice guidelines in oncology. *Journal of the National Comprehensive Cancer Network, 16*, 1362–1389. https://doi.org/10.6004/jnccn.2018.0083 (accessed on 21st July 2025).

11. Bianchi, M. G., Santos, A., & Cordioli, E. (2020). Benefits of teledermatology for geriatric patients: Population-based cross-sectional study. *Journal of Medical Internet Research, 22,* e16700. https://www.semanticscholar.org/paper/8c89351639550db9b964fbb8057252e78c4f7d47 (accessed on 21st July 2025).

12. Hildenbrand, C., Burgdorf, W. H., & Lautenschlager, S. (2001). Cowden syndrome-diagnostic skin signs. *Dermatology (Basel, Switzerland), 202*(4), 362–366. https://doi.org/10.1159/000051684(accessed on 21st July 2025).

13. Schaller, J., Rohwedder, A., Burgdorf, W. H., Itin, P. H., & Lautenschlager, S. (2003). Identification of human papillomavirus DNA in cutaneous lesions of Cowden syndrome. *Dermatology (Basel, Switzerland), 207*(2), 134–140. https://doi.org/10.1159/000071782(accessed on 21st July 2025).

14. Cocuz, I. G., Cocuz, M. E., Niculescu, R., Șincu, M. C., Tinca, A. C., Sabău, A. H., Chiorean, D. M., et al. (2021). The impact of and adaptations due to the COVID-19 pandemic on the histopathological diagnosis of skin pathologies, including non-melanocyte and melanoma skin cancers—A single-center study in Romania. *Medicina, 57,* 533. https://doi.org/10.3390/medicina57060533 (accessed on 21st July 2025).

15. Maniaci, A., La Via, L., Lavalle, S., Lentini, M., Pavone, P., Iannella, G., & Cocuzza, S. (2024). Presentation, Radiologic Features, and Treatment Options of Congenital Tongue Tumors: A Comprehensive Review. Annali italiani di chirurgia, 95 4, 481-496 .(accessed on 21st July 2025).

16. Sutedja, Eva Krishna; Gradia, Resti; and Latifah, Tri Aswila (2022) "Seborrheic Keratosis Profile at Dr. Hasan Sadikin Central General Hospital Bandung 2015-2019," Journal of General - Procedural Dermatology and Venereology Indonesia: Vol. 6: Iss. 2, Article 6. DOI: 10.7454/jdvi.v6i2.1005 Available at: https://scholarhub.ui.ac.id/jdvi/vol6/iss2/6(accessed on 21st July 2025).

17. Daniela Guerrero Carrillo, & Vianney Anguiano Carranza. (2024). Basal Cell Carcinoma with a Relationship in Dermatology and Plastic Surgery. *International Journal of Medical Science and Clinical Research Studies, 4*(01), 82–85. https://doi.org/10.47191/ijmscrs/v4-i01-18(accessed on 21st July 2025).

18. Guirguis, M., Arribas, E. M., Kapoor, M. M., Patel, M., Perez, F., Nia, E. S., Ding, Q., et al. (2024). Multimodality imaging of benign and malignant diseases of the nipple-areolar complex. *Radiographic: A Review Publication of the Radiological Society of North America, Inc., 44*(4), e230113. https://www.semanticscholar.org/paper/ef8553885cf4ce50d497d50eeb5ad1ce527f860b (accessed on 21st July 2025).

19. Heck, H. C., Van Poucke, L., Heck, B. E., Vasiloff, J., & Heck, B. E. (2024). Pedunculated osteochondroma presenting as verruca vulgaris: A diagnosis requiring a high index of suspicion: Case report. *Journal of Orthopedic Case Reports, 14,* 89–95. https://www.semanticscholar.org/paper/18a810f04edaecf9116272d26d0ff20b5c6792f6 (accessed on 21st July 2025).

20. Heller, G. (2020). Conservative management of a fourth ventricular epidermoid in a patient with Gardner syndrome. *Therapeutic Advances in Rare Disease, 1.* https://www.semanticscholar.org/paper/44d5155d063c2cf5d76fae37484fa671dc65a623 (accessed on 21st July 2025).

21. Karalis, V. (2024). The integration of artificial intelligence into clinical practice. *Applied Biosciences, 3,* 14–44. https://doi.org/10.3390/applbiosci3010002 (accessed on 21st July 2025).

22. Kocatürk, E., Kocatürk, A., & Kavala, M. (2014). Prevalence of skin diseases in female prisoners in Turkey: analysis of impact of prison conditions and psychological stress. *Acta dermatovenerologica Croatica : ADC, 22*(1), 26–31.(accessed on 21st July 2025).

23. Kotova, Tatyana Gennadyevna, Sergei Nikolaevich Tsybusov, Vladimir Ivanovich Kochenov, and Maksim Igorevich Tcyganov. 2018. 'Application of Cryogenic Methods in Skin Diseases of Different Etiology'. Dermatologic Surgery and Procedures. InTech. doi:10.5772/intechopen.70509.(accessed on 21st July 2025).

24. Li, Y., Wang, S., & Zhang, R. (2021). Epidermal cysts of the head and neck: A clinicopathologic analysis of 112 cases. *31*, 16–19. https://www.semanticscholar.org/paper/0b5d2375af100a329b1392abf44a5983dd6d8f5d (accessed on 21st July 2025).

25. Liopyris, K., Gregoriou, S., Dias, J., & Stratigos, A. (2022). Artificial intelligence in dermatology: Challenges and perspectives. *Dermatology and Therapy, 12*, 2637–2651. https://doi.org/10.1007/s13555-022-00833-8 (accessed on 21st July 2025).

26. Menzies, S. W., Kreusch, J., Byth, K., Pizzichetta, M. A., Marghoob, A., Braun, R., Malvehy, J., Puig, S., Argenziano, G., Zalaudek, I., Rabinovitz, H. S., Oliviero, M., Cabo, H., Ahlgrimm-Siess, V., Avramidis, M., Guitera, P., Soyer, H. P., Ghigliotti, G., Tanaka, M., Perusquia, A. M., ... Johr, R. (2008). Dermoscopic evaluation of amelanotic and hypomelanotic melanoma. *Archives of dermatology, 144*(9), 1120–1127. https://doi.org/10.1001/archderm.144.9.1120(accessed on 21st July 2025).

27. Meyer, T., & Stockfleth, E. (2024). Treatment and prevention of HPV-associated skin tumors by HPV vaccination. *Vaccines, 12*. https://www.semanticscholar.org/paper/364357e96704020200530f512c4c1d64fa516371 (accessed on 21st July 2025).

28. Fang, Wei-Cheng; Chou, Pei-Chien; Chiu, Li-Wen; Ke, Chiao-Li2; Cheng, Shih-Tsun. Dermoscopy as a Diagnostic and Monitoring Tool for Recurrent Extramammary Paget's Disease. Indian Journal of Dermatology 67(6):p 819-820, Nov–Dec 2022. | DOI: 10.4103/ijd.ijd_771_22 (accessed on 21st July 2025).

29. Northrup, H., Aronow, M. E., Bebin, E. M., Bissler, J. J., Darling, T. N., de Vries, P. J., Frost, M., et al. (2021). Updated international tuberous sclerosis complex diagnostic criteria and surveillance and management recommendations. *Pediatric Neurology, 123*, 50–66. https://doi.org/10.1016/j.pediatrneurol.2021.07.011 (accessed on 21st July 2025).

30. Northrup, H., Krueger, D. A., Roberds, S. L., Smith, K., Sampson, J. R., et al. (2013). Tuberous sclerosis complex diagnostic criteria update: Recommendations of the 2012 International Tuberous Sclerosis Complex Consensus Conference. *Pediatric Neurology, 49*, 243–254. https://doi.org/10.1016/j.pediatrneurol.2013.08.001 (accessed on 21st July 2025).

31. Oakley, A. (2017). *Dermatology Made Easy*. http://books.google.com/books?id=DYrTjgEACAAJ&dq=Benign+skin+tumors+and+cysts+in+dermatology+including+epidermoid+cysts,+pilar+cysts,+and+steatocystomas&hl=&source=gbs_api (accessed on 21st July 2025).

32. Olveres, J., González, G., Torres, F., Moreno-Tagle, J. C., Carbajal-Degante, E., Valencia-Rodríguez, A., Méndez-Sánchez, N., et al. (2021). What is new in computer vision and artificial intelligence in medical image analysis applications. *Quantitative Imaging in Medicine and Surgery, 11*, 3830–3853. https://doi.org/10.21037/qims-20-1151 (accessed on 21st July 2025).

33. Patnode, C. C. (2012). Identifying and managing keratoacanthoma. https://core.ac.uk/download/591546572.pdf (accessed on 21st July 2025).

34. Poalelungi, D. G., Mușat, C. L., Fulga, A., Neagu, M., Neagu, A. I., Piraianu, A. I., & Fulga, I. (2023). Advancing patient care: How artificial intelligence is transforming healthcare. *Journal of Personalized Medicine, 13*, 1214. https://doi.org/10.3390/jpm13081214 (accessed on 21st July 2025).

35. van der Velden, B. H. M., Kuijf, H. J., Gilhuijs, K. G. A., & Viergever, M. A. (2022). Explainable artificial intelligence (XAI) in deep learning-based medical image analysis. *Medical Image Analysis, 79*, 102470. https://doi.org/10.1016/j.media.2022.102470 (accessed on 21st July 2025).

36. Wei, M., Luo, Q., Li, W. J., Yan, H., Cao, X., & Li, X. (2022). [Reconstruction of facial skin defects by the V-Y subcutaneous pedicle flap]. *Zhonghua Er Bi Yan Hou Tou Jing Wai Ke Za Zhi = Chinese Journal of Otorhinolaryngology Head and Neck Surgery, 57*(6), 718–723. https://www.semanticscholar.org/paper/969439e9306bb786a00e82382323be52f0428032 (accessed on 21st July 2025).

PREMALIGNANT AND MALIGNANT SKIN TUMORS (BCC, SCC, MELANOMA)

2

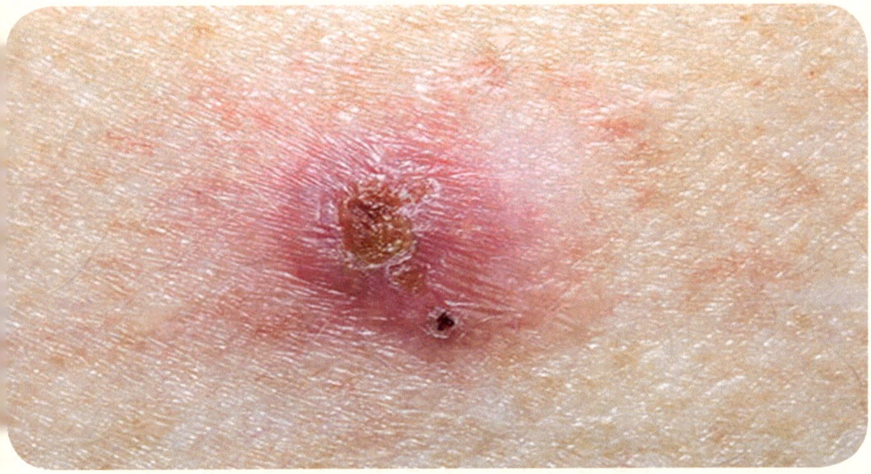

LEARNING OBJECTIVES

After studying this chapter, you will be able to:

1. Describe BCC, SCC, and Melanoma
2. Discuss risk factors associated with premalignant and malignant skin tumors
3. Understand symptoms and diagnosis of basal cell carcinoma (BCC), squamous cell carcinoma (SCC), and melanoma
4. Explain treatment options for premalignant and malignant skin tumors
5. Deal with effective prevention strategies for skin tumors
6. Focus on the prognosis for premalignant and malignant skin tumors

Introduction

The increased global incidence of skin cancer necessitates complete knowledge of its premalignant and malignant forms, particularly basal cell carcinoma (BCC), squamous cell carcinoma (SCC), and melanoma. Cutaneous tumors represent a significant public health concern due to widespread prevalence and associated morbidity and mortality. The most frequent type of cancer in the United States, skin cancer, presents unique diagnostic and treatment challenges. Skin Cancer. Causative elements for the development of skin tumors include ultraviolet (UV) radiation-associated environmental exposure, combined with genetic predisposition and lifestyle. Early diagnosis and intervention are crucial, as they significantly improve patient survival. This chapter is intended to evaluate the complexity of these cancers and to present details on their pathophysiology, risk factors, and diagnostic strategies that are essential for effective management. In the past few years, advances in diagnostic technology, such as optical coherence tomography (OCT), have revolutionized the clinical setting for the diagnosis of skin cancer. OCT facilitates advanced imaging of tissue architecture, thereby enabling differentiation between benign and malignant lesions. This novel imaging approach is very close to the resolution of histopathology, thus offering clinicians invaluable information at the time of diagnosis. As outlined in recent studies, OCT application in most epithelial tissues has proven effective and can distinguish between benign lesions and various cancers *in vivo*. The application of such technologies in clinical practice will be of paramount importance for improving diagnostic accuracy and ultimately guiding treatment decisions, thereby enabling timely interventions for patients with BCC, SCC, or melanoma. (Wessels et al., 2014). Appreciation of the function of such environmental agents as arsenic exposure emphasizes the multifaceted nature of skin carcinogenesis. Chronic arsenic ingestion has been associated with increased risk of skin cancer, with recent evidence pointing toward potential epigenetic alterations mediating such effect. Intersections between various carcinogenic pathways reveal such hidden mechanisms that are not only genetic but also epigenetic, involving dysregulation of microRNAs in arsenic tumors. These alterations can be utilized as biomarkers for early detection or therapeutic drugs, uncovering the contribution of environmental poisons to the causation and course of skin cancers. This molecular information enriches the prevention and treatment strategy, providing new avenues for investigation that may introduce precious advances in the war against skin cancer. The union of epigenetics and environmental science creates an essential foundation for controlling both BCC and SCC successfully, as well as gaining insight into the severe consequences of melanoma (Al-Eryani & Laila, 2017).

Significance of Understanding Skin Tumors

It is essential to understand skin tumors to facilitate early diagnosis and effective management, particularly for premalignant and malignant lesions such as basal cell carcinoma (BCC), squamous cell carcinoma (SCC), and melanoma. Skin tumors can develop in different ways, typically depending on their type and etiology, and thus awareness is crucial. Early recognition of abnormal skin appearance can lead to timely interventions, significantly improving patient outcomes. Moreover, public health education regarding the dangers of sun exposure and tanning beds can reduce the incidence of these tumors, in accordance with preventive dermatology objectives. Because of the growing incidence of skin cancer around the globe, both patients and health care providers must embrace awareness with regard to skin tumor characteristics to facilitate timely diagnosis and therapy. The complexity of skin tumor pathogenesis requires a broad understanding of its mode of action at the biological level. Research has demonstrated that both environmental and genetic stimuli are implicated in the development of these malignancies. For example, chronic exposure to certain carcinogens, such as arsenic, has been demonstrated to be a significant risk factor for the causation of skin cancer, as evidenced by the identification of epigenetic changes involved in carcinogenesis in arsenic-induced skin cancer (Al-Eryani & Laila, 2017). These findings help to underscore the need to inform clinical practice with scientific evidence. Through knowledge of the underlying mechanisms by which skin tumors form, clinicians and researchers can develop targeted therapeutic interventions and prevention strategies to improve patient treatment and mitigate the burden of skin cancer as a public health problem. Beyond clinical significance, the study of skin tumors offers strong potential for developing research and treatment protocols on which to build. As skin tumors become increasingly heterogeneous and present in varying forms, scientific investigation to characterize their distinct molecular patterns becomes imperative. The use of advanced diagnostic techniques—such as identifying microRNA expression changes as markers of cancer progression—can improve the efficacy of treatment strategies (Al-Eryani & Laila, 2017). This shifting landscape requires continuous education and training for clinicians to recognize and value skin tumors. Lacking a clear understanding of tumor biology and individual risk factors, treatment protocols will be less effective, ultimately influencing survival rate and the quality of life for skin cancer patients (Figure 2.1).

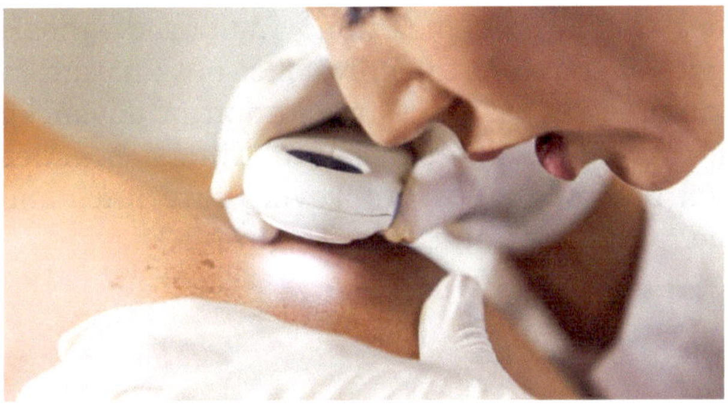

Figure 2.1. Understanding skin tumors is crucial for early detection and effective treatment.

Source: https://www.tru-skin.com/getmedia/a33bd602-dfbf-46c1-84eb-d89f495f3960/importance-skin-cancer-screening-hero.jpg?width=720&height=400&ext=.jpg.

Overview of Premalignant and Malignant Types

The classification of skin tumors spans a continuum from benign and premalignant types to malignant types, each with different features and clinical significance. Premalignant lesions, such as actinic keratosis and Bowen's disease, are of particular significance in the progression to skin cancer. These lesions arise primarily from chronic sun exposure, implying disruption of normal keratinocyte function, and are a potential precursor to malignancy. Actinic keratosis, for example, most often presents as rough, scaly lesions on sun-damaged skin and has the potential to progress to SCC if left untreated. Early detection and management of these premalignant lesions are important because they serve as early indicators of subsequent malignancies and inform the next level of clinical intervention required. On the other hand, malignant skin tumors, such as basal cell carcinoma (BCC), SCC, and melanoma, are a more advanced state of skin pathology. BCC, the most common skin cancer, is observed with uncontrollable basal cell growth and tends to be pearly nodules or open sores. In contrast, SCC arises from keratinocytes, can present as nodular, hard, red nodules or scaly plaques, and can metastasize; thus, it requires early diagnosis. Melanoma, while less common, is referred to as the most dangerous type of skin cancer due to its aggressiveness and rapid spread. Understanding the morphological and molecular characteristics of such tumors not only facilitates accurate diagnosis but also highlights the need for personalized treatment modalities that may include surgical excision, immunotherapy, or targeted therapy regimens. Recent research has unraveled the molecular mechanisms involved in both premalignant and malignant transformation of skin cells. Studies have shown that chronic exposure to arsenic causes meaningful epigenetic changes that potentially fuel skin carcinogenesis, emphasizing the development of microRNA (miRNA) deregulation as a contributor to skin cancers (Al-Eryani & Laila, 2017). In addition, therapies such as cryotherapy have become viable treatments for premalignant lesions and early-stage malignancies, indicating a shift toward less aggressive practices in dermatology (Akarsu, S., & Kamberoglu, I. 2018). Through continued study of these evolving treatment modalities and their mechanisms, clinicians will be better able to predict disease course and implement proactive patient management to offset the risks associated with these diverse skin tumors. Such reports emphasize the need for a coordinated strategy for the management of both premalignant and malignant cutaneous diseases and for optimizing overall patient care.

2.1. BCC, SCC, and Melanoma

Learning Outcome

1. Describe basal cell carcinoma (BCC).
2. Define squamous cell carcinoma (SCC).
3. Understand melanoma, a malignant skin tumor.

Skin tumors are usually classified into two types: benign and malignant; the latter is associated with adverse health outcomes. Among all malignancies, basal cell carcinoma (BCC) and squamous cell carcinoma (SCC) are the most frequently occurring forms of non-melanoma skin carcinoma. BCC arises from basal cells of the epidermis with slow growth and low metastatic likelihood. In contrast, SCC arises from squamous cells and, though similarly slowly growing, is more capable of invasion and metastasis than BCC. Both may develop as a result of chronic exposure to ultraviolet (UV) radiation, underscoring the imperative for prevention in at-risk individuals. The benign overall appearance of these skin cancers often leads to misdiagnosis, underscoring the need for effective diagnostic techniques to distinguish malignant from benign lesions. Melanoma, the most dangerous skin cancer, arises from melanocytes, the pigment-producing skin cells. This type of cancer is much more harmful than BCC or SCC and thus placing greater importance on early detection and treatment. Unlike non-melanoma skin cancers, melanoma can have a dramatic metastasis to remote sites in the body, with typically catastrophic results if not identified early in its development. Melanoma risk factors are multifaceted, consisting of genetic predispositions, previous sunburn, and the development of dysplastic moles. Surveillance is particularly important in high-risk individuals, such as organ transplant recipients, who have an extremely heightened risk of melanoma due to immunosuppression. Education and sensitization efforts with focused attention can lead to early referral and improved outcomes among at-risk patients (Chundydyal, 2015). Innovative diagnostic techniques are essential to improve early detection rates of skin tumors, particularly of melanomas and non-melanoma skin cancers. OIDRS research shows possible advancements in this regard. This non-invasive method provides fast, real-time assessment of skin lesions with high sensitivity and specificity for the detection of malignant tumors (Garcia-Urib et al., 2012). It can reduce the need for invasive biopsies with definitive diagnostics. It can also identify malignant and non-malignant skin lesions, making diagnosis more effective. As the prevalence of skin cancers continues to rise, the integration of advanced diagnostic technologies into clinical practice will be essential for improving cure rates and overall patient outcomes (Figure 2.2).

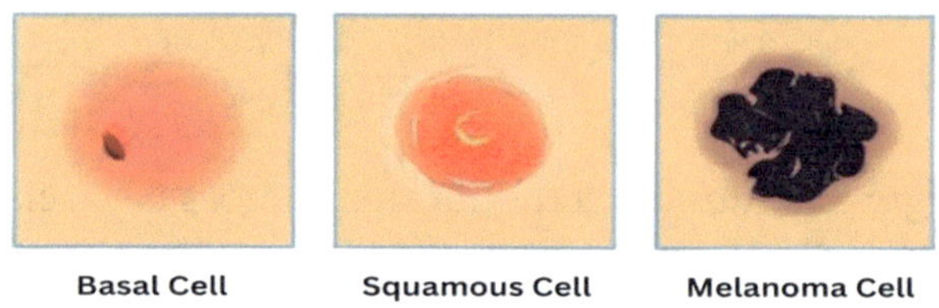

Figure 2.2. Types of skin cancer.

Source: https://coloradospringsdermatologyclinic.com/wp-content/uploads/Understand-the-Types-of-Skin-Cancer.png.

2.1.1. Basal Cell Carcinoma (BCC)

Basal Cell Carcinoma (BCC) is the most frequent skin cancer and arises predominantly from basal cells in the epidermis. The malignancy is more strongly associated with prolonged exposure to ultraviolet (UV) light radiation, generally sunlight. Consistent with this, the disease affects more fair-skinned individuals who are habitually sun-exposed with no protective measures. In contrast to more aggressive skin cancers, BCC generally grows slowly and rarely metastasizes to distant sites. Yet, it can cause extensive local invasion and subsequent morbidity if not treated, with resultant destruction of adjacent tissues and structures. Hence, understanding the pathophysiology of BCC is crucial because early detection and treatment can significantly alter clinical outcomes and reduce negative impacts on the patient's quality of life. Regarding diagnosis, the traditional method is a full clinical examination followed by a biopsy to determine the presence of carcinoma histologically (Figure 2.3).

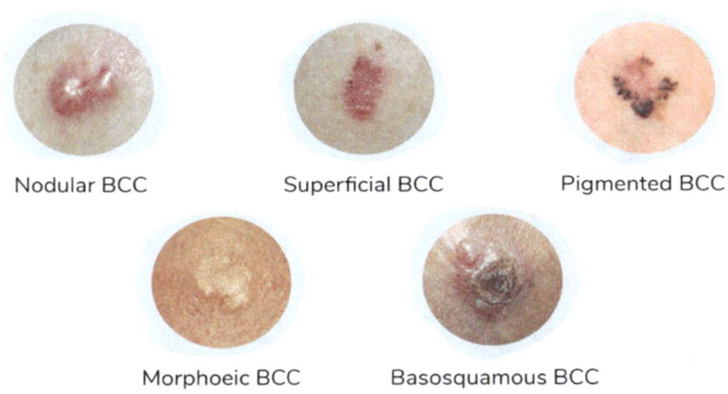

Figure 2.3. Types of basal cell carcinoma.

Source: https://miiskin.com/wp-content/uploads/2020/04/basal-cell-carcinoma-types.png.

New advances in diagnostic techniques, such as oblique incidence diffuse reflectance spectroscopy (OIDRS), have emerged as promising non-invasive tools for the detection of BCC. OIDRS is extremely sensitive and specific, with 92% specificity for the separation of pigmentation-free basal cell carcinomas from benign dermatological conditions , such as actinic keratoses. By facilitating earlier diagnosis, these advances are poised to reduce the use of more invasive tests and expedite treatment initiation, ultimately improving patient outcomes. The use of OIDRS in clinical settings represents a major turning point in dermatological diagnostic science, propelling the trend toward more patient-oriented care. Treatment for BCC ranges from excision to topical therapy and cryotherapy, depending on the size, site, and histological nature of the tumors. Cryotherapy or local freezing therapy has also gained wider acceptance as an effective and less disruptive treatment in suitable patients, especially superficial BCC or those with intolerance to surgery. This method, which has a brief recovery period and acceptable side effects, allows for the treatment of more than one lesion in a single sitting. Moreover, the excellent cosmetic outcome typical of cryotherapy makes it an appealing choice for multiple skin lesions in elderly patients who seek effective, non-surgical treatments. As the incidence rate of BCC is on the rise, especially among elderly individuals, awareness and utilization of diverse treatment modalities are increasingly essential in managing this common skin cancer (Garcia-Urib et al., 2012; Akarsu & Kamberoglu, 2018) (Figure 2.4).

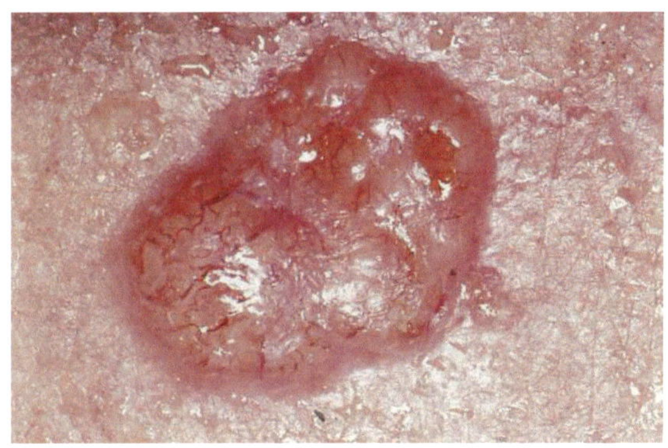

Figure 2.4. Basal cell carcinoma on the patient's back.

Source: https://upload.wikimedia.org/wikipedia/commons/4/4f/Basal_cell_carcinoma.jpg.

2.1.2. Squamous Cell Carcinoma (SCC)

Squamous Cell Carcinoma (SCC) is the most prevalent form of non-melanoma skin cancer, based primarily on the transformation of squamous cells present within the epidermis. Its development is primarily attributable to prolonged exposure to ultraviolet (UV) light, which induces direct DNA damage and mutations that promote malignancy. Squamous Cell Carcinoma pathogenesis is complex and involves many genetic and molecular alterations. Recent studies have determined that these mutations, together with other risk factors , such as immunosuppression and exposure to carcinogenic agents, may cross-talk to drive SCC onset and progression. Thus, familiarity with the molecular intricacies of SCC is essential for effective prevention and treatment, particularly among patients with high-risk factors (Ugo et al., 2018). Alongside its biological and genetic substrates, SCC exhibits a specific epidemiological pattern. Of particular note is that it demonstrates trends in incidence that imply variations according to population characteristics, such as age, sex, and geographic location. For instance, research indicates an increase in the incidence of SCC, particularly among older adults and immunocompromised individuals (Figure 2.5).

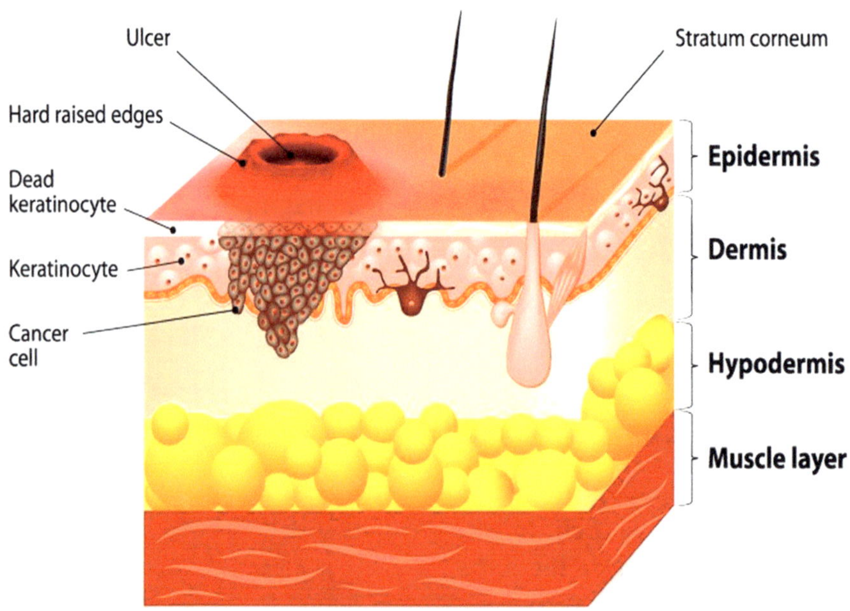

Figure 2.5. Squamous cell carcinoma (SCC).

Source: https://www.news-medical.net/image-handler/picture/2021/4/shutterstock_241007965.jpg.

From a phenotypic characteristic perspective, risk factors are particularly robustly correlated with SCC. Evidence suggests patients with a family history of skin cancers, high counts of nevi, or certain skin types are at higher risk for the development of SCC (Han et al., 2014). This new awareness underscores the importance of regular dermatological examination, particularly among high-risk populations, to enable early detection and treatment and thereby optimize patient outcomes. Clinical presentations of SCC can vary widely and may be scaly, erythematous patches, open ulcers, or protuberant masses with a central crust. The majority are localized and, if early diagnosed, have very good prognoses. There is a minority of SCCs that, left untreated, will metastasize and result in extensive morbidity. The treatment armamentarium for SCC includes surgical excision, cryotherapy, and topical chemotherapeutic agents, depending on the size and location of the tumors. New novel therapies with targeted agents and immunotherapy are also being explored, broadening the arsenal against SCC (Ugo et al., 2018). With increasing incidence rates, particularly in regions where sunlight prevails, public health campaigns targeting awareness, prevention, and early detection are crucial for SCC control and for relieving its health system burden (Figure 2.6).

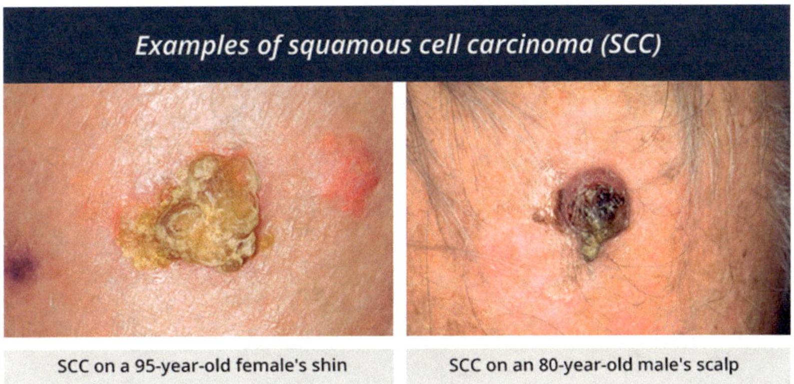

Figure 2.6. Examples of squamous cell carcinoma (SCC).

Source: https://media.healthdirect.org.au/images/inline/original/scc-examples-2ad126.jpg.

2.1.3. Melanoma

Melanoma, a malignant skin cancer caused by melanocytes, is a significant public health issue due to its rising incidence and mortality potential. Though it accounts for a smaller proportion of skin cancers than basal cell carcinoma (BCC) and squamous cell carcinoma (SCC), melanoma is the cause of most skin cancer deaths. The primary causative risk factors for the onset of melanoma include long exposure to ultraviolet (UV) radiation, a history of sunburn, and genetic predisposition. An early diagnosis is critical because melanoma advances rapidly into other organs, making therapy difficult and having a detrimental effect on prognosis (Figures 2.7 and 2.8).

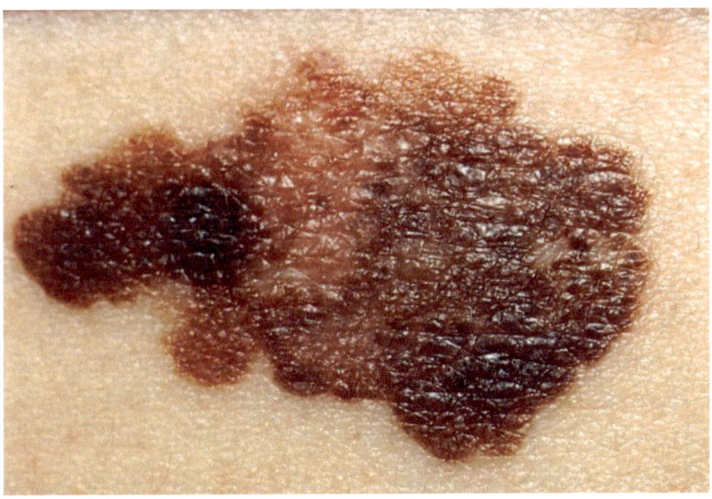

Figure 2.7. This slide shows a melanoma on a patient's skin.

Source: https://upload.wikimedia.org/wikipedia/commons/thumb/6/6c/Melanoma.jpg/800px-Melanoma.jpg.

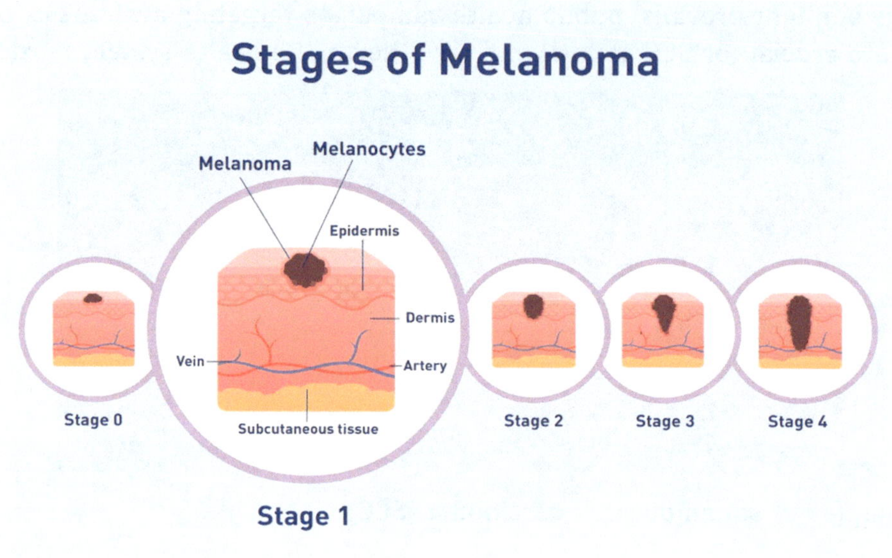

Figure 2.8. Stages of melanoma.

Source: https://melanomafocus.org/wp-content/uploads/2022/04/Stage-1-diagram-1024x675.png.

The clinical evaluation typically involves visual inspection followed by a confirmatory biopsy to assess malignancy and stage, which are pivotal for planning therapeutic intervention and improving patient outcomes. Treatment of melanoma is varied, paralleling the heterogeneity of its pathology and potential for progression. Surgical removal remains the cornerstone of therapy for local melanoma, allowing one to cure the tumor while at the same time getting informative staging data through sentinel lymph node biopsies. In advanced disease, where there has been metastasis, adjuvant forms of therapy in the guise of immunotherapy and targeted therapy have been useful forms of therapy. Of particular note, agents such as checkpoint inhibitors, which suppress immune activity, have revolutionized the management of metastatic melanoma. However, despite all these advancements, premalignant and malignant lesion separation is mostly based on timely identification and early clinical intervention. Of key importance, as identified by studies, is the need for expanded training among health practitioners, particularly in diagnosing malignant skin lesion characteristics, which can lead to timely referral to dermatology as well as slowing the progression of the disease (Viguier et al., 2015). Furthermore, the implications of melanoma extend far beyond individual cases to broader public health concerns. With the incidence of melanoma continuing to climb, especially among young adults and some demographic populations, it is crucial that there are educational and preventive measures underway at the community level. Education on sun protection, routine skin examination, and identification of melanoma warning signs is central to early detection and intervention in the population. Moreover, specialized educational programs for healthcare professionals, particularly in primary and rheumatology care, are required to equip them with the necessary competencies to accurately differentiate between benign and malignant skin lesions. As evidenced by recent research, promoting diagnostic capabilities through specialized training can substantially enhance early detection of malignant skin cancers, thereby improving patient outcomes and survival rates (Viguier et al., 2015).

Test Your Knowledge

1. What are the key differences in appearance between basal cell carcinoma (BCC), squamous cell carcinoma (SCC), and melanoma?
2. How does squamous cell carcinoma (SCC) typically spread compared to basal cell carcinoma (BCC)?

2.2. Risk Factors

Learning Outcome

1. Describe UV radiation exposure.
2. Understand the relationship between genetic predisposition and the development of skin tumors.
3. Explain the role of environmental factors in the development of skin tumors.

It is essential to know the risk factors of premalignant and malignant skin cancers, that is, basal cell carcinoma (BCC), squamous cell carcinoma (SCC), and melanoma, to prevent them as well as to detect them early. The most crucial environmental risk factor for the three mentioned skin cancers is ultraviolet (UV) radiation from sunlight exposure. Long-term exposure to UV causes DNA damage in the cells of the skin, and this results in mutations that can eventually result in tumor formation. Furthermore, sporadic high sun exposure, particularly causing sunburns, has been linked to elevated melanoma risk. The double nature of UV exposure proves the need for protective interventions , such as the use of sunscreen and protective clothing, to limit exposure. Increasing public awareness of preventive methods is crucial in preventing the spread of these skin cancers. Additionally, certain populations and inherited factors are significant in determining individuals' susceptibility to skin tumors. For instance, individuals who have light-colored eyes, light-colored hair, and fair skin are susceptible to skin cancer since they do not have adequate protective melanin. Additionally, a history of skin cancer within the family is indicative of increased risks, which, in turn, implies a genetic factor in susceptibility. Conditions , such as xeroderma pigmentosum, which undermine skin competence in repairing UV irradiation-induced DNA damage, significantly enhance the risk for skin cancers. Skin aging also undermines skin resistance and regenerative capacity, adding further risk factors. Combined, awareness of these demographic and genetic determinants is essential for clinicians to identify populations at risk and implement targeted screening and education programs. The role of immunosuppression in increasing vulnerability to skin carcinomas is a significant line of investigation. Inflammatory rheumatism patients, particularly those being treated with tumor necrosis factor (TNF) blockers, bear a much higher incidence of skin cancers than does the general population. Immunomodulation in this instance is harmful as it can make the body's capacity for identifying and eliminating developing cancer cells useless, allowing tumor development to occur. Thus, it is important for healthcare providers to be vigilant for the initial presentation of skin cancers in immunosuppressed patients, so that they can promptly refer them to dermatologists for assessment and management. Emerging diagnostic tools , such as optical coherence tomography (OCT), offer promising tools for *in vivo* differentiation of benign versus malignant lesions, emphasizing the incorporation of sophisticated diagnostic methods into routine clinical practice to better identify at-risk patients and coordinate their care (Wessels et al., 2014; Viguier et al., 2015) (Figure 2.9).

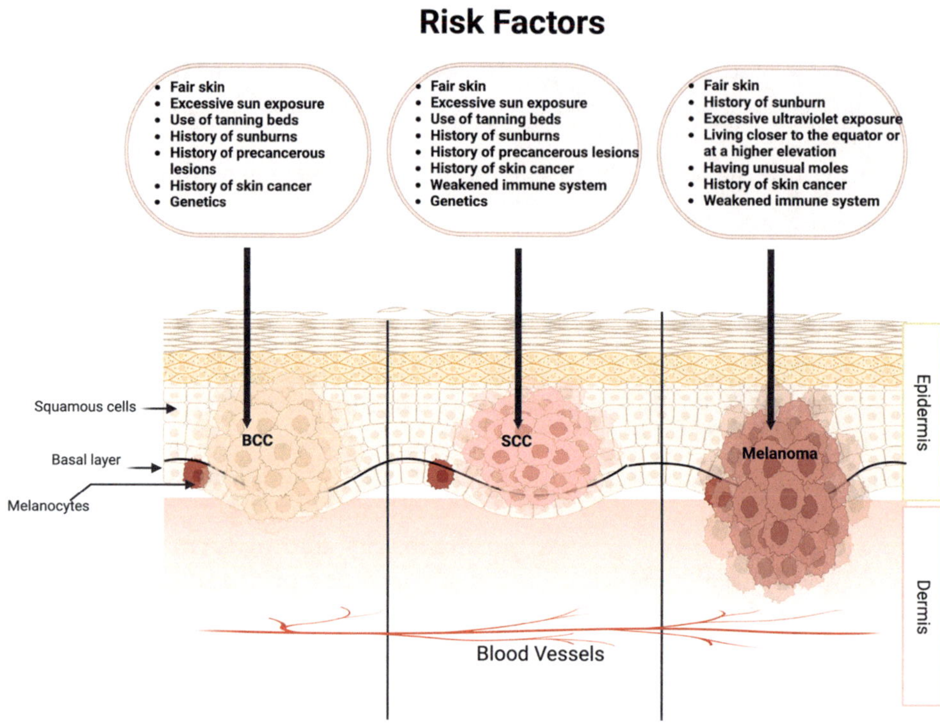

Figure 2.9. Risk factors for the most common types of skin cancer. BCC: basal cell carcinoma; SCC: squamous cell carcinoma.

Source: https://www.researchgate.net/publication/372741916/figure/fig1/AS:11431281210578891@1702055257160/Risk-factors-for-the-most-common-types-of-skin-cancer-BCC-basal-cell-carcinoma-SCC.tif.

2.2.1. UV Radiation Exposure

Understanding exposure to UV radiation is necessary to put its role in the etiology of premalignant and malignant skin tumors, primarily basal cell carcinoma (BCC), squamous cell carcinoma (SCC), and melanoma, into perspective. UV radiation is divided into UVA, UVB, and UVC, with UVB being the primary contributor to skin damage and carcinogenesis. Long-term exposure to UV radiation causes changes in the cellular composition of the skin, which initiates a chain of molecular reactions that may lead to cellular mutations. These mutations are most problematic for people with fair skin, as this subgroup is more prone to skin damage and, ultimately, tumor formation. Furthermore, cumulative UV exposure may significantly increase the risk of several skin cancers, underscoring the importance of preventive interventions against UV exposure among individuals at risk of skin malignancies. The link between actinic keratoses and UV radiation exposure identifies a crucial step in carcinogenesis to SCC. Actinic keratoses are benign intraepithelial neoplasms resulting from chronic sun exposure and reflect the skin's response to prolonged UV insult. As noted, the atypical keratinocyte's abnormal proliferation that defines these lesions, if left untreated, can progress to squamous cell carcinoma. The mechanism is facilitated by disruption of normal apoptotic mechanisms in photoexposed skin, thereby allowing abnormal keratinocytes to survive and continue to proliferate. Therefore, successful treatment of actinic keratoses is not only crucial for SCC prevention but also for the identification of individuals at risk for violent skin malignancies. Emphasis on early detection and ongoing follow-up can prevent the progression of such lesions toward invasive carcinoma and thus reduce the burden of skin cancer. Phototherapy, as used in dermatology, illustrates the delicate balance between therapeutic efficacy and the risk of exposure to UV radiation.

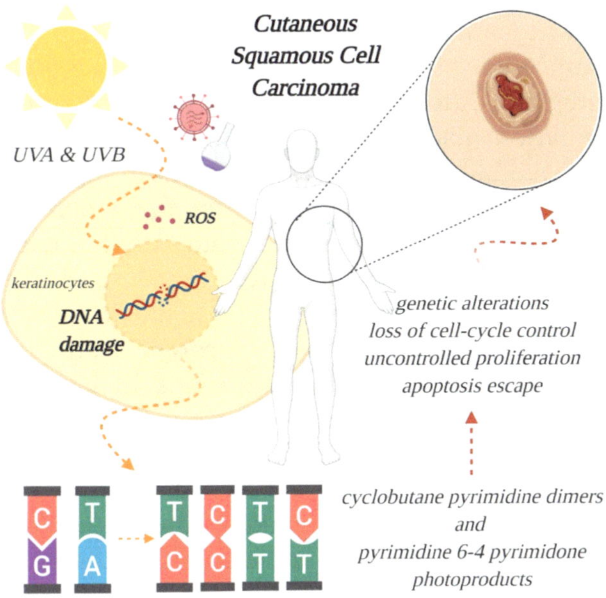

Figure 2.10. Effect of ultraviolet radiation on the genetic material of epidermal keratinocytes, from which cutaneous squamous cell carcinoma (SCC) originates. Excessive absorption of ultraviolet (UV) light generates oxidative stress through the formation of reactive oxygen species (ROS) and breaks the double helix, leading to aberrant binding of pyrimidines and further genetic alterations, culminating in tumor formation.

Source: https://www.researchgate.net/publication/342938293/figure/fig1/AS:11431281213036960@1702927535314/Effect-of-ultraviolet-radiation-on-the-genetic-material-of-epidermal-keratinocytes-from.tif.

Though ultraviolet B and A radiation therapies are deemed safe in terms of non-melanoma skin cancer induction, they continue to be the subject of research and concern for their carcinogenic potential. Patients receiving these therapies should be informed about potential side effects, including erythema, xerosis, and long-term effects such as photocarcinogenesis (Coelho , 2016). To eliminate these effects, clinicians recommend broad photoprotection practices, including a decrease in exposure to direct sunlight and the use of protective skincare habits. In addition, promotion of lifestyle change—like the use of phytochemical antioxidants—actually increases protective strategies against cancers of the skin (Coelho & Apetato, 2016). Regular dermatological follow-ups are essential for patients undergoing phototherapy to allow early identification of any developing skin lesions (Figure 2.10).

2.2.2. Genetic Predisposition

The relationship of genetic susceptibility and the development of skin tumors, such as basal cell carcinoma (BCC), squamous cell carcinoma (SCC), and melanoma, has been of considerable interest in the past few years. Genetic factors play a role in determining a person's susceptibility to these cancers, primarily in combination with environmental exposures such as ultraviolet radiation from the sun. For instance, research has demonstrated that some people with certain genetic markers are at a higher risk of acquiring such cancers. This complex interaction necessitates the search for intrinsic genetic mechanisms, as genetic susceptibility may present as early-onset, aggressive skin cancer. With physicians and researchers striving to characterize these genetic components, they are beginning to reveal potential pathways that someday will guide aimed prevention strategies and customized treatment protocols, reducing skin tumor incidence in genetically predisposed populations (Dlugosz et al., 2002). Within the context of BCC, genetic susceptibility is a significant consideration in its pathogenesis. All the epidemiologic studies describe four main risk factors: exposure to ultraviolet radiation, increasing age, male sex, and one's inherent ability to tan. One of the most intriguing aspects of the genetic predisposition to BCC is the identification of individual genes that have been discovered to be associated with the disease. The patched gene (PTCH), for example, has been shown to influence BCC risk, particularly in individuals with the rare condition known as Gorlin syndrome. While mutations in the PTCH gene have received significant attention, ongoing investigations continue to explore other genes, such as variants in the melanocortin 1 receptor (MC1R) gene, which have been associated with pigmentation and UV sensitivity (de Zwaan et al., 2008). Recognition of this polygenic pattern is key to the formulation of cancer-preventive interventions tailored to individuals at risk.

Outside of BCC, it is crucial to consider the role of genetic predispositions in SCC and melanoma too. Aggregation patterns of a familial nature suggest the existence of an inherited factor in these skin malignancies, with studies reporting a greater prevalence among first-degree relatives of the patient. Young patients' siblings, mothers, and fathers can have their risk of developing SCC and melanoma significantly elevated. This familial aspect is consistent with the concept that shared genetic susceptibilities, possibly supplemented by shared environmental exposures, underlie elevated incidence rates of skin cancers.

Furthermore, phenotypic risk factors—for example, skin type, pigmentation, and response to sunlight exposure—complement genetic susceptibilities, providing a multidimensional model of susceptibility. This evolving body of evidence clarifies cancer biology complexities and highlights the need to balance genetic information with preventive strategies in clinical practice and, therefore, create possible windows for future approaches toward skin cancers (Dlugosz et al., 2002; de Zwaan et al., 2008).

2.2.3. Environmental Factors

The role of environmental factors in the pathogenesis of skin tumors, including basal cell carcinoma (BCC), squamous cell carcinoma (SCC), and melanoma, is intricate and of great importance. Forensic radiation, most specifically ultraviolet (UV) radiation, is the foremost risk factor, with its capacity to induce DNA damage in skin cells linking to BCC and SCC. Chronic sun exposure produces mutations of the tumor suppressor p53 gene, which is vital for genomic integrity. Outdoor occupational exposure to UV radiation also increases the incidence of UV-induced skin cancers, as residents in high-UV-index areas experience a corresponding increase in the incidence of these malignancies. The wide variety of skin tumor types underscores the necessity for multifaceted public health measures to prevent exposure to UV through protective attitudes and awareness campaigns. In addition to UV radiation, certain environmental toxins play a significant role in the etiology of skin cancers. Arsenic is one such substance employed in tainted water for drinking and implicated in inducing skin malignancies, particularly in cases of chronic exposure. Data indicate that chronic arsenic intake is associated with the development of skin lesions that progress to malignancy, reflecting the intricate interaction between environmental carcinogens and genes. Researchers have identified striking epigenetic changes, such as variations in microRNA expression, that are crucial to arsenic-induced carcinogenesis. This new evidence underscores the multifaceted nature of environmental exposures and their interactions with cellular processes that drive skin cancer, and suggests that multiple mechanisms of interaction could ultimately promote tumor growth (Al-Eryani & Laila, 2017). Understanding of environmental causes extends beyond individual carcinogens and calls for a bigger picture of lifestyle and social determinants influencing the risk of skin cancer. For instance, demographic factors age, skin type, and socioeconomic position may interact with environmental exposure, dictating the overall vulnerability of the skin to tumors. Significantly, BCC, the most common type of skin cancer, influences the health environment; as research investigates its pathogenesis, discoveries regarding targeted treatments in light of environmental risk factors are emerging. A comprehensive knowledge of BCC allows for the possibility of having informed measures of prevention that account for environmental impacts on skin health. As researchers continue to study this dynamic topic, it is increasingly necessary to develop a public health model that accounts for environmental impacts on skin cancers to reduce their rates and improve outcomes among affected groups (Fang et al., 2022).

Test Your Knowledge

1. How does UV radiation exposure contribute to the development of premalignant and malignant skin tumors?
2. How does genetic predisposition influence the risk of developing malignant skin tumors?
3. What environmental factor is known to increase the risk of developing skin cancer?

2.3. Symptoms and Diagnosis

Learning Outcome

1. Understand the common symptoms of skin tumors.
2. Describe diagnostic methods utilized in the identification of premalignant and malignant skin tumors.
3. Explain the importance of early detection of premalignant and malignant skin tumors.

The clinical presentation of premalignant and malignant skin neoplasms, including basal cell carcinoma (BCC), squamous cell carcinoma (SCC), and melanoma, plays a primary role in early recognition and effective treatment. BCC typically appears as a pearly or waxy nodule with central ulceration, typically on sun-exposed skin. Conversely, SCC can present as a firm red nodule, scaling patch, or non-healing ulcer, suggestive of invasion of adjacent tissues. Melanoma, the most dangerous form, usually develops from an existing mole or as a new brown spot that is asymmetrical, with an irregular border and irregular coloration. Recognition of such symptoms enables early clinical evaluation, leading to a more accurate differential diagnosis that accounts for other skin lesions and diseases, ultimately optimizing treatment outcomes for the affected patients. The diagnostic process of skin tumors relies on a careful study of the patient's medical history, physical examination, and above all, dermatoscopy. Skin biopsy remains the gold standard for any final diagnosis, allowing histopathological examination of suspect lesions. In melanoma, the Breslow thickness, as a prognostic determinant, can be determined from a biopsy. Additionally, advanced imaging modalities such as sentinel lymph node biopsy and positron emission tomography (PET) scans may stage malignancies and evaluate for potential metastasis. Histological diagnosis further distinguishes invasive from non-invasive cancers, dictating ensuing therapeutic management and follow-up protocols. Therefore, an understanding of these diagnostic techniques is crucial for clinicians tasked with managing and preventing disease progression in skin tumors. Risk factors of skin cancers are also integral to the diagnostic paradigm. Specifically, ultraviolet (UV) exposure has been significantly identified as a key etiological factor for both BCC and SCC, while the association of melanomas with chronic sun exposure and intermittent severe sun exposure is most disturbing. Those with a history of previous immunosuppression, such as thiopurine treatment or anti-TNF therapy, are more susceptible to non-melanoma skin cancers, and hence the importance of regular dermatological follow-up in such patients is all the more significant (Magro et al., 2013). Studies have shown that patients exposed to causes like arsenic exposure can also develop a unique process of carcinogenesis in the skin, whose miRNA expression changes may serve as a biomarker and therapeutic target for arsenic-induced tumors (Al-Eryani & Laila, 2017). This understanding of such risk factors thus informs diagnosis and prevention among vulnerable populations.

2.3.1. General Symptoms of Skin Tumors

The appearance of skin tumors, both premalignant and malignant tumors, is usually followed by a variety of symptoms. Some of the most typical symptoms of the tumors are changes in the appearance of the skin, that is, new lesions or alterations in existing moles. Basal cell carcinoma (BCC) may manifest as a pearl or opalescent bump, while squamous cell carcinoma (SCC) may manifest as a hard red nodule or scaly lesion that persists and grows with time. Melanoma, the more serious skin cancer, is indicated by changes in the size, shape, or color of pigmented moles, usually displaying asymmetry and irregular edges. Identification of these initial symptoms is important for early intervention since early diagnosis can make an enormous difference in prognosis and survival (Figure 2.11).

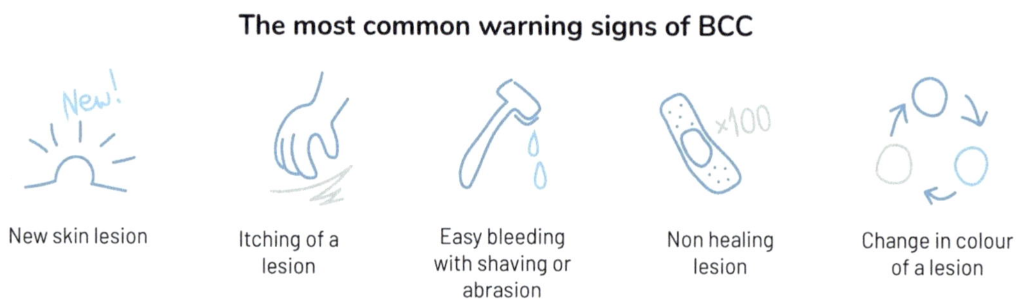
The most common warning signs of BCC
New!
x100
New skin lesion
Itching of a lesion
Easy bleeding with shaving or abrasion
Non healing lesion
Change in colour of a lesion

Figure 2.11. The most common warning signs of BCC.

Source: https://miiskin.com/wp-content/uploads/2020/04/guide-basal-cell-carcinoma-symptoms-signs-infographic.jpg.

Other than clinical growths, clinical symptoms of itching, bleeding, or oozing from the skin lesion, most especially in SCC and melanoma, may be accompanied by the patient. Clinical symptoms most often indicate a transition from a premalignant to a more malignant state, warranting further clinical evaluation. For instance, actinic keratosis, which is a type of precancerous lesion secondary to sun damage, can predict the development of SCC and presents as a consequence of rough, scaly plaques. Ulceration of tumors of the skin, particularly in its advanced form, indicates the need for patients to observe chronic lesions that fail to heal. Early detection, along with awareness of these alarming signs, is key to reducing the burden of skin cancer. Some groups are at increased risk of skin tumor formation and, as a result, may show symptoms earlier than others. For example, individuals with a prior history of immunosuppressive treatment, such as patients treated with thiopurines for inflammatory bowel disease, have been found to be at an increased risk for the development of skin cancers, including the non-melanoma type. This, therefore, places importance on organized dermatological follow-up and education on sun protection measures. In addition, maintaining an effective screening process for individuals at risk can lead to earlier detection of skin tumors and improved treatment outcomes. As patients become more educated about the common symptoms of skin tumors, they can better communicate with healthcare professionals, which can subsequently lead to earlier, curable diagnoses (Magro et al., 2013; Al-Eryani & Laila, 2017) (Figure 2.12).

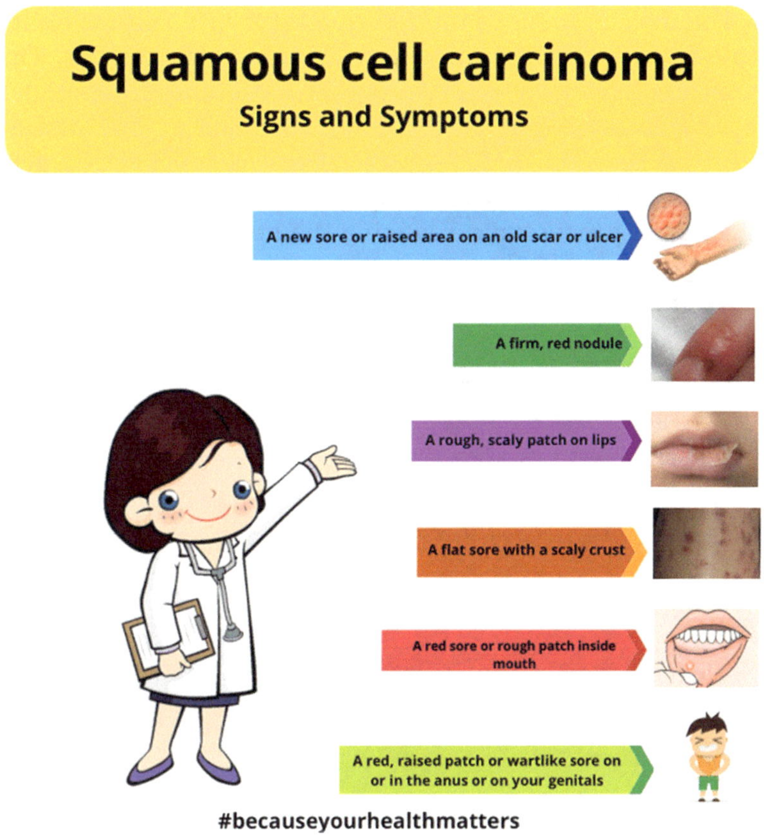

Figure 2.12. Common signs and symptoms of squamous cell carcinoma (SCC).

Source: https://www.nirujahealthtech.com/wp-content/uploads/2020/04/squamous-cell-1-1.png.

2.3.2. Diagnostic Methods

Diagnostic methods used in premalignant and malignant cutaneous tumor detection, such as Basal Cell Carcinoma (BCC), Squamous Cell Carcinoma (SCC), and Melanoma, are critical in the early and appropriate treatment of the disease. The traditional methods primarily involve clinical observation and histopathological examination, in which tissue biopsies are taken for microscopic analysis. Although these methods are considered the gold standard, they can be invasive and cause patient discomfort. Moreover, they are very time-consuming to process and analyze, thereby delaying diagnosis and treatment. Such constraints are being overcome by advances in non-invasive methods that provide immediate, accurate assessment that complements traditional methods and enhances diagnostic capability in clinical practice. Optical Coherence Tomography (OCT) is a new technique that visualizes tissue at high resolution in cross-sectional form without biopsy. By measuring backscattered near-infrared light, OCT both qualitatively and quantitatively reports tissue architecture, enabling medical professionals to effectively differentiate benign from malignant lesions. The utility of OCT is not confined to cutaneous application, as application in the diagnosis of other epithelial malignancies, like oral cavity and esophageal malignancies, is also possible. The growing evidence supporting OCT as an important diagnostic tool highlights its potential to improve patient outcomes through earlier diagnosis and more patient-focused diagnostic processes (Wessels et al., 2014). The development of the Oblique Incidence Diffuse Reflectance Spectroscopy (OIDRS) system is another important advance in skin cancer diagnostics. This technology allows clinicians to obtain spectral data from skin lesions in real time, distinguishing benign disease and all melanoma stages from nonpigmented carcinomas such as BCC and SCC and their benign counterparts. The system has been shown to be highly sensitive and specific, achieving 90% accuracy for melanoma detection and 92% accuracy for nonpigmented carcinomas in blinded clinical studies. By streamlining the diagnostic process and reducing the need for invasive tests, OIDRS represents a leap in non-invasive diagnosis of skin cancer, thereby meeting contemporary clinical demands to enhance patient comfort and speed up treatment (Garcia-Urib et al., 2012) (Figure 2.13).

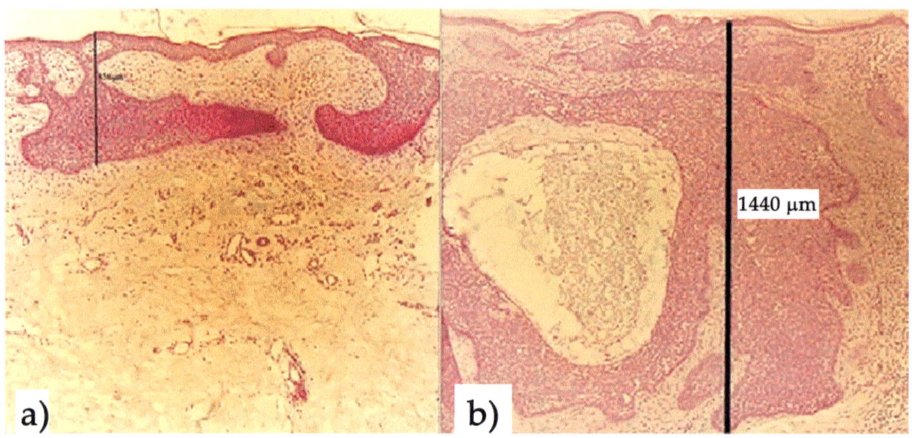

Figure 2.13. Basal cell carcinoma (BCC) histopathology: a) thin BCC. H&E stain, ×50 original magnification; b) thick BCC. H&E stain, ×50 original magnification.

Source: https://www.researchgate.net/profile/Artur-Bezugly/publication/338050569/figure/fig1/AS:837875197280256@1576776422556/Basal-cell-carcinoma-BCC-histopathology-a-thin-BCC-H-E-stain-50-original.png.

2.3.3. Importance of Early Detection

Early detection of premalignant and malignant skin tumors like basal cell carcinoma (BCC), squamous cell carcinoma (SCC), and melanoma is crucial in improving patient outcomes and reducing mortality. Early detection of these conditions enables early intervention, which significantly affects the effectiveness of treatment modalities. For instance, non-surgical treatment of BCC and SCC, in their early diagnosis, spares the need for more invasive surgeries and consequent complications. The stage of melanoma is also greatly dependent on how early the disease is recognized, and survival decreases significantly with increasing disease stage. Thus, awareness and information about early warning signs, such as variation of the mole or other skin abnormalities, can allow individuals to seek medical treatment in time, saving lives and healthy skin. In addition to raising public awareness, educating physicians is an important part of promoting early detection of skin cancer. As research on French rheumatologists shows, targeted online training significantly improved their diagnostic competence in distinguishing benign from malignant skin lesions (Viguier et al., 2015). This finding directs the need for systematic training modules that provide healthcare professionals with the skill set required to identify skin cancers at earlier stages. These programs benefit not only the professional's diagnostic skills but also bridge the clinical practice and new dermatological knowledge. Consequently, the incorporation of continuous medical education and training programs for physicians is essential to enhance early detection, thereby facilitating better management of skin cancers and ultimately improving patient care. Moreover, the measures for early detection can be cost-saving in reducing the economic burden of treating advanced skin cancer. The financial costs to patients and healthcare providers increase exponentially with the advancing stage of cancer, requiring intense treatments, extended inpatient care, or even palliative therapy during terminal stages. The literature asserts that early intervention reduces overall treatment costs and improves resource allocation within the healthcare system, allowing for more effective use of medical resources in areas of need (Nemazannikova et al., 2019). Furthermore, early intervention programs usually promote less invasive treatments, such as topical chemotherapy or laser treatment, which are also cost-effective and less taxing to patients. The introduction of a wide-screening program and a public health program in this manner not only enhances the quality of care delivered but can also yield considerable economic dividends while strengthening the culture of preventive health care.

Test Your Knowledge

1. What are the common symptoms of basal cell carcinoma (BCC)?
2. How does squamous cell carcinoma (SCC) typically present on the skin?
3. Which diagnostic methods are commonly used to confirm the diagnosis of skin cancer, such as BCC, SCC, or melanoma?

2.4. Treatment Options

Learning Outcome

1. Discuss surgical interventions in the management of premalignant and malignant skin.
2. Describe non-surgical treatments for non-surgical treatments.
3. Understand emerging therapies for premalignant and malignant skin tumors.

The treatment of premalignant and malignant skin tumors, such as basal cell carcinoma (BCC), squamous cell carcinoma (SCC), and melanoma, is multifaceted and includes varied modalities depending on tumor characteristics and patient factors. Cryotherapy is increasingly the choice for the management of superficial skin malignancies, particularly in elderly patients with multiple lesions, but who are not cooperative with major surgery. The technique is characterized by comfort, speed, and painlessness, usually requiring no anesthesia, and is therefore particularly ideal for day-case treatment. Of note, cryotherapy has provided outstanding cosmetic results and is regarded as useful in the treatment of such tumor precursors as actinic keratosis and Bowen's disease, which have the potential to develop into more virulent tumors. Better comfort for the patient and quick recovery times make cryotherapy the preferred option in the general dermatological treatment algorithms context (Akarsu & Kamberoglu, 2018).

Apart from cryotherapy, there are options among available surgery modalities for the treatment of skin tumors, particularly the invasive ones , such as BCC and SCC. Surgical excision remains the gold standard, allowing complete removal of the tumor along with an extra margin of normal tissue. Mohs micrographic surgery is an advanced surgical technique that involves real-time intraoperative analysis of tumor margins, significantly reducing the likelihood of recurrence. It is especially helpful in tumors located in anatomically complex regions , such as the face and ears, where cosmetic integrity is greater than necessary. In the case of slowly growing tumors, curettage and electrosurgery may be used, offering a less invasive excision with acceptable aesthetic results. Surgical choice is highly dependent upon the tumor characteristics, patient status, and site of the lesion (Sand et al., 2008). Systemic modalities, including chemotherapy and radiation, play roles in the management of more advanced skin cancers, most notably melanoma. Systemic treatment is optimally reserved for metastatic disease or if there are not many surgical alternatives due to tumor size or location. Targeted therapies and immunotherapy have revolutionized cancer therapy modalities in the last decade, with the promise of improved outcomes for patients with advanced melanoma. The development of drugs that target tumor-specific genetic mutations is a shining example of this move towards precision medicine. Furthermore, in case conventional treatment is contraindicated or ineffective, newer modalities , such as laser treatment and photodynamic treatment provide new modes of management. Combining all these different treatment modalities provides for individualized therapy, improving general patient care and prognostic results for patients diagnosed with skin cancers (Akarsu & Kamberoglu, 2018) (Figure 2.14).

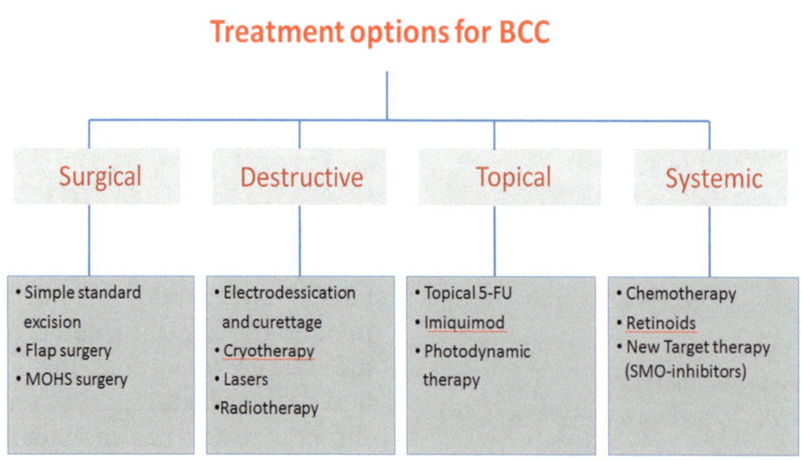

Figure 2.14. Treatment options for BBC.

Source: https://www.researchgate.net/publication/320173589/figure/fig1/AS:932473441644545@1599330401954/nterventions-for-Basal-cell-carcinoma-BCC-by-treatment-modality.png.

2.4.1. Surgical Interventions

Surgery is a cornerstone in the management of premalignant and malignant cutaneous neoplasms like basal cell carcinoma (BCC), squamous cell carcinoma (SCC), and melanoma. Choice of surgery largely relies on the size, depth, and site of the tumors, apart from an overall evaluation of the patient's health. For instance, Mohs micrographic surgery, a sensitive procedure with stepwise excision of cancerous skin one area at a time, is particularly applicable to BCC and SCC on cosmetically significant areas. By facilitating immediate inspection of tumor margins, Mohs surgery significantly minimizes the local recurrence risk and optimizes cosmetic outcome. This approach emphasizes the importance of individualized strategies in surgical treatment, demonstrating that tailored therapies significantly affect patient outcomes and satisfaction. In organ transplant recipients (OTR), the implication of surgical therapy takes on more complexity because they are more susceptible to skin cancers. Research has shown that surgical referral is likely to lead to delays in the timely diagnosis and treatment, with significant portions of the patient ultimately being diagnosed upon referral for unrelated dermatologic complaints, that is, rash or acne (Chundydyal, 2015). This serves to highlight a very urgent need for enhanced risk stratification and referral for OTR and highlights the very considerable influence surgical procedures are likely to have on the effective treatment of skin malignancies. By optimizing referral patterns and improving access to surgical dermatology services, clinicians may reduce the tumor burden in high-risk patient populations, thereby improving patient outcomes. While surgical procedures vary in their methods and applications, they become increasingly effective when coupled with intensive preoperative assessment and postoperative management. This is especially true with melanoma, where early surgical excision contributes significantly to survival. It has been established through evidence that early surgery can notably decrease the risk of mortality in high-risk patients (Fang et al., 2022). Moreover, postoperative surveillance is important for identifying potential recurrence or metastasis, necessitating interprofessional collaboration among surgical dermatologists, oncologists, and primary care providers. This overall strategy not only enables the management of surgical complications but also treats patients as a whole throughout their continuum of care, thereby achieving optimal outcomes and quality of life for those battling these cancers (Figure 2.15).

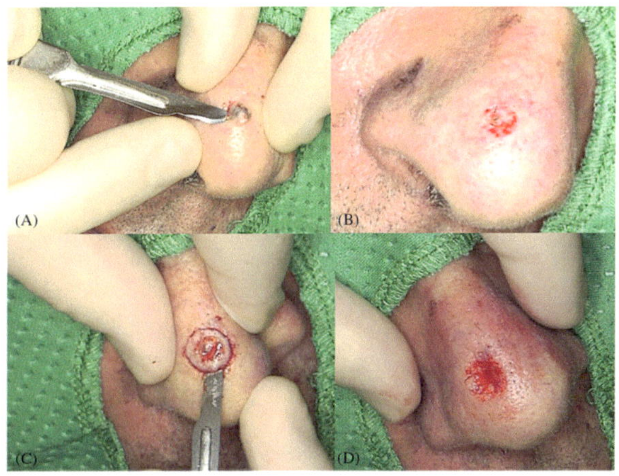

Figure 2.15. A multiphase MOHS micrographic surgery procedure performed on a basal cell carcinoma of the nose: A, B, a 30° to 45° angle incision with a circular shape around the lesion; C, horizontal cutting; D, surgical defect after tissue excision.

Source: https://www.researchgate.net/publication/341299951/figure/fig1/AS:11431281173882158@1689060064288/A-multiphase-MOHS-micrographic-surgery-procedure-performed-on-a-basal-cell-carcinoma-of.png.

2.4.2. Non-Surgical Treatments

Treatment of premalignant and malignant skin tumors basal cell carcinoma (BCC) and squamous cell carcinoma (SCC), now includes a variety of nonsurgical treatments. These are particularly valuable in patients who cannot undergo surgery due to medical conditions or who prefer the least invasive means. Topical chemotherapeutic agents 5-fluorouracil (5-FU) and imiquimod are increasingly used to treat superficial BCC and actinic keratosis, a precursor to SCC. These agents selectively kill cancer cells, thereby sparing surrounding normal tissue. Photodynamic therapy (PDT) is another modality used, in which light-activatable drugs are administered to induce tumor cell death, and it has the potential to be an ideal option for superficial skin cancers. Thus, such non-surgical treatments not only provide acceptable alternatives but also enhance patients' quality of life by reducing the physical and psychological burden of prolonged surgical treatments. For melanoma, the most malignant of skin cancers, non-surgical treatments provide dramatic advances in therapeutic approaches. Immunotherapy has transformed the treatment of melanoma by harnessing the body's own immune system to recognize and kill cancer cells. Medicines , such as pembrolizumab and nivolumab, which are checkpoint inhibitors, have proven to be phenomenal at fighting late-stage melanoma. These medicines block proteins that put the brakes on immune responses, enhancing the body's ability to attack melanoma cells. Besides, targeted therapies like BRAF and MEK inhibitors also offer other avenues for therapy in the situation of patients bearing specific genetic mutations. This multipronged approach not only improves overall survival but also allows for tailored treatment strategies created to address each individual patient's own tumor pattern.

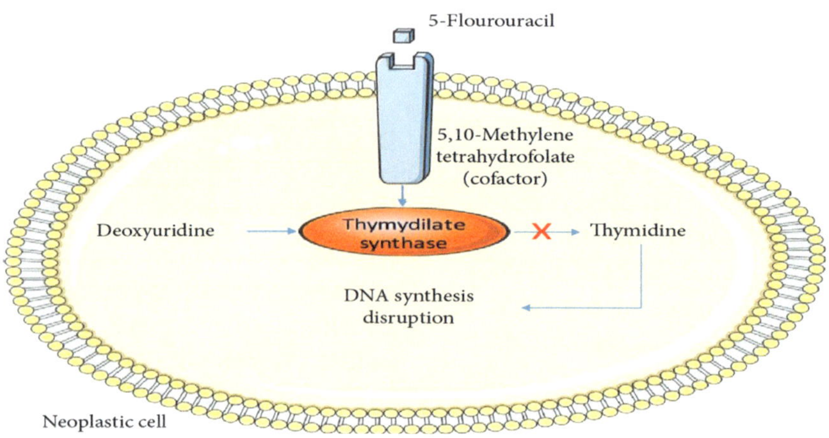

Figure 2.16. 5-Fluorouracil mechanism of action.

Source: https://www.researchgate.net/publication/330294486/figure/fig2/AS:1086076915585035@1635952323892/5-Fluorouracil-mechanism-of-action.jpg.

Furthermore, the application of ultrasonography in the assessment and management of skin tumors cannot be overemphasized. Although predominantly a diagnostic tool, ultrasound also has the potential to direct non-surgical treatment. For instance, preoperative imaging using varying frequencies clarifies tumor form and size and thus facilitates the exercise of choosing the treatment. It has been shown that ultrasound can determine tumor characteristics, such as depth of invasion and vascularization, which are vital in choosing appropriate non-surgical therapeutic regimens. Furthermore, as the literature shows, non-invasive techniques , such as elastography can assess the stiffness of the lesions and therefore help attain a better understanding of their aggressiveness. Overall, complementary imaging modalities enhance the effectiveness of non-surgical therapy and facilitate the development of integrated treatment strategies for patients with premalignant and malignant skin tumors (Tama et al., 2023; Stawarz et al., 2025) (Figure 2.16).

2.4.3. Emerging Therapies

The climate of new therapies for premalignant and malignant cutaneous tumors, notably basal cell carcinoma (BCC), squamous cell carcinoma (SCC), and melanoma, is considerably influenced by developments in molecular biology and genetics. Data gathered from proteomic and genomic studies have helped uncover novel biomarker signatures that can be of help in the early diagnosis and targeted therapy of these skin malignancies. Specifically, proteomic profiling of keratinocytes has characterized the significant alterations in patterns of protein expression that occur as development proceeds from normal to dysplastic and malignant states. Besides informing improvements in risk estimation, they also form the rationale for the design of new therapeutics that could end up improving patient outcomes and limiting the psychological and economic burdens of these neoplasms (Boda et al., 2017). Besides the identification of new biomarkers, research on the genetic origins of skin cancers has greatly helped with potential treatments. For instance, the elucidation of biochemical melanoma, BCC, and SCC pathways has opened doors to targeted interventions that attempt to impair malignant cell survival and growth pathways. These new approaches include the utilization of small-molecule inhibitors and monoclonal antibodies that act on proteins that are overexpressed or mutated. By tailoring treatments to the genetic profile of every tumor, physicians hope to optimize the quality of the treatment outcomes and minimize toxic side effects, enhancing patients' quality of life through more effective cancer therapies. These developments represent a dramatic shift from traditional broad-spectrum methods toward more precision-oriented approaches required in the battle against these prevalent skin cancers (Dlugosz et al., 2002). Moreover, the addition of immunotherapy as a mode of therapy for skin tumors is another area of promise for new treatments. Immunotherapeutic agents, such as checkpoint inhibitors, have revolutionized the treatment of advanced melanoma, demonstrating the promise to induce the body's immune response against cancer cells efficiently. The medications act by blocking inhibitory pathways that downregulate T cells from attacking tumor cells, thereby reactivating the immune system against cancerous growth. As ongoing research unravels the fueling immunogenic responses in skin cancers, widening the use of immunotherapy to SCC and BCC could, in the future, transform the treatment landscape for these cancers. Such breakthroughs, combined with effective prevention measures that reduce exposure to UV radiation, have the potential to significantly reduce the incidence and impact of skin cancers in the coming years (Dlugosz et al., 2002).

Test Your Knowledge

1. What is the most common surgical treatment for basal cell carcinoma (BCC) and squamous cell carcinoma (SCC)?
2. What is the role of topical treatments in treating premalignant or early-stage skin cancers?

2.5. Prevention Strategies

Learning Outcome

1. Implement effective sun protection measures in the prevention of premalignant and malignant skin tumors.
2. Explain the importance of regular skin examinations for the prevention of premalignant and malignant skin tumors.
3. Focus on public awareness campaigns.

Effective prevention strategies for skin tumors, particularly basal cell carcinoma (BCC), squamous cell carcinoma (SCC), and melanoma, play a crucial role in reducing incidence as well as mortality from these cancers. Prevention primarily relies on sun protection, which is essential because the etiology of skin tumors is linked to ultraviolet (UV) radiation. Individuals are urged to wear protective caps like broad-spectrum sunscreens with high SPF, protective clothes, and avoid sun exposure during the morning hours. Additionally, community public health campaigns that educate people on the risks of excessive sunbathing and tanning beds have been crucial in reducing risk factors. Furthermore, there has been an increased emphasis on wearing wide-brimmed hats and sunglasses outdoors. With continued research highlighting the link between UV exposure and skin cancer, the integration of these preventive measures into one's routine is a crucial step in minimizing the incidence of both premalignant and malignant skin tumors. Apart from sun protection, regular dermatological checkups are a significant step in preventing skin cancer among high-risk individuals. For instance, organ transplant recipients (OTRs) have heightened vulnerability to skin cancers as a result of immunosuppressive therapy, which calls for careful monitoring of the skin. In a study of OTRs, it was found that most patients referred for skin issues were subsequently diagnosed with malignant lesions in a matter of months, reflecting the urgency of proper and prompt referrals to dermatology experts (Chundydyal, 2015). With the implementation of a risk-stratification system that identifies high-risk patients and provides instant dermatological consultations, rates of early diagnosis and patient outcomes can improve. This preventive strategy is one aspect of reducing the burden of skin tumors and treating larger numbers of people at greater risk promptly. New treatments and technologies, such as phototherapy, are also an integral part of the prevention and treatment of skin tumors. While useful in the treatment of most skin ailments, phototherapy must be balanced against risks and benefits, such as the induction of skin cancer. In spite of problems with the carcinogenic risk of UV radiation, studies have shown that most patients treated with UV phototherapy are not at increased risk for the occurrence of non-melanoma skin cancer (Coelho & Apetato, 2016). In order to more effectively enhance the safety of phototherapy, employing preventive measures , such as restricting concurrent sun exposure and topical antioxidants, might help restrict adverse effects. As the landscape of dermatological treatments evolves, combining new preventive strategies with established interventions will be crucial to effectively control and prevent skin tumors.

2.5.1. Sun Protection Measures

The employment of proper sun protective measures is of utmost significance in the prevention of premalignant and malignant skin neoplasms, particularly basal cell carcinoma (BCC), squamous cell carcinoma (SCC), and melanoma. The ultraviolet (UV) radiation of the sun is a well-documented environmental carcinogen for these neoplasms. Education on the use of sunscreen is of utmost importance; broad-spectrum sunscreens that protect against UVA and UVB rays should have at least 30 SPF. Secondly, one should reapply sunscreen every two hours, as well as after swimming and perspiration. By minimizing exposure to direct sunlight and encouraging the use of protective clothing, brimmed hats, and UV-blocking sunglasses, one can significantly lower the risk of acquiring skin cancer. These preventive measures not only protect the skin from harmful UV radiation but also help maintain overall AZand immunity. Among the various methods of sun protection, the innovative incorporation of photoprotective measures as part of dermatologic procedures is most noteworthy. While treatments , such as phototherapy have therapeutic benefits, they also contain risks, including skin injury and indirect carcinogenesis from UV exposure. Evidence shows that short- and long-term side effects of phototherapy could include issues like dyspigmentation and xerosis, which highlight the necessity of stringent protection measures (Coelho & Apetato, 2016). Those who are treated with such therapy must attempt to decrease concurrent exposure to the sun and implement new photoprotective measures, for instance, using phytochemical antioxidants. By focusing on sun protection, phototherapy patients can minimize risks through the assistance of an integrative approach in the treatment of both diseases and treatment side effects involving the skin. The importance of risk stratification and referral at an early stage in high-risk populations, such as organ transplant recipients (OTRs), cannot be stressed enough while planning sun protection. OTRs carry a substantially increased risk of skin cancers using immunosuppression regimens that put them under very close dermatologic surveillance. Research has established correlations between the reasons for referral to specialty skin dermatology clinics and cancer diagnosis, identifying the significance of greater awareness of alterations in the skin (Chundydyal, 2015). With most patients diagnosed with premalignant or malignant lesions upon follow-up referrals for seemingly benign symptoms, there is a significant requirement for enhancing education regarding sun protection among patients as well as practitioners. A good risk stratification strategy, along with excellent sun protective practices, can significantly improve outcomes in high-risk groups and ultimately reduce the incidence of skin tumors (Figure 2.17).

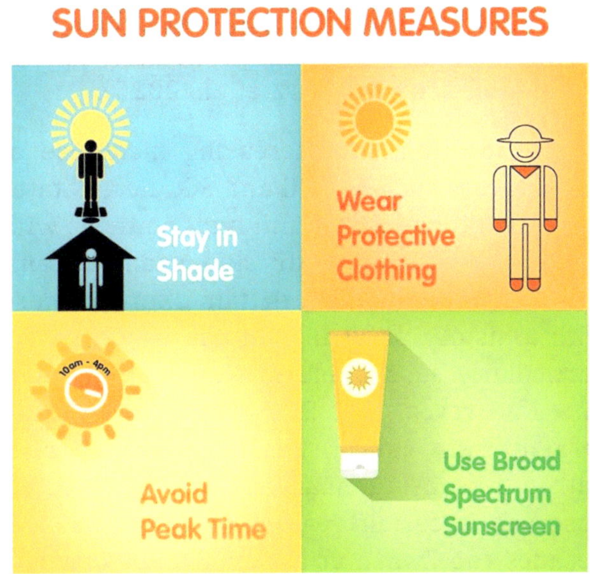

Figure 2.17. The implementation of effective sun protection measures is paramount for preventing premalignant and malignant skin tumors.

Source: https://i.pinimg.com/736x/e8/2d/38/e82d389711ac9edbbc1c4dcb5cbe6eb4.jpg.

2.5.2. Regular Skin Examinations

In premalignant and malignant skin tumors, such as basal cell carcinoma (BCC), squamous cell carcinoma (SCC), and melanoma, regular skin examination becomes a necessary part of skin health care. These screening tests play a crucial role in early detection, significantly improving the outcomes of treatment. Skin screening enables clinicians to recognize suspicious lesions and changes in the skin that may be a harbinger of malignancy. For instance, actinic keratoses, precursors to SCC, can often be diagnosed upon normal examination and hence are suitable for early treatment. This anticipatory process not only enables early diagnosis but also educates patients regarding their skin health, stimulating self-examination and detection of suspicious alterations. The integration of regular examinations into patient care models points to the important role played by preventive health practices in the fight against the threat of skin cancers, particularly among risk populations (Stawarz et al., 2025).

In addition, the increasing incidence of skin cancers such as BCC and SCC necessitates strengthening public health interventions, with an emphasis on regular skin examinations. Notably, individuals with fair skin or those with a history of significant sun exposure are particularly susceptible to skin malignancies. The data reveal that BCC, the most common form of skin cancer, has been on the rise, with a 1 to 2% annual increase in incidence observed in certain regions over the past two decades (de Zwaan et al., 2008). Regular skin checkup enables premalignant irregular growth patterns to be identified early before they can progress to malignancy, hence eliminating the possibility of developing advanced skin cancers (de Zwaan et al., 2008). The practice reinforces a preventive culture that protects not only the health of the people but also reduces the total societal and economic burdens of advanced skin cancers. Through proper education and screening procedures, healthcare systems can better combat the increasing rates of incidence of these skin cancers. In the long term, periodic skin examinations offer a multifaceted benefit as a diagnostic and educational tool for patients regarding the prevention of skin cancer. Beyond the mere detection of probable malignancies, these examinations allow patients to actively maintain surveillance of their own skin. Encouragement of skin self-examinations reinforced by clinical assessment is central to raising awareness and encouraging early intervention. This is particularly necessary for those who are presenting with risk factors for skin cancers, for example, sunburn history, outdoor occupations, or skin cancer family history (Stawarz et al., 2025). By strengthening early skin screening practices, medical practitioners can reduce the incidence and impact of premalignant and malignant cutaneous neoplasms, ultimately improving patient outcomes and public health.

2.5.3. Public Awareness Campaigns

Public health campaigns are needed to disseminate information about premalignant and malignant skin tumors, including basal cell carcinoma (BCC), squamous cell carcinoma (SCC), and melanoma. Through media sources, such campaigns aim to educate the public about the risks of exposure to ultraviolet (UV) radiation, the importance of routine skin checks, and early detection protocols. Effective campaigns can contribute effectively towards reducing melanoma occurrence, as experienced in areas like Australia, where skin cancer continues to increase year after year. Educational programs may emphasize the epidemiological risk factors of skin cancer, including UV radiation and genetics, thereby sensitizing individuals to sun protection strategies and regular dermatological check-ups, and generally enhance health outcomes as well as reduce healthcare expenses related to skin tumor control. New technologies have also revolutionized information delivery for public awareness campaigns. For instance, mHealth app development has facilitated easier access to screening tools and education for skin cancer. Research has indicated that it is possible for AI algorithms to identify individuals who are at greater risk of skin cancer through facial recognition technology to facilitate early interventions (Sangers, 2024). These technologies not only raise public awareness of skin cancer but also facilitate measures of public engagement with preventive health initiatives. Studies have shown that the attitude of the population as a whole towards mHealth tools for screening reflects a growing awareness and acceptance of using technology as a part of normal healthcare. By incorporating these new technologies, campaigns can target young people who are more likely to use digital media, thereby enlarging their audience and improving the effectiveness of their message. Moreover, targeted public education campaigns can be of significant utility in addressing particular demographic problems and beliefs leading to skin cancer underdiagnosis. Targeted campaigns to groups with traditionally poor sun-protective habits or lower awareness of genetic risks related to skin tumors may reduce differences. Because family aggregation of skin cancers has been documented, programs must outline the hereditary risks and encourage family conversations about sun protection (de Zwaan et al., 2008). Updating these campaigns periodically in accordance with changing social norms and technology ensures their effectiveness and relevance. By creating a culture of awareness and anticipatory care, these initiatives not only aim to decrease the prevalence of BCC, SCC, and melanoma but also help create a sustainable approach to public health focused on education and prevention.

Test Your Knowledge

1. What are the most effective sun protection measures to prevent skin tumors like basal cell carcinoma (BCC) and squamous cell carcinoma (SCC)?
2. Why is it important to conduct regular skin self-examinations, and how often should they be done?
3. How can public awareness campaigns help reduce the risk of melanoma and other skin cancers?

2.6. Prognosis and Outcomes

Learning Outcome

1. Understand survival rates for BCC, SCC, and melanoma.
2. Describe factors influencing prognosis.
3. Explain the long-term effects of treatment.

The prognosis for premalignant and malignant skin tumors, including basal cell carcinoma (BCC), squamous cell carcinoma (SCC), and melanoma, is mostly determined by early diagnosis and treatment. BCC and SCC, which account for most skin cancers, can be cured in most cases if diagnosed in time. Otherwise, late diagnosis may cause increased morbidity due to local invasion or metastasis. Understanding the mechanisms of carcinogenesis in skin is important for its curative outcome improvement; this includes examining the function of risk determinants , such as exposure to ultraviolet (UV) radiation and genetic predisposition. The wealth of scientific literature on skin cancers also points to the importance of aggressive monitoring and patient education towards early intervention and diagnosis, which ultimately maximizes prognosis and reduces complications in advanced disease (Hasan et al., 2023). In recent years, advancements in treatment modalities have improved the prognosis in patients with skin tumors. Traditional therapies, such as surgical excision and cryotherapy, are now being complemented by new therapies , such as photodynamic therapy (PDT) and targeted therapy targeting molecular pathways of tumor growth. For instance, daylight photodynamic therapy (dPDT), which utilizes the natural sunlight, has proved to be a very efficient, non-invasive, and improved option for the treatment of superficial cutaneous cancers, particularly in actinic keratosis patients (Chaw-Lee et al., 2020). In addition, their use in clinical practice is reflective of an interdisciplinarity in oncology, which ensures the individualization of intervention according to patient profiles. This care model, which is patient-centered, enhances overall treatment outcomes and disease management concepts in different populations and risk groups. Moreover, the prognosis of malignant melanomas remains an area of ongoing investigation because of their aggressive nature as well as the risk of early metastasis. Statistically, melanoma also has a poor prognosis over BCC and SCC since survival rates vary dramatically when the cancer is advanced and involves the lymph nodes or distant organs. Advances in immunotherapy and targeted therapies have introduced new treatment modalities for advanced melanoma, improving long-term survival rates for many patients. These newer treatment paradigms also emphasize the importance of genetic profiling and biomarker studies in predicting patient responses to therapy. Being at the forefront of a powerful and multi-pronged therapeutic weapons platform also helps to counteract the issue of drug resistance that can arise through traditional treatments, thereby optimizing patient prognosis in the event of this deadly skin cancer (Hasan et al., 2023).

2.6.1. BCC, SCC, Melanoma Survival Rates

Knowledge of skin cancer survival rates is important in the setting of premalignant and malignant tumors, particularly basal cell carcinoma (BCC), squamous cell carcinoma (SCC), and melanoma. BCC, the most frequent malignant skin tumor, has a very high survival rate, typically above 90% (Paolino et al., 2017).

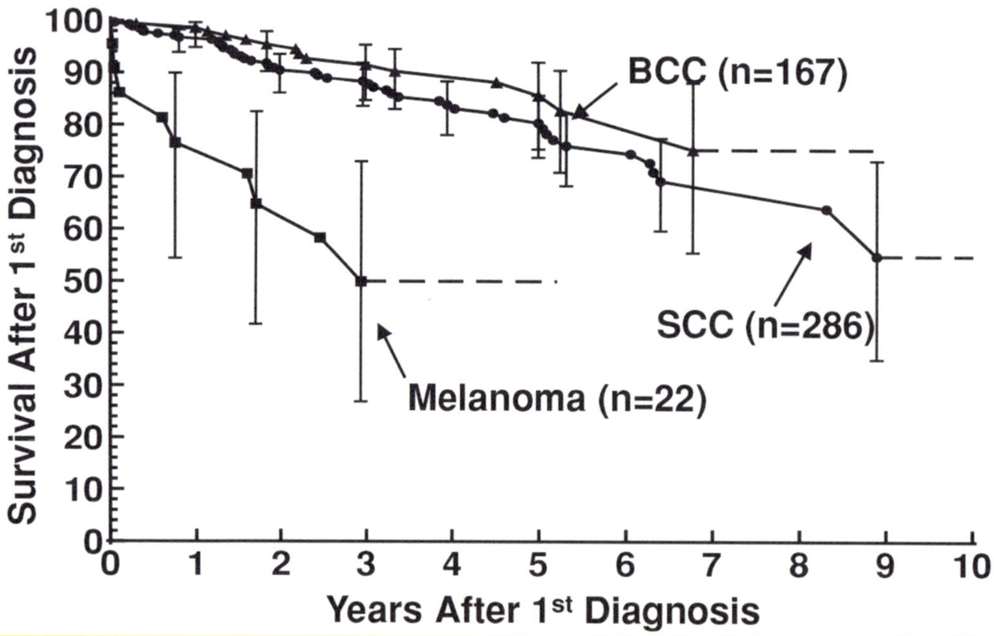

N (SCC)	286	249	199	158	112	78	51	29	15	6	1
N (BCC)	167	139	109	78	54	34	18	9	4	-	-
N (melanoma)	22	15	11	6	4	3	-	-	-	-	-

Figure 2.18. Survival (%) after diagnosis of BCC, SCC, and melanoma.

Source: https://www.researchgate.net/publication/51456939/figure/fig1/AS:281831564955688@1444205289467/Survival-after-diagnosis-of-BCC-SCC-and-melanoma-The-three-curves-are-not.png.

The favorable prognosis is due to its typically local behavior, so surgical interventions are effective. While it has a very good rate of cure, the rising incidence of BCC requires close follow-up, especially in those with significant risk factors. While the majority of BCC cases can be controlled, early detection still remains crucial in the prevention of complications of advanced disease. SCC, on the other hand, has a more complex survival curve. Whilst generally with good outcomes, SCC survival rates can also be quite variable based on numerous factors , such as tumor size, location, and depth of invasion.

The potential for metastasis, particularly in high-risk cases, requires a more aggressive treatment and follow-up protocol. In a recent study, individuals who had been treated for SCC have been found to have increased secondary tumor formation risk with a notable 26% recurrence rate during the first year following primary diagnosis (Katz et al., 2002). This increased surveillance and treatment reflect the need for close management in patients with a predisposition to multicentric lesions, ultimately affecting long-term survival rates. Melanoma is the most hazardous form of skin cancer because it tends to metastasize early on. Melanoma mortality rates are far below BCC and SCC rates, particularly at advanced stages. Five-year survival for localized melanoma is as high as 98%, but falls dramatically to only 23% when the disease is diagnosed at the distant metastasis stage, highlighting the importance of early diagnosis (Paolino et al., 2017). Tumor thickness and ulceration are key determinants of prognosis. Thus, comprehensive public health policy with the inclusion of skin cancer awareness and regular screening is paramount in the improvement of survival for melanoma, showing that while improvement in treatment has optimized survival, early detection remains the key to successful combat of this carcinomatous skin tumor (Figure 2.18).

2.6.2. Factors Influencing Prognosis

The fate of premalignant and malignant cutaneous neoplasms, including basal cell carcinoma (BCC), squamous cell carcinoma (SCC), and melanoma, is dictated by a variety of factors. Tumor stage at the time of diagnosis is one such pivotal determinant since early lesions may have a better prognosis than advanced tumors. For instance, the five-year survival rate for melanoma may vary significantly based on the difference between localized cancer and metastatic cancer.

Furthermore, variables tumor histological characteristics and the presence of certain biomarkers also enter the picture. Identification of mutations in genes of prime importance provides information on tumor behavior and potential for treatment response, thereby determining long-term survival outcomes. Patient-specific variables , such as age and health status, add to this situation, with younger patients and lower comorbidity having improved prognoses. Another key factor affecting prognosis is the type of treatment that is used for skin tumors. Surgical removal remains the mainstay of treatment for most skin cancers, including BCC and SCC, and can yield excellent results.

However, the effectiveness of systemic therapies like immunotherapy and targeted therapy of melanoma depends upon the genetic composition of the tumors. Evidence demonstrates that certain mutations, such as those in the BRAF gene, can predict response to targeted therapy and hence guide treatment choices, ultimately affecting prognosis. Furthermore, early treatment is important; even temporary delays in treatment will lead to tumor growth and metastasis, drastically compromising the prognosis of the patients. Clinicians and patients must be informed about such conditions and their treatment to effectively manage the skin cancer prognosis process. Environmental and lifestyle factors also play an important role in the prognosis of skin tumors. For instance, ultraviolet (UV) radiation is a confirmed risk factor for the induction and development of skin cancers like melanoma.

Total sun exposure, particularly during childhood and adolescence, has been shown to be linked with elevated melanoma risk and may have a detrimental effect on survival status. In addition, other environmental exposures, such as arsenic, are involved in skin carcinogenesis, highlighting the importance of external risk factor information (Al-Eryani & Laila, 2017). Lifestyle aspects, such as smoking and diet, can also contribute to these risks and may be pushed by cancer into the body, influencing the body's ability to fight cancer. Therefore, improving prognostic outcomes for patients with premalignant and malignant skin tumors requires education on prevention and risk reduction.

2.6.3. Long-Term Effects of Treatment

The treatment of premalignant and malignant skin tumors, such as basal cell carcinoma (BCC), squamous cell carcinoma (SCC), and melanoma, involves modalities with significant long-term implications for which one has to exercise caution. Phototherapy, specifically with ultraviolet (UV) radiation, is used frequently due to its efficacy; however, it is not risk-free. UV radiation over the long term has been associated with several harmful effects, such as color alterations of the skin, photoaging, and potential photocarcinogenesis. While most studies report that patients with ultraviolet B (both narrowband and broadband) and ultraviolet A1 phototherapy have no elevated risk of melanoma or non-melanoma skin malignancy, continued surveillance as well as dermatological assessment remains necessary for the prompt identification of secondary malignancies as well as for changes in the skin following treatment (Coelho & Apetato, 2016). This warning underscores the need for patient-specific treatment protocols and patient education on long-term follow-up.

Cryotherapy, a second well-liked treatment option for premalignant and malignant lesions, has certain advantages but its own set of long-term effects. The localized freezing effect effectively destroys the target cell's integrity, thereby promoting rapid recovery without any unwanted effects. However, because patients may receive multiple sessions to address recurrent lesions or other skin conditions, there is a possibility of a cumulative effect that should be addressed. Long-term outcomes vary and comprise improved cosmetic results for lentigo maligna and actinic keratosis, and hence cryotherapy is a first-line treatment in older patients who may be compliant with other treatments (Akarsu & Kamberoglu, 2018; Akarsu).

But therapists must remain vigilant for the development of hypopigmentation, scarring, or other adverse effects seen with repeated cryotherapy, and thus the need for an individualized treatment timing and method approach based on the patient's unique skin properties and treatment course. It is relevant that long-term side effects are considered in decision-making about the treatment of skin tumors, particularly given the potential psychological and social effects. They need to be informed about the permanence and stability of some treatment outcomes and the need for sustained skin care and sun avoidance after treatment.

Moreover, an active management plan must include routine follow-up visits to screen for recurrence or new lesions, along with counseling regarding lifestyle modifications to avoid additional risks of skin damage. Evaluation of long-term treatment effects should not be only oriented towards physical results but also directed at the psychosocial impact on patients, such as body image issues that may arise from scarring or skin texture change. As caregivers, creating an open line of communication with patients about what they anticipate and worry about is important in facilitating their overall well-being throughout treatment.

Test Your Knowledge

1. What are the survival rates for basal cell carcinoma (BCC) and squamous cell carcinoma (SCC)?
2. How does the stage of melanoma affect its prognosis?
3. What factors influence the prognosis of squamous cell carcinoma (SCC)?

SUMMARY

The growing incidence of premalignant and malignant skin neoplasia, including basal cell carcinoma (BCC), squamous cell carcinoma (SCC), and melanoma, necessitates an active and informed reaction by health practitioners. New evidence indicates alarming trends for these cancers, including rising increases for premalignant lesions , such as actinic keratosis (AK) and Bowen's disease, which reflect the mounting public health problem. Among 571,057 dermatology outpatients in 1991–2006, 2,598 were diagnosed with premalignant or malignant lesions, underscoring the importance of effective screening and early detection to address this risk. The data highlight the importance of regular follow-up and intervention to avoid the risks of the development of skin cancer, especially in high-risk populations. Furthermore, the need for training and education among medical professionals in the diagnosis and management of skin cancer cannot be overstated. A study demonstrated that online training significantly improved rheumatologists' diagnostic competency in skin tumors. Trained clinicians were found to be significantly better at discriminating between benign and malignant lesions. This has a direct impact on patient outcomes because timely referral and correct diagnoses are critical in the fight against skin cancers. Therefore, introducing educational programs to identify and manage cutaneous malignancies is not only beneficial but also necessary to improve patient care. Finally, it is the broad-based effort of public awareness, professional education, and comprehensive healthcare strategies that will combat the dangers of premalignant and malignant skin tumors. Continued rates of rising incidence, particularly in risk populations, for instance, patients on immunomodulatory therapy, reinforce the need for vigilance. As illustrated by the increasing prevalence of skin cancers in recent years, the development of an informed health care workforce can lead to greater awareness of skin lesions and better overall management. With public health still being challenged by skin cancer, promoting interdisciplinary teamwork towards education and advocacy will be important in limiting the effects of these cancers on individuals and society at large.

An understanding of the mechanisms of premalignant and malignant skin tumors, such as basal cell carcinoma (BCC), squamous cell carcinoma (SCC), and melanoma, is crucial for effective treatment as well as disease prevention. Arsenic has been identified as a critical risk factor for skin cancer, particularly with its long-term ingestion via drinking water. Evidence indicates that this metalloid has the potential to enhance carcinogenesis by epigenetic changes, that is, microRNA expression modification. These changes have been shown to associate with the lesion stage and phenotype of the skin lesions, suggesting that tracking microRNA profiles could not only improve our understanding of arsenic-induced skin cancer but also potentially form a platform for biomarker and target identification. These results underscore the complexity of developing successful prevention measures for individuals at high risk for skin cancers with environmental etiology, illuminating an important area for ongoing research and clinical investigation (Al-Eryani & Laila, 2017).

In organ transplant recipients (OTR), the incidence of skin cancer is a public health concern. The referral indicator to a specialized dermatology clinic can serve as a highly predictive marker for diagnosis and management of non-melanoma skin cancers. A patient history review in a transplant dermatology clinic revealed appalling statistics; that is, 26% of patients who were referred with a "lesion of concern" were found to have skin cancer on follow-up over a period of six months. Conversely, patients who were referred for less benign issues like "rash/acne" also continued to have high incidence rates of skin cancer diagnoses, showing that less salient symptoms must be a priority to notice. These findings highlight the importance of enhancing risk stratification standards and early referral, which would substantially improve outcomes in those patients already at risk for developing skin cancers due to immunosuppressive treatments required post-transplantation (Chundydyal, 2015). In conclusion, the complexities of the etiology and diagnosis of premalignant and malignant skin cancers require a multidisciplinary approach. The implications of environmental carcinogen exposure, including arsenic, underscore the need for additional research into molecular and epigenetic markers that would facilitate early detection and therapy. Meanwhile, for groups at risk like OTR, timely and appropriate referrals to dermatological care could be crucial to improving skin cancer outcomes. : A convergent understanding of these factors not only improves patient management but also stimulates the development of education programs aimed at preventing skin tumors. Ultimately, the creation of an inclusive approach that integrates research and clinical practice is necessary in addressing the increasing prevalence and enhancing prognoses for those afflicted with BCC, SCC, and melanoma.

KEY TERMS FROM THIS CHAPTER

- Biomarkers
- Carcinogenic agents
- Chronic exposure
- Clinical intervention
- Diagnostic methods
- Epigenetic changes
- Genetic mutations
- Genetic susceptibility
- Histopathological examination
- Cancer progression
- Carcinoma
- Chronic sun exposure
- Cryotherapy
- DNA damage
- Genetic determinants
- Genetic predisposition
- Health system
- Immunotherapeutic agents

CRITICAL THINKING QUESTIONS

1. **Which of the following is the most common risk factor associated with the development of basal cell carcinoma (BCC), squamous cell carcinoma (SCC), and melanoma?**
   a. Smoking
   b. Chronic sun exposure and ultraviolet (UV) radiation
   c. High-fat diet
   d. Viral infections
2. **A patient presents with a pearly, translucent nodule with telangiectasia on the face. Which skin tumor is most likely?**
   a. Squamous cell carcinoma (SCC)
   b. Melanoma
   c. Basal cell carcinoma (BCC)
   d. Actinic keratosis
3. **A pearly, translucent nodule with telangiectasia is most characteristic of which tumor?**
   a. Melanoma
   b. Squamous Cell Carcinoma (SCC)
   c. Kaposi Sarcoma
   d. Basal Cell Carcinoma (BCC)
4. **What is the primary treatment option for localized squamous cell carcinoma (SCC) of the skin?**
   a. Chemotherapy
   b. Surgical excision with clear margins
   c. Radiotherapy alone
   d. Topical corticosteroids
5. **Which prevention strategy is most effective in reducing the risk of premalignant and malignant skin tumors?**
   a. Taking vitamin supplements
   b. Avoiding all physical activity outdoors
   c. Using antibacterial soaps daily
   d. Regular use of sunscreen and protective clothing

Short Answer Questions

1. What are the major risk factors associated with the development of premalignant and malignant skin tumors like BCC, SCC, and melanoma?
2. How do the clinical presentations of basal cell carcinoma (BCC), squamous cell carcinoma (SCC), and melanoma differ?
3. What diagnostic methods are used to confirm the presence of BCC, SCC, and melanoma?
4. What are the primary treatment options available for premalignant lesions and malignant skin tumors , such as BCC, SCC, and melanoma?
5. What effective prevention strategies can individuals adopt to reduce their risk of developing skin tumors?
6. Why is early detection crucial for the prognosis of malignant skin tumors like melanoma?

Answer to Critical Thinking Questions

1. (b); 2. (c); 3. (d); 4. (b); 5. (d)

REFERENCES

1. Akarsu, S., & Kamberoglu, I. (2018). Cryotherapy for common premalignant and malignant skin disorders. In *InTech eBooks*. https://doi.org/10.5772/intechopen.70286Al-Eryani & Laila, "MiRNA expression changes in arsenic-induced skin cancer in vitro and in vivo." (2017). Electronic Theses and Dissertations. Paper 2767. https://doi.org/10.18297/etd/2767(accessed on 21st July 2025).

2. Magro, F., Peyrin-Biroulet, L., Sokol, H., Aldeger, X., Costa, A., Higgins, P. D., Joyce, J. C., Katsanos, K. H., Lopez, A., de Xaxars, T. M., Toader, E., & Beaugerie, L. (2014). Extra-intestinal malignancies in inflammatory bowel disease: results of the 3rd ECCO Pathogenesis Scientific Workshop (III). *Journal of Crohn's & colitis*, *8*(1), 31–44. https://doi.org/10.1016/j.crohns.2013.04.006(accessed on 21st July 2025).

3. Viguier, M., Rist, S., Aubin, F., Leccia, M. T., Richard, M. A., Esposito-Farèse, M., Gaudin, P., Pham, T., Richette, P., Wendling, D., Sibilia, J., Tubach, F., & Club Rhumatismes et Inflammation (2015). Online training on skin cancer diagnosis in rheumatologists: results from a nationwide randomized web-based survey. *PloS one*, *10*(5), e0127564. https://doi.org/10.1371/journal.pone.0127564(accessed on 21st July 2025).

4. Valejo Coelho, M. M., & Apetato, M. (2016). The dark side of the light: Phototherapy adverse effects. *Clinics in dermatology*, *34*(5), 556–562. https://doi.org/10.1016/j.clindermatol.2016.05.005(accessed on 21st July 2025).

5. Nemazannikova, N., Blatch, G. L., Dass, C. R., Sinclair, R., & Apostolopoulos, V. (2019). Vitamin D enzymes (CYP27A1, CYP27B1, and CYP24A1) and receptor expression in non-melanoma skin cancer. *Acta biochimica et biophysica Sinica*, *51*(4), 444–447. https://doi.org/10.1093/abbs/gmy170(accessed on 21st July 2025).

6. Sand M, Sand D, Brors D, Altmeyer P, Mann B, Bechara FG. Cutaneous lesions of the external ear. *Head Face Med*. 2008;4:2. Published 2008 Feb 8. doi:10.1186/1746-160X-4-2(accessed on 21st July 2025).

7. Boda, D., Caruntu, C., Constantin, C., Ilie, M., et al. (2017). Squamous cell carcinoma: Biomarkers and potential therapeutic targets. https://core.ac.uk/download/322432937.pdf (accessed on 21st July 2025).

8. Bottoni, U., Cantisani, C., Didona, D., & Paolino, G. (2018). Non-melanoma skin cancer pathogenesis overview. https://core.ac.uk/download/153368939.pdf (accessed on 21st July 2025).

9. Paolino, G., Donati, M., Didona, D., Mercuri, S. R., & Cantisani, C. (2017). Histology of Non-Melanoma Skin Cancers: An Update. *Biomedicines*, *5*(4), 71. https://doi.org/10.3390/biomedicines5040071(accessed on 21st July 2025).

10. Garcia-Uribe, A., Zou, J., Duvic, M., Cho-Vega, J. H., Prieto, V. G., & Wang, L. V. (2012). In vivo diagnosis of melanoma and nonmelanoma skin cancer using oblique incidence diffuse reflectance spectrometry. *Cancer research*, *72*(11), 2738–2745. https://doi.org/10.1158/0008-5472.CAN-11-4027(accessed on 21st July 2025).

11. Chundydyal, S. (2015). Skin cancer outcomes as a function of referral reason in solid organ transplant recipients. https://core.ac.uk/download/232768708.pdf (accessed on 21st July 2025).

12. Wessels R, De Bruin DM, Faber DJ, Van Leeuwen TG, Van Beurden M, Ruers TJ. Optical biopsy of epithelial cancers by optical coherence tomography (OCT). *Lasers Med Sci.* 2014;29(3):1297-1305. doi:10.1007/s10103-013-1291-8(accessed on 21st July 2025).
13. de Zwaan, S. E. (2008). The genetics of basal cell carcinoma of the skin. https://core.ac.uk/download/41232211.pdf (accessed on 21st July 2025).
14. Dlugosz, A., Merlino, G., & Yuspa, S. H. (2002). Progress in cutaneous cancer research. https://core.ac.uk/download/82724432.pdf (accessed on 21st July 2025).
15. Han, J., Qureshi, A. A., & Zhang, M. (2014). Heterogeneity in host risk factors for incident melanoma and non-melanoma skin cancer in a cohort of US women. https://core.ac.uk/download/28947660.pdf (accessed on 21st July 2025).
16. Hasan, N., Nadaf, A., Imran, M., Jiba, U., Sheikh, A., Almalki, W. H., Almujri, S. S., et al. (2023). Skin cancer: Understanding the journey of transformation from conventional to advanced treatment approaches. *Molecular Cancer, 22.* https://doi.org/10.1186/s12943-023-01854-3 (accessed on 21st July 2025).
17. Katz, K. A., Marcil, I., & Stern, R. S. (2002). Incidence and risk factors associated with a second squamous cell carcinoma or basal cell carcinoma in psoralen + ultraviolet A light-treated psoriasis patients. https://core.ac.uk/download/pdf/82138241.pdf (accessed on 21st July 2025).
18. Lee, C. N., Hsu, R., Chen, H., & Wong, T. W. (2020). Daylight photodynamic therapy: An update. *Molecules, 25,* 5195. https://doi.org/10.3390/molecules25215195 (accessed on 21st July 2025).
19. Fang, Wei-Cheng; Chou, Pei-Chien; Chiu, Li-Wen; Ke, Chiao-Li2; Cheng, Shih-Tsun. Dermoscopy as a Diagnostic and Monitoring Tool for Recurrent Extramammary Paget's Disease. Indian Journal of Dermatology 67(6):p 819-820, Nov–Dec 2022. | DOI: 10.4103/ijd.ijd_771_22 (accessed on 21st July 2025).
20. Park, C. J., Chun, Y. S., Chung, J., de Vries, E., Diepgen, T., Yu, D. S., Cho, E. A., et al. (2010). Recent trend in the incidence of premalignant and malignant skin lesions in Korea between 1991 and 2006. https://core.ac.uk/download/pdf/8414049.pdf (accessed on 21st July 2025).
21. Sangers, T. (2024). Exploring artificial intelligence and mobile health in skin cancer care: From development to implementation. https://core.ac.uk/download/621176488.pdf (accessed on 21st July 2025).
22. Stawarz, K., Gałązka, A., Misiak-Gałązka, M., Durzyńska, M., Gorzelnik, A., Bieńkowska-Pluta, K., Korzon, J., et al. (2025). Advances in skin ultrasonography for malignant and benign tumors of the head and neck: Current insights and future directions. *Journal of Clinical Medicine, 14.* https://www.semanticscholar.org/paper/d669d2c28ecee876ba6e0e4c309423290543c631 (accessed on 21st July 2025).
23. Tamaș, T., Dinu, C., Lenghel, L., Boțan, E., Tamas, A., Stoia, S., Leucuța, D., et al. (2023). High-frequency ultrasound in diagnosis and treatment of non-melanoma skin cancer in the head and neck region. *Diagnostics, 13.* https://www.semanticscholar.org/paper/6b9702c1e77a3452b623cfc0191c9dc4d0980c57 (accessed on 21st July 2025).

CUTANEOUS LYMPHOMAS AND METASTATIC SKIN DISEASES

3

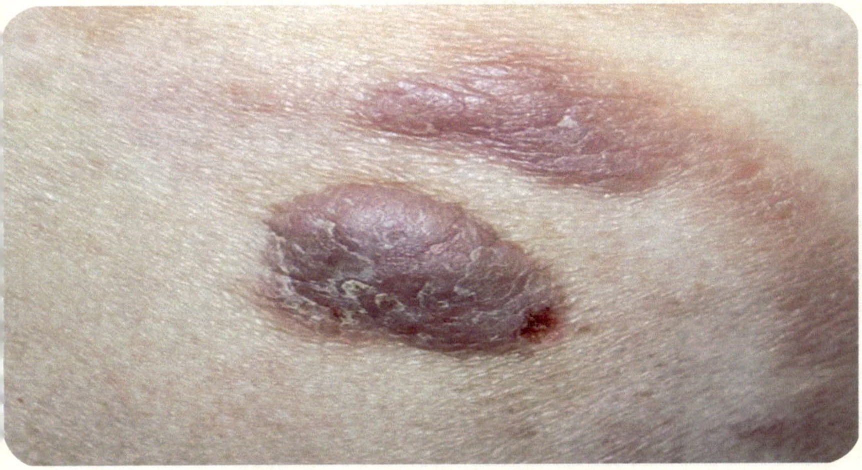

Introduction

The increasing frequency of skin lymphomas and skin metastases highlights the need for improved understanding of these complex disorders. Skin cancer, in the form of the most common type of malignancy globally, is a clinically heterogeneous collection of malignant neoplasms, with cutaneous lymphomas being an unusually challenging subtype due to their pathological heterogeneity. The interplay between the environmental exposures and genetic susceptibilities, such as exposure to ultraviolet (UV) radiation, has been implicated in the etiology of skin malignancies. Although the diagnosis of non-melanoma skin cancers (NMSCs) like basal cell carcinoma and squamous cell carcinoma is frequent, cutaneous lymphomas are a reminder of the pressing need for targeted research and therapeutic advancements. Overall, the rising incidence of skin cancer, combined with the aging population, has prompted a need to revisit existing public health policy and resource planning to address these growing challenges (Kohnehshahri et al., 2023).

LEARNING OBJECTIVES

After studying this chapter, you will be able to:

1. Explain the types of cutaneous lymphomas
2. Understand the pathophysiology of cutaneous lymphomas
3. Discuss how to diagnose cutaneous lymphomas
4 Deal with treatment options for cutaneous lymphomas
5. Describe metastatic skin diseases
6. Focus on the diagnosis and management of metastatic skin diseases

Under this complex scenario, the role of immunological factors cannot be overstated. Immunocompromised hosts, be they hosts of primary immunodeficiency or secondary disease, such as HIV, are at risk of cutaneous malignancy, including very aggressive skin lymphomas. Human papillomavirus (HPV) is a prime agent in this regard and is responsible for skin carcinogenesis to a large extent in immunocompromised hosts. Mechanisms of tumor development triggered by HPV are not yet clearly defined and, therefore, raise a tremendous amount of scientific curiosity. Because many current treatment options still fail this delicate population, overcoming the barriers posed by immunosuppression is important for achieving better outcomes. With these factors in mind, research into novel therapeutic modalities, like RNA-based approaches for gene targeting, bodes well in attacking recalcitrant forms of skin cancer (Hewavisenti et al., 2023). As we unravel the intricacies of cutaneous lymphomas and metastatic skin diseases, the necessity for a multidisciplinary treatment strategy becomes evident to enhance survival rates as well as the quality of life of patients. The advent of immunotherapies, exemplified by the invention of monoclonal antibodies, foretells the guard changing at the gate of treatment strategies, making interventions more targeted and more effective. Clarification of the root etiologies of skin cancers, from environmental causatives to immune evasion strategies, is crucial for the best management plans. In addition, the integration of advances in genetics and technology will enable the development of new biomarkers that inform therapeutic choices and facilitate earlier detection of these neoplasms. Consequently, coordinated research and clinical activities are necessary to alleviate the public health burden of cutaneous lymphomas and metastatic skin malignancies (Kohnehshahri et al., 2023).

Definition of Cutaneous Lymphomas

The realm of cutaneous lymphomas, which is a heterogeneous group of skin-predominant malignancies, consists of a number of histological and clinical subtypes. They are characterized by the proliferation of lymphocytes, primarily T-cells or B-cells, within the epidermis and dermis. To understand the definition of cutaneous lymphomas, it is important to appreciate their distinction from other skin illnesses, particularly metastatic disease arising from systemic cancers. Cutaneous lymphomas are categorized, which is important in that not only does it influence diagnostic examinations, but also therapeutic regimens as well as prognostic outcomes. The categorization enables the identification of unique subtypes, which are of utmost importance for administering customized therapeutic regimens that can optimize patient outcomes. The distinction from other skin dermatoses as well as metastatic diseases of the skin poses one of the greatest challenges in the diagnosis of cutaneous lymphomas. Lesions are common in patients who may have presentation that is a mimic of benign dermatoses, and hence, a careful clinical and histopathological workup has to be done. The application of diagnostic modalities , such as immunohistochemistry and genetic studies is important to establish definitive diagnoses. ALCL, especially the ALK-negative type, is a classic example of diagnostic vagueness because it can present as other skin malignancies. A sharp awareness of such nuances is critical for both dermatologists and oncologists. An integrated diagnosis minimizes the possibilities of misdiagnosis, ultimately leading to more effective treatment protocols for cutaneous lymphoma patients (Ferreri et al., 2012).

Cutaneous lymphoma research has pointed to the significance of new therapeutic strategies, specifically those that target specific genetic and molecular pathways. Recent work underscores the value of histone deacetylase (HDAC) inhibitors, which have garnered interest as anti-neoplastic agents owing to their control of gene expression patterns and remodeling of chromatin (Milazzo et al., 2020).

Such a novel therapeutic approach reflects the evolving landscape of oncologic treatment. Utilization of targeted therapy, along with conventional chemotherapy protocols, depicts a more tailored approach to treating cutaneous lymphomas. These developments not only improve the effectiveness of therapy but also open the doors to individualized medicine, tailoring to a patient's tumor's unique genetic makeup. As research continues, the treatment and management of cutaneous lymphomas will surely evolve, promising improved patient care (Figure 3.1).

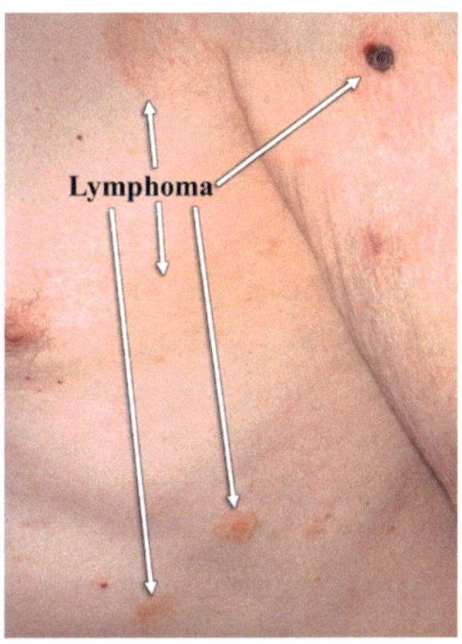

Figure 3.1. Illustration of cutaneous lymphomas.

Source: https://acadderm.com/wp-content/uploads/2023/01/Lymphoma4Samlaska-683x1024.jpg.

Overview of Metastatic Skin Diseases

The metastatic cutaneous disease syndrome is characterized by the invasion of the skin by malignant cells from a distant site, typically indicating advanced malignancy within the systemic circulation. It can be expressed in a variety of ways, including metastasis of melanoma, carcinoma of the breast, and lymphomas, each with different clinical characteristics and importance. Cutaneous metastatic illnesses typically arise from malignancies that predominantly involve internal sites and extend to the epidermal structures via lymphatic or hematogenous routes. Significantly, their onset can radically alter a patient's prognosis, serving as an indicator of cancer progression and in most instances inducing more aggressive treatment measures. It is crucial to identify and properly diagnose these disorders since the skin is not only a site for metastasis but is also an active participant in the body's immune response to internal malignancies. Among the various forms of skin disease that can be metastatic, cutaneous lymphomas, including Sézary syndrome and MALT lymphoma, are distinctive because they have distinct immunologic and histopathologic features. Sézary syndrome, a subtype of cutaneous T-cell lymphoma, is particularly virulent and is characterized by erythroderma, lymphadenopathy, and an intravascular malignant T-cell growth. Some inflammatory markers , such as IL-1B and IL-18, have been shown recently to determine disease severity and prognosis in patients. The imbalance of these cytokines, particularly the higher levels of IL-18 across different skin layers, illustrates the complex interplay between the tumor microenvironment and the immune system. Understanding the processes behind is not just beneficial in terms of diagnosis but also for possible targeted treatment and management of the patient (Manfrere et al., 2023). In MALT lymphoma, cutaneous lesions can be challenging to diagnose because their histopathology overlaps with that of other granulomatous skin diseases. Granulomatous reaction in the skin can confound the clinical presentation and camouflage the malignancy. As pointed out in some examples, immunohistochemistry (IHC) and immunoglobulin heavy-chain gene rearrangement analysis are essential diagnostic tools that can determine the presence and the degree of MALT lymphoma even when primary skin lesions are discovered to have non-specific granulomatous alterations. Furthermore, current evidence suggests that granulomatous reactions that are developed in the setting of MALT lymphoma can lead to a better prognosis as a sign of a beneficial immune response in the skin. Therefore, correctly categorizing the nuances of cutaneous lymphomas remains of first-order importance to better enhance early detection and improve therapeutic optimization (Scarfi et al., 2019) (Figure 3.2).

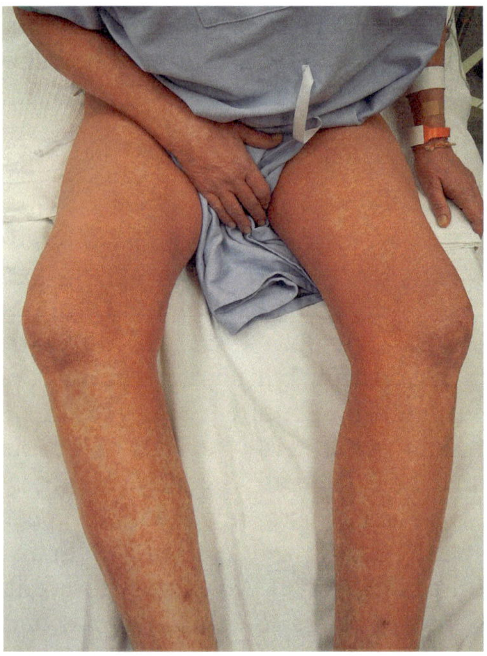

Figure 3.2. The bright red rash of Sezary syndrome.

Source: https://upload.wikimedia.org/wikipedia/commons/thumb/a/a1/Sezery2.jpg/800px-Sezery2.jpg.

Importance of Studying These Conditions

Research into cutaneous lymphomas and metastatic skin disease is critical to advancing care for skin cancer patients, particularly in treatment effectiveness and patient outcomes. Incidence of conditions , such as cutaneous squamous cell carcinoma (cSCC) is on the rise globally, and due to this, making evidence-based guidelines is critically important to optimize patient care. Successful management relies on integrating clinical evidence from systematic reviews and large datasets, as highlighted by the British Association of Dermatologists (BAD) guidelines (Keohane et al., 2020). By comprehensively reviewing the epidemiologic trends, risk factors, and treatment strategies, clinicians cannot only enhance diagnostic methods but also offer patients timely interventions specific to their unique presentations of these diseases. In addition, above and beyond statistics, the significance of learning about cutaneous lymphomas and metastatic skin diseases is based on the ethical obligation healthcare workers have towards their patients. Setting guidelines and recommendations on the basis of the latest evidence—like those for the management of higher-risk cSCC—ensures that clinicians can deliver care that is proportionate to patient value and requirement (Keohane et al., 2020). This is particularly relevant as skin disease can have psychological and emotional weights that affect individuals, and therefore, there must be a more multifaceted approach to both medical and psychosocial management. The delineation of treatment approaches also facilitates interdisciplinary cooperation among multiple care teams, in which all elements of patient health are addressed. The research into immunotherapies and associated toxicities offers a valuable dimension to the study of cutaneous lymphomas and metastatic skin neoplasms. Of specific interest, improved cancer therapy with checkpoint inhibitors and adoptive cell transfer has revolutionized management options and improved patient outcomes. Nevertheless, each of these therapies has a distinct toxicity profile that must be addressed in a specialized and knowledgeable fashion. Identification of these side effects, as well as their mechanisms of action, not only adds to the quality of the care delivered but also facilitates developing robust guidelines that incorporate the new evidence into clinical practice. Ultimately, learning about these conditions creates a greater awareness of the benefit of both practitioners and patients, resulting in more effective treatment guidelines and potentially improved overall results.

3.1. Types of Cutaneous Lymphomas

Learning Outcome

1. Understand primary cutaneous T-cell lymphomas.
2. Describe primary cutaneous B-cell lymphomas.
3. Discuss other rare forms of cutaneous lymphomas.

Skin lymphoma is diverse, encompassing two broad categories: primary and secondary cutaneous lymphomas. Primary cutaneous lymphomas occur predominantly in the skin and are distinct entities with characteristic histologic and clinical features. Cutaneous T-cell lymphomas (CTCLs) constitute the largest share, with mycosis fungoides and Sézary syndrome as the most common variants. These disorders are caused by the malignant growth of T-cells in the skin, with manifestations ranging from cutaneous lesions to systemic disease in advanced stages. Secondary cutaneous lymphomas, by contrast, present on the skin as a skin manifestation of cutaneous lymphoma, hematogenously seeding from some other site within the body. These distinctions are crucial to recognize, as they affect disease prognosis, treatment decisions, and ultimately patient management in the clinical setting. Aside from the primary and secondary cut, cutaneous lymphomas can be further classified based on their histological features and cellular origin. For instance, B-cell lymphomas, although less common than T-cell lymphomas, include primary cutaneous follicle center lymphoma and primary cutaneous diffuse large B-cell lymphoma, leg type. Both are distinguished by typical morphological features that are most significant for accurate diagnosis and treatment planning. The molecular signature of such lymphomas has also become increasingly significant, with advances in immunophenotyping and genetic profiling giving insight into their neoplastic and chronic inflammatory processes. The regulatory pathway of the malignancies NF-kB and JAK-STAT, is involved in pathogenesis in cutaneous lymphomas and hence a therapeutic target for new therapies and clinical treatment (Zhao et al., 2021). The modalities for the treatment of cutaneous lymphomas are as diverse as the diseases themselves, from superficial to systemic chemotherapy and targeted biologic therapies. Localized disease is characterized by radiation therapy, particularly in early-stage disease, whereas advanced disease could necessitate systemic therapies, such as brentuximab vedotin or emerging immunotherapies directed against cancer stem cells. The concept of targeting cutaneous lymphoma stem cells is gaining momentum, as they have been found to be the cause of recurrence and resistance to conventional therapies. Recent research emphasizes that factors in the tumor microenvironment, such as inflammatory cytokines and extracellular matrix constituents that interact with cancer stem cells, promote drug resistance and survival (Yang et al., 2020). Together, these observations underscore the heterogeneity of cutaneous lymphomas and the need for tailored treatment approaches to reduce their impact on patients' health and quality of life.

3.1.1. Primary Cutaneous T-Cell Lymphomas

Primary cutaneous T-cell lymphomas (CTCLs) constitute a unique category of lymphoproliferative diseases involving the skin, largely distinguished from systemic lymphomas with potential for cutaneous disease. Mycosis fungoides is the most common CTCL and traditionally presents as patches and plaques that eventually evolve into more aggressive disease forms, including tumor-stage disease. Unlike metastatic skin diseases, and thus due to remote malignancies, CTCL is due to the skin's own malignancy of T-cells. The pathogenesis of CTCL is composed of complex interactions between the host microenvironment and malignant T-cells, leading to chronic inflammation and immune dysregulation. This interaction contributes to the disease's course and resistance to conventional therapies, underlining the need for specifically targeted treatment modalities that can specifically address the unique characteristics of these skin tumors. The therapeutic landscape of primary cutaneous T-cell lymphomas has expanded in the last few years with the introduction of new treatments that attack the molecular and immunologic components of the illness. Among the new methods under development are antibody-drug conjugates (ADCs), which have been described for their potential to deliver cytotoxic drug molecules to cancer cells specifically with impunity to normal tissue. An ADC is a monoclonal antibody conjugated to an immensely potent cytotoxic drug, thus harnessing the selective targeting ability of antibodies for the efficient killing of cancer cells (Fu et al., 2022). This modality represents a milestone in the handling of CTCL challenges , such as treatment resistance and unfavorable response to standard treatments. Further, the incorporation of immunotherapies that leverage the body's immune system presents encouraging potential for the maximization of therapeutic outcomes and survival advantages in CTCL patients with advanced disease. Evidence also supports the pivotal role of inflammation in tumour growth and treatment response in primary cutaneous T-cell lymphomas. Inflammation in CTCL can create a tumor microenvironment that fosters survival and growth of the tumor, which becomes resistant to treatment (Zhao et al., 2021). Signaling pathways , such as nuclear factor kappa B (NF-kB) and Janus kinase/signal transducers and activators of transcription (JAK-STAT) were discovered to play a central role in the inflammatory mechanisms that lead to malignancy. Cognizance of the crosstalk between tumorigenesis and inflammation is crucial for the design of novel therapeutic regimens. Current research is aimed at efficient modulation of the pathways, which may enhance the anti-tumor immune response and also reduce resistance to therapy. Therefore, the treatment of the inflammatory milieu in CTCL presents a promising way of improving patient prognosis and further understanding the intricate relationship between skin lymphomas and their systemic signs (Figure 3.3).

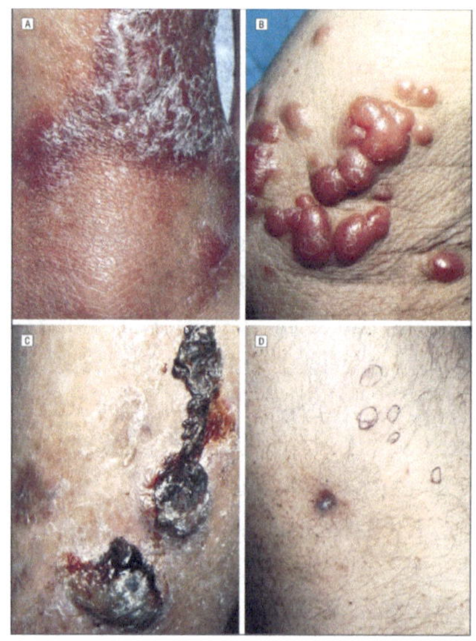

Figure 3.3. Clinical spectrum of patient 2 with cutaneous T-cell lymphoma. A, A scaly plaque on the ankle resembles mycosis fungoides. B, Multiple pink to plum-colored tumors on an upper extremity. C, Characteristic ulcerated tumors covered with hemorrhagic crust. D, Indurated subcutaneous nodules on a thigh.

Source: https://www.researchgate.net/profile/Elaine-Jaffe/publication/12393214/figure/fig1/AS:340695631056896@1458239576167/Clinical-spectrum-of-patient-2-with-cutaneous-T-cell-lymphoma-A-A-scaly-plaque-on-the.png.

3.1.2. Primary Cutaneous B-Cell Lymphomas

Clinical presentation of primary cutaneous B-cell lymphomas (CBCL) encompasses a few subtypes that are characterized by different clinical and biological features. Widely categorized into three main groups—follicle center lymphoma (pcFCL), marginal zone lymphoma (pcMZLPD), and diffuse large B-cell lymphoma, leg type (DLBCL-LT)—these possess very different conduct and prognosis. pcFCL and pcMZLPD are typically indolent, with over 70% long-term survival for pcFCL, while DLBCL-LT, being aggressive in nature, is reflected to have a drastically lower five-year relapse-free survival of only 23%. Identifying these distinctions is significant for the development of effective management plans, which may include localized therapy for less aggressive subtypes and systemic therapy for more advanced stages of the disease, thereby enabling a subtype-focused treatment approach. Effective management of primary cutaneous B-cell lymphomas often relies on the integration of clinical characteristics with treatment approaches. In the case of pcFCL and pcMZLPD, dermatologic treatments , such as excision and intralesional corticosteroids have proven to be useful, with studies touting their superb TTNT compared to other treatments. In contrast, individuals with DLBCL-LT usually require more intense systemic treatments , such as chemotherapy and immunotherapy in order to achieve substantial clinical responses. This disparity in the treatment approach underscores the need for precise diagnosis because timely and correct classification of the type of lymphoma largely decides the clinical outcome. Moreover, new therapies, which target cancer-specific proteins or modulate the immune system, will enhance therapy and improve patients' quality of life as research in this field proceeds further (Barbati & Charli-Joseph, 2025). The need for ongoing research into primary cutaneous B-cell lymphomas can be overstressed. Despite advances, much remains unknown regarding the optimal management of these rare diseases. Insights into the distinctive immunological and molecular features of each subtype may identify new directions in personalized therapies that could improve patient prognosis and survival rates (Barbati & Charli-Joseph, 2025). Additionally, urgency must be placed on investigating issues of health equity, as current studies often do not enroll diverse patient groups in a representative manner. As clinicians and researchers seek to understand the pathophysiology and treatment responses in primary CBCL, inclusive research designs will be essential. It is through this commitment to a complete investigation that therapies not only become better, but all patients with these diseases are equally accorded access to improved treatments and optimized care outcomes (Figure 3.4).

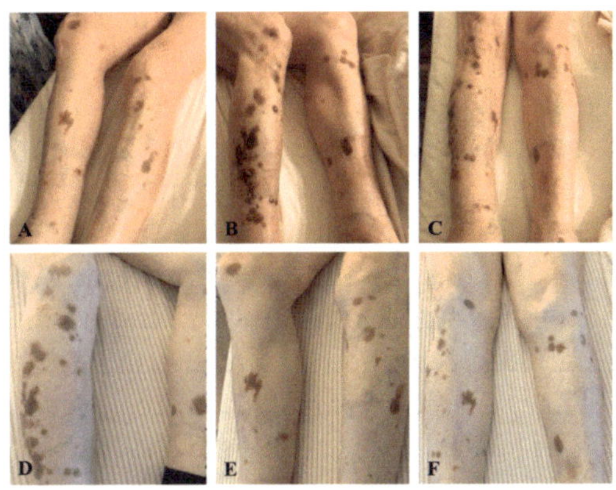

Figure 3.4. The clinical picture of primary cutaneous diffuse large B-cell lymphoma, leg type and its response to treatment. (A-C) Multiple violaceous, raised skin lesions involving the right lower extremity, before starting ibrutinib therapy. (D-F) Dissipating skin lesions approximately six months after initiating ibrutinib therapy.

Source: https://www.researchgate.net/publication/342220816/figure/fig1/AS:903226056515585@1592357281488/The-clinical-picture-of-primary-cutaneous-diffuse-large-B-cell-lymphoma-leg-type-and-its.png.

3.1.3. Other Rare Forms of Cutaneous Lymphomas

Among the diverse population of uncommon cutaneous lymphomas, angiosarcoma is a highly aggressive malignancy arising from endothelial cells. Angiosarcoma is a common form of cutaneous lymphoma that often occurs in the skin and soft tissues and has a poor prognosis with an extremely low five-year survival rate of approximately 9% (Yamakawa et al., 2025). Angiosarcoma pathogenesis is complex and often involves multiple recurrent genetic alterations that support tumorigenesis. Progress in the molecular characterization of the disease has offered promise for the development of targeted therapies, but the efficacy of these treatments in the context of metastatic disease is not guaranteed. A multidisciplinary management approach—combining surgical, radiologic, and systemic therapies—underscores the challenges of managing this rare dermatological disease, calling for novel research designs to maximize patient outcomes. Another highly prevalent type in the class of cutaneous lymphomas is primary cutaneous B-cell lymphoma (PCBCL), which has several subtypes, including primary cutaneous follicle center lymphoma and primary cutaneous marginal zone lymphoma. The classification and diagnosis of these lymphomas are intricately associated with histopathologic evaluation and immunohistochemistry, which provide relevant information regarding the driving force of the illness (Hristov et al., 2025). Local therapy in the form of radiotherapy has been effective in patients with cutaneous lesions limited in extent, resulting in adequate control over the disease. In spite of this, the variability of patient response necessitates risk-adapted therapy based on consideration of disease spread and specific histopathology. This stratification is crucial to the individualization of treatment modalities such that patients receive the best available level of care for their respective prognoses. Cutaneous lymphomas also include the less frequent entities, such as lymphomatoid papulosis, which is a relapsing papule or nodule on the skin and is a CD30-positive lymphoproliferative disorder. The disease has a massive overlap with other cutaneous T-cell lymphomas, and thus, diagnostic methods and therapeutic treatment are challenging. An accurate classification relies heavily on histopathological and immunophenotypic assessment, indicating an imperative diagnostic method (Hristov et al., 2025). Treatment of lymphomatoid papulosis is generally dermally oriented, but the disease's variability may necessitate a systemic strategy in more extensive presentations. Understanding the characteristic features and management regimens of rare skin lymphomas, such as lymphomatoid papulosis, is essential to improve overall care for dermatology and oncology patients, as clinicians are now confronted with the heterogeneity of this spectrum of disease (Figure 3.5).

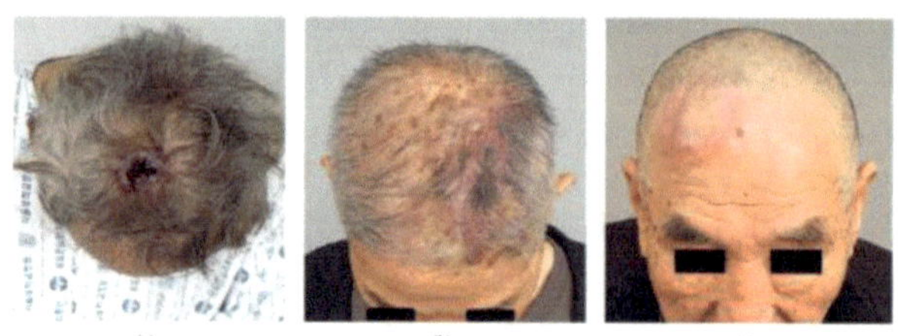

Figure 3.5. Three different types of scalp angiosarcoma. (a) ulcer type (b) bruise type (c) nodular type.

Source: https://upload.wikimedia.org/wikipedia/commons/b/b2/Three_types_of_scalp_angiosarcoma.jpg.

Test Your Knowledge

1. What is the most common type of primary cutaneous T-cell lymphoma (CTCL)?
2. What are the common clinical features of primary cutaneous B-cell lymphomas (CBCL)?

3.2. Pathophysiology of Cutaneous Lymphomas

Learning Outcome

1. Describe genetic mutations and their role
2. Explain how the immune system plays a pivotal role in the pathogenesis and progression of cutaneous lymphomas and metastatic skin diseases
3. Discuss the environmental factors in the development of cutaneous lymphomas and metastatic skin diseases

The pathophysiology of cutaneous lymphomas, and CTCL in particular, is multifaceted and involves genetic, immunologic, and environmental factors. CTCL represents a heterogeneous group of malignancies characterized by the infiltration of malignant T cells into the skin. The interaction between external stimuli, such as infection or chemical exposure, and genetic changes is a critical factor in the etiology of the disease. It is currently understood that inflammation is a critical driver of CTCL development, and cytokines such as IL-9 play central roles in this process. The microenvironment of the tumour is supportive of lymphocyte proliferation and activation, which is likely to transform benign T-cells into malignant forms, therefore highlighting the complexity of the disease's pathophysiologic processes (Attrish et al., 2025). Recent studies point to the antioxidant response pathway in CTCL, with special emphasis on glutathione synthetase (GSS) as a critical enzyme.

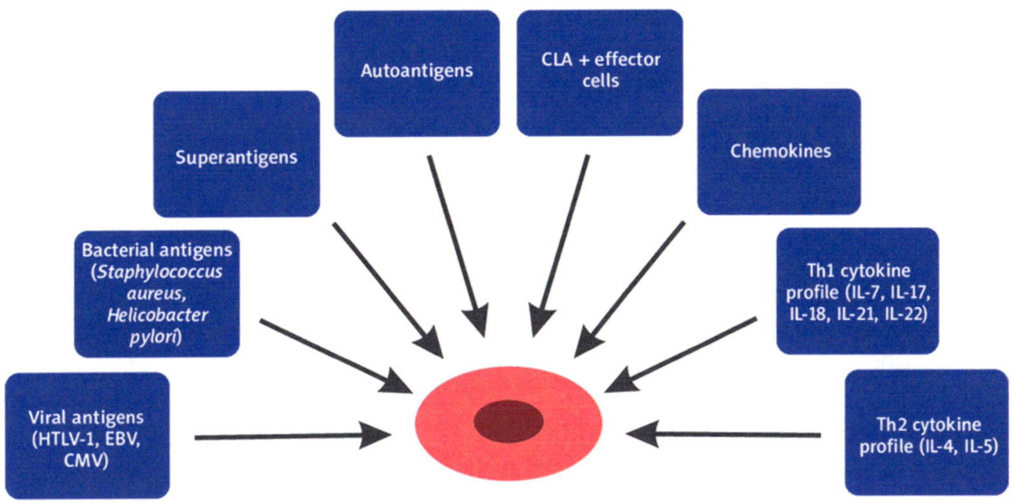

Figure 3.6. Pathogenesis of cutaneous T-cell lymphoma.

Source: https://www.researchgate.net/publication/284670171/figure/fig1/AS:616826237120513@1524074243228/Pathogenesis-of-cutaneous-T-cell-lymphoma.png.

Elevated GSS levels have been correlated with oxidative stress responses in lymphoma cells, conferring survival and proliferation on cells. Upon IL-9 stimulation, research has found increased glutathione metabolism, which enables malignant T cells to survive under unfavorable conditions. The regulation of antioxidant signaling not only affects tumor development but also reveals potential therapeutic weaknesses.

Inhibition of GSS, for example, has been shown to be promising in depleting this antioxidant, leading to increased generation of reactive oxygen species (ROS) and subsequent cell death. Therefore, the comprehension of these metabolic changes is useful in understanding how to utilize weaknesses in CTCL to ensure therapeutic intervention (Attrish et al., 2025). Imaging is focal to the clinical management of cutaneous lymphomas to gauge the extent of disease and treatment. Staging entails a comprehensive strategy that evaluates lymphatic involvement, perineural spread, and metastatic nodal disease, which contribute to the dermatologic malignancy's clinical picture. Follow-up imaging with contrast-enhanced CT and PET/CT scans is vital for the measurement of disease progression and the detection. These imaging methods not only enhance the understanding of the local presentation of cutaneous lymphomas but also provide critical information on potential metastatic spread. Thus, inclusion of radiologic evaluations in the management plan is essential, as although cutaneous lymphomas are primarily dermatologic in nature, they can have significant systemic implications that necessitate a multidisciplinary approach (Figure 3.6).

3.2.1. Genetic Mutations and Their Role

The landscape of cutaneous lymphomas and metastatic skin disease is highly influenced by genetic mutations that are involved in the pathogenesis of these conditions. Cellular processes are disrupted by mutations, leading to uncontrollable proliferation of cells, cell differentiation, and survival of cells of the skin that result in malignancies , such as lymphomas. Recent advances in genetic sequencing technologies have enabled researchers to detect mutations associated with various skin cancers, thereby improving our understanding of their molecular basis. For instance, mutations in the TP53 and BRAF genes have been linked to cutaneous T-cell lymphoma (CTCL) and melanoma, respectively. Such observations not only illustrate the complexity of disease progression but also open doors to specific therapies, and thus, identification of genetic alterations comes to assume pivotal importance in clinical management of cutaneous lymphomas and metastatic skin conditions. Advances in molecular diagnostics have further underscored the importance of genetic mutations in cutaneous lymphomas by enabling early diagnosis and personalized therapy regimens. Technologies , such as next-generation sequencing (NGS) now facilitate large-scale profiling of tumor DNA and identification of the disease-causing mutations. The application of such methods has been the most important factor in distinguishing between subtypes of skin cancer, thereby informing therapeutic treatment. Most notably, the identification of actionable mutations may lead to the use of targeted agents, thereby improving the prognosis of metastatic skin disease. Moreover, genetic information on germline mutations in patients will inform risk assessment and prophylactic treatment for hereditary skin cancer syndromes in families. Under these conditions, the incorporation of genetic testing into routine clinical practice represents a paradigm shift toward personalized medicine, whereby the patient is provided with optimal and appropriate treatment. Despite the potential therapeutic applications of genetic mutations, their association with increased risks of secondary malignancies has prompted significant clinical consideration. As noted within studies evaluating the long-term effect of therapies like PUVA, a strong correlation between follow-up skin cancers and immunosuppressive treatment has been reported. The inherent genetic makeup of the tumors in many cases often expresses mutations suspected to be the consequence of prior therapy, further elevating risk in the patient. For example, cumulative exposure to UV light, an essential component of PUVA treatment, causes mutagenic changes in skin cells, increasing the incidence of non-melanoma skin cancers, including squamous and basal cell carcinomas. Therefore, the monitoring of genetic mutations associated with therapeutic interventions not only facilitates the understanding of disease development but is also critical in assessing the long-term health of the patients that have undergone treatment for cutaneous lymphomas and metastatic dermatological conditions, a factor that illustrates the delicate interface between genetics and clinical therapeutic interventions (Väkev, 2006; Gabriel et al., 2024).

3.2.2. Immune System Involvement

The immune system plays a key role in the pathogenesis and evolution of cutaneous lymphomas and metastatic skin disease. Most notably, skin cancers , such as cutaneous squamous cell carcinoma (cSCC) often arise in the setting of a dysregulated immune response. Ultraviolet radiation has been extensively implicated as an etiological factor in genetic alterations in epithelial cells that precede cSCC. However, recent research indicates that interactions between the immune system and the skin microbiota are equally crucial. Notably, symbiotic to pathogenic ratios of microbes , such as *Staphylococcus aureus,* can have major impacts on immune system responses. These can range from alterations in cytokine profiles with pro-tumorigenic or anti-tumorigenic consequences. Understanding these complex interdependencies is essential to developing novel therapeutic strategies that leverage the immune system's capacity to combat skin cancers, as outlined in existing literature (Zhang et al., 2025). The therapeutic landscape for metastatic skin disease, particularly with the advent of immune checkpoint inhibitors, also underscores the significance of immune system dynamics. Agents like nivolumab have revolutionized treatment by reactivating the immune system against tumor cells. However, their use for administration has also been associated with various immune-mediated side effects, implying an uncontrolled immune reaction not only against tumors but also against the patient's own healthy tissues. For instance, in a case of a patient treated with nivolumab, an inflammatory cascade with elevated levels of cytokines was revealed, pointing towards a hybrid inflammatory response. This reflects the dual role of the immune system in being able to recognize and destroy tumor cells while at times being responsible for generating pathological immune responses that manifest through various organ systems (Khizha et al., 2025). The study reflects the intricacy of immune interactions within the context of cutaneous lymphomas and metastatic skin disease in the clinical environment. The integration of immune system involvement into the analysis of cutaneous lymphomas and metastatic skin disease presents challenges and opportunities for new treatment approaches. Immunotherapeutic considerations, in turn, informed by a sensitization to immune-mediated mechanisms, can yield better control of such diseases. For instance, the targeting of specific cytokines involved in the inflammatory process potentially enhances therapeutic effectiveness with decreased toxicity. Further, identification of the intricate interaction between immune function and skin microbials might offer scope for adjunctive therapies to augment the immune system's power to combat malignancies. The multi-dimensional concept of immune system involvement in dermatological disease thus illustrates the imperative for ongoing research and clinical trials devoted to the unveiling of new therapeutic modalities while carefully navigating the thin line of immune control (Zhang et al., 2025).

3.2.3. Developmental Factors Due to the Environment

Environmental factors play a pivotal role in cutaneous lymphomas and metastatic skin diseases, ranging from an enormous spectrum of influences that go from chemicals to physical agents. Ultraviolet radiation is among the strongest causative factors, as long-term exposure can induce mutations in epidermal cells, ultimately resulting in cancers such as melanoma and non-melanoma skin cancers.

Additionally, the role of environmental toxins, such as industrial chemicals and heavy metals, has gained prominence in the past few years. These toxins have been noted to provoke inflammatory responses and build a pro-tumoral microenvironment. The interaction between environmental stressors and genetic components underscores the importance of understanding these factors in skin cancers, thereby informing preventive strategies and treatment. The inflammatory response due to environmental exposure is highly linked with cutaneous lymphoma onset and advancement, particularly in cutaneous lymphomas. Experiments proved that continued inflammation due to long-term exposure to toxic substances can offer a pro-tumoral microenvironment that favors tumor growth. Pro-inflammatory mediators , such as cytokines and chemokines, play significant roles in sustaining cellular proliferation and survival and avoiding anticancer immune responses. These pathways, including nuclear factor kappa B (NF-κB) and Janus kinase/signal transducer and activator of transcription (JAK-STAT), have been shown to be pivotal in the regulation of the relationship between tumorigenesis and inflammation (Zhao et al., 2021). Hence, the targeting of inflammatory pathways may offer novel therapeutic targets in an effort to restore homeostasis and negate the adverse effects of environmental stress on dermal health. In addition to UV exposure and chemical pollutants, lifestyle and socioeconomic status have a major influence on the incidence and severity of cutaneous lymphomas. For instance, those with limited access to healthcare services will be affected by late diagnosis and prognosis. In addition, exposure to protective measures, including sunscreen and protective clothing, is influenced by socioeconomic status. Geographic variations in UV radiation exposure also increase the incidence of skin cancer across populations and underscore the importance of public health initiatives for prevention and education. By examining the interaction of several environmental factors and their cumulative impact on the skin, researchers can identify high-risk groups and inform interventions that can counteract these external forces (Fu et al., 2022).

Test Your Knowledge

1. What role do genetic mutations play in the development of cutaneous T-cell lymphomas (CTCL)?
2. How does the immune system contribute to the pathogenesis of cutaneous lymphomas?
3. What environmental factors have been associated with an increased risk of developing cutaneous lymphomas?

3.3. Diagnosis of Cutaneous Lymphomas

Learning Outcome

1. Discuss clinical evaluation in diagnosing cutaneous lymphomas and metastatic skin diseases.
2. Explain biopsy and histopathological examination.
3. Describe advanced imaging techniques.

Cutaneous lymphomas are inherently complex and require a multidimensional approach to achieve accurate diagnosis and guide treatment. Initial evaluation will most likely begin with a comprehensive clinical evaluation of the skin, with lesions being very differently presented, from plaques to nodules. A high clinical suspicion is appropriate, particularly when chronic wounds are present and unresponsive to conventional therapy. In these cases, differentiation between malignant and benign wounds is critical. Skin biopsy is an important diagnostic test; it allows for histological analysis, which may provide definite information about the character of the lesions. The importance of early biopsy cannot be overstressed, as earlier intervention can significantly improve patient outcome, especially in patients with advanced disease (Fang et al., 2024). Immunohistochemistry is also a crucial element in cutaneous lymphoma diagnosis, through the identification of certain cell types and markers that accompany lymphoma subtypes. In primary cutaneous anaplastic large-cell lymphoma (PC-ALCL), recent experience has shown that unusual cellular morphology complicates diagnosis. For instance, large atypical cells with characteristic features can cause clinicians to initially suspect metastatic carcinoma. Characterization by complex immunohistochemical staining with markers , such as CD30 and CD45 aids in distinguishing from the other cutaneous cancers, including metastatic forms (Lee et al., 2021). Use of an extended panel of immunostains is crucial, which not only facilitates the characterization of lymphoma subtypes but also provides insight into their biologic behavior and potential response to treatment. Diagnostic concerns extend beyond labeling the cutaneous lymphomas to encompass the process of staging, which is vital in formulating treatment regimens. The extent of the disease, particularly if compounded by systemic significance, calls for detailed evaluation of clinical history as well as additional imaging as would be necessitated. Staging helps shed light on whether the lymphoma is still confined to the skin or has progressed to more serious, systemic patterns. In more advanced cases, treatment plans can be transitioned to palliative care focused on symptom control and comfort. The requirement for the integration of clinical, histological, and immunophenotypic data reflects the multifaceted nature of diagnosing cutaneous lymphomas, allowing physicians to develop the optimal treatment strategies for their patients (Fang et al., 2024) (Figure 3.7).

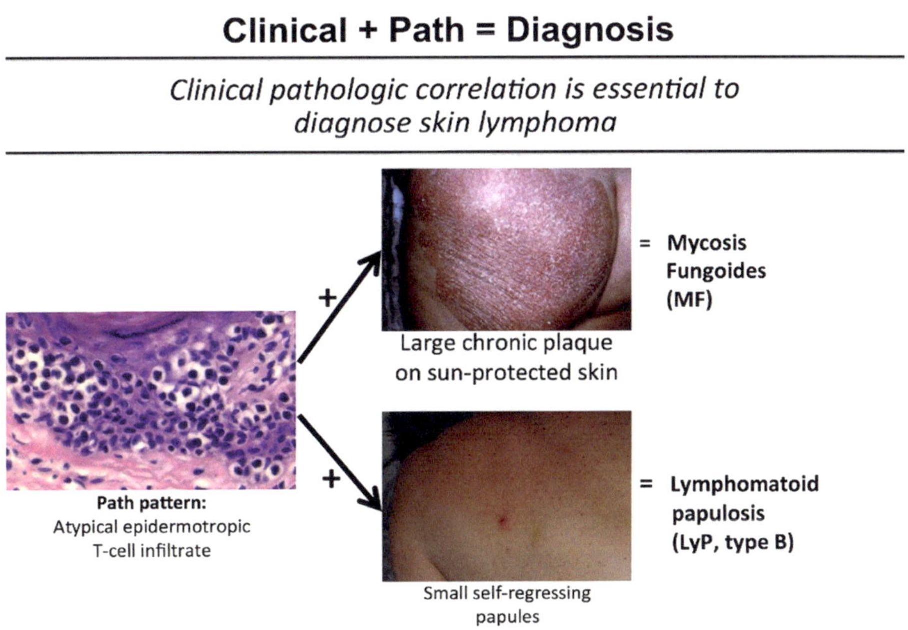

Figure 3.7. The diagnosis of cutaneous lymphomas is inherently complex, often requiring a multifaceted approach to ensure accurate diagnosis and effective treatment.

Source: https://www.surgpath.theclinics.com/cms/10.1016/j.path.2014.02.007/asset/80429f8f-787a-4f0f-9300-edc7b95782d6/main.assets/gr1_lrg.jpg.

3.3.1. Clinical Evaluation and History

Careful clinical evaluation is most critical in the diagnosis of cutaneous lymphomas and metastatic skin disease because these lesions are likely to have nonspecific dermatologic findings. The entire patient history is initially required to disclose potential risk factors, previous malignancies, and any hereditary tendencies towards skin disease. For instance, the patient's medical history examined might be discovered to contain earlier treatments with tyrosine kinase inhibitors (TKIs), which lead to some skin eruptions , such as acquired ichthyosis. This scenario, which is aware of the temporal order of skin changes relative to treatment initiation, is highly informative and guides subsequent diagnostic procedures, such as biopsy and histological evaluation. The timeliness of their identification plays a major role in intervention modalities; hence the importance of careful history-taking in patient management (Munera-Campos et al., 2020).

Physical examination also acts to bridge the clinical evaluation by identifying typical features of cutaneous lymphoma-related skin lesions. For example, the occurrence of multiple erythematous plaques or nodules can suggest subclinical neoplastic activity. In horses with lymphoma, as in clinical experience, lesions may present as progressive subcutaneous nodules that enlarge without other signs of systemic disease. These thus need to be ruled out from more common disease conditions , such as insect hypersensitivity or infection. Since cutaneous lymphoma is rare, dermatological assessments need to be a full-body examination to ascertain the size of lesions, particularly in the areas that drain lymph. Accurately identifying the nature of such lesions through thorough examination is fundamental to formulating an effective treatment plan (Santos et al., 2017).

Histopathological examination of biopsies remains the cornerstone for diagnosing cutaneous lymphomas and metastases. The histological patterns that are observed can provide certain clues as to the nature of the lymphoma and its behavior. For instance, the presence of atypical lymphocytes in a biopsy not only makes the diagnosis but can also point to potential directions of disease progression. Where lesions are disseminated in cutaneous lymphoma in equines, prognosis depends on early detection of metastasis to organs within. Therefore, an integrative approach including clinical history, physical examination findings, and histopathology is crucial in the management of cutaneous lymphomas and in guiding further therapeutic interventions. The interactive dynamic among these factors underscores the value of a multidisciplinary approach to the evaluation and management of skin lymphomas (Santos et al., 2017) (Figure 3.8).

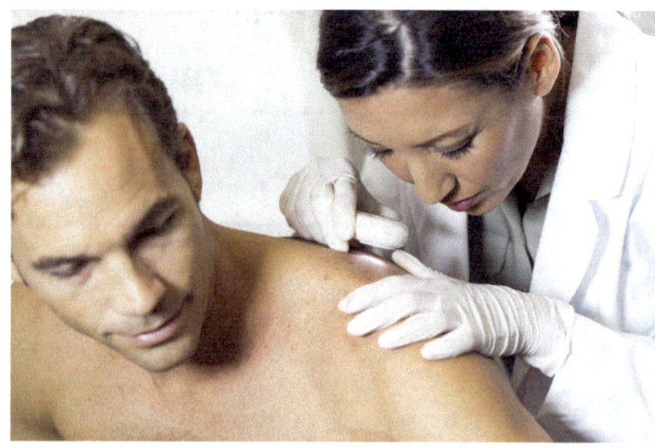

Figure 3.8. Doctor examining a male patient's skin for cutaneous lymphomas.

Source: https://domf5oio6qrcr.cloudfront.net/medialibrary/10036/doctor-examining-male-patients-skin.jpg.

3.3.2. Biopsy and Histopathological Examination

Biopsy and histopathologic examination are very important in the diagnosis of cutaneous lymphomas and metastatic skin diseases. A biopsy is a technique in which a small skin tissue sample is removed and then examined by histopathology. The test is employed to distinguish between a number of skin conditions that present with superimposing symptoms but require various treatment regimens. For instance, as pointed out in recent literature, clinical misdiagnosis may lead to inappropriate therapy, which emphasizes the significance of histopathologic confirmation. Punch biopsy, commonly employed in outpatients, facilitates immediate tissue specimen procurement, ultimately aiding in the correct diagnosis and treatment of various skin diseases and ensuring effective patient management and use of resources. By correlating histological examination with clinical history, the dermatopathologist can have a significant effect on the treatment outcome of patients with cutaneous lymphomas and other skin conditions (Kantibhai et al., 2025). Histopathological examination plays a twofold role in the diagnosis of cutaneous lymphomas: facilitating appropriate classification of the disease and shaping the treatment plan. Primary cutaneous lymphomas are a heterogeneous group of lymphomas requiring meticulous evaluation of skin biopsies by immunohistochemical staining combined with histopathological analysis. Differential diagnosis of primary cutaneous and systemic lymphomas is based on correlating clinical features and histological findings observed in biopsy specimens. The specific histopathological characteristics are not only important in the establishment of the diagnosis but also serve as important prognostic indicators, particularly in the delineation of primary cutaneous B-cell lymphomas (Hristov et al., 2025). This multifaceted perspective illustrates the crucial role of careful histopathological examination in the provision of an integrated picture of the disease and a subsequent therapy. The effects of biopsy and histopathologic examination go beyond diagnosis and also play a heavy role in the treatment of patients with skin cancers. Risk stratification through histopathology is critical, particularly in the differential diagnosis between various forms of primary cutaneous lymphomas, such as B-cell and T-cell lymphomas. Histopathology decides the appropriate management. For example, solitary lesion patients may be subjected to localized methods of treatment, such as radiation therapy, whereas widely cutaneous-involvement patients are going to require systemic therapies. Hence, familiarity with the histopathological characteristics of these conditions not only paves the way for treatment but is also an enabler of individualized, risk-adapted treatments (Hristov et al., 2025). The intense scrutiny inherent in histopathological research defines its key role in enhancing clinical outcomes and advancing the overall body of knowledge regarding cutaneous lymphomas and metastatic skin disorders (Figure 3.9).

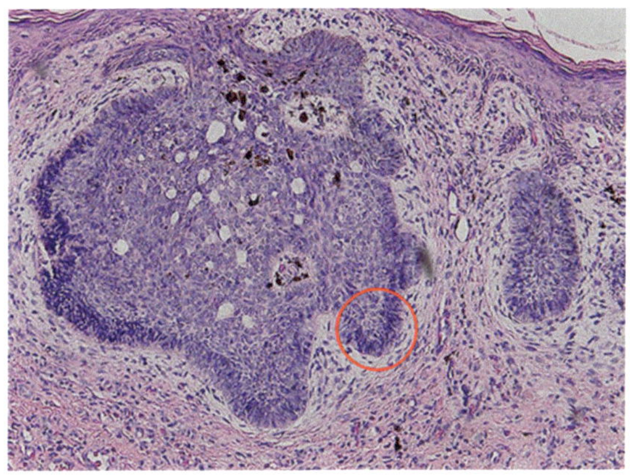

Figure 3.9. Histopathological examination showing that the tumor cells formed a palisading structure (red circle) (Hematoxylin-eosin stain, 100x magnification).

Source: https://www.researchgate.net/publication/372076626/figure/fig3/AS:11431281256484779@1719536216621/Histopathological-examination-showing-that-the-tumor-cells-formed-a-palisading-structure.jpg.

3.3.3. Advanced Imaging Techniques

The employment of advanced imaging modalities has revolutionized the diagnostic profile of cutaneous lymphomas and metastatic skin cancers. Traditional imaging techniques are often not sufficient in providing the desired resolution of detail in the complex vascular and anatomical structure of the skin. MRI, CT, and PET are newer technologies that have proven to be useful tools in detecting more precise localization and characterization of lesions. With their potential for high-resolution imaging, these techniques can demonstrate the extent of skin involvement, invasion into surrounding tissue, and even distant metastasis. These advances make possible ever more refined appreciation of disease progression, so critical in the development of effective regimens of therapy individualized for a patient. The application of imaging techniques in the therapy of cutaneous lymphomas also plays a secondary function of improving decision-making for therapy. For instance, imaging can guide biopsies such that it is possible to sample the most representative areas of a tumor and consequently improve diagnostic accuracy. Additionally, imaging assessment of treatment response allows clinicians to monitor changes in tumor size and metabolic activity that can indicate the success of a given administered therapy. Such information is important, particularly with treatments becoming more innovative and new immunotherapies being at the forefront. As the NCCN Guidelines highlight, soft tissue sarcomas are treated by a multidisciplinary program with an emphasis on the imaging component in evaluating the response to therapy and adjusting management plans appropriately when necessary (Margaret et al., 2022).

In addition to conventional modalities, emerging imaging devices , such as high-frequency ultrasound and optical coherence tomography (OCT) are also beginning to play a central role in the evaluation of cutaneous lymphomas. These emerging techniques offer real-time, high-resolution images of skin tumors, with the option of careful examination of epidermal and dermal layers. Moreover, since they are non-invasive, the pain and risk of complications of conventional biopsy procedures are reduced. Further, integration of molecular imaging techniques is on the horizon, with the potential for visualization of tumor-specific biomarkers that can lead to more efficient and targeted therapies. With greater research in this area, the role of advanced imaging in maximizing therapeutic response and outcomes in cutaneous lymphomas and metastatic skin cancers is underscored (Anand et al., 2022) (Figure 3.10).

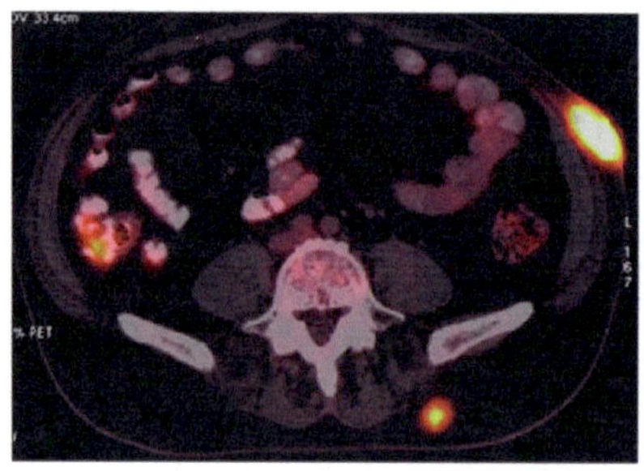

Figure 3.10. T cell cutaneous lymphoma showing intense FDG uptake in a skin lesion and subcutaneous nodules in a 62-year-old man.

Source: https://www.researchgate.net/profile/Raghava-Kashyap/publication/51832615/figure/fig15/AS:670543451799559@1536881425633/T-cell-cutaneous-lymphoma-showing-intense-FDG-uptake-in-a-skin-lesion-and-subcutaneous.png.

Test Your Knowledge

1. What aspects of clinical history are important when evaluating a patient for possible cutaneous lymphoma?
2. Why is a skin biopsy essential in diagnosing cutaneous lymphomas?
3. What imaging studies are used to assess the extent of disease in suspected cutaneous lymphoma cases?

3.4. Treatment Options for Cutaneous Lymphomas

Learning Outcome

1. Describe topical therapies in the management of cutaneous lymphomas and metastatic skin diseases.
2. Understand systemic treatments for cutaneous lymphomas and metastatic skin diseases.
3. Focus on radiation therapy in the management of cutaneous lymphomas and metastatic skin diseases.

The treatment landscape for cutaneous lymphomas, particularly cutaneous T-cell lymphoma (CTCL), has been highly dynamic in recent years, reflecting the complexity of the disease and the advent of diverse therapeutic modalities. The diverse symptoms depicted by the patients have led to a multidisciplinary approach. Topical therapies, such as corticosteroids and retinoids, are commonly used in initial treatment strategies, particularly for localized lesions. However, for more advanced phases or more severe forms like mycosis fungoides, systemic therapy becomes necessary. These can include phototherapy, employing ultraviolet light to treat skin conditions extensively, and systemic agents specifically directed against the underlying malignancy. With the limitations of conventional methods, research has gone on to seek new immunotherapies and applications of biomarkers that might allow more customized medical strategies, holding the future of treatment in a positive context of hope for enhancement. There is increasing evidence for the role of biomarkers in the optimization of treatment in cutaneous lymphomas, particularly in therapy response and prognosis. One interesting biomarker is the neutrophil-to-lymphocyte ratio (NLR), which has been found to be a potential predictor of response to treatment in various cancers, including skin non-melanoma cancers. Current systematic reviews suggest that, despite the remaining uncertainty on the prognostic significance of NLR in cutaneous lymphomas, that is, CTCL, its usefulness is gaining attention (Seretis et al., 2024). Such knowledge regarding the implications of such biomarkers may encourage clinicians to tailor treatment choices more appropriately according to the patient's personal profile. This personalized approach is pivotal to managing the nuances of cutaneous lymphomas, leading to more effective and targeted treatments. Directed treatments have been noted as an emerging promise for treating cutaneous lymphomas, with JAK inhibitors as a landmark development. Research has established that cancerous T cells in CTCL release an abundance of cytokines that damage skin barrier integrity and enhance disease progression (Gluud et al., 2022). Notably, clinically proven JAK inhibitor, Tofacitinib, has been effective in amplifying the expression of critical skin proteins, thereby reinforcing the integrity of the skin barrier. This mechanism addresses not only the expressions of disease but also the pathophysiologic mechanisms underlying them. Working on these agents highlights the importance of an opposing philosophy of both symptom management and disease-modifying therapy in planning overall care regimens for cutaneous lymphoma patients with advanced disease. Further studies will increasingly entail the incorporation of such new therapies, reorienting the standard of care for these patients.

3.4.1. Topical Therapies

Topical treatments have emerged as a key component in the management of cutaneous lymphomas and metastatic skin malignancies, providing localized treatment modalities with diminished systemic side effects. Topical treatments consist of a variety of agents, such as corticosteroids, chemotherapy creams, and biologics, each of which is formulated to treat specific cutaneous malignancy presentations and subtypes. The primary goal of treatment with topical therapy is control of the local disease, symptom alleviation, and improvement of quality of life in patients. Because of the heterogeneity and complexity of cutaneous lymphomas, treatment needs to be individualized to yield maximal effect. For example, topical corticosteroids reduce inflammation and induce temporary remission in inflammatory dermatoses and are also used as adjuvants when combined with systemic medications. While topical medications play a vital role in the treatment of conditions, such as cutaneous B-cell lymphomas, they are not similarly effective in all malignancies. The variable response of cutaneous lymphomas to local therapy necessitates diligent patient evaluation to determine the most appropriate regimen. For example, topical chemotherapy using drugs like imiquimod or 5-fluorouracil can be used to effectively manage localized disease and can be particularly useful in non-melanoma skin cancers.

The drug must be used carefully, since such agents may induce local irritation or other side effects. Most importantly, advances in the molecular analysis of skin cancers have created new possibilities for combining topical treatment with systemic therapy and demonstrating that improved treatment regimens based on genetic tumor profiles are possible. Topical treatment of cutaneous lymphomas and metastatic skin cancer is also supported by ongoing research with new formulations and delivery systems. Topical biologics, for example, are being explored for their ability to harness immune response effectively against cancer cells without excessive systemic exposure. These new treatments would give a more specific, more effective treatment for metastatic skin patients, particularly those not eligible for surgery. Moreover, studies indicate that the combination of topical and systemic therapy could be synergistic and lead to improved outcomes in advanced skin cancers. With the ongoing evolution of science, the evolution of multimodal therapeutic regimes with the incorporation of topical therapy is a rich research area for optimizing the treatment of cutaneous lymphomas and metastatic skin malignancies (Figure 3.11).

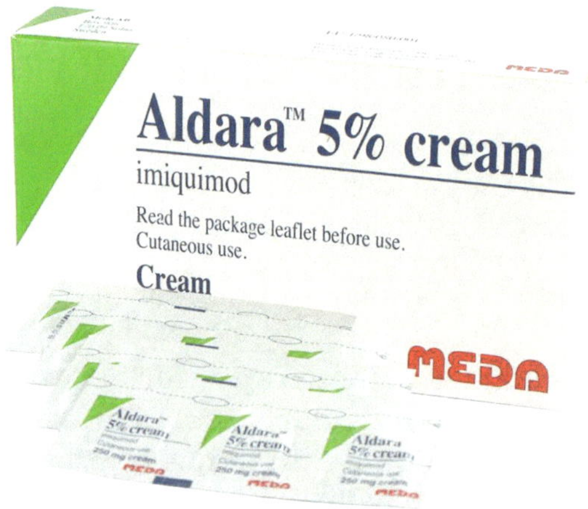

Figure 3.11. Imiquimod cream.

Source: https://www.rebeccaayers.co.nz/images/dmImage/StandardImage/aldara.jpg.

3.4.2. Systemic Treatments

Systemic therapy for cutaneous lymphomas and metastatic skin diseases has evolved significantly, reflecting the complexity and heterogeneity of such conditions. Systemic agents are intended to target disseminated malignant cells beyond the skin, offering more universal treatment than localized approaches. Systemic agents include chemotherapeutic agents, immunotherapy, and targeted therapies, each with unique mechanisms of action. For example, chemotherapy can have a broad cytotoxic effect, such as in aggressive cutaneous lymphomas. However, the challenge in most instances is to achieve a therapeutic balance that balances efficacy with minimal side effects; as such, patient selection is essential. The integration of systemic treatments into an international management strategy has revolutionized care, enabling the personalization of interventions to individual patient characteristics and disease presentations, thereby improving patient outcomes and quality of life. Immunotherapy, a significant advancement in the therapeutic process, harnesses the body's own immune system to actively combat malignant cells. Medications , such as immune checkpoint inhibitors have gained attention for their ability to revive T-cell activity against the tumor. In cutaneous lymphomas, treatments directed at the programmed death cell protein 1 (PD-1) pathway have been encouraging, particularly in refractory disease. These medications have the capability to generate durable responses, including in those who are resistant to conventional therapy. Moreover, the safety profile of these immunotherapeutic agents is typically good, allowing for maintenance therapy. However, monitoring for immune-related adverse effects is essential because they complicate treatment. With ongoing research on combination strategies, the potential for improved efficacy and tolerability marks a new era for the systemic treatment of these disabling cancers. The evolving landscape of targeted therapies has also significantly contributed to the systemic treatment paradigm for cutaneous lymphomas and skin metastases. Targeted therapies target distinct molecular pathways that govern the growth and survival of cancer cells and are more specific, causing less damage to surrounding normal tissues. For instance, small-molecule inhibitors that disrupt activities , such as Hedgehog and other processes have emerged as effective therapies for certain skin cancers. This reflects an improved understanding of the pathogenic pathways underlying diseases, as evidenced by recent studies of the genomic profiles of cutaneous cancers. However, challenges remain, including the emergence of drug resistance and patient outcome heterogeneity. While scientists seek new targets and treatment combinations, the aim is not only to enhance efficacy but also to improve quality of life in such difficult-to-treat patients (Sol et al., 2024; Cedirian et al., 2025) (Figure 3.12).

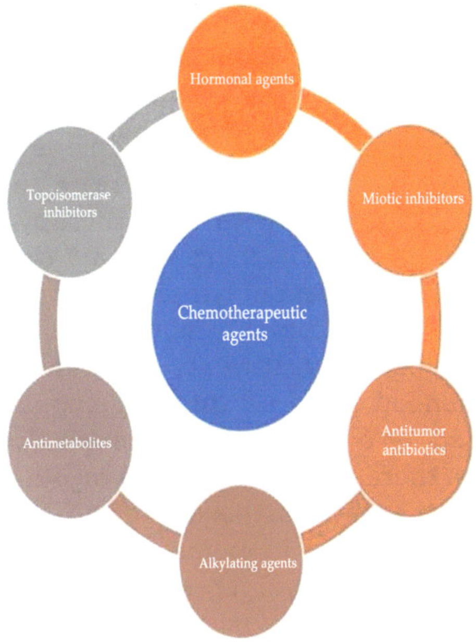

Figure 3.12. Types of chemotherapeutic agents.

Source: https://scienceinfo.com/wp-content/uploads/2023/09/Chemotherapeutic-agents.jpg.

3.4.3. Radiation Therapy

Radiation therapy remains a cornerstone of therapy for cutaneous lymphoma as well as metastatic skin disease. The procedure involves the use of high-energy radiation to interfere with the cancer cells' DNA so that they cannot divide and live. In PCALCL, in particular, local radiation is usually utilized because the disease tends to remain localized to the skin. The concentrated quality of radiation therapy decreases exposure to nearby healthy tissue, which can be crucial in saving patients from the unwanted side effects of unnecessary radiation. Radiation therapy is also particularly well suited for lesions localized because they would pose a greater risk had they been approached surgically or when the overall health of the patient would not allow more aggressive therapy. The effectiveness of radiation therapy in this context not only underscores its importance but also its ability to complement good patient outcomes. In the therapeutic setting, radiation therapy is usually combined with other therapy modalities, which complement the overall efficacy against cutaneous lymphomas. For example, systemic therapies , such as chemotherapy may be administered along with radiotherapy given for local disease if there is any potential systemic involvement of lymphoma not evident on imaging. A combined modality is a more comprehensive treatment regimen and is recommended based on studies demonstrating improved progression-free survival when radiation therapy is administered together with systemic therapy. Furthermore, the palliative role of radiotherapy in metastatic skin diseases cannot be overstated, as it provides prompt relief from symptoms such as pain and ulceration, which can significantly affect a patient's quality of life. The synergy between radiotherapy and systemic therapy mirrors a multidisciplinary treatment regimen of utmost importance in managing these advanced diseases. As cutaneous lymphoma biology continues to evolve, so does radiotherapy. New evidence points to an increasing recognition of the potential for extracutaneous dissemination, as seen in the few cases of PCALCL with gastric metastasis (Khrais et al., 2022). Such findings raise questions about traditional beliefs regarding the virulence of these cancers. In addition, with increased rates of nonmelanoma skin cancers in immunocompromised populations, particularly those with HIV, it is evident that patient-specific radiation protocols and dosimetry are needed to manage the toxicities of treatment (Garlassi et al., 2012). This shift in mentality must be met through an interdisciplinary effort by oncologists, dermatologists, and radiation therapists to individualize therapies based on each individual's history and presentation. Lastly, as new evidence emerges, radiation therapy will continue to be an integral part of optimizing patient treatment in the context of cutaneous lymphomas and metastatic skin cancers (Figure 3.13).

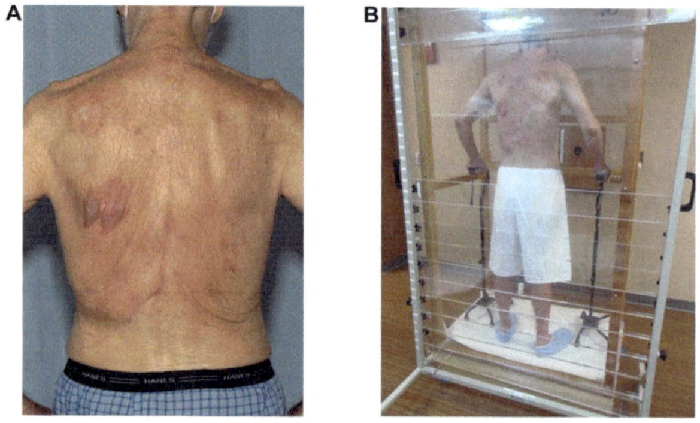

Figure 3.13. A patient with cutaneous T cell lymphoma involving the thorax who received subtotal skin electron beam therapy (STSEBT).

Source: https://ar.iiarjournals.org/content/anticanres/44/4/1491/F1.large.jpg?width=800&height=600&carousel=1.

Test Your Knowledge

1. What topical therapies are commonly used to treat early-stage cutaneous T-cell lymphoma (CTCL)?
2. Which systemic treatments are used for advanced or refractory cutaneous lymphomas?

3.5. Metastatic Skin Diseases: Overview

Learning Outcome

1. Explain the definition and types of metastatic skin diseases.
2. Describe common primary cancers that metastasize to the skin.
3. Focus on the epidemiology of cutaneous lymphomas.

Metastatic skin disease is a variety of disorders in which malignant cells metastasize to the skin from other primary sites and account for a great deal of morbidity in affected individuals. These manifestations can be secondary to a wide variety of cancers, most importantly breast, lung, and melanoma, these being notorious for their cutaneous metastasizing potential. Metastatic skin lesions clinically usually present as plaques, nodules, or ulcerations that can have a similar appearance to benign dermatoses and can be deceptively diagnosed. Due to their superficial location, the lesions may result in heterogeneous histopathological reactions and make diagnosis challenging, requiring comprehensively executed pathological evaluations to differentiate them from primary cutaneous neoplasia. Accurate identification and effective treatment of metastatic cutaneous diseases are necessary since they tend to reflect the overall health status of the underlying malignancy and indicate a deteriorating prognosis of the disease. Their interdependence with metastatic skin cancers is also noteworthy, which shows the complexity of skin involvement with systemic malignancies. Cutaneous lymphomas, especially those that are lymphoproliferative disorders, can follow behavior patterns similar to metastasis. For instance, Sézary syndrome, a severe cutaneous T-cell lymphoma, is characterized by an inflammatory disease in which cytokines IL-1β and IL-18 are important in the pathology, indicating the role of the immune environment in affecting the skin (Manfrere et al., 2023). Moreover, the systemic presentation of MALT lymphoma, characterized by granulomatous skin infiltrates, underscores how lymphomatous phenomena may mimic the behavior of metastatic disease (Scarfì et al., 2019). Knowledge of such parallels is important for clinicians to formulate appropriate diagnostic and therapeutic maneuvers for patients with skin presentations. A systemic approach to metastatic skin disease is critical, particularly as the treatment modalities become increasingly advanced to target underlying malignancies more directly. As needed, multimodal treatments are applied from systemic therapy to localized dermatological interventions based on the nature and distribution of the primary neoplasm with accompanying skin signs. For instance, therapies like R-CHOP have been effective in the management of lymphoma skin presentation, stressing a well-informed assessment of cutaneous and systemic disease (Scarfì et al., 2019). Additionally, future immunotherapies and targeted therapies may be promising for the management of complicated cases of metastatic skin disease, enhancing the quality of life and survival of patients. Thus, an interdisciplinary system involving dermatological, oncologic, and immunologic knowledge continues to be necessary in order to optimize outcomes in affected individuals.

3.5.1. Definition and Categories of Metastatic Skin Disorders

Metastatic cutaneous diseases are a severe category of skin diseases in which malignant cells infiltrate the skin from primary malignancies outside the body. This process is mainly seen in breast, lung, and melanoma cancers, so the clinician must identify and diagnose such malignancies at an early stage. The skin most frequently presents as a distant organ where metastatic cells reside with varied morphology mimicking benign cutaneous lesions. The appearance could be nodules, plaques, or ulcerations, and as such, the assessment should be done carefully and methodically. It is important to distinguish metastatic from primary skin neoplasms, as this distinction not only facilitates accurate diagnosis but also informs treatment strategies that can differ dramatically depending on the behavior and location of origin of the primary malignancy. Some metastatic skin diseases can be classified based on their original sites. Breast cancer cutaneous metastases may have unique characteristics, such as firm, subcutaneous nodules called cutaneous carcinomas. Similarly, melanoma metastases are pigmented lesions, but there can also be non-pigmented lesions. Heterogeneity supports well-integrated clinical and, in some cases, histological evaluation to identify the cancer type involved. Skin lesions in metastasis of squamous cell carcinoma may be indurated and keratinizing and can be challenging to treat, as some of them can be aggressive in nature and require surgery. As modalities of treatment have become sophisticated, identification of the primary source of the skin metastasis remains a bedrock of patient care. Management of metastatic cutaneous disorders is optimally managed with a multidisciplinary approach, particularly in keeping with available treatment options for the primary malignancy. Resection remains a common practice, although systemic therapy like immunotherapy is increasingly employed, particularly for tumors like melanoma, for which immune checkpoint inhibitors have been found to be incredibly beneficial. The role of thorough histopathological evaluation cannot be overstated, as it informs risk stratification and guides appropriate lines of management. For metastatic cutaneous squamous cell carcinoma, guidelines allow for an integrated approach through clinical oncologists, dermatologists, and surgical teams to devise customized care. This collective effort is essential for addressing the unique challenges of metastatic skin cancers, underscoring the need for ongoing research to further optimize treatment protocols and improve patient outcomes (Keohane et al., 2020) (Figure 3.14).

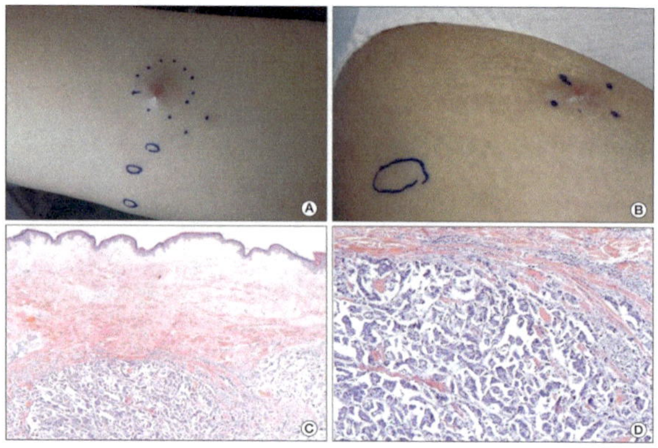

Figure 3.14. Skin lesions due to metastatic adenocarcinoma of the ovary in the right thigh (A) and right inguinal area (B) with multiple lymphatic spaces in the dermis infiltrated by metastatic adenocarcinoma.

Source: https://www.researchgate.net/publication/229157470/figure/fig1/AS:216382600945678@1428601040897/Skin-lesions-due-to-metastatic-adenocarcinoma-of-the-ovary-in-the-right-thigh-A-and.png.

3.5.2. Common Primary Cancers That Metastasize to the Skin

Skin is a common location for metastasis of primary cancer, particularly those of internal organ origin. Carcinoma metastases, including breast and lung carcinoma, are most commonly noted in the skin due to the large vascular supply and lymphatic drainage pathways of the skin. The metastatic lesion may present with mixed morphology, including nodules, plaques, or ulcerations, and is therefore more challenging to diagnose and treat. Breast cancer, for example, is known for cutaneous metastasis, and this can happen years later after the initial diagnosis. Early detection typically results in good control, but the late presentation of skin metastases may indicate advanced disease, in which treatment becomes increasingly less feasible and more complex. Hence, it is important to comprehend the kinetics of such metastatic processes in the treatment of cutaneous metastatic disorders, and close monitoring in high-risk groups is stressed. Melanoma is another significant source of skin metastases. Melanoma is an extremely aggressive cutaneous cancer that can also arise from pre-existing melanoma lesions. Unlike nonmelanoma skin cancers, which do not spread and are curable, melanoma has a propensity to metastasize to various cutaneous sites as new pigmented lesions or inflammatory nodules. This aggressive nature makes it a must that such patients are followed carefully after treatment because early lesions in the skin may precede systemic disease. Treatment now employs immunotherapy and targeted therapy with a favorable impact on advanced melanoma. However, the formation of resistant lesions remains a major challenge. Therefore, it is necessary to understand the biological mechanism of melanoma and its metastatic capacity to improve prognostic outcomes in patients suffering from it and guide future treatment.

Apart from melanoma and breast carcinoma, other tumors like lung cancer and colorectal cancer are most frequently implicated in skin metastasis. Lung cancer, and small cell lung carcinoma in particular, may lead to cutaneous manifestations, typically indicative of an advanced state of the disease. Skin lesions may result from both direct extension from structures within and hematogenous metastasis. Similarly, colorectal cancer, particularly the advanced varieties, has a propensity for skin metastasis as well as systemic dissemination. Metastatic skin lesions from such sites typically indicate a poor prognosis and require aggressive therapeutic interventions. New developments in immunotherapy may provide additional therapeutic options in such cases. As additional research emerges that unravels the complexity of skin-metastasizing cancers, clinicians can better tailor treatment regimens and make informed palliative care decisions based on an emerging understanding of such cancers as theorized in (Melgaard et al., 2025) and the compelling observations of cutaneous T-cell lymphomas in (Wang et al., 2024) (Figure 3.15).

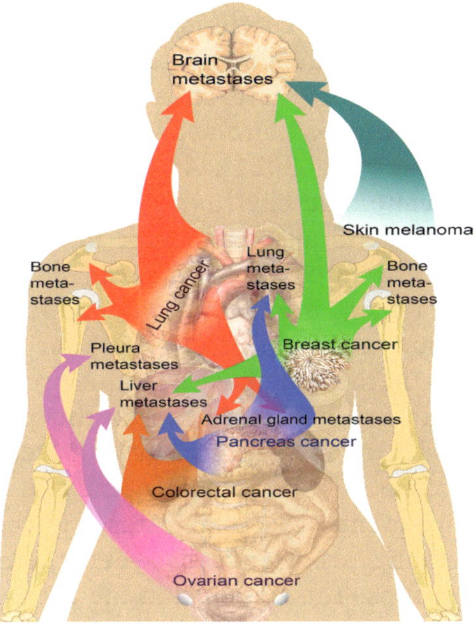

Figure 3.15. Metastasis sites for common cancers.

Source: https://upload.wikimedia.org/wikipedia/commons/7/7e/Metastasis_sites_for_common_cancers.svg.

3.5.3. Epidemiology and Prevalence

The epidemiology of cutaneous lymphoma reveals significant trends in incidence and prevalence that warrant close attention. Cutaneous lymphomas, a heterogeneous group of malignancies with a primary origin in lymphoid tissue within the skin, exhibit bimodal incidence across populations and age groups. Mycosis fungoides, the most common subtype, is discovered to have an elevated prevalence among elderly patients, more significantly among men than women. The longitudinal analysis of trends, it reveals that the incidence of non-Hodgkin lymphoma, including cutaneous forms, continues to exhibit an increasing trend. The cause of the rise has to do with the enhanced diagnostic methods coupled with possibly a growing prevalence of underlying risk factors, such as immunosuppression and certain infections. These patterns highlight the importance of continuous monitoring and study of the epidemiology of these diseases, particularly with reference to changes in population composition and availability of health care (Islami et al., 2021). An understanding of the epidemiologic environment of metastatic skin diseases is also important in mitigating their health impacts. Metastatic cutaneous lesions, which are secondary deposits of malignancy in the skin from a primary tumor elsewhere in the body, have a unique prevalence based on the characteristics of the primary cancer, such as incidence rates and treatment modalities. For instance, melanoma and breast cancer frequently cause metastases in the skin with varying prevalence between racial and ethnic groups. The rise in skin metastases can follow the hike in survival rates among patients with advanced cancers, who then can develop cutaneous manifestations. Epidemiological surveillance is crucial in such cases, as it enables timely interventions, appropriate treatment regimens, and improved patient outcomes. Furthermore, these results provide beneficial information that can be used to shape public health policy and clinical practice for skin cancer screening and treatment (Robb et al., 2020). The interconnection between epidemiology, prevalence, and survivorship forms the core of building our body of knowledge concerning cutaneous lymphomas and metastatic skin disease. Analysis of demographic data indicates disparities in incidence and outcomes across geographic, socioeconomic, and racial groups. For example, certain groups may be at higher risk for developing specific types of cutaneous lymphoma depending on environmental exposure or genetic predisposition. Moreover, with advancements in treatment paradigms, survival rates for some groups are improving, indicating the pressing need for equal access to healthcare across various groups. This dynamic epidemiological setting demands an integrated approach, bridging research evidence to practice in clinical oncology and public health. Ultimately, a close examination of the epidemiological data on these illnesses can significantly enhance prevention, early detection, and effective treatment protocols for various groups (Islami et al., 2021).

Test Your Knowledge

1. What is the definition of metastatic skin disease?
2. What are the most common primary cancers that metastasize to the skin?
3. How do cutaneous metastases typically present clinically?

3.6. Diagnosis and Management of Metastatic Skin Diseases

Learning Outcome

1. Understand diagnostic imaging and biopsy techniques.
2. Describe treatment strategies for metastatic skin lesions.
3. Focus on the integration of palliative care into the treatment plan for patients with cutaneous lymphomas and metastatic skin diseases.

Diagnosis of metastatic skin disorders requires careful consideration of imaging, history, and clinical presentation. Metastatic cutaneous disease presentations in the skin can be an infiltrate, plaque, or nodule, and commonly complicate the diagnosis. Diagnosis is typically made by a biopsy that provides histological findings necessary to distinguish primary cutaneous lesions from metastatic cutaneous disorders, such as lymphomas. Furthermore, imaging tests, including ultrasound and magnetic resonance imaging, are crucial for defining the extent of the disease and planning therapeutic interventions. The American Cancer Society projections of cancer incidence and mortality emphasize the increasing sophistication in oncologic diagnoses, where early diagnosis is the most critical aspect. With increasing incidence rates of melanoma, breast, and colorectal cancers, attention to multidisciplinary diagnostic interventions is essential to have timely and specific detection of metastatic skin disease (Rebecca et al., 2024).

Treatment consists of multiple therapeutic interventions, typically guided by tumor status, location, and extent of metastasis. Localized treatments, such as surgery and radiation therapy, may be employed for superficial or localized metastases. For patients with systemic disease, systemic modalities, including chemotherapy, targeted therapy, and immunotherapy, are used. The NCCN guidelines provide a general framework for treatment plans by type of soft tissue sarcoma and cutaneous lymphoma, highlighting the importance of personalization in clinical choice (Margaret et al., 2022). Immunotherapies have introduced a new dimension to management options, with the potential to improve outcomes in patients for whom traditional chemotherapeutic regimens are no longer available. Informed, participative discussion between patients and clinicians is required to identify optimal modalities in the context of patient quality of life. Progress in molecular oncology is transforming the diagnostic and management paradigm for metastatic cutaneous malignancy, enabling targeted therapies that improve patient outcomes. Implementation of genomic profiling in clinical practice enables tailored therapeutic plans targeting the individual mutations that drive tumor growth. This model of precision medicine has been particularly successful in metastatic melanoma, where BRAF- and MEK-targeting treatments have produced substantial improvements in survival. Challenges remain, however, particularly around the lack of access to advanced treatments. The American Cancer Society's reports demonstrate ongoing disparities in cancer mortality across different population groups, reinforcing the need for policies of equal access to new treatments. Further research and investment are needed to expand therapeutic options and improve availability, thereby addressing the evolving metastatic skin disease management landscape (Rebecca et al., 2024).

3.6.1. Diagnostic Imaging and Biopsy Approaches

The accurate diagnosis of cutaneous lymphomas and metastatic skin cancers hinges to a significant extent upon the use of effective diagnostic imaging and biopsy techniques. Imaging modalities , such as magnetic resonance imaging (MRI), computed tomography (CT), and positron emission tomography (PET) play crucial roles in determining the extent of disease and whether lymphatics are involved. These imaging modalities enhance the clinician's capacity to differentiate between primary and secondary lymphoproliferative disorders, which is of great significance given the varying prognostic implications placed upon their presentation. For instance, disseminated lesions are often indicative of a more aggressive disease course for which urgent treatment is necessary. Additionally, imaging enables visualization of deep tissue engagement, which aids in planning biopsies under surgical cover, which are critical for accurate diagnosis (Zanardi, 2025). In the context of histopathological diagnosis, the choice of biopsy technique greatly affects the level of accuracy. Excisional, incisional, and punch biopsies are commonly employed techniques with specific indications based on presentation. Excisional biopsies are particularly favored when the lesion is focal and help in the acquisition of a satisfactory tissue sample, allowing for sound histopathological examination. Punch biopsies, however, offer another option that is not so invasive and yet well-suited to small lesions without being insufficient to establish the underlying pathology. The findings on histopathology from these biopsies, such as the identification of specific markers like CD30 in Anaplastic Large Cell Lymphoma, are crucial to differentiate between various cutaneous neoplasms (Fang et al., 2024). Systematically derived biopsy specimens directly inform treatment protocols and improve overall patient outcomes. Moreover, adjunctive molecular techniques have become a standard component of the diagnostic strategy for cutaneous lymphomas and metastatic skin disease. These techniques include fluorescence *in situ* hybridization (FISH) and polymerase chain reaction (PCR), which are valuable for ascertaining genetic alterations and clonal proliferation in lymphoma. Such molecular data facilitates the discrimination of indolent and aggressive lymphoma subtypes, impacting therapy. For instance, the identification of specific genetic markers determines the eligibility of patients for targeted therapy, altering the management approach from the use of traditional chemotherapy to more personalized regimens. By combining molecular diagnostics with imaging and histopathology, clinicians can achieve an all-around picture of the disease, enhancing diagnostic accuracy and therapeutic efficacy (Fang et al., 2024; Zanardi, 2025) (Figure 3.16).

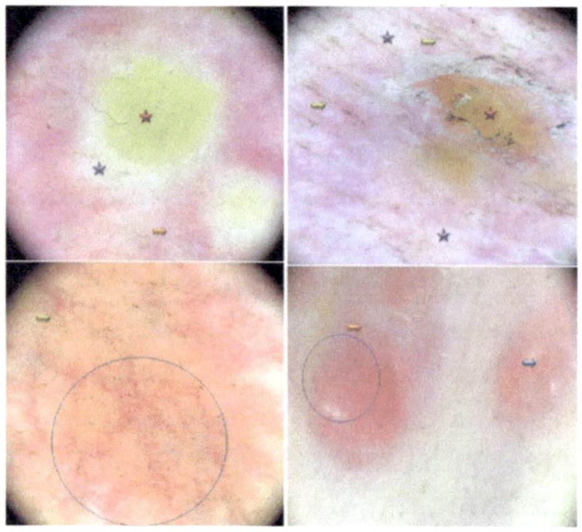

Figure 3.16. Dermoscopic image of the skin metastases.

Source: https://www.researchgate.net/publication/327823425/figure/fig4/AS:675645369634816@1538097817072/Case-2-Dermoscopic-image-of-the-skin-metastases-Linear-irregular-arborizing-and.png.

3.6.2. Treatment Strategies for Metastatic Skin Lesions

Treatment of metastatic cutaneous lesions is problematic in the clinical setting, largely due to the variability of cutaneous malignancies and variable sensitivity to therapy. Current treatment is multimodal, comprising local therapy, systemic therapy, and novel targeted therapies.

Local therapies, such as surgical excision and radiation, remain the cornerstones for isolated lesions. Local therapies are inadequate, however, for diffuse disease. Systemic therapy has grown more sophisticated, with immunotherapy playing a more significant role as it has the potential to harness the body's own immune system against cancer cells. In particular, immune checkpoint inhibitors have been remarkably effective in metastatic melanoma. Even with such progress, knowledge of prognostic factors, such as the neutrophil-to-lymphocyte ratio (NLR), is critical, as it can inform treatment decisions and patient monitoring, thereby optimizing therapeutic outcomes, particularly for advanced non-melanoma skin cancers (Seretis et al., 2024).

Emerging targeted therapies, particularly those employing novel strategies such as targeted protein degradation (TPD), are transforming treatment paradigms for metastatic skin lesions. TPD is a novel mechanism that redirects cellular processes to eliminate disease-causing proteins, holding new promise for conventionally undruggable oncogenic targets in patients. For example, in the treatment of cutaneous T-cell lymphoma, agents like KT-333 exploit this process by degrading transcription factors like STAT3, a key mediator of tumor growth and survival. Clinical trials have shown early evidence of antitumor activity with low toxicity, thereby realizing the promise of TPD in redefining treatment paradigms and improving therapeutic ratios (Mainolfi, 2024). Targeted therapies not only optimize efficacy but also minimize the side effects typically seen with conventional chemotherapies, with added specificity in treating metastatic lesions. The intersection of novel biomarkers and therapies is of utmost significance in individualizing therapy in metastatic skin lesions. As research continues to uncover the molecular mechanisms of cutaneous lymphomas and metastatic skin diseases, biomarkers NLR are increasingly coming to the forefront for stratifying patients and guiding subsequent individualized interventions. Identification of high-risk patients might lead to more aggressive therapies or new trial opportunities, and perhaps spare those with a more favorable prognosis from more severe interventions. In addition, combination regimens that combine immunotherapy with TPD may exhibit synergistic activity, further enhancing therapeutic efficacy. The way is long to complete and efficient control of metastatic skin disease, and it needs constant refinement of approach and firm dedication to research in this dynamic field.

3.6.3. Palliative Care Considerations

The integration of palliative care into the treatment of patients with cutaneous lymphomas and metastatic skin cancers significantly enhances quality of life. Palliative care is focused on alleviating suffering and psychological care, particularly for the gravely ill patient. Given that the conditions typically present themselves through disabling skin manifestations , such as pruritus, pain, and cosmetic disability, palliative overall management is essential. Through the application of therapeutic modalities like topical and systemic therapy, pain can be significantly reduced. Generally, symptom relief through the application of agents such as imiquimod can ease symptoms while simultaneously addressing psychological burdens imposed by disfiguring lesions, thereby contributing to patient satisfaction and higher compliance with treatment regimens (Flindris et al., 2025). Also, early detection of palliative care needs can lead to more effective interventions. This is particularly relevant with skin metastases, which might be a symptom of advanced disease and cause distress. The use of a multidisciplinary model of collaboration among oncologists, dermatologists, and palliative care specialists increases the likelihood that patients discuss their care goals and treatment preferences early in their disease trajectory. The tacit management of symptoms, together with truthful communication, can support the coping strategies of the patient in the face of severe illness. The identification of the psychological significance inherent in the diagnosis of cutaneous lymphomas or metastases gives an opening to supportive care strategies tailored according to the individual patient's needs, ultimately enhancing the entire care experience (Alhashimalsayed et al., 2025). Lastly, caregiver support and family dynamics cannot be adequately overstressed in the case of cutaneous condition patients in palliative care. Involving the family in the care process enhances the facilitation of a caring environment and shared decision-making that is critical to improving patient well-being. It is important to comprehend the emotional and physical load that can influence patients and their caregivers; thus, incorporating educational materials and psychosocial services into the care plan can improve outcomes. These factors, being considered, not only improve the quality of life of the patients but also improve the strength of the caregivers, enabling them to cope with changing needs with emerging cutaneous diseases. By giving precedence to this entire-patient viewpoint, palliative care itself then becomes an indispensable aspect of treating cutaneous lymphomas and metastatic skin diseases, raising both care and compassion in the treatment agenda.

Test Your Knowledge

1. What diagnostic technique is essential for confirming metastatic skin disease?
2. Which imaging modalities are commonly used to assess the extent of disease in patients with cutaneous metastases?
3. When is radiation therapy indicated in the management of metastatic skin lesions?

SUMMARY

The research on cutaneous lymphomas and metastatic skin diseases points to the complexity and the need for better treatment methods. Clinical trials, particularly those investigating novel therapies , such as oncolytic virotherapy using Talimogene laherparepvec (T-VEC), have yielded promising results. Cutaneous lymphomas and non-melanoma skin cancers are often refractory to standard treatments, which provides the rationale for introducing new modalities. With T-VEC causing clinical reactions in a great number of injected tumors, this is proof of the capacity to improve patient results by way of augmented immune stimulation (Ramelyte et al., 2023). This calls for a paradigm shift in interest in the creation of integrating immunotherapy into standard treatment protocols for such neoplasms, hence reiterating the demand for increased research in the area. Furthermore, insights into the molecular mechanisms of metastatic skin cutaneous melanoma (SKCM) can also be used to inform strategies for improving treatment strategies. The discovery of CEBPB as a key biomarker linked to an active immune environment provides a unique window of opportunity to delineate more accurate prognostic assessment and respond accordingly with treatments. As SKCMs outcome is influenced by parameters , such as lymphocytic infiltration and inflammatory pathways, a focus on these molecular predictors can be a game-changer in the stratification of patients in the clinical setting (Yang et al., 2022). With accurate selection of patients having a high risk of aggressive disease onset, health care providers can implement personalized treatment regimens that are in line with the specific biological behavior of the involved tumors, thus optimizing therapeutic efficacy. In short, the areas of overlap between cutaneous lymphomas and metastatic cutaneous diseases demand a coordinated approach with new treatment modalities as well as improved knowledge of the underlying biological drivers. The promising results emanating from studies into the application of T-VEC and such critical biomarkers as CEBPB attest to the worth of continued investment in research and clinical trials. As our understanding of immune responses and tumor microenvironments continues to evolve, it will lead to increasingly more effective and targeted therapies, ultimately resulting in enhanced survival and better quality of life for such difficult skin malignancies. Treatment in the future of this disease will not only rely on new drugs but also on an overall understanding of the relationship between immunology and oncology.

The cutaneous lymphoma group encompasses several skin cancers that are primarily characterized by the fact that they develop from lymphocyte cells. Among them, cutaneous T-cell lymphoma (CTCL) is a critical but rare group, where the T-cell malignant proliferation leads to skin manifestations and systemic illnesses. An essential aspect of CTCL pathology is the activity of the JAK/STAT signal pathway, which plays an important role in the proliferation and survival of cells. When this pathway is abnormally stimulated, it may augment the progression of CTCL. Recent advances in treatment approaches highlight the potential of JAK inhibitors, such as ruxolitinib and cerdulatinib, which suggest targeting this abnormal pathway. Although initial studies are promising, with tolerable side effects, researchers remain cautious, as potential side effects could worsen the disease in certain patients; thus, further studies are required to identify optimal therapeutic applications (Kashyap et al., 2025). Primary cutaneous B-cell lymphomas, however, constitute a distinct group of lymphoproliferative neoplasms with characteristic clinical behaviors and inherent biology. The large cutaneous diffuse large B-cell lymphoma leg type (pcDLBCL-LT) is highly aggressive, whereas primary cutaneous follicle center lymphoma (pcFCL) and primary cutaneous marginal zone lymphoma (pcMZL) are more indolent at presentation. Recent single-cell RNA sequencing studies account for the differential transcription among these lymphoma subtypes, highlighting the manner in which their molecular characteristics reflect their clinical course. Specifically, whereas pcMZL and pcFCL retain ongoing germinal center responses typical of antigen recognition, pcDLBCL-LT lacks such features to establish its malignancy. Such an understanding is very important to clinicians because it forms the foundation for prognosis and therapeutic protocols tailored to the individualized biological behavior of each lymphoma subtype (Griss et al., 2024). The pleiotropic nature of cutaneous lymphoma clinical presentations and the heterogeneous behavior underscore the necessity for individualized diagnosis and treatment approach. The unravelling of mechanisms of causation, such as the JAK/STAT pathway in CTCL and the antigen-driven germinal center immune responses that are unique in primary cutaneous B-cell lymphomas, enhanced the understanding of disease pathogenesis alongside therapeutic targets. With advances in research, treatment paradigms are developing to keep pace with the demands of personalized patient profiles, particularly with the emergence of targeted therapies. The possibility of combining molecular profiling techniques promises improved prognostication and guiding clinicians toward optimum management in patients with these complex skin disorders. In summation, the attempt to understand cutaneous lymphomas continues to evolve, highlighting the tango of scientific inquiry and clinical practice (Griss et al., 2024; Kashyap et al., 2025).

KEY TERMS FROM THIS CHAPTER

- Atypical cells
- Breast carcinoma
- Cutaneous lymphomas
- Erythroderma
- Histopathological examination
- Immune interactions
- Immunohistochemistry
- Immunotherapies
- Lymphadenopathy
- Benign wounds
- CD30-positive lymphoproliferative disorder
- Cutaneous T-cell lymphomas (CTCLs)
- Genetic predisposition
- Human papillomavirus (HPV)
- Immune response
- Immunophenotypic assessment
- Intravascular malignant T-cell growth
- Lymphoma subtypes

CRITICAL THINKING QUESTIONS

1. **Which of the following is the most common type of primary cutaneous T-cell lymphoma?**
   a. Sézary syndrome
   b. Mycosis fungoides
   c. Anaplastic large cell lymphoma
   d. Peripheral T-cell lymphoma, NOS
2. **Which clinical sign is most associated with Sézary syndrome rather than mycosis fungoides?**
   a. Erythematous patches on the trunk
   b. Pruritus
   c. Generalized erythroderma with lymphadenopathy
   d. Hypopigmented patches
3. **Which immunohistochemical marker is typically positive in cutaneous T-cell lymphoma?**
   a. CD3
   b. CD20
   c. CD138
   d. S100
4. **Which internal malignancy most frequently metastasizes to the skin?**
   a. Colon carcinoma
   b. Renal cell carcinoma
   c. Breast carcinoma
   d. Prostate carcinoma
5. **A rapidly growing, firm, red skin nodule in a patient with known lung cancer is most likely:**
   a. Primary skin lymphoma
   b. Dermatofibroma
   c. Basal cell carcinoma
   d. Metastatic carcinoma

Short Answer Questions

1. What is the most common type of primary cutaneous T-cell lymphoma, and how does it typically present?
2. How does Sézary syndrome differ from mycosis fungoides in terms of clinical features and severity?
3. Which diagnostic techniques are essential for confirming cutaneous lymphoma?
4. What treatment options are available for early-stage cutaneous lymphomas?
5. What are metastatic skin lesions, and how do they differ from primary skin cancers?
6. Which primary cancers are most likely to metastasize to the skin?
7. How are metastatic skin lesions diagnosed and confirmed?
8. What are common management strategies for cutaneous metastases, especially in advanced disease?

Answer to Critical Thinking Questions

1. (b); 2. (c); 3. (a); 4. (c); 5. (d)

REFERENCES

1. Alhashimalsayed, Z., & McIntosh, K. (2025). A250 ESOPHAGOGASTRIC JUNCTION OUTFLOW OBSTRUCTION SECONDARY TO METASTATIC SQUAMOUS CELL CARCINOMA A CASE REPORT AND REVIEW OF THE LITERATURE. *Journal of the Canadian Association of Gastroenterology*, *8*(Supplement_1), i103–i104. https://doi.org/10.1093/jcag/gwae059.250Anand, U., Dey, A., Singh Chandel, A. K., Sanyal, R., Mishra, A., Pandey, D. K., De Falco, V., et al. (2022). Cancer chemotherapy and beyond: Current status, drug candidates, associated risks and progress in targeted therapeutics. *Genes & Diseases, 10*, 1367–1401. https://doi.org/10.1016/j.gendis.2022.02.007 (accessed on 21st July 2025).

2. Attrish, D., Dhamija, B., Mukherjee, D., Sawant, V., Sharma, N., Shet, T., Jain, H., et al. (2025). Abstract 1545: IL-9-mediated glutathione synthetase (GSS) expression modulates anti-oxidant response in cutaneous T cell lymphoma (CTCL). *Cancer Research*. https://www.semanticscholar.org/paper/3107e255a3b834ae8dda15670b4c88d621a15710 (accessed on 21st July 2025).

3. Gabriel, J. A., Weerasinghe, N., Balachandran, P., Salih, R., & Orchard, G. E. (2024). A Narrative Review of Molecular, Immunohistochemical and In-Situ Techniques in Dermatopathology. *British journal of biomedical science, 81*, 13437. https://doi.org/10.3389/bjbs.2024.13437(accessed on 21st July 2025).

4. Barbati, Z., & Charli-Joseph, Y. (2025). Unveiling primary cutaneous B-cell lymphomas: New insights into diagnosis and treatment strategies. *Cancers, 17*. https://www.semanticscholar.org/paper/c3b29196fceabe18e87c715b0c84fd3ace93c00d (accessed on 21st July 2025).

5. Cankaya, R., Kleiner, P. L., Hilke, F., Moritz, R. K. C., Eigentler, T., Schlaak, M., & Dobos, G. (2025). How to treat primary cutaneous B cell lymphoma–Results from a monocentric cohort study on 98 patients. *Journal der Deutschen Dermatologischen Gesellschaft = Journal of the German Society of Dermatology: JDDG*. https://www.semanticscholar.org/paper/4e7eeb3412de8ac0bacb2ec76bb6a29f7b6dc86a (accessed on 21st July 2025).

6. Cedirian, S., Zengarini, C., Lepri, M., Piraccini, B., & Pileri, A. (2025). Cutaneous adverse events related to skin lymphoma therapies. *Italian Journal of Dermatology and Venereology, 160*(3), 225–233. https://www.semanticscholar.org/paper/de80c51d84eb9fe5e17bb09c4dfe6f3111d35ead (accessed on 21st July 2025).

7. Fang, L., Simman, R., Workman, L., Ayoub, S., & Bratton, C. (2024). Malignant wound etiology, diagnosis and management: A case series and literature review. *Journal of Wound Care, 33*(2), 102–117. https://www.semanticscholar.org/paper/a69cb6856a23f4a47fcea2c70529826723d99696 (accessed on 21st July 2025).

8. Ferreri, A. J. M., Govi, S., Pileri, S., & Savage, K. J. (2012). Anaplastic large cell lymphoma, ALK-negative. *Critical Reviews in Oncology/Hematology, 85*, 206–215. https://doi.org/10.1016/j.critrevonc.2012.06.004 (accessed on 21st July 2025).

9. Flindris, S., Margioula-Siarkou, C., Margioula-Siarkou, G., Gouta, C., Styliara, E. I., Navrozoglou, I., Petousis, S., et al. (2025). Cutaneous metastasis of triple negative breast cancer: A case report and review of literature. *Cureus, 17*. https://www.semanticscholar.org/paper/eafd6f489b74b5654f1194af064c79266c6a8adc (accessed on 21st July 2025).

10. Fu, Z., Li, S., Han, S., Chen, S., & Zhang, Y. (2022). Antibody drug conjugate: The "biological missile" for targeted cancer therapy. *Signal Transduction and Targeted Therapy, 7*. https://doi.org/10.1038/s41392-022-00947-7 (accessed on 21st July 2025).

11. Garlassi, E., Harding, V., Weir, J., Francis, N., Nelson, M., Newsom-Davis, T., & Bower, M. (2012). Nonmelanoma skin cancers among HIV-infected persons in the HAART era. *Journal of Acquired Immune Deficiency Syndromes, 60*(2), e63–e65. https://www.semanticscholar.org/paper/7faeb9e57e8ce3ee025d5885d77ea37df653d2b7 (accessed on 21st July 2025).

12. Gluud, M., Pallesen, E. M. H., Buus, T. B., Gjerdrum, L., Lindahl, L., Kamstrup, M., Bzorek, M., et al. (2022). Malignant T cells induce skin barrier defects through cytokine-mediated JAK/STAT signalling in cutaneous T-cell lymphoma. *Blood*. https://www.semanticscholar.org/paper/5cf009ce197341e7ee9b95dca0d6be52fc320fad (accessed on 21st July 2025).

13. Griss, J., Gansberger, S., Oyarzun, I., Drach, M., Nguyen, V., Shaw, L., Mann, U., et al. (2024). Indolent primary cutaneous B-cell lymphomas resemble persistent antigen reactions without signs of dedifferentiation. *bioRxiv*. https://www.semanticscholar.org/paper/14cab528204df10567ef54b0616fd553bcd4dbde (accessed on 21st July 2025).

14. Hadavani, D. K., Dharaiya, C. M., Faldu, B. R., Soni, K., & Goswami, H. (2025). Histopathological study of cutaneous lesion by punch biopsy. *International Journal of Scientific Research*. https://www.semanticscholar.org/paper/7a2cdda43e7f3a1c8db311eb2f7f654d004148ca (accessed on 21st July 2025).

15. Hewavisenti, R., Arena, J., Ahlenstiel, C., & Sasson, S. C. (2023). Human papillomavirus in the setting of immunodeficiency: Pathogenesis and the emergence of next-generation therapies to reduce the high associated cancer risk. *Frontiers in Immunology, 14*. https://doi.org/10.3389/fimmu.2023.1112513 (accessed on 21st July 2025).

16. Hristov, A., Tejasvi, T., & Wilcox, R. A. (2025). Mycosis fungoides, Sézary syndrome, and cutaneous B-cell lymphomas: 2025 update on diagnosis, risk-stratification, and management. *American Journal of Hematology*. https://www.semanticscholar.org/paper/66d13edca528f925813514e85fc2ee2447173108 (accessed on 21st July 2025).

17. Islami, F., Ward, E., Sung, H., Cronin, K. A., Tangka, F. K. L., Sherman, R., Zhao, J., et al. (2021). Annual report to the nation on the status of cancer, part 1: National cancer statistics. *JNCI Journal of the National Cancer Institute, 113*, 1648–1669. https://doi.org/10.1093/jnci/djab131 (accessed on 21st July 2025).

18. Kashyap, A., Dai, J., & Ni, X. (2025). Therapeutic targeting of the Janus kinase/signal transducer and activator of transcription pathway in cutaneous T-cell lymphoma. *Cancers, 17*. https://www.semanticscholar.org/paper/77818acdef99d479ba873aa4b9e7390f69bf53d0 (accessed on 21st July 2025).

19. Keohane, S., Botting, J., Budny, P. G., Dolan, O. M., Fife, K., Harwood, C. A., Mallipeddi, R., et al. (2020). British Association of Dermatologists guidelines for the management of people with cutaneous squamous cell carcinoma 2020. *British Journal of Dermatology, 184*, 401–414. https://doi.org/10.1111/bjd.19621 (accessed on 21st July 2025).

20. Khizha, V. V., Kozlova, D. I., Sholokhov, G. V., Kuzin, S. O., & Khaimanova, D. G. (2025). Plasma cytokine levels in a patient with multiple immune-mediated adverse events on the background of nivolumab therapy for metastatic skin melanoma. *Cytokines and Inflammation*. https://www.semanticscholar.org/paper/d9935a81840137fcc1f731ec56364d68908afb38 (accessed on 21st July 2025).

21. Khrais, A., Abboud, Y., Le, A., Patel, P., & Vossough-Teehan, S. (2022). Primary cutaneous anaplastic large cell lymphoma with gastric metastasis. *Cureus, 14*. https://www.semanticscholar.

org/paper/e1bcc1ea5e554532dc464d4e80423d8168105df7 (accessed on 21st July 2025).

22. Kociol, R. D., Cooper, L. T., Fang, J. C., Moslehi, J. J., Pang, P. S., Sabe, M., Shah, R. V., et al. (2020). Recognition and initial management of fulminant myocarditis. *Circulation, 141*. https://doi.org/10.1161/cir.0000000000000745 (accessed on 21st July 2025).

23. Kohnehshahri, M. K., Sarkesh, A., Khosroshahi, L. M., HajiEsmailPoor, Z., Aghebati-Maleki, A., Yousefi, M., & Aghebati-Maleki, L. (2023). Current status of skin cancers with a focus on immunology and immunotherapy. *Cancer Cell International, 23*. https://doi.org/10.1186/s12935-023-03012-7 (accessed on 21st July 2025).

24. Lee, J., Jiang, H., & Gru, A. (2021). Primary cutaneous anaplastic large-cell lymphoma with aberrant cytokeratin expression: An unusual mimicker of poorly differentiated carcinomas. *Journal of Cutaneous Pathology, 49*, 306–309. https://www.semanticscholar.org/paper/6b2fdd63d04c98e1a8bfee60f4cbbae738b946a8 (accessed on 21st July 2025).

25. Mainolfi, N. (2024). Abstract SY12-01: Targeting validated but un-drugged oncogenes with small molecule protein degraders. *Cancer Research*. https://www.semanticscholar.org/paper/10134be020bd7be48872c56cce748d4428daa5b3 (accessed on 21st July 2025).

26. Manfrere, K. C., Torrealba, M. P., Ferreira, F. M., Alho de Sousa, E. S., Miyashiro, D., Teixeira, F. M., Custódio, R. W. A., et al. (2023). Imbalanced IL-1B and IL-18 expression in Sézary syndrome. *International Journal of Molecular Sciences, 24*. https://www.semanticscholar.org/paper/e25f687786795cd735cb3e9fbd5c5e0bb36a342c (accessed on 21st July 2025).

27. McGrail, D. J., Pilié, P. G., Rashid, N. U., Voorwerk, L., Slagter, M., Kok, M., Jonasch, E., et al. (2021). High tumor mutation burden fails to predict immune checkpoint blockade response across all cancer types. *Annals of Oncology, 32*, 661–672. https://doi.org/10.1016/j.annonc.2021.02.006 (accessed on 21st July 2025).

28. Melgaard, K. E., Lonkvist, C. K., Nielsen, A. L., Nielsen, D., & Eefsen, R. (2025). Long-term data from patients who received pembrolizumab in locally advanced or metastatic cutaneous squamous cell carcinoma. *Case Reports in Oncological Medicine, 2025*. https://www.semanticscholar.org/paper/71d377d3507669a181f3dd4a1ca54a27e2701b47 (accessed on 21st July 2025).

29. Milazzo, G., Mercatelli, D., Di Muzio, G., Triboli, L., De Rosa, P., Perini, G., & Giorgi, F. M. (2020). Histone deacetylases (HDACs): Evolution, specificity, role in transcriptional complexes, and pharmacological actionability. *Genes, 11*, 556. https://doi.org/10.3390/genes11050556 (accessed on 21st July 2025).

30. Munera-Campos, M., Carrascosa, J., Quer, A., & Ferrándiz, C. (2020). Ichthyosiform eruption and facial erythema secondary to ponatinib therapy. *JDDG: Journal der Deutschen Dermatologischen Gesellschaft, 18*. https://www.semanticscholar.org/paper/7a5b7c00ee301d9c6f4ccea5d4467cc1506b41db (accessed on 21st July 2025).

31. Overfield, C. J., Rhyner, P. A., Hall, M. R., & Bhatt, A. (2024). More than skin deep: Imaging of dermatologic disease in the head and neck. *Radiographic, 44*(12), e240052. https://www.semanticscholar.org/paper/1da03d4f387ec7d658df433592bd723394781481 (accessed on 21st July 2025).

32. Ramelyte, E., Pawlik, L., Turko, P., Sella, F., Roshardt Prieto, N. M., Stäger, R., Maul, J., et al. (2023). Intralesional oncolytic virotherapy with talimogene laherparepvec in patients with cutaneous lymphomas and non-melanoma skin cancers. *Journal of Clinical Oncology*. https://

www.semanticscholar.org/paper/ab2bf225c086954c31355996cf3983a3e12efe80 (accessed on 21st July 2025).

33. Santos, F., Wouters Ugolini, L., Oliveira, H., Machado, T. P., & Alves, L. P. (2017). Linfoma cutâneo em equino Quarto de Milha. *Acta Scientiae Veterinariae*. https://www.semanticscholar.org/paper/7b2250ea97a41919b6c89ca7a2daa612eabefa44 (accessed on 21st July 2025).

34. Scarfì, F., Melotti, B., Veronesi, G., Ravaioli, G., Baraldi, C., Lambertini, M., Patrizi, A., et al. (2019). Sweet syndrome in metastatic melanoma during treatment with dabrafenib and trametinib. *Australasian Journal of Dermatology, 60*. https://www.semanticscholar.org/paper/5e973070e803a6db5c1eaafbd9a5fcd640cb481c (accessed on 21st July 2025).

35. Seretis, K., Sfaelos, K., Boptsi, E., Gaitanis, G., & Bassukas, I. (2024). The neutrophil-to-lymphocyte ratio as a biomarker in cutaneous oncology: A systematic review of evidence beyond malignant melanoma. *Cancers, 16*. https://www.semanticscholar.org/paper/a4e22b7d777dd326755207b88032a88fdb7af057 (accessed on 21st July 2025).

36. Siegel, R. L., Giaquinto, A. N., & Jemal, A. (2024). Cancer statistics, 2024. *CA: A Cancer Journal for Clinicians, 74*, 12–49. https://doi.org/10.3322/caac.21820 (accessed on 21st July 2025).

37. Sol, S., Boncimino, F., Todorova, K., Waszyn, S., & Mandinova, A. (2024). Therapeutic approaches for non-melanoma skin cancer: Standard of care and emerging modalities. *International Journal of Molecular Sciences, 25*. https://www.semanticscholar.org/paper/716865fa6df622ed6605c32d8077bd7784509712 (accessed on 21st July 2025).

38. Väkevä, L. (2006). The risk of cancer associated with immunosuppressive therapy for skin diseases. https://core.ac.uk/download/14918245.pdf (accessed on 21st July 2025).

39. von Mehren, M., Kane, J. M., Agulnik, M., Bui, M. M., Carr, J. R., Choy, E., Connelly, M., et al. (2022). Soft tissue sarcoma, version 2.2022, NCCN clinical practice guidelines in oncology. *Journal of the National Comprehensive Cancer Network, 20*, 815–833. https://doi.org/10.6004/jnccn.2022.0035 (accessed on 21st July 2025).

40. Wang, C., Wolfe, A., Geng, X., & Wilcox, R. A. (2024). Single cell atlas of cutaneous T cell lymphomas reveals XPO1 dependency. *Blood*. https://www.semanticscholar.org/paper/4978aaf80a56ab3ba5a88072408c752ef8c234dd (accessed on 21st July 2025).

41. Yamakawa, K., Ogata, D., Namikawa, K., Nakano, E., Yamaguchi, Y., & Yamazaki, N. (2025). A review of cutaneous angiosarcoma: Epidemiology, diagnosis, prognosis, and treatment options. *Japanese Journal of Clinical Oncology*. https://www.semanticscholar.org/paper/5606519d0cad39682f60d5be5da8944d7f2a0994 (accessed on 21st July 2025).

42. Yang, J., Xu, Y., Xie, K., Gao, L., Zhong, W., & Liu, X. (2022). CEBPB is associated with active tumor immune environment and favorable prognosis of metastatic skin cutaneous melanoma. *Frontiers in Immunology, 13*. https://www.semanticscholar.org/paper/f321c704b56f1545c563f1b3b3866f1f8f68e443 (accessed on 21st July 2025).

43. Yang, L., Shi, P., Zhao, G., Xu, J., Peng, W., Zhang, J., Zhang, G., et al. (2020). Targeting cancer stem cell pathways for cancer therapy. *Signal Transduction and Targeted Therapy, 5*. https://doi.org/10.1038/s41392-020-0110-5 (accessed on 21st July 2025).

44. Zanardi, P. I. (2025). An ALK-positive anaplastic large cell lymphoma with striking cutaneous manifestations and diagnostic insights. *Journal of Dermatology Research*. https://www.semanticscholar.org/paper/4f4564d6ba937cd46e616503c64d9324d77f225a (accessed on 21st July 2025).

45. Zhang, Z., Liang, L., Jiang, X., Shan, J., Li, S., Liu, J., Dong, Q., et al. (2025). Skin microbiome influences the progression of cutaneous squamous cell carcinoma through the immune system. *World Journal of Surgical Oncology, 23*. https://www.semanticscholar.org/paper/b6153681153d2c0828c006930a97384d2bdc281a (accessed on 21st July 2025).

46. Zhao, H., Wu, L., Yan, G., Chen, Y., Zhou, M., Wu, Y., & Li, Y. (2021). Inflammation and tumor progression: Signaling pathways and targeted intervention. *Signal Transduction and Targeted Therapy, 6*. https://doi.org/10.1038/s41392-021-00658-5 (accessed on 21st July 2025).

PHOTODERMATOSES AND UV-INDUCED SKIN DISORDERS

4

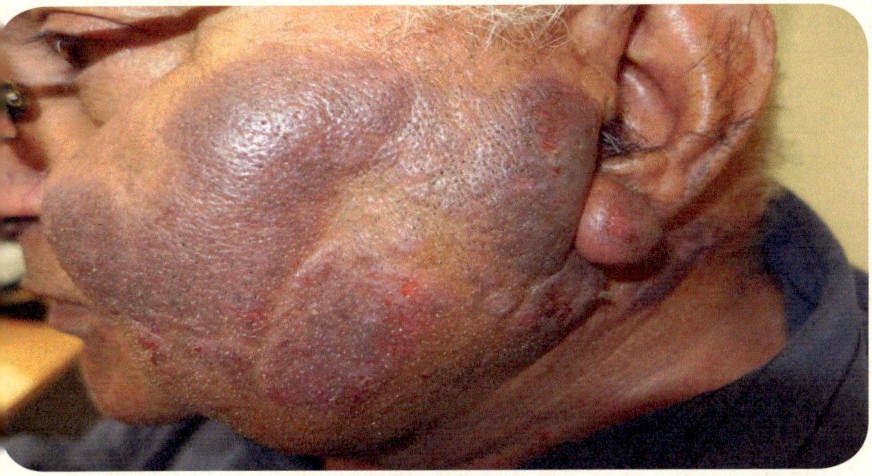

LEARNING OBJECTIVES

After studying this chapter, you will be able to:

1. Explain the types of photodermatoses
2. Understand the mechanisms of UV-induced skin damage
3. Describe risk factors for photodermatoses
4. Discuss symptoms associated with photodermatoses
5. Define effective treatment options for photodermatoses and ultraviolet (UV)-induced skin disorder
6. Focus on effective prevention strategies for photodermatoses and UV-induced skin disorders

Introduction

The photodermatoses and disorders of the skin caused by UV point towards the importance of understanding the impact of ultraviolet radiation on human health. The photodermatoses, which comprise a large number of inflammatory skin diseases prompted by sun exposure, are a significant topic in dermatology. They could range from the very benign sunburn to as severe as systemic lupus erythematosus, which illustrates the varying degrees of photosensitivity among patients. It should be noted that despite the well-established deleterious effects of UVR, the mechanisms through which they provoke lesions in the skin are still the subject of continued research. A review of lupus erythematosus illustrates that the detrimental effects of UVR on patient populations were recognized over a hundred years ago. This context calls to mind recent studies with a view to developing targeted treatment plans and diagnostic standards for victims of such illnesses (Walchner et al., 1997). In addition, the focus of UV light includes not only UVA and UVB but also newly emerging factors , such as infrared radiation

(IR) and visible light (VIS). Current research indicates that such diversified types of radiation have the potential to worsen the pathogenesis of photodermatoses, making it necessary to evolve with a deeper insight into the way the skin responds to sun exposure. For example, dermatoses caused by long-term exposure to UV radiation can cause complications like skin cancer and photoaging, which illustrates the urgent necessity for an effective prevention protocol. Furthermore, outstanding developments in photoprotection, such as in the form of natural products like Fernblock®, suggest possible therapeutic avenues and management. Fernblock®, a substance that is derived from the fern Polypodium Leucotomos, suggests promise in both topical and oral supplement forms for skin health with a safety profile that would favor ongoing clinical use (Rodríguez-Luna et al., 2023). The interaction of environmental and susceptibility factors makes a multidisciplinary treatment essential in both assessment and treatment of photodermatoses. Skin type, geographic location, and individual history of UV exposure are major predictors of the severity of sunburn. As awareness of these skin conditions increases, further research into their etiology and treatment awaits more refinement. Understanding the role of various factors in cutaneous reactions to UV radiation is critical for clinicians who wish to provide the best therapy to affected individuals. Additionally, scientists are challenged to unravel the molecular processes underlying photosensitivity to formulate new therapeutic strategies. These would not only mitigate the suffering caused by photodermatoses but also support public health programs aimed at reducing UV-induced dermatoses across populations.

Definition of Photodermatoses

Photodermatoses are a heterogeneous group of skin disorders that are characterized by abnormal reactions to UV light exposure. They are caused by a broad spectrum of pathophysiological mechanisms that may be genetic, immunological, or environmentally influenced. The most common manifestation is the development of inflammatory reactions, such as erythema or rashes, in the photosensitive person. Because these conditions develop particularly following sun exposure, they usually result in severe distress and sequelae, including permanent skin changes and even malignancies. Defining the photodermatoses will assist investigators in better understanding the triggers of these exaggerated cutaneous reactions, enabling them to explore new and more effective intervention modalities for these patients. The prime example of photodermatoses is Xeroderma pigmentosum (XP, a rare genetic disorder with hypersensitivity to the sun and a heightened risk of skin cancer. XP patients obtain abnormal skin responses, that is, severe sunburn or color changes in the skin, within a few hours of sun exposure, highlighting the genetic causation of photodermatoses. XP is caused by DNA repair gene mutations for UV-induced damage and has a wide range of clinical presentations, including premature skin cancers. XP has historically been important in advancing our knowledge of photodermatoses, both for the unique clinical presentation and for its implications regarding UV safety and prevention. Such understanding sets XP apart from other disorders of this type, enabling appropriate diagnosis and management for those affected (Lehmann et al., 2011). Another frequent example of photodermatoses is related to systemic lupus erythematosus (SLE), in which photosensitivity is the primary element in exacerbating skin lesions. Skin reactions caused by UV radiation occur in patients with lupus, pointing to the interconnectedness of systemic diseases and localized photodermatoses. The photoinduced harmful effects manifest as rashes or lesions and have a significant effect on patients' quality of life. It led to the standardization of procedures for the diagnosis and classification of photosensitive disorders in such patients. Under controlled test conditions, physicians are better equipped to diagnose the distinct manifestations of lupus and thus employ more targeted therapeutic interventions. UV protection and patient education are still stressed in managing these conditions effectively (Walchner et al., 1997) (Figure 4.1).

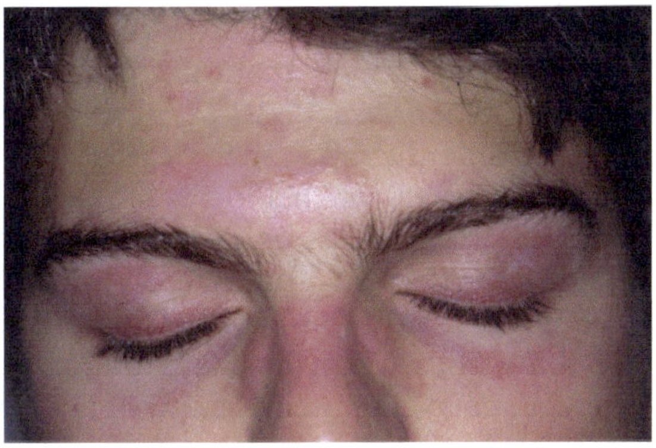

Figure 4.1. Photodermatoses caused by sun or ultraviolet (UV) radiation exposure.

Source: https://medizinonline.com/wp-content/uploads/2013/09/aaa6.png.-e5aec0_831.png.

Importance of Understanding UV-Induced Skin Disorders

The relevance of familiarity with UV-induced dermatoses is underscored by the increasing number of cases involving conditions , such as photosensitivity, photoaging, and skin cancers. These diseases are not only caused by acute UVR exposure but also by chronic cumulative exposure to UVR over the course of years. The effects of solar radiation are not restricted to immediate reactions, such as sunburn; they encompass long-term alterations in the skin's structure and function. Research has indicated that even after exposure to UV has ceased, the damage to DNA continues in skin cells, leading to increased susceptibility to malignancies and other skin ailments. Awareness of these diseases is thus imperative, along with the development of effective prevention, early detection, and treatment strategies, ultimately reducing the public health burden of skin disorders attributable to UV exposure. Moreover, the development of targeted photoprotection technologies is essential for reducing the risk of UV-induced skin disease. The new study indicates the use of natural products as oral and topical agents for photoprotection. Of specific significance are extracts like Fernblock®, which are derived from the fern Polypodium leucotomos, and have possessed a good safety and high efficacy profile in the treatment of a number of skin diseases worsened by sunlight (Pandey et al., 2023).

These advances underscore the importance of identifying mechanisms of UV-induced damage and harnessing natural resources for therapeutic use. By incorporating these interventions and strategies into public health programs, it is possible to promote healthier behaviors and reinforce individuals' protective measures against the adverse effects of UV radiation, thereby fostering an active skin-care culture. Besides, information on UV-induced skin diseases also incorporates the wider contexts of environmental factors, which are essential in today's discussion of skin health. The interactions of UV radiation with other lights , such as visible and infrared radiation, have been brought to light, illustrating further intricacies in reactions by the skin (Pandey et al., 2023). Furthermore, the reactive oxygen species (ROS) generated during such exposures may lead to oxidative stress, thus further complicating skin integrity and health (Pandey et al., 2023). An understanding of the phenomena, therefore, enables the development of broad-spectrum photoprotection products that are effective in addressing multiple light-induced effects on the skin. As continued research continues to unveil the intricate work of UV exposure, individuals must be as educated as possible and utilize protection measures, hence building a society in which the importance of skin health protection is determined and accorded its deserved significance.

4.1. Types of Photodermatoses

Learning Outcome

1. Describe polymorphous light eruption.
2. Define solar urticarial.
3. Discuss chronic actinic dermatitis.

Photodermatoses are a heterogeneous group of skin conditions induced by ultraviolet (UV) radiation and manifest in various forms that can significantly affect an individual's health. The most prevalent forms include polymorphous light eruption (PLE), actinic keratosis, and solar urticaria. PLE is characterized by a pruritic rash appearing on the sun-exposed areas after the first exposure to the sun during the spring season. In contrast, actinic keratosis is characterized by scaly, rough lesions on sun-exposed areas and serves as a precursor to skin carcinoma. Solar urticaria is characterized by hives induced by UV exposure and can significantly compromise quality of life. These conditions highlight the significant burden imposed by UV radiation on skin health and warrant awareness and preventive behaviors among affected groups. Together, the identification and definition of these specific types underpin effective therapeutic approaches to photodermatoses. Beyond the individual details of the various photodermatoses, hereditary and familial elements also contribute to susceptibility to these UV-induced conditions. For example, individuals inherit a predisposition to photoallergic responses that exacerbate conditions such as PLE. Increased sensitivity to sunlight is also caused by drugs, leading to photodermatoses in susceptible individuals. Some common day-to-day drugs, particularly antihypertensive medications, have been reported to produce increased sensitivity to sunlight, rendering their patients all the more challenging to treat (Pandey et al., 2023). This relationship between genetics, drug consumption, and the environment necessitates an integrative approach to treatment as well as risk control. By identifying patients at high risk based on genetic susceptibility and medication use, health care providers can tailor preventive interventions to reduce UV-induced skin diseases and enhance patients' quality of life. The increasing prevalence of photodermatoses is underscored by the global rise in UV radiation exposure and by the complex interactions of UV radiation with environmental and lifestyle factors. As the world's climate warms, increased levels of UV radiation may further exacerbate prevalent skin diseases and contribute to the etiology of new diseases. In addition, the economic costs of managing these skin diseases underscore their relevance to the public health debate. For instance, while photodermatoses lack the life-threatening results of cutaneous cancers, they still take a very heavy toll on patients' quality of life and incur gigantic costs in medical treatment (Zaid et al., 2022). In addition to ongoing studies on potential treatments and prevention, public sensitization campaigns and education interventions are paramount for informing the public about photodermatoses. This multi-disciplinary approach will ultimately assist in reducing the incidence of these disorders and circumscribing their impact upon affected individuals.

4.1.1. Polymorphous Light Eruption

Polymorphous light eruption (PLE) is the most common idiopathic photodermatosis, with clinical presentations that often mimic other cutaneous diseases. The disorder is more frequent in young adults, with a marked female predominance, and usually presents after sun exposure, particularly after prolonged exposure in winter or after a decrease in regular sunlight exposure. Clinical presentations can include erythematous papules, plaques, or vesicles, which can appear on skin-exposed areas , such as the neck, arms, and upper back. A cross-sectional study demonstrated that in 98.5% of PLEs, pruritus was a common complaint, and the most frequently observed morphological type was plaque PLE, occurring in 35.7% of cases (Patil et al., 2023). Awareness of these clinical findings is required for accurate diagnosis and effective treatment of PLE. The pathophysiology of PLE includes complex immunological responses to UV radiation that lead to abnormal skin cell migration and cytokine production. PLE has been reported to involve changes in the migration of Langerhans cells, which play a significant role in controlling immune responses and maintaining skin integrity. A study demonstrated that following UV-B exposure, PLE patients had decreased expressions of pro-inflammatory cytokines , such as TNF-alpha and IL-4, demonstrating their impaired immune response in the skin. Most significantly, this reduced cytokine expression also appears to be associated with the diminished inflammation of neutrophils in affected skin, leading to defective Langerhans cell function and insufficient T(H)2 response that can exacerbate symptoms of PLE (Wendy Kölgen et al., 2004). Research into these immune mechanisms further illuminates the disorder's etiology.

Treatment of PLE is typically preventive and symptomatic and may require a multimodal approach. Patients are advised against exposure to the sun, particularly during peak sun hours, and are instructed to wear protective clothing and apply broad-spectrum sunscreen to reduce the risk of symptom development. In addition to photoprotection, antihistamines are often prescribed for pruritus, whereas topical corticosteroids can be applied to minimize inflammation during exacerbation. In chronic conditions, controlled phototherapy with UV radiation can develop tolerance over time and reduce the severity of subsequent eruptions. Overall knowledge of the clinical presentation and underlying immunopathophysiologic mechanisms enhances the capacity of healthcare professionals to tailor effective management plans for patients with PLE, ultimately improving their quality of life in the context of this destructive disease (Figure 4.2).

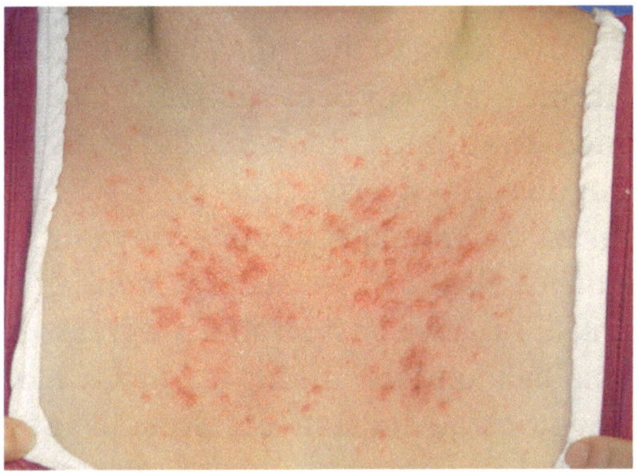

Figure 4.2. Polymorphic light eruption on the chest.

Source: https://upload.wikimedia.org/wikipedia/commons/a/a9/Polymorphic_Light_Eruption_on_the_chest.jpg.

4.1.2. Solar Urticaria

Solar urticaria, a type of photodermatosis, is an acute hypersensitivity reaction to ultraviolet (UV) radiation. Symptoms , such as erythema, pruritus, and whealing typically occur in patients within minutes of sun exposure. Solar urticaria can occur in healthy individuals with no apparent history of such a reaction; therefore, it is not easy to diagnose and treat (Figure 4.3).

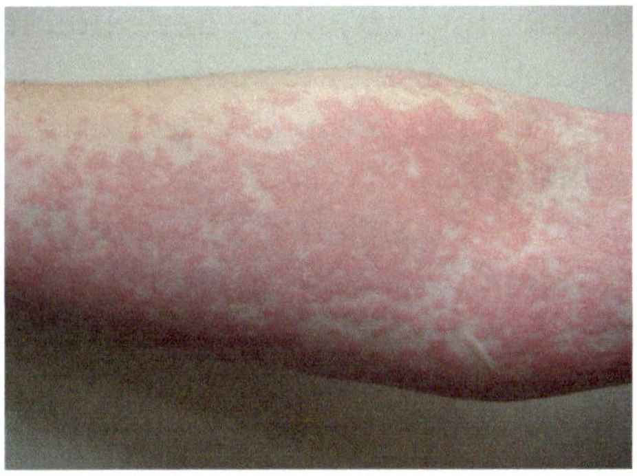

Figure 4.3. Formation of wheals on the arm.

Source: https://upload.wikimedia.org/wikipedia/commons/thumb/6/63/EMminor2010.JPG/800px-EMminor2010.JPG.

The pathophysiology of solar urticaria involves triggering mast cells in the skin, with the release of histamine and other inflammatory mediators, leading to the clinical manifestations. The immediate hypersensitivity reaction indicates that patients with solar urticaria may require highly rigorous photoprotection measures to manage their symptoms and maintain quality of life. Management of solar urticaria has made considerable progress, driven by enhanced understanding of individualized photoprotection measures. Recent studies emphasize the importance of personalized sun protection in relation to an individual's characteristics, such as skin phototype, genetic predisposition, and environmental determinants. This advancement in personal photoprotection balances efficacy with individual patient requirements, particularly in cases of photodermatoses such as solar urticaria. Recent investigations show that some pharmaceutical actives and antioxidants have the potential to mitigate UV-induced skin damage and lead to better outcomes in patients. These strategies emphasize not only the use of topical medication and physical barriers but also lifestyle modifications that are required in preventing relapses and managing the disease adequately (Gracia et al., 2024). Besides, the prophylactic application of antioxidants and photoprotective agents is central in managing the oxidative stress of solar urticaria. Induction of reactive oxygen species (ROS) following exposure to UV is a significant skin inflammation and cell damage, aggravating the condition. Incorporation of antioxidants in sunscreen formulations has been hopeful in preventing visible light-induced oxidative damage (Pandey et al., 2023). Antioxidants , such as vitamins E and C not only suppress the formation of free radicals but also help to reduce sun-induced erythema and pigmentary changes. As the field of solar urticaria and its mechanisms of action continues to grow, such photoprotection breakthroughs could significantly benefit the management of this challenging disease, enhancing patients' quality of life while reducing side effects from sunlight (Figure 4.4).

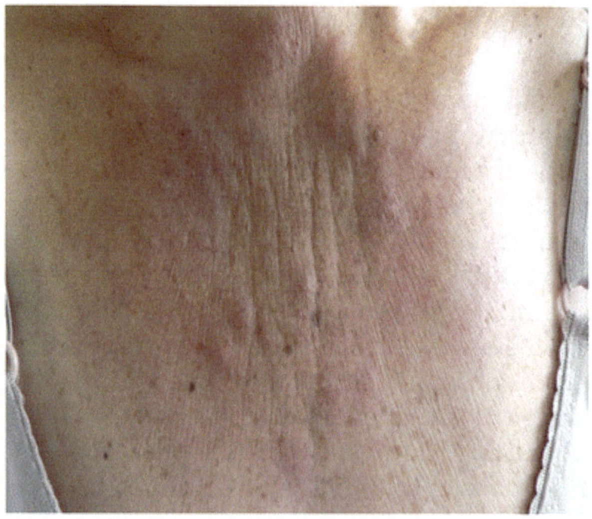

Figure 4.4. Solar urticaria. A 66-year-old female patient with solar urticaria. Observe the lesions on sun-exposed areas ("V" of the neck).

Source: https://www.researchgate.net/publication/318170222/figure/fig3/AS:962671792893969@1606530249723/Solar-urticaria-A-66-year-old-female-patient-with-solar-urticaria-Observe-the-lesions.gif.

4.1.3. Chronic Actinic Dermatitis

Chronic actinic dermatitis (CAD) is among the most challenging of the photodermatoses, a distinct inflammatory skin disorder characterized by heightened sensitivity to ultraviolet (UV) radiation. CAD typically affects elderly people, particularly those with actinically damaged skin. Upon exposure to UV radiation, the subjects develop an inflammatory reaction that persists even after cessation of exposure to UV radiation, thus ultimately illuminating the immunological underpinnings of CAD. The clinical presentations typically include erythema, vesicles, and scaling patches, which primarily occur on sun-exposed regions of the body. Since it is a chronic disease, CAD often needs to have a multifaceted treatment protocol, which in certain circumstances might include photoprotection and immunomodulator treatments in order to minimize inflammation and ensure healing of the skin. The pathogenesis of chronic actinic dermatitis is mostly immune-mediated processes that are triggered by UV radiation. One of the salient features of CAD is the participation of photoallergic reactions, wherein photosensitizers in the skin, sensitized by exposure to UV, react with proteins to produce complex antigens. Immunological activation may result in widespread skin lesions, which show how CAD belongs to a larger group of photoallergic dermatoses. Notably, while single photo allergens in CAD can be unknown in some cases, correlations with some chemicals and drugs have been made. The significance of these interactions underscores the importance of establishing the patient's history to identify potential triggers that may exacerbate CAD symptoms and to improve disease control (Krolo et al., 2008). Recent research has investigated the impact of optical radiation environments on the sensitivity of skin, with significant relevance to chronic actinic dermatitis. Work emanating from within the Photobiology Unit has revealed the heterogeneity of the response of normal and diseased skin towards artificial sources of UV, with implications for the requirement of accurate measurement technology in the assessment of UV exposure level and its associated risks. Moreover, it has been observed that standard predictive models may not reveal the intrinsic vulnerabilities of pathological skin conditions, such as CAD. This data makes a revision of safety standards on UV exposure necessary and results in an emphasis on the way proper protective measures, including protective clothing and photoprotection, need to be utilized for preventing unwanted effects induced by natural and artificial sources of light (Oliver, 2006) (Figure 4.5).

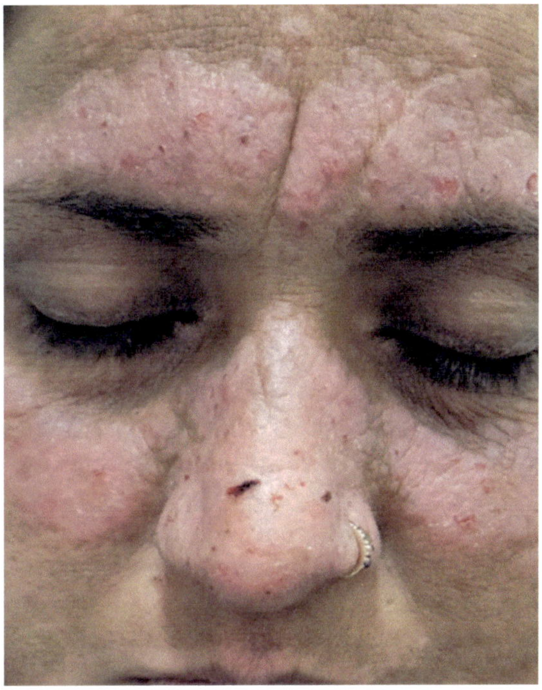

Figure 4.5. Chronic actinic dermatitis in the form of multiple, well-defined erythematous plaques on the forehead, malar area of cheeks, nose, and philtrum.

Source: https://www.researchgate.net/publication/342138797/figure/fig1/AS:11431281173700948@1689028705025/A-Chronic-actinic-dermatitis-in-the-form-of-multiple-well-defined-erythematous-plaques.png.

Test Your Knowledge

1. What are the typical clinical features of polymorphous light eruption (PMLE)?
2. How does solar urticaria differ from other photodermatoses in terms of onset and symptoms?
3. What are common sites of involvement in chronic actinic dermatitis (CAD)?

4.2. Mechanisms of UV-Induced Skin Damage

Learning Outcome

1. Understand the relationship between DNA damage and repair mechanisms.
2. Discuss the role of reactive oxygen species.
3. Describe the immune system response to UV exposure.

It is important to clarify UV-induced harm processes of skin in order to better understand pathogenesis of certain photodermatoses and skin diseases. The most significant risk of ultraviolet radiation (UVR) is its penetration of the skin and damage to cellular integrity. Direct DNA damage by UVR results in formation of pyrimidine dimers, which, if not repaired properly, result in mutation. In addition to the immediate DNA damage, UV exposure stimulates the generation of reactive oxygen species (ROS) and reactive nitrogen species (RNS), which can cause injury to cellular structures , such as proteins, lipids, and other DNA, causing an inflammatory cascade. The cascade not only causes the clinical manifestations of cutaneous diseases, such as skin diseases, but also melanizes pigmentation as a protective response to prevent further UV-induced injury. Thus, unmasking of such underlying molecular mechanisms explains why UV exacerbates chronic actinic dermatitis and solar urticaria and implies the need for effective photoprotection measures. The action of UV radiation on the skin is mediated by intricate biochemical mechanisms that may initiate a cascade of deleterious effects. Delayed onset of DNA damage following the first UV exposure means that cellular responses can persist even after exposures have ceased. Research demonstrates that even weeks following the cessation of UVR exposures, DNA repair mechanisms remain overwhelmed, leading to further cellular stress and even increased risk for skin cancers. Along with the direct mutagenic effect, inflammation caused by UV is also responsible for the majority of skin damage through cytokine release and immigration of immune cells. In addition to promoting further progression of skin damage, the inflammatory response also exacerbates photodermatoses, indicating that treatments that prevent these activities are required.

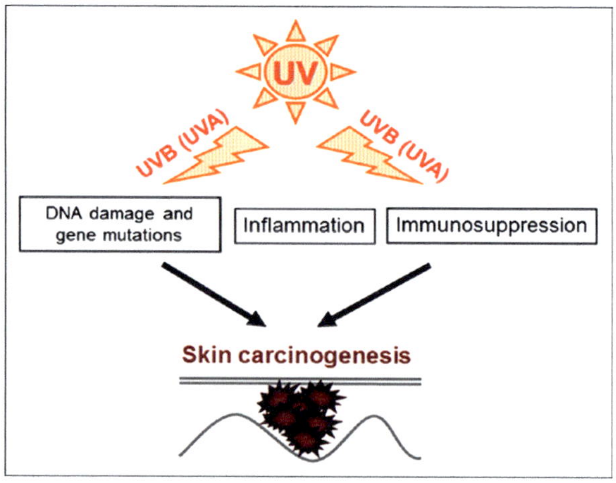

Figure 4.6. UV-induced carcinogenesis in the skin. UV radiation is carcinogenic because it induces DNA damage, gene mutation and chronic inflammation and has immunosuppressive effects on the skin.

Source: https://www.researchgate.net/profile/Tadamichi-Shimizu/publication/221919677/figure/fig1/AS:305317561815043@1449804787512/UV-induced-carcinogenesis-in-the-skin-UV-radiation-is-carcinogenic-because-it-induces.png.

Therefore, an understanding of these biological pathways can be used to formulate new treatment regimens to combat UV-induced diseases. New photoprotection modalities point towards reversal of UV-induced pathways of skin damage. Emerging technologies suggest that natural agents, such as those with Fernblock®, offer topical as well as systemic protection against UV-induced damage. The purified Polypodium leucotomos extract has been found to be effective in preventing photodermatoses by fortifying cellular defenses and enhancing DNA repair mechanisms. Moreover, the use of antioxidants in sunscreens has shown positive effects in the prevention of UV and visible light irradiation-induced oxidative injury. The combined use of antioxidant sunscreens that act on ROS and RNS, along with conventional UV blockers, forms the basis of complete photoprotection. Thus, with the enhanced understanding of UV damage to skin, it is the need of the day to develop new protective agents to guard against and cure photodermatoses and other dermatoses (Pandey et al., 2023; Rodríguez-Luna et al., 2023) (Figure 4.6).

4.2.1. DNA Damage and Repair Mechanisms

Cross-talk between DNA damage and repair processes is critical to the pathophysiology of photodermatoses and disorders associated with UV-induced skin damage. Ultraviolet radiation (UVR) in sunlight is a prominent environmental agent that causes DNA damage, most commonly in the form of pyrimidine dimers, which may lead to mutations if not repaired. Nucleotide excision repair (NER) is the prime mechanism for the removal of these UV-induced lesions. This complex mechanism involves recognition of damaged DNA, excision of the lesion, and DNA synthesis, mediated by enzymes and proteins that maintain genomic stability. A deficiency in these repair mechanisms can result in the accumulation of mutations, thereby increasing the risk of skin diseases such as melanoma and squamous cell carcinoma. These processes must be unraveled in the design of effective photoprotective strategies and treatment modalities in high-risk populations. Beyond conventional DNA repair pathways, the cellular response to UV-induced damage also involves intricate signaling pathways that regulate the repair process. A mechanism is the induction of the NRF2 transcription factor that coordinates the expression of genes involved in antioxidant defense and cytoprotection. As highlighted by recent studies, NRF2 activation can enhance cellular resistance to the harmful effects of UVR and thereby provide an adjunctive protective pathway against photocarcinogenesis. Such protection is particularly important in photodermatosis, where exposure to UV induces skin hypersensitivity. Targeting NRF2 and elucidating its role in inhibiting DNA damage may reveal new therapeutic approaches for treating patients with UV-induced skin disease. Therefore, ongoing investigation in this area will be key to optimizing levels of protection against long-term injury. Furthermore, advances in pharmacological enhancement of DNA repair mechanisms offer promising avenues for prevention of the deleterious action of UV radiation. Natural products the fern extract Fernblock®, have emerged as effective agents of topical and systemic photoprotection. As suggested by more recent evidence, this extract not only protects against solar damage immediately, such as sunburn and inflammation, but may also improve the natural DNA repair capacity of the skin. Such addition of naturally occurring photoprotective agents may have major implications for clinical photodermatosis treatment and provide an added advantage for at-risk patients with skin cancers and other UV-induced conditions. By utilizing these multi-modal approaches, dietary supplementation and local treatment, the potential for enhancement of DNA repair mechanisms emphasizes the worth of such comprehensive treatments in the prevention of UV-induced skin diseases, ultimately translating into an improved clinical practice in dermatology.

4.2.2. Role of Reactive Oxygen Species

The role of reactive oxygen species (ROS) in unravelling photodermatoses and UV-induced cutaneous disorders cannot be overemphasized. When the skin is exposed to UV light, it generates a number of ROS that cause oxidative stress, subsequently damaging cellular structures, such as proteins, lipids, and DNA. The resulting oxidative damage triggers inflammatory responses that contribute to skin diseases such as solar urticaria and chronic actinic dermatitis. As ROS accumulate, they drive the pathophysiology of these diseases by modulating cellular signal transduction pathways, potentially leading to further sensitization of the skin and long-term effects. Therefore, the understanding of the mechanistic actions of ROS in skin pathologies is critical in designing specific therapeutic interventions that reverse their harmful effects and preserve skin integrity, as explicated in recent evidence demonstrating that antioxidants can scavenge these harmful species effectively to reverse oxidative stress (Pandey et al., 2023).

Current evidence highlights the importance of antioxidants in preventing UV-induced ROS and preserving skin health. When added to topical formulations, such as sunscreens, antioxidants, such as vitamins C and E, can quench ROS and thereby minimize the development of photodermatoses. Indeed, recent progress in cosmetic dermatology is directed towards encapsulating these compounds in order to optimize efficacy and UV stability. Specifically, studies have shown that topical combinations of these antioxidants not only protect against erythema but also inhibit hyperpigmentation in at-risk skin types. Improvements in products such as pigmented sunscreens or antioxidant-containing ones reflect the heightened sensitivity regarding the need for global photoprotection interventions. Not only does such an intervention cure current skin disease, but it also protects against the onset of future disease, elucidating the multifaceted role ROS has in the preservation of skin health and disease management (Pandey et al., 2023).

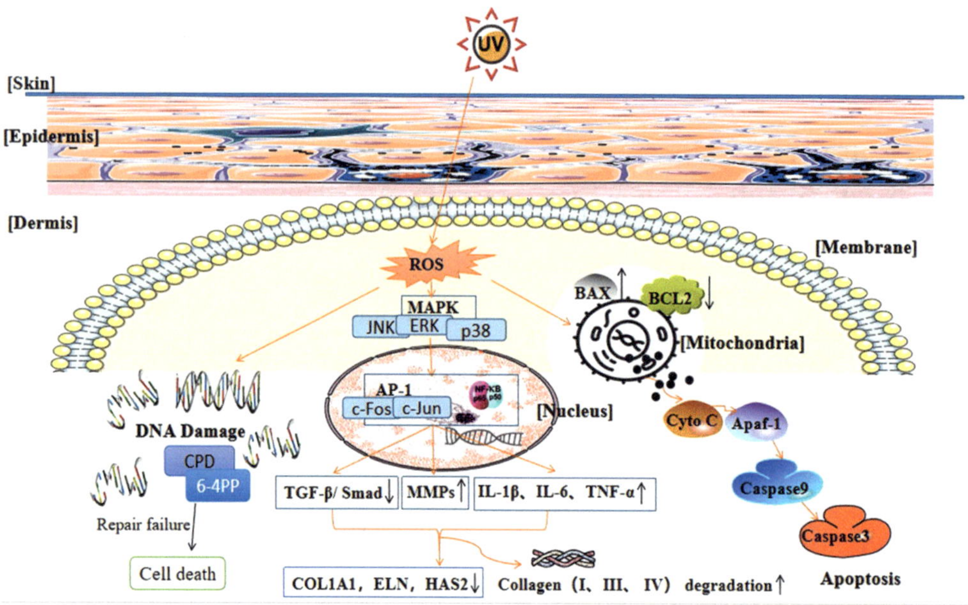

Figure 4.7. Signaling pathways of reactive oxygen species (ROS) in ultraviolet (UV)-induced skin photodamage.

Source: https://www.researchgate.net/publication/377361213/figure/fig4/AS:11431281217287987@1705116301573/Signaling-pathways-of-reactive-oxygen-species-ROS-in-ultraviolet-UV-induced-skin.png.

In addition, triggering endogenous defense mechanisms is a promising strategy for counteracting ROS-mediated injury caused by UV exposure. The transcription factor NRF2 is a key cellular defense component that controls the expression of antioxidant-producing genes and cytoprotective genes. By activating NRF2, scientists aim to enhance the skin's resilience to UV-induced oxidative stress. These pharmacological treatments are not only of potential use in averting photocarcinogenesis but also in the management of photodermatosis, as their capacity to overexpress protective proteins that neutralize ROS makes them worthwhile. The addition of natural and synthetic NRF2 activators to dermatological treatments underscores a prophylactic approach in dermatological treatments aimed at preventing both acute and cumulative damage to the skin by UV radiation. This shifting perspective considers the relevance of continued research into photodermatosis mechanisms and the therapeutic application of NRF2 pathways for optimal protection of the skin (Figure 4.7).

4.2.3. Immune System Response to UV Exposure

The immune response to ultraviolet (UV) irradiation is a complex interplay of protective and harmful mechanisms that critically affects skin health. UV radiation, particularly UVA, induces a range of physiological changes that modulate immune responses. While immunosuppression caused by UV exposure has certain benefits, such as tolerance to the allergen or suppression of certain autoimmune disorders, it also leads to an increased vulnerability to disease from infection or to skin cancer cell proliferation. Recent research, as illustrated in assessments by the Environmental Effects Assessment Panel, portrays the two sides of UV-induced immune modulation where excessive exposure weakens the skin's immune defense with a resultant high rate of skin cancers, especially melanoma and keratinocyte cancer among vulnerable populations (Rachel et al., 2023). Thus, understanding this delicate balance is central to developing strategies to optimize skin protection against immune alterations induced by UV radiation. Also, the generation of reactive oxygen species (ROS) by UV radiation is another central factor in the immune response. UVA radiation penetrates deeply into the skin and generates ROS that initiate oxidative stress and consequent inflammatory reactions. The cellular damage ultimately results in a cascade of biological effects, including mutations and apoptosis, which can significantly alter immune function (Françoise Bernerd et al., 2022). Particularly, this oxidative stress is very likely to exacerbate photoimmunosuppression, with increased risk of photoallergic reaction and inflammatory dermatosis. This link underscores the importance of multilayer photoprotection procedures that include not only UVB but also UVA protection, since both spectra are harmful. Thus, this dual approach can help to minimize the adverse impacts on the immune function of the skin while allowing the beneficial effects of controlled sun exposure. In the framework of photodermatoses, the immune reaction to UV light is paramount in the pathogenesis and regulation of most skin disorders. Polymorphous light eruption and solar urticaria illustrate how immune dysfunction induced by UV radiation can lead to heightened reactivity and inflammation. Current evidence suggests that patients with photodermatoses may respond differently to UV-induced immunosuppression, and that a more complex interaction among UV exposure, immune tolerance, and cutaneous reactions may be involved (Rachel et al., 2023). Clinicians need to consider such interactions when developing effective treatment plans that may involve immunomodulatory therapies or increased protective care. Comprehending the immune system's reaction to UV exposure not only helps in treating current skin conditions but also guides measures against future instances of photodermatoses and UV-related skin ailments.

Test Your Knowledge

1. What type of DNA damage is most commonly caused by ultraviolet B (UVB) radiation?
2. How do reactive oxygen species (ROS) contribute to UV-induced skin damage?

4.3. Risk Factors for Photodermatoses

Learning Outcome

1. Describe genetic predisposition associated with photodermatoses and UV-induced skin disorders.
2. Understand environmental factors in the exacerbation of photodermatoses and UV-induced skin disorders.
3. Explain the relationship between lifestyle choices and ultraviolet (UV) exposure in understanding the incidence and severity of photodermatoses and UV-induced skin disorders.

The course of photodermatoses is strongly correlated with a risk factor complex, the primary component of which is ultraviolet (UV) radiation. Contact with UV light, particularly with ultraviolet A (UVA) and ultraviolet B (UVB) radiation, has been identified as leading to various dermatological diseases, including photoaging and pigmentary changes. Individuals with lighter skin color are particularly susceptible because they have lower melanin levels, which serve as an inherent defense against ionizing radiation. Moreover, excessive sun exposure with inadequate protection can exacerbate these disorders. While public awareness about the threat posed by UV radiation is rising, the quality and consistency of photoprotection measures, such as the application of sunscreens, remain poor among different populations. Therefore, it is crucial to recognize and understand these risk factors to effectively prevent photodermatoses, particularly among individuals at higher risk due to skin type or lifestyle.

Skin type and ethnicity are other key factors in deciding the risk of photodermatoses. Individuals with skin of color possess unique characteristics that provide a certain level of defense against UV damage a higher eumelanin-to-pheomelanin ratio. Despite these protection mechanisms, they are vulnerable to UV-induced cutaneous diseases like photodermatoses. To their misfortune, there exists a paradox where individuals with dark skin are less likely to follow photoprotective behaviors, for example, sunscreen application on a daily basis, since they are not conscious or feel that they are vulnerable. This gap is likely to lead to a greater incidence of photo-exacerbated pigmentary disorders in these populations. In contrast, educational programs specifically targeted at these populations are urgently needed to raise awareness of UV exposure risk across skin types and promote healthy photoprotection behaviors among them (Krutmann et al., 2022). Geographic location and season of the climate also significantly affect the risk of photodermatoses. People dwelling in regions with higher UV index levels, particularly those near the equatorial regions, are more likely to be at risk. High-intensity UV radiation can lead to more incidents of skin disease, particularly for those individuals who do not exercise protective behaviors. In addition, some activities that favor prolonged periods of exposure to sunlight, such as sporting activities and occupations, increase this susceptibility. In light of this, public health responses need to incorporate protection against these risks, especially where UV radiation is otherwise elevated. Seasonal fluctuations also require a responsive strategy, as individuals tend to reduce sun protection when it's cold and perceive the risk as lower. Educational campaigns should therefore emphasize the importance of sun protection and protective behaviors like broad-spectrum sunscreen that blocks both UVA and UVB radiation throughout the year (El-Zahraa et al., 2021).

4.3.1. Genetic Predisposition

By examining photodermatoses and UV-induced skin diseases, it is theoretically possible to assess the effect of genetic predisposition on susceptibility to these diseases. Genetic predisposition refers to the inherited likelihood of acquiring specific traits or diseases, which can significantly influence an individual's response to ultraviolet (UV) rays. Such genetic predisposition is particularly relevant for conditions polymorphous light eruption (PLE), which primarily affects fair-skinned individuals. Vulnerability to the effects of developing such disorders is heightened by genetic factors that affect skin pigmentation, immune response, and DNA repair systems. The interaction between one's genetic susceptibility and exposure to UV light intensifies the severity and incidence of photodermatoses, which brings into focus the need for individuals to realize their genetic susceptibility in taking measures against UV-induced dermatoses. Complicating the interplay between genetics and photodermatoses is the need to examine specific genetic mechanisms underlying these disorders. For instance, individuals with genetic variation in proteins involved in the skin's protective system may be more sensitive to UV radiation. It has been shown that the NRF2 pathway activation leading to the overexpression of cytoprotective proteins could have protective effects against some of the damage caused by UV radiation. By learning more about how genetic predispositions impact these pathways, scientists will be able to design targeted therapeutic interventions. Examination of individual genetic markers could not only be applied to the identification of at-risk individuals but also help in developing tailored treatment regimens for the management of UV-induced skin disease, thus adding a genetic component to preventative dermatology. Despite significant progress in elucidating genetic susceptibility to photodermatoses, gaps remain. While it is currently understood that certain genetic predispositions confer greater susceptibility, the genes and their mutations, in most cases, have yet to be fully characterized. For example, interindividual variation in responses to UVA and UVB radiation suggests that genetic factors may modulate the action spectrum of diseases such as PLE, but no comprehensive study has examined this. One of the basic requirements is further studies to explain such relationships, particularly in facilitating diagnostic tools and preventive strategies. Through the stimulation of increased awareness of genetic predisposition in the context of photodermatoses, clinical management of UV-associated skin disease can be optimized, leading to enhanced patient outcomes through tailored interventions and management of high-risk populations (Figure 4.8).

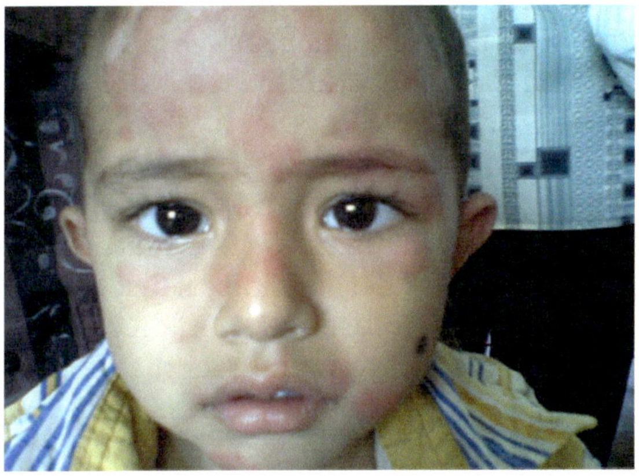

Figure 4.8. Multiple weals on face, demonstrating a clear genetic influence.

Source: https://www.researchgate.net/profile/Sahana-Srinivas-2/publication/232916934/figure/fig6/AS:297133661016076@1447853593921/Urticaria-multiple-weals-on-face.png.

4.3.2. Environmental Factors

The environmental determinants are the central mechanisms to induce exacerbation of photodermatoses and UV radiation-induced disorders. Of the determinants, the amount and duration of exposure to ultraviolet (UV) radiation are the major causes of skin injury. Due to increased urbanization and urban growth, land-use changes and atmospheric conditions have altered the levels of UV radiation. Specifically, global phenomena such as ozone layer depletion increase UV radiation at Earth's surface, leading to increased sunburns, photoaging, and skin cancer. In addition, reflective surfaces, including water, sand, and even snow, have the potential to amplify UV exposure, affecting susceptible populations. All these environmental problems must be addressed by public health programs that aim to reduce the burden of UV-related skin diseases and promote effective sun protection habits, especially among sensitive groups such as outdoor workers and children. The combination of environmental pollutants with UV radiation further complicates the case of photodermatoses. Airborne toxins, including particulate matter and volatile organic compounds, have the potential to increase the sensitivity of the skin and inflammatory reactions when synergistically coupled with UV radiation. This synergy often leads to exacerbated skin afflictions, such as eczema and contact dermatitis. People living in urban areas, where pollution is elevated, have a higher incidence of dermatological disorders due to UV exposure, according to studies. Further, the presence of these pollutants may alter the efficacy of local treatments, such as sunscreens, which can diminish their sun-protective effect against UV radiation. It is essential to understand the complex relationship between environmental pollutants and UV exposure to establish integrative prevention and management approaches for photodermatoses, tailoring public health interventions in a bid to prevent these risks as efficiently as possible. Over the past few years, heightened awareness of climate change and its potential health impacts has underscored the role of environmental factors in skin disease. Climate change and increased temperatures can influence UV radiation exposure and alter the distribution of photodermatoses. For example, warmer climates may lead to prolonged outdoor exposure, thereby increasing people's exposure to sunlight and UV radiation and increasing the risk of UV-related diseases. Furthermore, habitat alteration and alterations in biodiversity could affect the availability of natural photoprotecting compounds, such as polyphenols in plants, which have proven to decrease UV damage. The therapeutic potential of these natural products, such as the administration of rosehip oil rich in bioactive compounds, indicates their need for study concerning naturally integrated skin care applications. By incorporating environmental sensitivities and skin health, stakeholders can better plan preventive measures against photodermatoses and advocate for sustainable lifestyles that promote overall well-being in a changing environment.

4.3.3. Habits of Lifestyle and UV Exposure

The relationship between lifestyle and exposure to ultraviolet (UV) radiation is significant in explaining the onset and severity of photodermatoses and other UV-triggered skin diseases. The daily routine of individuals, outdoor activity rates, and sun protection significantly influence their total exposure to harmful UV radiation. People who engage in outdoor games or outdoor recreations without sun protection are likely to receive greater exposure to UV, thus exposing them to skin diseases like actinic keratosis and melanoma. In turn, inadequate knowledge of the ill effects of exposure to UV can lead to incorrect sun protection practices, such as neglecting to use sunscreen or protective clothing, to further heighten the possibility of skin damage and disorder due to overexposure to UV radiation.

Among the strongest lifestyle determinants of UV exposure is the behavior of tanning, either by sunbathing or the use of bed tanning. The pursuit of tanned skin has been a culturally ingrained want, often associating a garment's bronzed look with beauty and good health. The practice, however, too frequently results in increased exposure to UV radiation from both natural sunlight and artificial light. Reports indicate that regular users of tanning beds may be at increased risk for the incidence of skin cancers, particularly melanoma, due to the intense UV emissions that these machines emit. Moreover, chronic sunbathing leads to changes in the skin, such as premature aging and photodermatoses, as the skin's cellular matrix responds adversely to repeated UV exposure, underscoring the need for effective public health measures to promote healthier sun exposure behaviors. Furthermore, dietary matters and nutrition also play a critical role in the way our skin responds to UV exposure. Vitamins , such as antioxidants in fruits and vegetables can fortify skin defense mechanisms against UV ray damage. For instance, vitamins C and E have worked in preventing skin damage resulting from oxidative stress due to exposure to UV rays. Conversely, an inadequate diet that lacks protective vitamins can predispose individuals to increased skin damage and related conditions. Additionally, dietary hydration levels can influence skin barrier function; therefore, adequate intake of vitamins and minerals is essential. Essentially, maintaining a propositive lifestyle pattern, such as an optimum diet and sound sun protection, is key in minimizing the risk of photodermatoses as well as sun-sickness skin diseases, considering the interconnectedness of health behaviors and skin health in the case of UV exposure.

Test Your Knowledge

1. How does genetic predisposition contribute to the development of photodermatoses like polymorphous light eruption (PMLE)?
2. Which environmental factors can increase the likelihood or severity of photodermatoses?

4.4. Symptoms and Diagnosis

Learning Outcome

1. Describe common symptoms of photodermatoses.
2. Explain diagnostic methods and tools.
3. Differentiate between types of skin disorders.

The spectrum of symptoms of the photodermatoses is extremely variable, depending on the specific disorder and on the mechanisms involved. For instance, erythema and blistering, as typically seen in solar urticaria, may progress to severe manifestations, such as increased sensitivity to sunlight observed in disorders such as xeroderma pigmentosum. Symptoms typically develop within a short period following sun exposure, with the immediate effects, such as swelling and itching, developing in some people, while others develop more delayed effects, such as skin cancers and hyperpigmentation. Accurate detection of such symptoms is crucial, especially among vulnerable populations , such as children, in which the symptoms may be indicative of more serious systemic diseases (Sjerobabski-Masnec et al., 2010). Awareness of this heterogeneity will be useful for early diagnosis of photodermatoses and underscore the importance of early medical intervention to prevent the aggravation of skin lesions. Photodermatoses are primarily diagnosed clinically by taking a patient history and documenting the symptoms. A complete evaluation typically involves identifying the patterns of cutaneous responses to UVA/UVB radiation exposure, taking the medical history for any predisposing conditions, and excluding other dermatoses. Diseases xeroderma pigmentosum are diagnosed based on a combination of clinical presentation and supportive tests, including cell assays for defective DNA repair, which are foundational for elucidating the pathology of UV-induced damage (Lehmann et al., 2011). The presence of characteristic markers skin changes at early onset and a history of sunburn, can also direct the process of diagnosis. Accurate diagnosis is not only important for the successful management of such disorders but also to provide prognostic information that can direct treatment and prevention efforts. Beyond the standard clinical examination, advances in genetic sequencing and molecular diagnostics have improved the accuracy of photodermatoses diagnoses. Techniques , such as DNA mutation analysis enable clinicians to identify the specific genetic mutations causing such conditions as xeroderma pigmentosum and other inherited photodermatoses. Such a gene-oriented approach can be applied to both the care of individual patients and general family screening regimens, allowing high-risk individuals to implement prevention strategies against UV exposure (Lehmann et al., 2011). Moreover, early detection of symptoms has been associated with better outcomes, thereby preventing the emergence of skin malignancies and other complications. Increased awareness of symptoms and early diagnosis support patient treatment and public health efforts to reduce the incidence of serious UV-induced skin disorders.

4.4.1. Symptoms of Photodermatoses

Photodermatoses are a group of skin conditions that result from exposure to ultraviolet (UV) light, with a range of signs and symptoms that can significantly impair quality of life in affected individuals. They are often characterized by an inflammatory response that can take the form of erythema, or redness of the skin, that typically develops within hours of UV exposure. In addition to erythema, patients may experience pruritus (itching), which increases discomfort and can lead to secondary skin irritation. This redness is a direct consequence of the skin's immune response against UV-induced injury, reflecting the critical role of keratinocytes, the most common cell type in the epidermis, in modulating skin defense mechanisms. Consequently, identification of these early signs may enable prompt intervention and control, which is critical for individuals who are more susceptible to UV light and those at risk of photodermatoses.

Other than erythema and pruritus, photodermatoses can also manifest as vesicular eruptions, which are small, fluid-filled vesicles that form as a result of severe inflammatory reactions. The vesicles would eventually rupture, resulting in weeping lesions and crusting that reflect ongoing skin damage. Another important symptom is desquamation, or peeling of the skin, that may occur as the skin attempts to heal from the inflammation. Symptoms might be more pronounced in darker skin, which may also exhibit changes in pigmentation from UV exposure. This condition underscores the need for tailored educational interventions on skin protection and care procedures for each skin type, given that photodermatoses-induced lesions may vary in appearance and severity by skin type. Furthermore, individuals may experience the longer-term consequences of photodermatoses, such as dyspigmentation resulting from cumulative or repeated UV exposure. This can present as hyperpigmentation, an increase in pigmentation of the skin resulting from overproduction of melanin, or hypopigmentation, a decrease in skin pigmentation due to loss of melanin. The presence of such symptoms is not only cosmetically unpleasant but also indicates underlying damage to skin health. Interestingly, individuals with color in their skin possess unique features, in that they possess greater levels of melanin, which can alter their perception of photodermatoses. Evidence highlights that although melanin has some protective effect against UV damage, it fails to protect individuals entirely from the adverse effects of UV exposure, such as induction of pigmentary disorders (Krutmann et al., 2022). This dichotomy between risk and protective factors highlights the complexity of managing symptoms in photodermatoses and the value of photoprotective education, as well as the specificity of therapeutic interventions.

4.4.2. Diagnostic Methods and Tools

One of the major factors in the treatment of photodermatoses and UV dermatoses is the effective diagnostic methods and strategies employed by physicians. Diagnosis is crucial, as reactions to UV radiation can vary widely among individuals, depending on skin type, underlying disease, and genetic factors. Normal clinical evaluation, along with appropriate patient histories and symptom reviews, constitutes the foundation for diagnosing the condition. In addition, advanced diagnostic techniques, such as photo testing play a very important role. Phototests typically involve exposing the skin to defined levels of UV light to quantify an individual's sensitivity and identify disorders such as solar urticaria and chronic actinic dermatitis, which are characterized by increased but inappropriate skin reactions to ultraviolet light.

They foster a deeper understanding of a patient's specific condition and inform subsequent treatment strategies. Photobiological testing has made it possible to develop new diagnostic instruments that tell us more about how exposure to UV produces varying results in various types of skin. A case in point is spectroradiometry, which is increasingly being utilized to test UV sources and offer critical information on the natural and artificial light environments (Oliver , 2006).

This device assesses the spectral power distribution of light sources and enables clinicians to measure potential harm from different types of UV radiation. In addition, research at Ninewells Hospital's Photobiology Unit emphasizes the requirement for testing artificial sources, such as sunbeds, which are most commonly used in cosmetic and therapeutic applications. With standardized measurement techniques and regulatory requirements, healthcare providers can enhance the assessment and risk reduction of such light sources to protect patients' safety. With continued advancements in diagnostic methods, the application of digital modalities, such as teledermatology, presents new possibilities for improved patient outcomes in patients with disorders resulting from exposure to UV light. With mobile technology, patients can take photographs and forward them to dermatologists for distant diagnoses and interventions at rapid speeds. This is highly effective in populations with limited access to specialist services (Oliver & Balachandran, 2006). Moreover, the use of artificial intelligence to examine patients at the outset enables the automation of the initial examination, providing clinicians with preliminary information that can guide subsequent diagnostic procedures. These advances in technology not only increase efficiency but also provide patients with individually tailored treatment plans based on their specific needs and skin types, thereby enhancing the quality of care for photodermatoses and UV-induced cutaneous disorders (Figure 4.9).

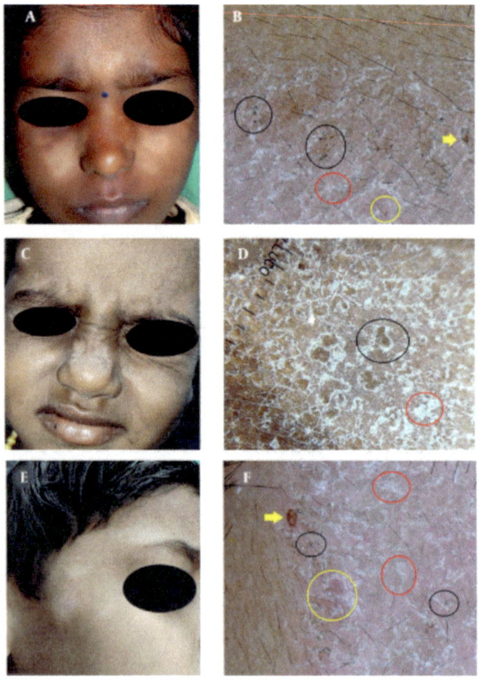

Figure 4.9. A, C, and E, Clinical images of polymorphous light eruption showing hypopigmented patches on the face; B, D, and F, Corresponding dermoscopy showing yellow clod signs (serocrusts) (yellow arrows), clustered red dots (yellow circles), and coarse brown scales (black circles). Note the coarse white scales (red circles) and the light brown background.

Source: https://www.researchgate.net/profile/Balachandra-Ankad/publication/358245398/figure/fig2/AS:11431281104753983@1670238044778/A-C-and-E-Clinical-images-of-polymorphous-light-eruption-showing-hypopigmented-patches.ppm.

4.4.3. Differentiating Between Types of Skin Disorders

Skin disease classification is complex due to the polyfactorial etiology of these conditions. Among them, photodermatoses constitute a distinct category, characterized by abnormal cutaneous reactions to UV light. Polymorphic light eruption (PLE) and solar urticaria are excellent examples of such conditions, manifesting as an eruptive rash or systemic hypersensitivity soon after sun exposure. Differentiation from other cutaneous conditions is necessary in order to treat them properly, because overlapping symptoms with non-photodermatosis conditions, such as contact dermatitis or psoriasis, are prevalent. Additionally, patients with systemic illnesses, that is, lupus erythematosus, show characteristic photosensitivity, expanding the range of symptoms caused by exposure to UV radiation. Detection of specific stimuli and reactions in photodermatoses enables appropriate therapeutic interventions, thereby improving patient outcomes (Walchner et al., 1997). Notably, UV radiation's impact on skin health extends beyond its immediate effects, with long-term consequences if not addressed appropriately. Photodermatoses, as a reaction to external stressors, typically become worse with prolonged sun exposure, leading to more severe dermatoses as well as increased risk for skin cancer. For instance, patients with lupus erythematosus develop an exacerbated response to UV radiation, thus requiring differential diagnosis in order to exclude other inflammatory cutaneous conditions in favor of photodermatosis. Studies indicate that controlled UV light exposure can demarcate unique characteristics of these skin diseases so that they can be diagnosed aptly and firmly suggest the integration of standardized test protocols in dermatology practice (Walchner et al., 1997). The segregation is of prime importance not only for classifying skin diseases but also for implementing appropriate prevention and treatment regimens. Furthermore, the development of protective pharmacological therapies against UV-induced cutaneous damage has become a priority research area in dermatology. Through an understanding of the barrier properties of the skin and the skin's response to UV radiation, researchers identify NRF2 activation as a protective process. Induction of cytoprotective proteins may enable protection of photodermatoses patients from the harmful effects of UV radiation. This line of research points to the importance of differentially treating according to the nature of dermatological disease. Additionally, because cutaneous and systemic diseases overlap, an appreciation of these nuances—particularly in photodermatoses—will guide research toward specific interventions and improvements in patient quality of life. Overall, advances in recognizing the distinguishing features of skin diseases will be key to dermatological well-being (Figure 4.10).

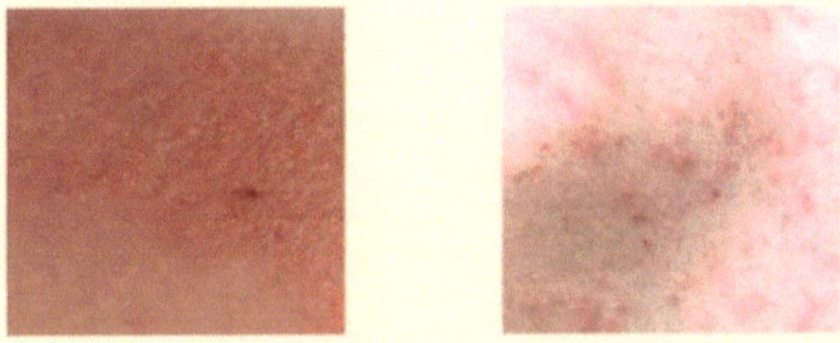

Figure 4.10. Solar urticaria vs PLE.

Source: https://knyamed.com/cdn/shop/files/solar-urticaria-vs-pmle-708x364.jpg?v=1716897593&width=600.

Test Your Knowledge

1. What are the typical symptoms of polymorphous light eruption (PMLE)?
2. What diagnostic tool is commonly used to confirm a photodermatosis and determine sensitivity to specific wavelengths of light?

4.5. Treatment Options

Learning Outcome

1. Discuss about topical therapies for management of photodermatoses and UV-induced skin disorders.
2. Understand the concept of phototherapy.
3. Focus on systemic treatments of photodermatoses and UV-induced skin disorders.

Effective therapeutic strategies for photodermatoses and ultraviolet (UV)-sensitizing diseases have also attracted increased interest, as their pathophysiology is better understood. One promising strategy is to apply topical and oral photoprotective substances, particularly those of natural origin. Fernblock®, an aqueous fern extract of the fern Polypodium leucotomos, has emerged recently as an interesting candidate, with outstanding safety and efficacy profiles in clinical practice. This extract not only protects against damage caused by harmful UV radiation but also facilitates photodynamic therapy (PDT) for actinic keratoses (AKs) and other diseases. Studies have demonstrated its effectiveness in relieving photodermatoses and associated inflammatory dermal diseases; thus, it is an essential component of the treatment kit for individuals with a predisposition to UV-induced damage (Rodríguez-Luna et al.,

2023). These advances underscore the need for integrating innovative therapies into multisector management regimens for such individuals. Apart from botanicals, the therapeutic potential of antioxidants in the management of sun-related skin disorders cannot be overstated. Reactive oxygen and nitrogen species (ROS and RNS) are, according to existing literature, significant causatives of skin damage brought about by UV and visible light irradiation. Therefore, the use of topical antioxidants in skin care is extremely critical. Studies have shown that plant-based antioxidants can effectively neutralize oxidative injury, thereby providing protection against solar urticaria and chronic actinic dermatitis, among other conditions. Furthermore, cosmetic products containing vitamins C and E, along with other active pharmaceutical ingredients (APIs), have been shown to neutralize free radicals and mitigate the deleterious effects of light exposure. These antioxidant-enriched creams not only impart photoprotection but also contribute to slowing down the skin aging process, and thus are relevant in the case of patients with the treatment of photodermatoses and allied disorders (Pandey et al., 2023).

Finally, the advent of tinted sunscreens and antioxidant-enriched preparations underscores the multidisciplinary nature of the treatment of photodermatoses. These proprietary products are designed to provide broad-spectrum protection against UV and visible light while simultaneously relieving environmentally induced oxidative stress. In patients with increased sensitivity, the synergy of VL-blocking agents and potent antioxidants is a synergistic approach for the reduction of erythema and pigmentation, particularly in sensitive skin. Recent advances in sunscreen technology have led to new strategies for enhancing photoprotection with more targeted treatments. As the number of researchers examining the application of antioxidants and radical scavengers in daily skincare increases, prospects are good for patients of photodermatoses and diseases induced by UV light (Pandey et al., 2023; Rodríguez-Luna et al., 2023) (Figure 4.11).

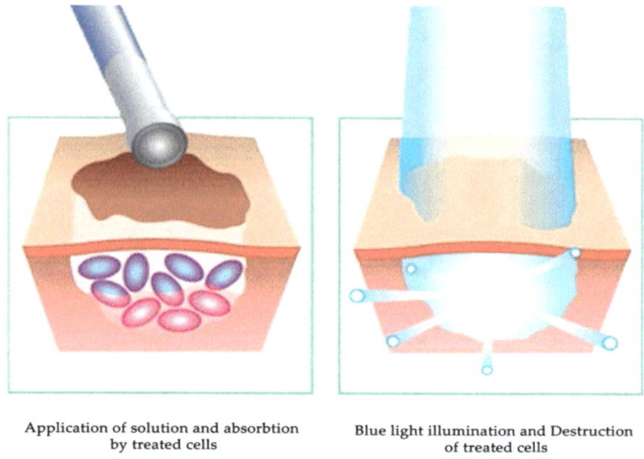

Figure 4.11. Complements photodynamic therapy (PDT).

Source: https://www.compdermcenter.com/wp-content/uploads/2016/02/Levulan-image-1.jpg.

4.5.1. Topical Therapies

Management of photodermatoses and skin disorders caused by ultraviolet radiation is frequently achieved with topical therapy aimed at mitigating the adverse effects of ultraviolet radiation. A major benefit of these treatments is the localized action, which permits focused treatment at the area of damage without a systemic effect due to oral medication. Various formulations, including creams, gels, and ointments, are available and can deliver the active constituents directly to the site of action. Natural extracts, notably, have been shown to protect against UV-induced cell damage in clinical studies. These include Prunus persica extracts. By activation of nuclear factor E2-related factor 2 (Nrf2), these treatments enhance the antioxidant defense system of the skin and resistance of cells to oxidative stress, suggesting a new future orientation for cosmetic and therapeutic applications for UV disorders (Kim et al., 2025).

In addition to natural extracts, traditional topical therapies , such as corticosteroids and calcineurin inhibitors have also been utilized to manage photodermatoses. They exert their effects through anti-inflammatory and immunomodulatory mechanisms, ultimately promoting the healing of skin lesions. Due to side effects and long-term therapy, there is an increased interest in synergizing these conventional therapies with complementary ones herbal supplements, in order to increase efficacy and reduce side effects. Recent studies have demonstrated that topical therapy with herbal extracts such as Aloe vera and Calendula officinalis significantly enhances skin healing when combined with routine treatments. These extracts not only help in reducing inflammation but also assist in the regeneration of skin integrity through an enhancement of antioxidant enzyme activities, thereby reversing the oxidative cutaneous damage after exposure to UV (Verma, S., & Vishwakant. , 2024). As demand for efficient and safe treatments for UV-induced skin disorders increases, the role of topical therapy in clinical practice warrants special consideration.

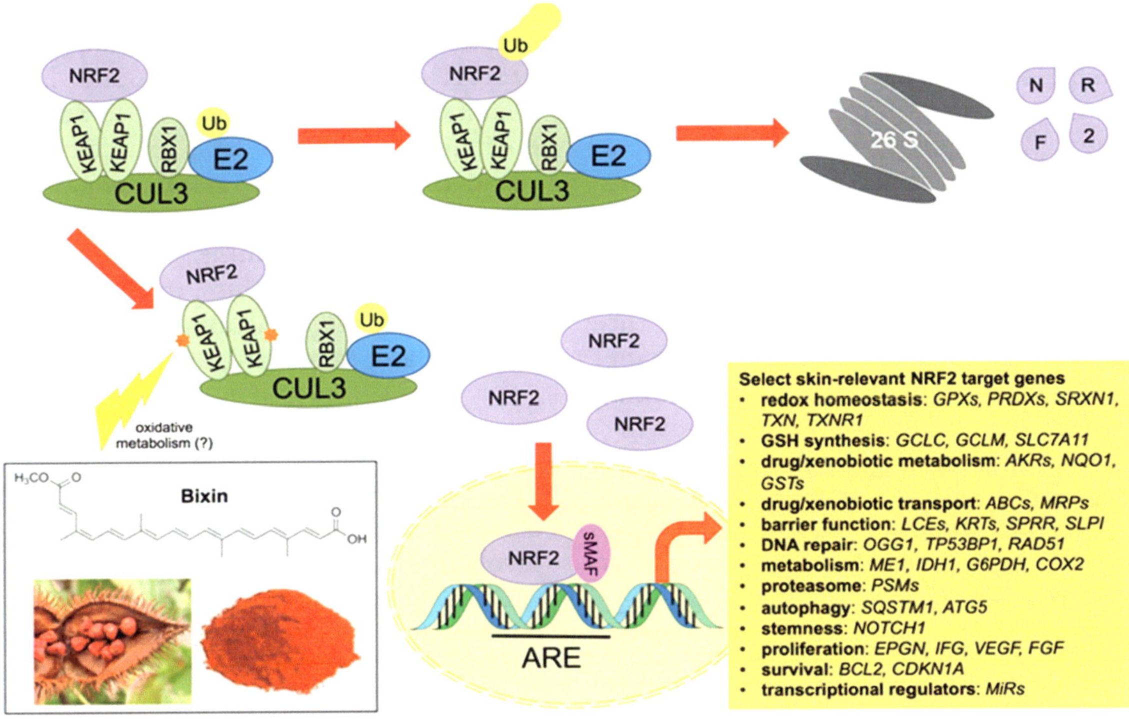

Figure 4.12. The nuclear factor-E2-related factor 2 (NRF2) pathway with a focus on skin barrier function and environmental stress protection.

Source: https://www.researchgate.net/publication/321909421/figure/fig1/AS:11431281212396210@1702617295661/The-nuclear-factor-E2-related-factor-2-NRF2-pathway-with-a-focus-on-skin-barrier.tif.

The hope of the therapy is the potential for multipronged protection against the multiplicity of mechanisms of UV damage. For instance, studies have shown that certain topical substances can inhibit lipid peroxidation and enhance the skin's natural repair mechanisms to avoid further progression of photodermatoses. Innovative formulation strategies that combine classic topical drugs with synergistic medicinal plant preparations could be a revolutionary approach in dermatology, not only treating acute manifestations but also protecting long-term skin integrity. Finally, a mechanistic understanding of how these treatments function could provide access to the identification of novel, patient-specific approaches to therapy and prevention of UV-induced skin disorders and help ensure that patients receive the best possible treatment (Verma, S., & Vishwakant. , 2024; Kim et al., 2025) (Figure 4.12).

4.5.2. Phototherapy

Phototherapy is a vital modality for managing photodermatoses and light-assisted skin diseases, with various wavelengths of light used to induce beneficial biological responses. Employing light from the ultraviolet (UV), visible, and infrared (IR) ranges, phototherapy effectively controls skin conditions, such as psoriasis, eczema, and vitiligo, as well as enhancing overall skin health. The mechanism of action is the activation of cellular pathways that enhance skin healing, quell inflammation, and potentially inhibit the formation of UV-induced skin cancers. Once again, patients often have sudden relief of symptoms and improvement in their well-being following phototherapy, emphasizing the therapeutic role of light in dermatology. The incorporation of antioxidant compounds into phototherapy treatment has become increasingly popular in improving the outcome of photodermatoses. One example is the extract of Polypodium leucotomos (PL), which is known to possess strong antioxidant effects that counteract the impact of UV-induced oxidative stress on cells in the skin. Besides neutralizing reactive oxygen species (ROS), PL also plays a role in repairing DNA and hence protecting the integrity of the skin from the harmful effects of UV light. This methodology is particularly pertinent to the reality that UV-induced photooxidative damage is a precursor of many skin diseases, including photoaging and skin cancers. The incorporation of PL into phototherapy regimens can complement traditional treatments by augmenting and supporting endogenous skin protection, as evidenced by clinical trials demonstrating efficacy against diseases such as actinic keratoses and other photodermatoses (Parrado et al., 2020). Further studies prove that chronic low-dose exposure to UV, a common method of phototherapy, can cause the adaptive antioxidant response of the skin and therefore enhance its resistance to photodermatologic disease. Studies have found that enzymes such as manganese superoxide dismutase (SOD2) and glutathione peroxidase (GPx1) play a significant role in protection mechanisms. When exposed to sublethal doses of UVA radiation, skin fibroblasts show enhanced expression and activity of SOD_2, leading to enhanced cellular protection against subsequent high-dose UV challenge (Wlaschek, M., & Scharffetter-Kochanek, K., 2004). This adaptive response also demonstrates the potential of phototherapy not only as a therapeutic modality but also as a means of retraining the skin's defenses against UV-induced injury, thereby manifesting the bivalent role of healing light in promoting recovery and enhancing skin resistance.

4.5.3. Systemic Treatments

The treatment of photodermatoses and skin diseases caused by ultraviolet exposure typically involves systemic therapy. Systemic therapies include numerous pharmacologic treatments designed to treat the internal and external symptoms of skin disease caused by ultraviolet radiation exposure. Among these therapies, immunosuppressive drugs corticosteroids and systemic retinoids have shown promise. Corticosteroids, on the other hand, may inhibit inflammation and reduce immune activity, providing relief in acute exacerbations of diseases such as polymorphous light eruption and lupus erythematosus. Systemic retinoids can also reorganize keratinocyte proliferation and differentiation, thereby playing a significant role in the treatment of dysregulated growth disorders. These therapies not only address the skin's surface but also shift the underlying immune reactions, presenting a more complete management approach. Beyond traditional pharmacologic treatment, more recent evidence has begun to look at the interaction between the gut microbiome and the skin, providing the avenue for novel systemic treatment approaches. The gut microbiome is a dynamic population of microorganisms that plays a significant role in immune function and overall skin health. Disruption, or dysbiosis, of this microbial community has the potential to exacerbate cutaneous conditions related to UV. Research has also shown that normalization of gastrointestinal microbiota balance through probiotic administration or dietary modification can improve symptoms in photodermatoses. This new field of research centers on the interplay between systemic and cutaneous well-being, opening new avenues for a therapy that integrates gut and skin treatments. In addition to pharmacologic treatments, systemic treatments also involve behavior and lifestyle changes, particularly with respect to exposure to UV. More and more evidence is found to indicate that UV radiation is capable of triggering physiological reactions, like increased appetite, through mechanisms involving p53 protein in epidermal keratinocytes. Systemic effects in this manner can direct treatment modalities involving dietary regulation and behavior modification on top of pharmacotherapy. By managing not just the symptoms of photodermatoses, but also the overall determinants of health affected by UV exposure, such as diet and mood, clinicians can optimize the effectiveness of treatments. This systematic review of systemic treatments represents a hopeful frontier in the treatment of photodermatoses, ultimately aiming for a synergistic effect in improving patient outcomes and quality of life (Parikh et al., 2023; Criton et al., 2024) (Figure 4.13).

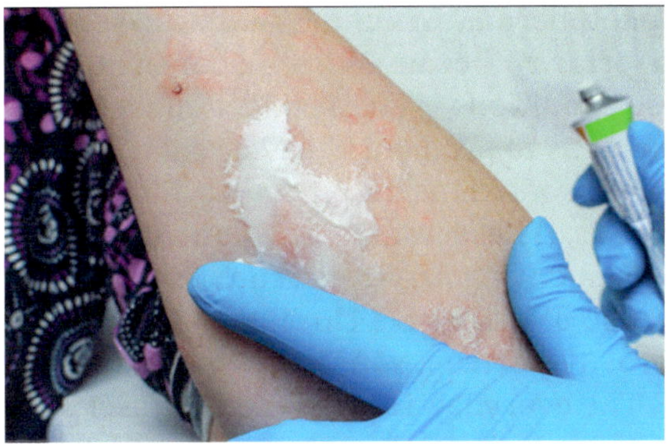

Figure 4.13. Using topical steroids.

Source: https://d8tzmbmuvomgp.cloudfront.net/medialibrary/pce-content/the-exchange/images/142/exchange-post-topical-steroids.png.

Test Your Knowledge

1. What topical treatments are commonly used for managing mild photodermatoses , such as polymorphous light eruption (PMLE)?
2. How can phototherapy be used as a preventive treatment for photodermatoses?

4.6. Prevention Strategies

Learning Outcome

1. Discuss sun protection measures.
2. Understand education and awareness campaigns.
3. Explain the role of dermatologists in the prevention of photodermatoses and UV-induced skin disorders.

Implementation of effective prevention strategies for photodermatoses and UV-induced conditions is a priority because the global incidence of these conditions is increasing. Public education campaigns to promote behavior changes related to sun protection are among the most crucial methods. These campaigns contribute to the public adopting practices , such as avoiding the sun, use of protective clothing, and application of broad-spectrum sunscreen with appropriate SPF. The everyday, regular use of sunscreen can effectively reduce exposure to UV radiation, the largest reason for skin damage and resultant cancer, with NMSC being one of the largest contributors (Asad et al., 2025). Furthermore, attention has to be given to the detrimental effect of UV radiation directed towards vulnerable individuals with light skin, history of family skin cancers, or past history of skin illness, thereby fostering a culture of prudent care of one's own skin well-being. Another extremely important element of prevention strategies is the growing role of oral supplements in enhancing photoprotection. Studies have shown that nicotinamide (NAM), a derivative of vitamin B3, is highly photoprotective, promoting DNA repair and preventing the formation of skin tumors (Pihl et al., 2024). When combined with other compounds , such as phloroglucinol, NAM has been shown to further augment its protective role against damage brought about by the ultraviolet spectrum. Because these supplements are increasingly accepted as adjuncts to topical sun-prevention regimens, they offer a new option for patients to enhance protection against skin disease. This multi-layered prevention approach combining lifestyle changes with nutritional therapy can give people more control over their skin's health and reduce the danger of UV exposure by a substantial amount. In addition to individual- and community-level interventions, policy-level initiatives for mass-scale UV protection are necessary. Laws, such as mandates of usage of UV protective measures in schools and outdoor environments, can significantly contribute towards public health security. In addition, unifying efforts with dermatological specialists in implementing measures for screening of skin on a regular basis can lead to improved therapeutic outcomes due to early diagnosis of UV-related alterations in the skin. Policymakers also need to encourage funding for research into new prevention technologies and treatments for photodermatoses. In incorporating these actions in public health policy, the impact of UV-induced skin diseases can effectively be reduced, fostering a healthier population in order to offset the detrimental effects of sun exposure (Asad et al., 2025).

4.6.1. Sun Protection Measures

Practical sun protection is essential for preventing the risk of photodermatoses and other skin diseases caused by ultraviolet radiation. These methods aim to reduce exposure to damaging ultraviolet light, which plays a central role in the etiology of most skin diseases. Central among these methods is the application of broad-spectrum sunscreens, which protect against UVA and UVB light. It is necessary for individuals, especially those with light-colored skin, to apply sunscreens with a high sun protection factor (SPF) on a regular basis, especially in the middle of the day. Furthermore, dermatological recommendations are to reapply sunscreen every two hours and more frequently when swimming or perspiring. However, it is worthy of note that darker-skinned people have a natural feeling of protection against exposure to the sun due to increased melanin content, and this might extend to carelessness with the use of sunscreen. Therefore, educating individuals across all skin types about the importance of sunscreen remains key to preventing skin diseases caused by UV exposure (Krutmann et al., 2022). In addition to sunscreen, protective clothing serves as a practical and efficient means of protection from UV radiation. Tight-weave clothing, wide-brimmed hats, and sunglasses with UV-blocking ability can significantly limit the degree of sun exposure. This complex prevention of photoprotection is required, as clothing can shield the skin not just from direct sun exposure but also reduce the risk of skin cancers, such as melanoma and non-melanoma skin cancers, that are most prevalent in people with high sun exposure. Further, shielding oneself from sun exposure during peak sun hours, typically between 10 a.m. and 4 p.m., is an essential preventive measure. By implementing these behavior modifications and using sunscreen, individuals can develop robust protective measures. The impetus to initiate such practices is strengthened by the increasing incidence of photodermatoses and UV-induced disorders worldwide, underscoring the importance of appropriate photoprotection for public health (Mohiuddin, 2019). Public education programs play an essential role in promoting effective sun protection behaviors among diverse populations. A crucial element of such campaigns is dispelling myths about UV radiation and its effects on diverse skin types. For instance, individuals with skin of color will tend to downplay their risk for UV-induced damage and associated skin disorders. As proposed in the literature, such a group may not delve so deeply into photoprotective practices and, consequently, be more likely to acquire pigmentary disorders and sun-induced alteration of the skin. Therefore, focused learning programs should encourage the importance of uniform sun protection practices, such as the frequent use of broad-spectrum sunscreens and protective clothing. Just as critical, these programs should encourage product innovation aimed at creating suitable sunscreens for every skin type, particularly increased cosmetic suitability for people with dark skin, to encourage a broader sun protection agenda (Krutmann et al., 2022) (Figure 4.14).

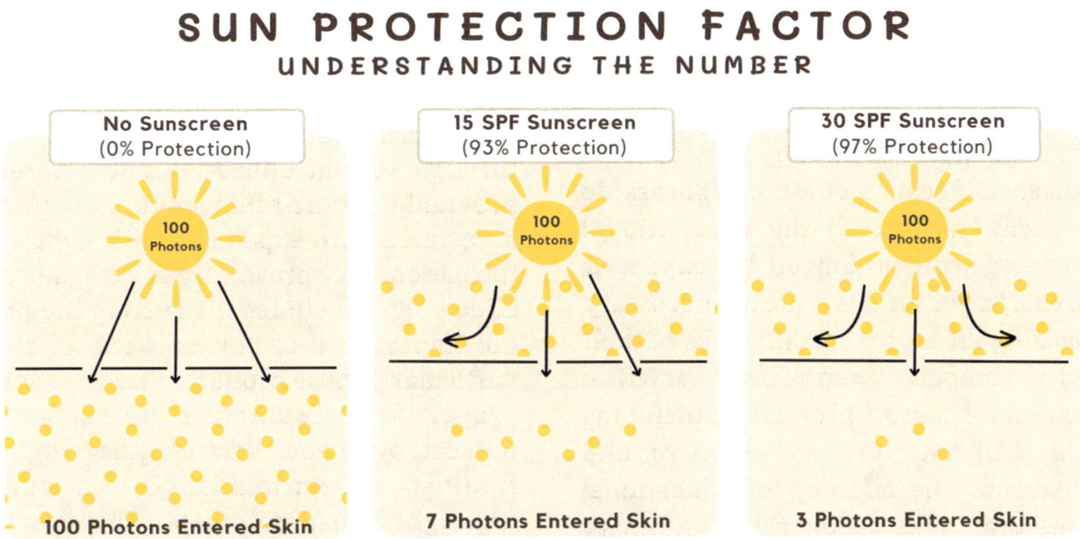

Figure 4.14. Sun protection factor (SPF).

Source: https://s.guavahealth.com/article-img/decoding-spf/spf-explained.png.

4.6.2. Education and Awareness Campaigns

Effective sensitization and education campaigns are crucial for addressing the high incidence of photodermatoses and other cutaneous disorders caused by UV exposure. The campaigns ought to offer information regarding the hazards of ultraviolet (UV) radiation, particularly among groups that tend to play down the risks. Despite some awareness among some sections Black African men, many remain ignorant, under the mistaken belief that sun protection is unimportant or only for women. This ignorance highlights the need for targeted educational interventions that get across the importance of sun protection for all, irrespective of gender and skin type. Knowledge that dark skin also requires protection from UV radiation is vital; educating the public about this can significantly reduce the risk of skin disease. This is due to overexposure to the sun, and therefore, a better skin culture in all populations (Mayeza, 2021).

In professional and business contexts, greater awareness of the risks of UV exposure is particularly important for outdoor workers. Studies have established that field labor exposes workers to considerable solar radiation, increasing vulnerability to adverse health consequences, including skin cancers and eye disease. Because outdoor laborers do not necessarily experience the occupational risks associated with prolonged UV exposure, education campaigns on this issue are necessary. By emphasizing the highly specific risks of their line of work, campaigns can provide practical recommendations for UV protection, including wearing appropriate protective attire and using sunscreen. The addition of educational components that make visible the preliminary signs of skin damage can enable workers to seek timely medical counseling and preventive care, ultimately developing a culture of safety and health in outdoor labor sectors (Modenese et al., 2018). Initiating comprehensive education and awareness campaigns demands collaboration between health professionals, schools, and community-based organizations. Engaging such stakeholders increases the likelihood of developing educational campaigns that impact diverse populations. Useful education may include workshops, seminars, and community outreach that not only present information but also encourage discussion and highlight the necessity of protecting oneself from the sun. It is important that these programs employ culturally relevant messages and practices that resonate with the target audience, resulting in high levels of participation and retention. Additionally, continuous monitoring of campaign effectiveness through analysis and feedback can help refine these programs and address emerging knowledge gaps. Later, these help foster an enlightened public that enables individuals to take preventive action against UV-induced skin diseases, thereby maintaining overall skin health (Mayeza, 2021).

4.6.3. Prevention Role of Dermatologists

Dermatologists play a vital role in preventing photodermatoses and UV-induced skin disease through patient education and awareness. By providing detailed information about the risks associated with exposure to UV light, they help the patient take preventive steps against harmful effects. This includes instructing the patient on the importance of constant use of sunscreen, particularly those products that have antioxidant properties to counteract the oxidative stress induced by various wavelengths of light. Recent findings on antioxidant-based sunscreens highlight dermatologists' responsibility to advise patients with scientifically validated products. While research confirms that visible light aggravates specific skin illnesses, it is the responsibility of dermatologists to remain vigilant while informing patients of the relevance of photoprotection by means of more than mere traditional UV shielding, thereby supporting an incredibly protective measure against photodermatoses and skin damage (Pandey et al., 2023). Further along the preventive spectrum, dermatologists are also engaged in developing and disseminating customized treatment guidelines for diverse skin colors. Patients of color represent a unique patient subgroup that requires special attention under the umbrella of photoprotection. With the increased prevalence of photoexacerbated pigmentary conditions in these groups, it is the responsibility of dermatologists to ensure that patients understand the necessity of broad-spectrum sunscreens that are effective protectants against both UVA and visible light. Despite the inherent protective properties conferred by melanin, it is known to dermatologists that dark-skinned persons are oftentimes susceptible to underdiagnosis and undertreatment and, as a result, lose out on the protective modalities against photodermatoses (Granger et al., 2023). Dermatologists are hence leaders in advocating for greater awareness and designing more suitable products appropriate to the aesthetic and protective needs of patients with multiethnic skin colors. Patient education and customized treatment regimens aside, dermatologists are also actively involved with pharmaceutical companies and researchers to advance the science of photoprotection. Such cooperation is instrumental in disseminating information on the progress of revolutionary sunscreen products, which are specifically formulated for diverse skin types and conditions. By encouraging research that keeps the particular challenge of diverse populations in its consideration, dermatologists help formulate products that not only protect against UV radiation but also consider visible light as well as any accompanying photodermatoses. This collaborative effort places dermatologists in the vanguard of using therapeutic agents, such as vitamin E and other antioxidants, in products so that dermatologists provide comprehensive solutions for the maintenance of healthy skin. By doing so, they demonstrate a commitment to preventive care that extends beyond the clinic, promoting healthier skin for all patients and addressing most emergent issues associated with UV disorders (Pandey et al., 2023).

Test Your Knowledge

1. What are the most effective sun protection measures for preventing photodermatoses?
2. How do public education and awareness campaigns help reduce the incidence of UV-induced skin disorders?
3. What role do dermatologists play in preventing UV-induced skin disorders in at-risk populations?

SUMMARY

In short, it is essential to know photodermatoses and UV ray-induced dermatoses to comprehend the relationship between ultraviolet radiation and skin pathology. The diseases indicate the skin's vulnerability to environmental factors, particularly UV radiation, which has been shown to be a catalyst for a range of dermatoses. The impact of such an interaction is noteworthy, particularly among those who have pre-existing diseases , such as lupus erythematosus. UV exposure among these patients can cause severe skin lesions; therefore, a personalized treatment and diagnostic plan that accounts for the patient's sun sensitivity is important. This calls for standard testing in order to accurately identify and type such photosensitivity disorders, which will ultimately lead to improved outcomes for the patients as well as improved management plans overall (Walchner et al., 1997). Furthermore, the capacity to develop effective photoprotection strategies remains a significant consideration for individuals at risk of UV-induced dermatological disease. Recent research underscores the need for universal protection beyond traditional sunscreen products, including natural agents with novel protective effects. As an example, Fernblock®, a sesquiterpene compound derived from the fern plant Polypodium leucotomos, has emerged as a significant contributor to photoprotection. Its efficacy has been demonstrated in clinical practice, particularly for the treatment of diseases such as actinic keratoses and photodermatoses. Such advancements not only provide increased protection against the toxic action of UV light but also open up new therapeutic possibilities for the management of inflammatory and pigmentary disease induced by sunlight exposure (Rodríguez-Luna et al., 2023). In conclusion, the intricate interaction of photodermatoses, UV exposure, and skin disease warrants ongoing research into new prevention and treatment methodologies. The cumulative data for the role of UV radiation in inducing chronic skin damage and systemic illnesses like lupus emphasize the necessity for combating such health conditions at both individual and public health levels. Given the growing recognition of the many causes of this spectrum of conditions, including the roles of infrared and visible radiation, it is essential that health practitioners adopt a multimodal approach. This includes not only short-term protective treatments but also informed patient education on UV risk and the benefits of natural protective measures in daily practice. Combined, these interventions can be capable of lessening the severity of UV skin diseases and enhancing the quality of life of individuals with such diseases.

The resemblance among photodermatoses and skin disorders caused by UV indicates the critical role that ultraviolet (UV) radiation plays in changing skin well-being. Photodermatoses, that is, diseases of the skin caused by exposure to UV light, illustrate the physiological effects of solar radiation on the skin. UVA radiation, particularly the longest wavelengths, penetrates deeply into the skin and causes various alterations at the cellular level. Specifically, these rays initiate the production of reactive oxygen species (ROS), leading to oxidative stress that can damage lipids, proteins, and DNA in skin cells. The impact of these changes is photosensitivity, inflammatory response, and ultimately skin cancer as well. The body's reactions to chronic UV exposure, such as heightened inflammation or immunosuppression, again demonstrate the clinical effects arising from sun exposure over long periods of time, as highlighted in prevailing literature (Françoise Bernerd et al., 2022).

Clinical manifestations of photodermatoses can range from mild to serious and play an important role in impacting the quality of life of patients. These conditions, like polymorphous light eruption and solar urticaria, are representative of acute reactions to UV exposure with manifestations like blisters and rashes when exposed to the sun. Chronic damage due to UV radiation results in more long-lasting problems in the form of photoaging and an increased risk of skin cancers like melanoma and non-melanoma types. The skin's natural barrier function is crucial in preventing the harmful effects of UV radiation, but this protection can be easily compromised by environmental factors such as pollution and visible light, which can accelerate skin symptoms. Moreover, recent studies indicate that the integration of natural products can provide therapeutic benefit for such conditions, as these products have been shown to reduce inflammation and enhance skin healing (Zaid NAM et al., 2022). Preventive measures are integral in controlling and mitigating the severity of photodermatoses. The most effective method of mitigation is general sun protection, including the use of broad-spectrum sunscreens that also cover UVA and UVB. Physical and clothing barriers may be employed to further protect, particularly for individuals with heightened light sensitivity. An understanding of the additive nature of UV damage necessitates mass education campaigns that unmask the risks of sun exposure. In addition to guard reactions, recent advances in understanding natural products have highlighted their therapeutic potential in combating skin diseases. In addition to being anti-inflammatory and antioxidant, they also demonstrate the capacity to interact favorably with skin cells, shaping future treatment possibilities (Zaid NAM et al., 2022). The intersection of prophylactic and therapeutic strategies should provide a way to more effectively treat UV-induced skin conditions in susceptible individuals.

KEY TERMS FROM THIS CHAPTER

- Actinic keratosis
- Antioxidant defense system
- Cell damage
- Chronic actinic dermatitis
- Corticosteroids
- DNA repair pathways
- Hypersensitivity reaction
- Inflammatory dermal diseases
- Inflammatory skin disorder
- Active pharmaceutical ingredients (APIs)
- Calendula officinalis
- Cellular structures
- Chronic actinic dermatitis (CAD)
- DNA repair mechanisms
- Glutathione peroxidase (GPx1)
- Immune function
- Inflammatory reaction
- Infrared radiation

CRITICAL THINKING QUESTIONS

1. **Which of the following is an example of an idiopathic photodermatosis?**
   a. Xeroderma pigmentosum
   b. Polymorphous light eruption (PMLE)
   c. Drug-induced photosensitivity
   d. Systemic lupus erythematosus (SLE)
2. **What is the primary mechanism by which ultraviolet (UV) radiation causes skin damage?**
   a. Enhanced collagen synthesis
   b. Activation of melanin-producing enzymes
   c. Generation of reactive oxygen species (ROS) leading to DNA damage
   d. Suppression of keratinocyte proliferation
3. **Which of the following is a significant risk factor for developing photodermatoses?**
   a. High melanin levels in the skin
   b. Use of broad-spectrum sunscreen
   c. Cold climate exposure
   d. Genetic disorders affecting DNA repair mechanisms
4. **A patient presents with itchy, red, scaly patches on sun-exposed areas of the skin. Which symptom is most commonly associated with photodermatoses?**
   a. Petechiae
   b. Blistering and pruritus after sun exposure
   c. Cyanosis of extremities
   d. Deep dermal ulcerations
5. **Which of the following is an effective prevention strategy for photodermatoses and UV-induced skin disorders?**
   a. Daily exfoliation of the skin
   b. Application of topical steroids before sun exposure
   c. Avoiding sun exposure during peak hours and using broad-spectrum sunscreen
   d. Increasing UV exposure gradually to develop tolerance

Short Answer Questions

1. What are the common types of photodermatoses, and how do they differ in presentation?
2. What are the key mechanisms by which ultraviolet (UV) radiation damages the skin?
3. Which risk factors increase susceptibility to photodermatoses?
4. What are the hallmark symptoms associated with photodermatoses?
5. What topical therapies are effective in managing mild to moderate photodermatoses?
6. How is phototherapy used in the prevention or treatment of photodermatoses?
7. Which systemic treatments are considered for severe or refractory cases?
8. What prevention strategies are recommended to reduce UV-induced skin disorders?

Answer to Critical Thinking Questions

1. (b); 2. (c); 3. (d); 4. (b); 5. (c)

REFERENCES

1. El-Aziz, F. E. A., & Ali, M. (2021). Towards study of UV-C radiation effect on earthworms and isopods via electron microscopy. *Egyptian Academic Journal of Biological Sciences. B, Zoology*, *13*(2), 33–46. https://doi.org/10.21608/eajbsz.2021.189084Abdul Kader Mohiuddin. (2019). Sunscreen and suntan preparations. *ARC Journal of Pharmaceutical Sciences*. https://www.semanticscholar.org/paper/a1b7bdb046659f358d7b9bf64680c22f9c46b1d1 (accessed on 21st July 2025).

2. Pandey, P., Sinha, S., & Akhade, K. S. (2023). Effects of visible lights, photodermatoses and role of antioxidants in skin health. *International Journal of Research in Medical Sciences*, *11*(11), 4272–4276. https://doi.org/10.18203/2320-6012.ijrms20233418 (accessed on 21st July 2025).

3. Araki, S. M., & Baby, A. (2025). New perspectives on titanium dioxide and zinc oxide as inorganic UV filters: Advances, safety, challenges, and environmental considerations. *Cosmetics*. https://www.semanticscholar.org/paper/75af2fa35274fc013e5ecffe553881c9f5507593 (accessed on 21st July 2025).

4. Oliver, H. E., & Balachandran, W. (2006). The impacts of optical radiation in the environment on skin: Hazards, measurement, regulation and protection. Brunel University School of Engineering and Design PhD Theses. https://core.ac.uk/download/40071864.pdf (accessed on 21st July 2025).

5. Bernerd, F., Passeron, T., Castiel, I., & Marionnet, C. (2022). The damaging effects of long UVA (UVA1) rays: A major challenge to preserve skin health and integrity. *International Journal of Molecular Sciences, 23*, 8243–8243. https://doi.org/10.3390/ijms23158243 (accessed on 21st July 2025).

6. Walchner, M., Messer, G., & Kind, P. (1997). Phototesting and photoprotection in LE. *Lupus*, *6*(2), 167–174. https://doi.org/10.1177/096120339700600212(accessed on 21st July 2025).

7. Cohen, G., Dinkova-Kostova, A. T., Gruzman, A., Hofmann, A., et al. (2022). NRF2 in dermatological disorders: Pharmacological activation for protection against cutaneous photodamage and photodermatosis. https://core.ac.uk/download/524920780.pdf (accessed on 21st July 2025).

8. Criton, V. J. S., & Joy, S. (2024). Beyond skincare routines: Follow your gut to healthy skin–A review of the interplay between gut microbiome and skin. *Journal of Skin and Sexually Transmitted Diseases*. https://www.semanticscholar.org/paper/72bb3f99065818af8abdcd511f69614726cfc306 (accessed on 21st July 2025).

9. Rodríguez-Luna, A., Zamarrón, A., Juarranz, Á., & González, S. (2023). Clinical Applications of *Polypodium leucotomos* (Fernblock®): An Update. *Life (Basel, Switzerland)*, *13*(7), 1513. https://doi.org/10.3390/life13071513(accessed on 21st July 2025).

10. Gracia-Cazaña, T., Aguilera, J., Navarro-Bielsa, A., González, S., Lim, H. W., & Gilaberte, Y. (2024). New trends on personalized sunscreens. *Photodermatology Photoimmunology & Photomedicine, 40*. https://doi.org/10.1111/phpp.12967 (accessed on 21st July 2025).

11. Granger, C., Krutmann, J., Lim, H. W., Morgado-Carrasco, D., et al. (2023). Photoprotection for people with skin of colour: Needs and strategies. https://core.ac.uk/download/555344410.pdf (accessed on 21st July 2025).

12. Hölzle, E., Lehmann, P., Plewig, G., von Kries, R., et al. (1987). Polymorphous light eruption. https://core.ac.uk/download/82014085.pdf (accessed on 21st July 2025).

13. Khan, A. U., Wang, Q., Roh, E., Dickinson, S. E., Wondrak, G. T., Curiel-Lewandowski, C., Bode, A. M., et al. (2025). TOPK drives IL19-mediated crosstalk between cancer cells and fibroblasts to promote solar UV-induced skin damage and carcinogenesis. *Cancers*. https://www.semanticscholar.org/paper/471a453e7e8746d7954af3ed743de3f8587c8f02 (accessed on 21st July 2025).

14. Kim, E. O., Lee, D., Jung, C. J., Yu, Y., Hong, M., Cho, I., & Ku, S. (2025). *Prunus persica* leaf extract mitigates ultraviolet-induced skin damage via activation of AMP-activated protein kinase. *Natural Product Communications, 20*. https://www.semanticscholar.org/paper/09603f4432e19c8a43e99797060e1fc29379ed7b (accessed on 21st July 2025).

15. Kölgen, W., van Meurs, M., Jongsma, M., van Weelden, H., Bruijnzeel-Koomen, C., Knol, E., van Vloten, W. V., et al. (2004). Differential expression of cytokines in UV-B-exposed skin of patients with polymorphous light eruption: Correlation with Langerhans cell migration and immunosuppression. *Archives of Dermatology, 140*(3), 295–302. https://www.semanticscholar.org/paper/126f325454d5b8b811fc10c9097d5298d0b02007 (accessed on 21st July 2025).

16. Krolo, I., Lugović Mihić, L., Šitum, M., Bulat, V., & Čavka, V. (2008). Allergic hypersensitivity skin reactions following sun exposure. https://core.ac.uk/download/14407093.pdf (accessed on 21st July 2025).

17. Krutmann, J., Piquero-Casals, J., Morgado-Carrasco, D., Granger, C., Trullàs, C., Passeron, T., & Lim, H. W. (2022). Photoprotection for people with skin of color: Needs and strategies. *The British Journal of Dermatology, 188*(2), 168–175. https://www.semanticscholar.org/paper/6e065350aeaac1324276934454d05838054038c7 (accessed on 21st July 2025).

18. Lehmann, A. R., McGibbon, D., & Stefanini, M. (2011). Xeroderma pigmentosum. *Orphanet journal of rare diseases, 6*, 70. https://doi.org/10.1186/1750-1172-6-70(accessed on 21st July 2025).

19. Mayeza, Z. E. (2021). Knowledge, attitudes and practices of Black African males towards the use of sun protection: A case study of a University of Technology in KwaZulu-Natal. https://doi.org/10.51415/10321/4047 (accessed on 21st July 2025).

20. Modenese, A., Korpinen, L., & Gobba, F. (2018). Solar radiation exposure and outdoor work: An underestimated occupational risk. *International Journal of Environmental Research and Public Health, 15*, 2063–2063. https://doi.org/10.3390/ijerph15102063 (accessed on 21st July 2025).

21. Mohd Zaid, N. A., Sekar, M., Bonam, S. R., Gan, S. H., Lum, P. T., Begum, M. Y., Mat Rani, N. N. I., et al. (2022). Promising natural products in new drug design, development, and therapy for skin disorders: An overview of scientific evidence and understanding their mechanism of action. *Drug Design Development and Therapy, 16*, 23–66. https://doi.org/10.2147/dddt.s326332 (accessed on 21st July 2025).

22. Neale, R. E., Lucas, R., Byrne, S. N., Hollestein, L. M., Rhodes, L. E., Yazar, S., Young, A. R., et al. (2023). The effects of exposure to solar radiation on human health. *Photochemical & Photobiological Sciences, 22*, 1011–1047. https://doi.org/10.1007/s43630-023-00375-8 (accessed on 21st July 2025).

23. Oargă (Porumb), D. P., Cornea-Cipcigan, M., Nemeș, S. A., & Cordea, M. (2025). The effectiveness of a topical rosehip oil treatment on facial skin characteristics: A pilot study on wrinkles, UV spots reduction, erythema mitigation, and age-related signs. *Cosmetics*. https://www.semanticscholar.org/paper/cff6a6bd59157747d3caf4d60265ddfaae20a2ee (accessed on 21st July 2025).
24. Oliver, H. E. (2006). The impacts of optical radiation in the environment on skin: Hazards, measurement, regulation and protection. https://core.ac.uk/download/337720.pdf (accessed on 21st July 2025).
25. Pandey, P., Sinha, S. P., & Akhade, K. S. (2023). Effects of visible lights, photodermatoses and role of antioxidants in skin health. *International Journal of Research in Medical Sciences, 11*, 4272–4276. https://doi.org/10.18203/2320-6012.ijrms20233418 (accessed on 21st July 2025).
26. Parikh, S., Parikh, R., Harari, M., Weller, A., Bikovski, L., & Levy, C. (2023). Skin epidermal keratinocyte p53 induces food uptake upon UV exposure. *Frontiers in Behavioral Neuroscience, 17*. https://www.semanticscholar.org/paper/14f1ca6e8d90c5a5f132635efed7d1ed9a0da9c9 (accessed on 21st July 2025).
27. Parrado, C., Nicolás, J., Juarranz, Á., & González, S. (2020). The role of the aqueous extract *Polypodium leucotomos* in photoprotection. *Photochemical & Photobiological Sciences, 19*, 831–843. https://www.semanticscholar.org/paper/3e68cd30cd73944c3a248d04d3399a0e85b655c9 (accessed on 21st July 2025).
28. Patil, N., Bubna, A., Krishnamoorthy, M., & Joseph, L. (2023). A clinicopathological study of polymorphous light eruption. *Clinical Dermatology Review, 7*, 215–222. https://www.semanticscholar.org/paper/16fb1fe1615741ea71c0b47ddae7ef72cff7e652 (accessed on 21st July 2025).
29. Pihl, C., Andersen, F., Bjerring, P., Haedersdal, M., & Lerche, C. (2024). Efficacy of combinational treatment versus nicotinamide monotherapy in the prevention of ultraviolet radiation-induced skin cancer. *Dermatology, 240*, 453–461. https://www.semanticscholar.org/paper/9792394537fc1ca837f38c25dd93873dd89df126 (accessed on 21st July 2025).
30. Reichrath, J., Vogt, T., Holick, M. F., & Friedrich, M. (2022). Abstracts of the joint international symposia “Vitamin D in prevention and therapy” and “Biologic effects of light.” *Anticancer Research, 42*, 2193–2222. https://doi.org/10.21873/anticanres.15702 (accessed on 21st July 2025).
31. Salman, S., Paulet, V., Hardonnière, K., & Kerdine-Römer, S. (2025). The role of NRF2 transcription factor in inflammatory skin diseases. *Biofactors (Oxford, England), 51*. https://www.semanticscholar.org/paper/818e62ca8cdc776c056ca2bac02808445d907965 (accessed on 21st July 2025).
32. Sjerobabski-Masnec, I., Kotrulja, L., Šitum, M., Poduje, S., & Ožanić-Bulić, S. (2010). Photosensitivity skin disorders in childhood. https://core.ac.uk/download/14422812.pdf (accessed on 21st July 2025).
33. Verma, S., & Vishwakant. (2024). Effects of herbal extracts on the healing of UV-induced skin damage in albino rats (*Rattus norvegicus*). *Journal for Research in Applied Sciences and Biotechnology*. https://www.semanticscholar.org/paper/fbe1e36f831d2a6e509978b2491b03309fbdcb85 (accessed on 21st July 2025).
34. Wlaschek, M., & Scharffetter-Kochanek, K. (2004). Adaptive antioxidant response and photoaging. *International Journal of Cosmetic Science, 26*, 107–108. https://www.semanticscholar.org/paper/bb77afca936d29f1947b70f17f59203945b06e90 (accessed on 21st July 2025).

OCCUPATIONAL SKIN DISEASES

5

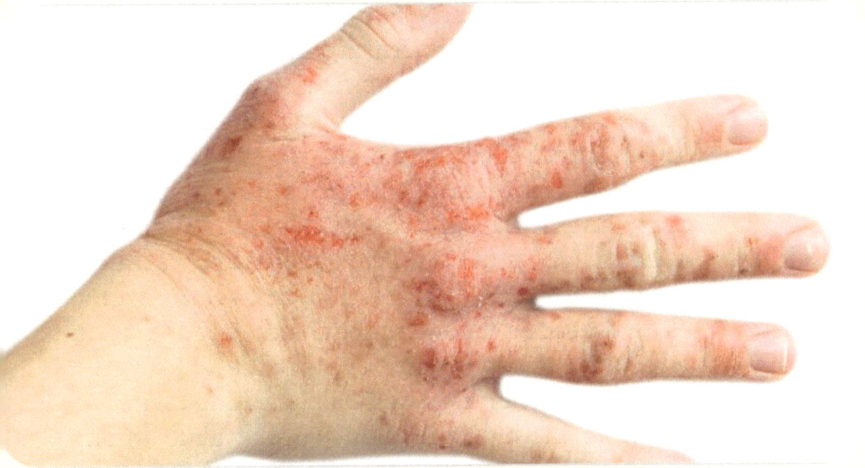

Introduction

Occupational dermatoses are a range of conditions that result from contact with various irritants and allergens in the occupational environment. The dermatoses, most commonly manifesting as dermatitis, can significantly impair an individual's quality of life and performance. The skin acts as the body's first line of defense against external agents and is therefore the most exposed to them. As businesses evolve and the workforce diversifies, understanding the myriad of reasons behind skin diseases in the workplace becomes crucial. With approximately 30% of all occupational injuries attributed to skin diseases, the stakes are high beyond employee health and reach into overall workplace safety and economic viability. Therefore, developing a comprehensive understanding of occupational skin diseases is essential for protecting workers and maintaining a healthy work environment. The chronic issue of occupational skin diseases is proof of the need for prevention and education. Employers and employees must be informed of the risks involving particular job activities that involve the handling of injurious materials or

LEARNING OBJECTIVES

After studying this chapter, you will be able to:

1. Explain the types of occupational skin diseases
2. Explain causes and risk factors associated with occupational skin diseases
3. Focus on populations at risk for occupational skin diseases
4. Understand the symptoms of occupational skin diseases
5. Define prevention strategies
6. Deal with treatment options for occupational skin diseases

repeated exposure to irritating chemicals. While protective measures have been implemented across most industries, the absence of specific guidelines creates gaps in protection and care practices. There are discrepancies in existing guidelines, and no universally followed standards for the prevention and management of these conditions. Eliminating these discrepancies is essential to preventing worker ill health and the economic costs associated with skin diseases. Safety culture and workplace training can significantly reduce occupational skin diseases and overall worker ill health. Furthermore, the socioeconomic effects of occupational dermatoses are far-reaching and necessitate a response by the employer and public health community that is multifaceted. Because the workers experience discomfort and, in severe cases, disfigurement or disability from skin conditions, the overall quality of life is lost for them. This impact is accompanied by increased healthcare costs and lost productivity, which can affect families and the healthcare system as well. Identification of this issue necessitates large-scale data collection and research to further elucidate the roles of the environment and chemicals in the development of skin diseases. According to existing research, an integrative approach that combines education, effective regulatory frameworks, and community awareness is essential. This technique has not only possible benefits for individual workers but also functions to enhance the general public health.(Montero et al., 2022; Rebecca et al., 2021)

Definition of Occupational Skin Diseases

Occupational skin diseases are a range of dermatoses that arise from exposure to hazardous chemicals and environmental factors in the workplace. They may present as irritant contact dermatitis, allergic contact dermatitis, or more severe skin conditions associated with certain occupational hazards. The underlying causes of these diseases are primarily chemical agents, mechanical irritants, and biological agents. Moreover, the work environment—humidity levels, temperature fluctuations, and exposure to light—can exacerbate preexisting skin conditions or cause new ones to develop. Occupational skin disease requires consideration not only of the nature of the irritants but also of the significant impact of occupational exposure on the overall condition of the skin and on worker productivity. Occupational skin diseases vary across sectors. For instance, workers in construction, manufacturing, and healthcare are typically exposed to specific irritants, including adhesives, solvents, and biological agents. Exposure of these chemicals to the skin might lead to inflammation, allergic contact dermatitis, and infection, and hence require special preventive methods. Furthermore, studies have indicated a correlation between chronic skin diseases and occupational exposure, in which individuals may experience aggravated symptoms when exposed over the long term. For example, the high prevalence of oily acne among workers exposed to hydrocarbons underscores the link between environmental exposures and skin. Thus, the description of the pathogenesis of these diseases requires careful assessment of both the causative factors and the exposure context, as evidenced by the association of technogenic effects with dermatopathology (Karpova et al., 2022).

Prevention and treatment of occupational dermatoses require concerted efforts of dermatologists and occupational health experts. Such interprofessional communication plays a critical role in identifying populations at risk and in implementing effective intervention policies. Informing staff about the risks associated with their work and educating them on appropriate protective measures can significantly reduce the incidence of such diseases. It is also essential to conduct regular inspections of workplace conditions alongside skin assessments to help prevent long-term complications. Research has shown that knowledge of autoimmune correlations, for example, in conditions like psoriasis, can also be helpful in understanding and treating occupational skin diseases. By promoting the culture of awareness and forethought care, the workplaces can minimize the dermatological impact on the workers and enhance health outcomes and productivity (Dvornikov et al., 2024) (Figure 5.1).

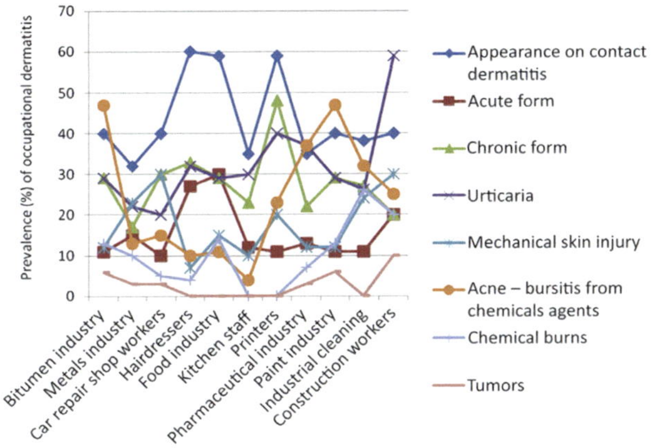

Figure 5.1. Types of enterprises with the highest prevalence of occupational skin diseases studied.

Source: https://www.researchgate.net/publication/257535873/figure/fig1/AS:203051009875975@1425422541738/Types-of-enterprises-with-the-highest-prevalence-of-occupational-skin-diseases-studied.png.

Importance of Studying Occupational Skin Diseases

Occupational skin disease is of greatest importance for a variety of reasons, primarily due to its prevalence within the workplace and ability to impact employee health and productivity dramatically. Skin diseases dermatitis, eczema, and contact allergy are readily provoked by exposure to chemicals, irritants, or allergens in nearly any occupation, from healthcare to manufacturing. Identification of such conditions not only facilitates care and recognition of affected workers but also enables employers to implement required preventive measures. Firms' identification of occupational skin disease etiology and risk factors can help develop healthier work environments and reduce healthcare costs associated with treatment and absenteeism. Another significant implication of research on occupational skin disease is the potential for early intervention and control. Research has established that early detection of symptoms is likely to improve health outcomes among affected workers, thereby preventing the progression of these conditions to later stages that may require extended medical care and work loss.

Detection of patterns and trends in occupational skin diseases also identifies areas of concern within specific industries, enabling targeted interventions to minimize risks. Moreover, skin care and protective equipment training, promoted through research and firm training initiatives, can be effective in increasing workers' knowledge and fostering a prevention culture. Finally, the overall applicability of research on occupational skin disease encompasses public health and policy considerations. By describing occupational skin disease work practice relationships, researchers can inform regulatory standards and guidelines that protect worker health. This aspect has gained prominence as more businesses recognize the value of investing in employee well-being programs. Additional investigation contributes to the body of knowledge that informs training for occupational safety experts and healthcare professionals. By doing so, it not only seeks to mitigate the economic effects of such conditions but also upholds employees' right to a healthy and safe working environment, which is necessary for overall public health (Burak, I. I., & Cherkasova, O. A., 2013; Office of Services et al., 1989).

5.1. Types of Occupational Skin Diseases

Learning Outcome

1. Understand allergic contact dermatitis.
2. Describe irritant contact dermatitis.
3. Focus on skin infections related to occupational exposure.

Occupational skin diseases are prevalent and are predominantly classified as irritant contact dermatitis, allergic contact dermatitis, and skin infections. Irritant contact dermatitis is characterized by skin inflammation due to immediate contact with causative agents, such as solvents, detergents, or chemicals that are characteristically used in industries. This condition typically occurs without prior sensitization and is therefore more common among workers in sectors such as construction and manufacturing, where there is regular exposure to irritants. Allergic contact dermatitis, on the other hand, results from a hypersensitivity reaction to some allergens, which can range from nickel in jewelry to perfumes in cosmetics. This condition normally requires pre-sensitization, it represents a repeat case for employees who have been exposed to allergens in their workplaces, normally leading to severe health impacts as well as excessive healthcare costs. Skin infections are among the most significant types of occupational skin diseases, further complicating the situation for infected employees. Bacterial infections, such as impetigo or folliculitis, would be more related to circumstances under which hygiene is not good or the integrity of the skin is broken, usually in occupations, such as food service or healthcare. Furthermore, fungal infections, such as ringworm or athlete's foot, thrive in warm, humid environments and pose particular risks to individuals who work in agricultural or damp settings. These infections not only result in discomfort and absenteeism but also lead to secondary infection or cross-transmission of disease to high-risk groups. Knowledge of specific occupational skin diseases and their causative factors is thus crucial for drafting prevention measures in at-risk industries. Technological development over the last few decades has resulted in enhanced detection and control of occupational skin diseases. For instance, machine learning algorithms are increasingly used in image classification to improve diagnostic precision, assisting in the identification of various skin conditions. It has been found that even when such algorithms efficiently categorize ailments within a particular population, they fail for irregular skin tones, particularly in the identification of skin cancer. Attempts to combine a greater number of skin types into training sets aim to close these gaps, thereby ensuring that diagnostic equipment is equitable across populations. By emphasizing the importance of inclusive healthcare solutions, these technological advancements can ultimately maximize occupational skin disease management and optimize worker health outcomes across industries (Bizel et al., 2024; Aboulmira et al., 2024).

5.1.1. Allergic Contact Dermatitis

Allergic contact dermatitis (ACD) is recognized as a significant concern within the broader category of occupational skin diseases, characterized by an inflammatory response following exposure to allergens. This immunologically mediated condition arises when individuals encounter specific substances that trigger an allergic reaction, distinguishing it from irritant contact dermatitis, which results from non-immunological mechanisms. In the workplace, ACD can result from exposure to numerous allergens, such as metals, rubber, perfumes, and preservatives, in workplace products. The duration of exposure and frequency, along with personal susceptibility, determine the incidence of the condition among workers from various sectors. Identification of the offending allergen is crucial for effective prevention and management, underscoring the importance of a thorough occupational history and patch testing for those involved. The increasing prevalence of allergic contact dermatitis in the workplace necessitates active prevention and early detection steps. Occupational physicians can play a key role in conducting risk assessments and recommending products with lower sensitization potential to minimize exposure to dermatologic hazards. Secondly, stimulation of protective behaviors, such as the use of non-irritating skin creams, is important for maintaining skin barrier integrity and for the prevention of dermatitis. Regular medical surveillance enables monitoring of employees' skin, and medical professionals can provide individual guidance on dermal protection and hygiene strategies. As emphasized in research, implementation of all-rounded preventative strategies can significantly reduce ACD incidence, ultimately providing a better workplace environment for risk groups (Filon et al., 2025).

Moreover, the COVID-19 pandemic has increased the rate of allergic contact dermatitis due to the resulting increased hand sanitizer and personal protective equipment, such as masks, usage. Workers, particularly from the health sector, have reported a higher incidence of skin disease due to such essential items, since chronic usage of alcohol-based hand sanitizers and prolonged use of face masks cause both irritant and allergic contact dermatitis. This realization highlights an immediate need for ongoing research and education on occupational dermatitis, especially as cases are anticipated to rise due to mandatory protective gear. Understanding the relationship between these products and ACD development will be essential in developing better prevention measures so that critical health and safety protocols do not inadvertently undermine skin wellness in the workplace (Esraa et al., 2024) (Figure 5.2).

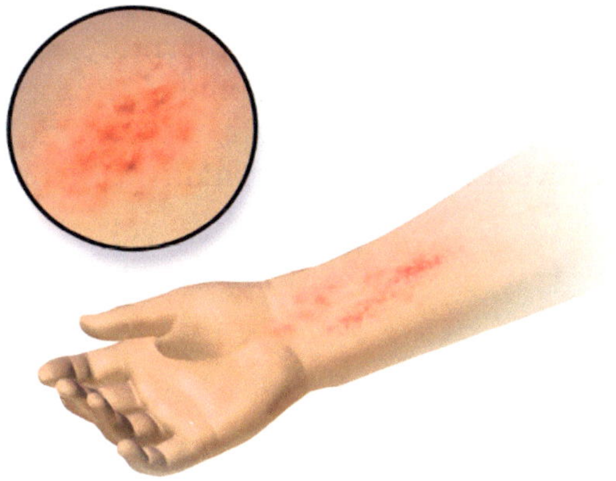

Figure 5.2. Illustration of allergic contact dermatitis.

Source: https://upload.wikimedia.org/wikipedia/commons/thumb/1/19/Blausen_0014_AllergicDermatitis.png./800px-Blausen_0014_AllergicDermatitis.png.

5.1.2. Irritant Contact Dermatitis

Irritant contact dermatitis (ICD) is a highly prevalent occupational cutaneous disorder characterized by skin inflammation following exposure to irritants. The disease is commonly observed among healthcare workers, cleaners, and construction workers and results from repeated contact with chemicals such as soaps, detergents, and solvents. Compared with immune-mediated allergic contact dermatitis, irritant contact dermatitis results from disruption of the skin barrier and the development of symptoms ranging from redness and swelling to itching and blistering. The pathophysiology of ICD underscores the importance of awareness of workplace exposure, particularly given that over 70% of contact dermatitis cases are irritant-type, posing a significant challenge for occupational health practitioners. Thus, early intervention and effective workplace practice are required to mitigate the risk of ultimately suffering from this condition. Prevention measures play a key role in controlling irritant contact dermatitis in the workplace. This includes implementing education and training initiatives that increase awareness of potential hazards associated with various substances used. Furthermore, the use of personal protective equipment (PPE), such as gloves and barrier creams, can significantly reduce direct contact with irritants (Figure 5.3).

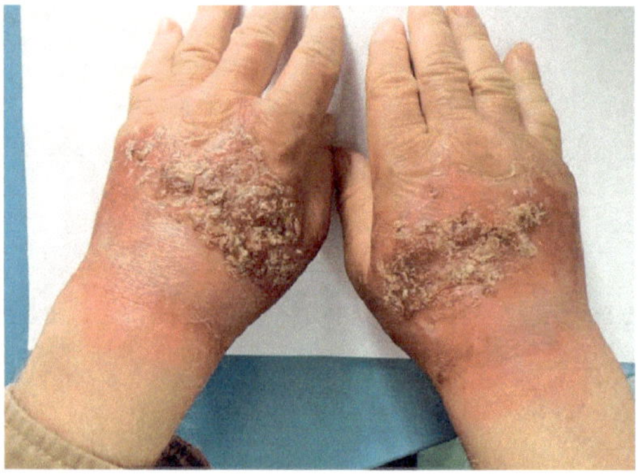

Figure 5.3. Acute irritant contact dermatitis with impetiginization.

Source: https://www.researchgate.net/profile/Liborija-Lugovic-Mihic/publication/333656538/figure/fig2/AS:767194111700994@1559924738537/Acute-irritant-contact-dermatitis-with-impetiginization.png.

Regular screening of employees also aids in early detection of signs and symptoms, facilitating early intervention and treatment. Interestingly, the utilization of non-invasive biomarkers is gaining importance in the discipline of dermatology, as they enable objective quantification of skin wellness. Hence, the ever-increasing need for research, both preventive and therapeutic in nature, to counteract the impact of irritant contact dermatitis so that employees remain healthy and productive in their work environment (Kezic et al., 2024).

The ongoing problem of irritant contact dermatitis has been brought under further consideration with the widespread use of hand sanitizers and personal protective equipment during the COVID-19 pandemic. Hand dermatitis has become a common consequence of heightened hygiene measures across industries, particularly in healthcare. Based on various studies, including systematic reviews of occupational contact dermatitis caused by similar agents, an increase in the prevalence of skin ailments is anticipated due to long-term exposure to irritants (Esraa et al., 2024). Hence, it becomes necessary to understand the implications of such changes for effective workplace health interventions. Research activities on the discovery of effective treatment protocols and the promotion of skin health by the early detection and better working conditions are critical in reducing the collective burden of occupational skin disorders, like irritant contact dermatitis (Figure 5.4).

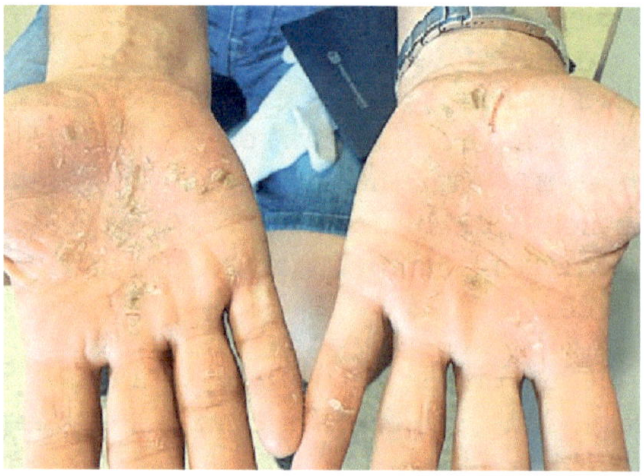

Figure 5.4. Chronic irritant contact dermatitis.

Source: https://www.researchgate.net/profile/Liborija-Lugovic-Mihic/publication/333656538/figure/fig4/AS:767194111684608@1559924738638/Chronic-irritant-contact-dermatitis.png.

5.1.3. Skin Infections Related to Occupational Exposure

Occupational skin infections are a significant health concern across most industries, and exposure to specific environments greatly increases the risk of infection. In particular, healthcare, aquaculture, and agriculture industries are usually exposed to skin infections resulting from occupational and environmental exposure. For instance, those in the aquaculture industry are always in wet and contaminated environments, exposing them to a high risk of acquiring skin infections. A questionnaire-based survey of aquaculture farm laborers found that 23% had skin infections, underscoring the urgent need to address this occupational health issue (Yalamanchi et al., 2022). Besides, the combination of work conditions, hygiene practices of individuals, and lack of proper safety precautions can cause the spread of such infections and, in turn, cause additional complicated health issues. Consequently, identifying the relationship between occupational exposure and skin infection is important for developing effective prevention strategies. Outside specific industries, the influence of climate change on occupational exposure further complicates the issue of skin infections among employees. Increasing temperatures and shifting environmental conditions can increase the intensity and severity of infections. Extensive heat stress can weaken the natural protections of the skin, exposing it to pathogens that thrive in hot temperatures. Furthermore, elevated levels of vector-borne infectious agents, driven by climate change, pose new challenges for workers across sectors, as reflected in the rising incidence of vector-borne illnesses. As elaborated in research on the effects of climate change, these changes pose significant occupational health threats and lead to skin diseases among vulnerable populations (R et al., 2022). Therefore, concerted efforts must be aimed at raising workers' awareness of the potential skin health risks associated with climate change and at implementing protective practices. Successful management of occupational skin infections requires short-term interventions in the workplace along with long-range strategic planning. Employers must give top priority to the implementation of protective measures specific to the hazards involved in their occupation. This entails providing appropriate protective equipment and conducting regular training on hygiene and safety protocols to reduce the incidence of skin infections. Additionally, ongoing observation and assessment of the work environment can help identify potential hazards and develop appropriate response strategies to minimize exposure risks. Collaboration between medical professionals and occupational health experts is needed during the development of education programs aimed at informing workers about the signs and symptoms of skin infections and the right times to visit a doctor. Through these combined efforts, it is possible to reduce the incidence of occupational dermatological infections and enhance workers' overall health at risk (Yalamanchi et al., 2022; R et al., 2022) (Figure 5.5).

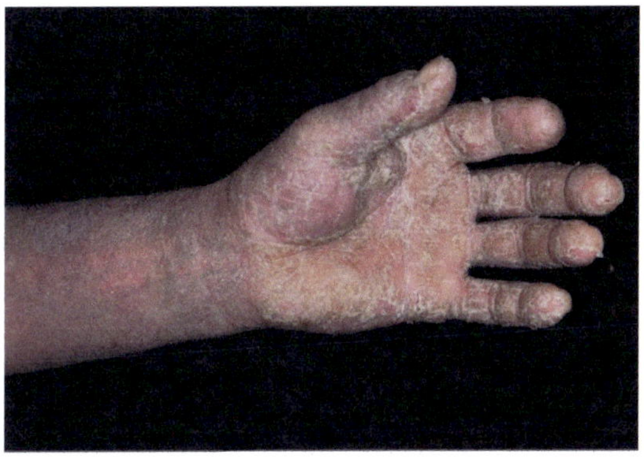

Figure 5.5. Figure showing occupational skin infection.

Source: https://occderm.asn.au/wp-content/uploads/2014/10/Manky-hands-good-photo.jpg.

Test Your Knowledge

1. What is the primary difference between allergic contact dermatitis and irritant contact dermatitis?
2. Name three common occupational allergens that can cause allergic contact dermatitis.

5.2. Causes and Risk Factors

Learning Outcome

1. Understand the role of chemical exposures in the workplace.
2. Describe physical factors contributing to skin diseases.
3. Discuss about biological agents and their impact on skin health.

Occupational skin diseases are caused by a wide range of factors and hazards that vary across workplaces. Chemical exposures, for instance, in the form of detergents, soaps, and solvents are among the most essential causes of skin diseases, such as allergic contact dermatitis and irritant contact dermatitis. For instance, workers in healthcare, manufacturing, and cleaning industries spend substantial time handling these substances, thereby increasing their risk of adverse skin reactions. The level and duration of exposure to irritants increase the risk; hence, occupational safety guidelines are required. In fact, compliance with personal protective equipment (PPE) use is largely lacking, underscoring the need for appropriate training and knowledge to mitigate such risks. Another highly significant factor in the causation of occupational skin diseases is the interaction between environmental factors and individual susceptibility.

Working conditions with high humidity, temperature fluctuations, or constant wet work exposure can compromise the skin barrier and increase susceptibility to damage and irritation. Individuals with pre-existing skin conditions and those with allergic reactions are also at higher risk, as more reactive skin is more susceptible to occupational exposure. For example, healthcare workers are continually exposed to potential irritants within patient care environments and consequently may have higher incidence rates of allergic contact dermatitis and disorders of similar cause (Kezic et al., 2024). Detection of these individual and environmental risk factors is important for developing targeted intervention strategies.

Lastly, recent advances in biomarker research have opened opportunities to enhance the detection and management of occupational skin disorders. As noted by recent studies, sampling from the stratum corneum may provide valuable information on the skin's response to various irritants and external stimuli. Not only can these biomarkers facilitate early diagnosis of the condition, but they can also distinguish among the various types of dermatitis, which can significantly impact treatment. The integration of advanced diagnostic equipment into workplace health services may facilitate more effective identification of susceptible individuals, thereby mitigating the impact of skin diseases on workers' health and productivity (Kezic et al., 2024). With these practices adopted by employers and physicians, the overall incidence of occupational skin diseases may decline substantially.

5.2.1. Chemical Exposures in the Workplace

Exposure to chemicals in the workplace is a major contributor to occupational skin disease, and dermatitis is the most prevalent type. The widespread use of industrial chemicals exposes workers to numerous substances, with minimal protection and risk awareness in most situations. For instance, studies have documented higher risks among workers in the chemical, petroleum, and food-processing sectors, where exposure to specific chemicals, such as metalworking fluids and organic solvents, is prevalent. This illustrates the necessity of targeted intervention programs to assess and manage risk to minimize exposure. Surveillance schemes, such as the Occupational Disease Surveillance System, employ historical claims data to identify high-risk groups and direct public health action to reduce dermatitis cases among workers (Shakik et al., 2019). In most cases, chemical safety in the workplace must be addressed through multidimensional measures, including employee training and stricter regulatory guidelines. Furthermore, the negative health effects of exposure to poisonous chemicals disproportionately affect vulnerable groups, including women and minority groups, in the workplace. The beauty and personal care industries, in particular, pose risks due to the widespread use of hazardous chemicals in everyday products (Figure 5.6).

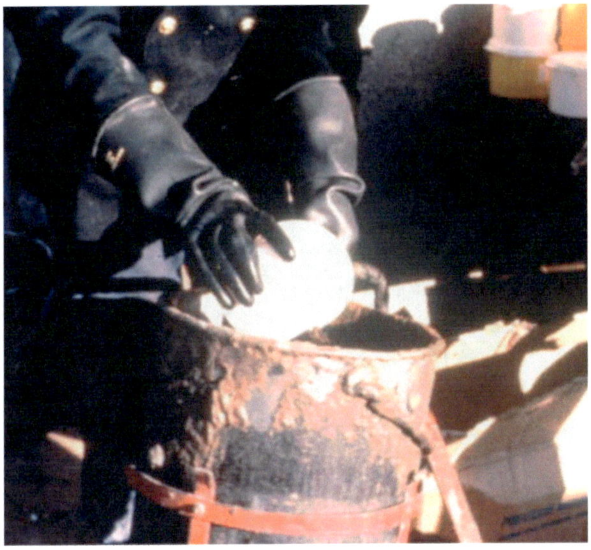

Figure 5.6. A worker is using solvents to clean sludge from a barrel.

Source: https://www.researchgate.net/profile/Sean-Semple-2/publication/8670725_Dermal_exposure_to_chemicals_in_the_workplace_Just_how_important_is_skin_absorption/links/00b7d5242ba6e80814000000/Dermal-exposure-to-chemicals-in-the-workplace-Just-how-important-is-skin-absorption.pdf?_tp=eyJjb250ZXh0Ijp7ImZpcnN0UGFnZSI6Il9kaXJlY3QiLCJwYWdlIjoicHVibGljYXRpb24ifX0.

Reproductive health professionals have complained about the impact of these chemical exposures on their ability to champion policy issues addressing environmental justice. The majority of cosmetic products contain toxicants identified as posing significant threats to health, including skin irritation and systemic disease. Immigrant workers and women of color employed in the beauty industry tend to have higher levels of exposure to such chemicals, further heightening the awareness of the link between socioeconomic standing and occupational health risks (Ami et al., 2017). Thus, the beauty industry is a classic case of the urgent need for strict controls and informed consumer behavior to mitigate the health impacts of such chemical exposures in work settings. Besides, awareness of workplace chemical exposure patterns is essential in designing effective prevention strategies. Workers are exposed to hazardous chemicals through skin contact, inhalation, or ingestion, depending on the nature of their workplaces. For instance, workers who handle cleaning chemicals and solvents are exposed to dermal and pulmonary routes, with potential long-term damage to skin health. Substantial evidence points to the role of environmental factors, such as inadequate ventilation and lack of protective gear, in fueling these hazards. Enhanced occupational health regulations, as recommended by health authorities, could improve working conditions and reduce rates of occupational skin diseases. Central to this discussion is the role of employers and employees, both, in observing and acting upon chemical hazards in terms of fostering a healthier, safer working environment with consideration to skin health as well as overall well-being (Shakik et al., 2019) (Figure 5.7).

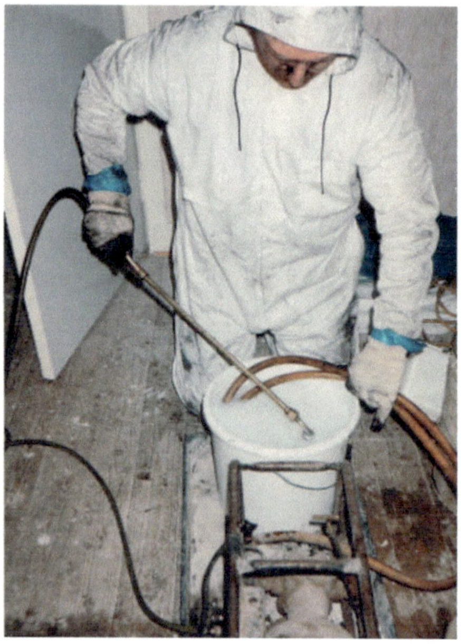

Figure 5.7. A worker in a coverall washing a spray lance.

Source: https://www.researchgate.net/profile/Sean-Semple-2/publication/8670725_Dermal_exposure_to_chemicals_in_the_workplace_Just_how_important_is_skin_absorption/links/00b7d5242ba6e80814000000/Dermal-exposure-to-chemicals-in-the-workplace-Just-how-important-is-skin-absorption.pdf?_tp=eyJjb250ZXh0Ijp7ImZpcnN0UGFnZSI6Il9kaXJlY3QiLCJwYWdlIjoicHVibGljYXRpb24ifX0.

5.2.2. Physical Factors Contributing to Skin Diseases

The interaction of physical factors with occupational skin diseases is complex and multidimensional. In these factors, exposure to abrasive materials can lead to dermatitis or eczema. Workers in manual-labor sectors, including construction and manufacturing, are often exposed to the risk of skin abrasion from friction or rubbing against rough surfaces. These abrasions can disrupt the skin barrier, leaving it vulnerable to allergens and irritants. Furthermore, the poor working conditions that certain ethnic groups have been exposed to, as indicated in (Clay et al., 2004), could mean that some populations have a higher likelihood of developing such skin conditions because they lack access to preventive measures and safety training. Thus, preventing such physical risks in occupational environments can be essential for reducing the incidence of skin disorders. Exposure to the environment, particularly near waste dumps or pollutants, is also a causative factor for occupational skin disorders. Studies have found that people living in the vicinity of landfills have a high incidence of skin disorders like irritations and dermatitis, which may be a result of toxicants in the environment and dust exposure. The phrases used by Al-Delaimy et al. (2014) are employed to explain the study, highlighting the connection between where people live and their exposure to environmental pollution, which increases their risk. In the workplace, this translates to those employees who unknowingly enter polluted environments or handle materials that are contaminated by toxic agents. Inhalation and contact with particulate matter are likely to trigger allergic reactions and exacerbate existing skin ailments, underscoring the need for comprehensive environmental health assessments in the workplace to safeguard employees' well-being. Notably, the contribution of water and humidity cannot be ignored while looking at physical determinants of skin disease in occupational environments. Prolonged exposure to water or wet conditions can cause skin maceration and increase susceptibility to dermatitis and fungal infections. Dry conditions, however, can cause skin desiccation and irritation, disrupting the barrier. Prolonged exposure to occupations where such conditions are experienced include agriculture or working under extreme weather conditions. As detailed by Clay et al. (2004), cultural and socioeconomic factors can affect how these workers maintain skin health, particularly when they lack access to protective gear or appropriate skin-care products. Consequently, training of employees on why they must keep their skin hydrated and wear protective devices becomes crucial to prevent occupational skin disorders.

5.2.3. Biological Agents and Their Impact on Skin Health

Exposure to biological agents in the workplace, including viruses, bacteria, and fungi, poses a significant risk to skin health and can lead to various dermatological conditions. Biological agents pose the greatest risk of skin disease to agricultural, food-processing, and healthcare workers. For instance, workers handling plant or animal products may develop hypersensitivity reactions or allergic dermatitis due to exposure to allergens present in these biologic agents. These conditions not only interfere with skin integrity but also reduce occupational productivity and overall quality of life. Socioeconomic impact further complicates the problem, as infected workers may lose their jobs or take extended medical leave, so effective prevention strategies for workplaces at risk are a priority. Management of skin health in occupational settings involves extensive knowledge of the types of biological agents workers may be exposed to. In particular, diseases such as occupational dermatitis and infections necessitate the implementation of stringent hygiene protocols and protective measures. Personal protective equipment (PPE) is the first line of defense against contact with biological agents harmful to the skin. Nevertheless, as noted by Gauci, M., & Vella, N. (1997), effective screening programs play a significant role in verifying the health appropriateness of workers for a specific occupation, ensuring that employees are properly aware of the risks and sufficiently healthy to perform their jobs without damaging their skin. Preventive screening, along with education about the hazards of biological exposure, can abolish or remarkably minimize the incidence of occupational skin diseases. Additionally, regular monitoring and assessment programs can address increasing risks associated with repeated contact with biological agents. According to Balla et al. (2017), repeated exposure to biological agents can enhance the likelihood of developing allergic reactions, which further evolve into more complex conditions , such as work-related rhinitis and dermatitis. These consequences can adversely affect the worker's health and performance. Hence, establishing a culture focused on awareness, training, and hazard management is essential to prevent skin diseases resulting from biological agents at work. Through this inclusion, employers can protect their workers while ensuring general occupational health and safety, promoting an improved working environment indirectly.

Test Your Knowledge

1. How do chemical exposures in the workplace lead to occupational skin diseases?
2. Name two physical factors in the workplace that can contribute to skin diseases and explain how.
3. What are the biological agents that affect skin health in occupational setting

5.3. Populations at Risk

Learning Outcome

1. Identify healthcare workers at risk of occupational skin diseases.
2. Focus on construction and manufacturing workers suffering from occupational skin diseases.
3. Define agricultural workers and exposure to pesticides.

Risk groups for occupational skin disease are typically defined by occupational exposure, demographics, and socioeconomic status. Healthcare workers, manufacturing, and construction workers are exposed to skin irritants and allergens that can produce dermatitis and eczema. Ethnic minority populations are likely to experience increased vulnerabilities due to a cluster of environmental factors along with limited access to health care resources. For instance, whilst UK South Asians overall are under-represented in the highest risk occupation categories, they experience higher levels of limiting long-term illness and self-assessed poor general health, suggesting that even in less hazardous environments, they are vulnerable to occupational skin diseases. Due to limited surveillance of these populations, little is known about the nature and extent of the risks to which they are exposed (Clay et al., 2004). In addition, ethnicity and race are significant demographic factors in understanding susceptibility to occupational skin disease. Research has revealed that ethnic groups have varying injury and illness rates in the workplace. For instance, although they tend to have overall lower injury rates, UK South Asians have increased chances of excluding themselves from work through sick leave when compared to Whites. This is exacerbated by systemic barriers to early medical treatment, which is paramount in mitigating the impact of skin diseases. Medical screening programs targeting particular occupational hazards must be prioritized to the highest level to effectively address the respective demands of these populations. These programs may not only increase awareness but also help prevent the aggravation of occupational skin diseases among vulnerable workers (Gauci, M., & Vella, N., 1997). Both prevention and targeted intervention are necessary to meet the needs of populations at risk. Occupational health promotion workshops among ethnic minorities can increase awareness and community-level engagement and encourage proactive health-seeking behaviors. Additionally, the establishment of ethnic minority health and safety Beacon sites could provide prime focal points for resource sharing and support for populations at risk. Increasing collection and monitoring of data on these groups is needed to develop effective public health interventions. Without a proper understanding of the unique occupational exposures of diverse worker groups, interventions may not be tailored, leaving numerous vulnerable workers without the protection they require against occupational skin disorders (Clay et al., 2004; Gauci, M., & Vella, N., 1997).

5.3.1. Workers in Healthcare Settings

The health care sector is widely recognized as a cornerstone of community health, with health care workers exposed to occupational hazards that increase their risk of occupational skin disease. Their work involves frequent contact with patients, biological materials, and various chemical agents, some of which are skin irritants that cause dermatitis. Healthcare workers, such as nurses and aides, continually expose themselves to disinfectants and antiseptics that, although necessary to prevent infection, can irritate or cause skin disease. With many people becoming healthcare workers, the mechanism of how occupational skin diseases develop in this setting is important to understand. Hence, developing particular prevention strategies is crucial to avoid such hazards and maintain long-term health among healthcare workers. Additionally, health workers are at the highest risk of contracting not only skin but also other contagious diseases that can complicate their work. For instance, research has shown that health workers are at risk of contracting tuberculosis even if they are based in areas of low incidence (Luca et al., 2017). This shows the overlap between respiratory and dermatological wellbeing, where compromised skin barriers expose them to infection. With effective screening methods, such as tuberculin skin test (TST) and subsequent more specific tests, where necessary, it is imperative to have stringent health surveillance among health care workers. Thus, an integrated approach to their health entails both occupational skin disease prevention as well as infectious disease monitoring, leading eventually to a healthier working environment. Moreover, healthcare inequalities among healthcare workers can significantly affect their overall well-being and job performance. Literature reveals that certain minority ethnic groups demonstrate special patterns of ill health, for example, limiting long-term sickness and variable levels of workplace injury (Clay et al., 2004). Such inequalities call for particular health promotion interventions, particularly among minority workers engaged in healthcare professions. By addressing the specific vulnerabilities of these groups, we can reinforce occupational health programs that meet not only skin health, but also the broader aspects of health risk. We can develop workshops and health campaigns for these population groups that will reduce occupational skin diseases and improve their work experience, ultimately resulting in a healthier better and fair work environment in healthcare (Figure 5.8).

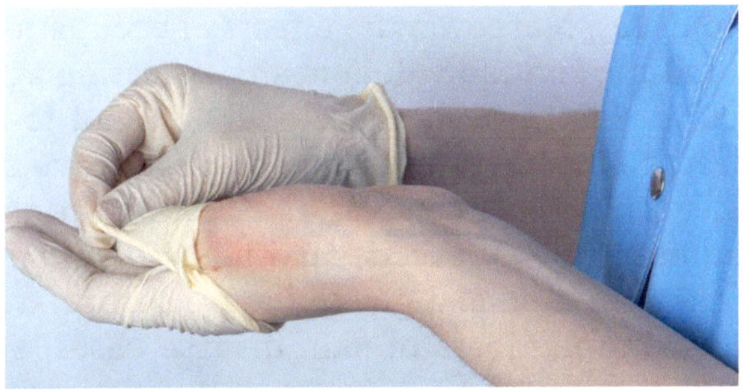

Figure 5.8. Gloves allergy.

Source: https://media.assets.medline.eu/www/media/amasty/blog/cache/B/A/1200/500/BAN_Gloves_Allergy.jpg.

5.3.2. Construction and Manufacturing Workers

The manufacturing and construction sectors are reported to involve high environmental exposure, a significant cause of occupational skin disease. Workers in these sectors are most likely to be exposed to various irritants, including metals, chemicals, and dust, which can lead to dermatitis and other skin-related issues. For example, a study reported that nine men employed in welding and grinding with nickel dust developed erythematous papules and intense itching, leading to allergic and irritant contact dermatitis attributable to these exposures (Kim et al., 2022). Such an incident highlights the importance of proper monitoring and safety measures to prevent skin-related health risks. Insufficient training and unsafe working conditions also increase the risk of such diseases, which require urgent attention from employers and policymakers. Despite the documented risks, the majority of construction and manufacturing workers report inadequate training in skin protection. According to statistics gathered within a five-year span, workers employed in the health and manufacturing sectors are more likely to receive skin protection training than their construction and service sector counterparts, with their relatively much lower percentages reported (Holness et al., 2020). This disparity starkly illustrates the workplace health education disparity that might put many at risk for skin occupational diseases. The inability to utilize proper personal protective equipment and identify hazardous chemicals can lead to more skin illnesses, which makes specific training programs imperative. Thus, improved workplace safety precautions and a comprehensive education on maintaining healthy skin is crucial in safeguarding the health of such employees. Moreover, the effects of occupational skin disorders in manufacturing and construction extend beyond individual health, affecting aggregate productivity and economic spending in these sectors. Skin disorders are likely to lead to absenteeism and decreased work effectiveness, with affected employees needing extended leave or treatment, eventually depleting healthcare systems and economic resources. The aforementioned nickel dust exposure case provides the utmost testimony to increased surveillance and monitoring practice in occupational health, guarding workers in time and giving them appropriate intervention and treatment (Kim et al., 2022). With increasing numbers of skin disease cases, strict protective measures and ongoing education for workers need to be prioritized. By addressing these issues holistically, industries can reduce the incidence of occupational skin diseases and promote a healthier workforce (Table 4.1).

Table 4.1. Distribution of Skin Diseases Among Construction

workers (n=140).

Disease	Frequency	Percentage
Work place injuries	40	28.6
Respiratory problems	64	45.7
Occupational skin diseases	110	78.6
Musculoskeletal disorders	46	32.8
Others	44	31.4

Source: https://www.researchgate.net/profile/Ruksana-Hamid/publication/349925992/figure/tbl5/AS:999490295189506@1615308464785/Distribution-of-skin-diseases-among-construction.png.

5.3.3. Agricultural Workers and Exposure to Pesticides

Farm workers are often exposed to multiple pesticides, a practice that raises significant concerns regarding occupational skin disease. The application of these chemicals is essential for crop protection and yield enhancement; nevertheless, health risks associated with pesticide exposure must not be underestimated. Skin diseases acquired through immediate or inadvertent contact can range from mild irritation to full-blown dermatosis. Moreover, prolonged exposure is likely to exacerbate such conditions, leading to chronic diseases that primarily affect the quality of life among exposed workers. Understanding the dynamics of pesticide exposure is significant because it not only places populations at risk but also guides interventions to reduce injuries among farm workers, which is crucial for ensuring sustainable agricultural practices. Beyond skin diseases, pesticide exposure may also lead to a range of broader health consequences. The character of these chemicals usually makes them as possible endocrine disrupters and neurotoxicants, and hence there are concerns of systemic health effects aside from dermal manifestations. Extended studies indicate that chronic exposure may give rise to severe health afflictions, such as cancers, reproductive illnesses, and autoimmune diseases. Furthermore, workers often lack appropriate protective equipment and training, further increasing their vulnerability. Efforts to enhance education and access to resources within the agricultural community are crucial in minimizing risks associated with pesticide exposure. These efforts will contribute to safer handling standards and lay the groundwork for adopting integrated pest management techniques, ultimately building a healthier work environment. Although the risks of pesticide exposure are substantial, there is growing interest in preventive measures to protect farmers' health. Raising awareness campaigns regarding the manifestations of pesticide-caused skin diseases and the importance of preventive measures can enable workers to make well-informed decisions regarding their own health. Imposing regular skin health checks and providing personal protective equipment will also reduce the incidence of occupational skin disease in this population. Reporting and case documentation programs that encourage the reporting of skin reactions play a critical role in determining the extent of the problem. As pointed out in various other environmental studies, the connection between pesticide application and health impact highlights the need to adopt sustainable practices for pesticide application, which would significantly promote the well-being of farm workers as well as the overall environment (Ferronato, N., & Torretta, V., 2019; Ali et al., 2019) (Figure 5.9).

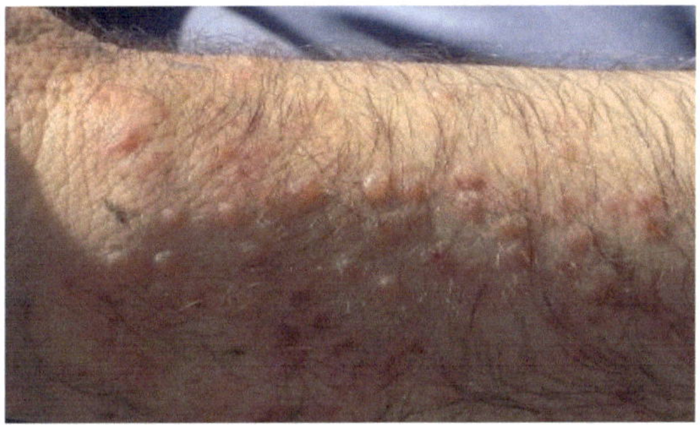

Figure 5.9. Rashes on the hands of a farmer.

Source: https://www.researchgate.net/publication/350177228/figure/fig2/AS:1017248277880832@1619542297039/Rashes-on-the-hands-of-a-farmer-in-Fereydoon-Kenar-town-north-of-Iran.jpg.

Test Your Knowledge

1. Why are healthcare workers particularly susceptible to occupational skin diseases like contact dermatitis?
2. What types of skin diseases are commonly seen in construction and manufacturing workers?
3. How does pesticide exposure affect agricultural workers' skin health?

5.4. Symptoms and Diagnosis

Learning Outcome

1. Describe common symptoms of occupational skin diseases.
2. Explain diagnostic methods for occupational skin diseases used by healthcare professionals.
3. Explain the importance of early detection and intervention.

In occupational skin diseases, understanding the symptoms and accurate diagnosis are essential to facilitate appropriate management and cure. Occupational skin diseases may present in diverse ways, depending on the type of irritant or allergen involved. Symptoms can be anything from erythema, pruritus, blistering, and desquamation of the skin in severe cases. For instance, a person exposed to chemical irritants may develop localized dermatitis with inflammation and redness. Early detection of such symptoms is critical in order to prevent progression to chronic conditions, including extensive lesions and scarring. Regular screening and surveillance of workers in high-risk occupations are preventive measures that enable early treatment and reduce morbidity from such conditions. Diagnosing occupational skin disease requires an integrated approach that incorporates clinical examination and a comprehensive medical history. Dermatologists typically rely on the patient's occupational history, considering exposure to specific chemicals, allergens, or irritants that may have caused the patient's symptoms. For instance, contact with substances , such as latex or certain industrial chemicals can result in specific allergic responses, such as when a nurse exhibits symptoms credited to latex after being exposed in the clinical setting, which were diagnosed using advanced devices , such as ImmunoCap (Crivellaro et al., 2020). In addition, patch testing can identify specific contact allergens that induce contact dermatitis and thereby inform appropriate management strategies. A detailed analysis of working conditions and a multidimensional diagnostic approach can improve diagnostic accuracy and lead to more effective treatment interventions. Knowledge of the clinical manifestations and diagnostic approaches to occupational dermatoses also derives from clinical reports that describe severe cases and their management. For instance, a case of severe poisoning following dermal exposure to monomethylamine highlighted multiple symptoms , such as nausea, confusion of consciousness, and multi-system dysfunction, which highlighted the need for early diagnosis and treatment (Zuo et al., 2025). Such case reports are of particular significance in shedding light on the clinical manifestations of toxic exposure and accentuating the importance of recognizing patterns of symptoms pertaining to occupational exposures. By applying appropriate diagnostic procedures and drawing on published findings, medical personnel are better able to understand the complexities of occupational skin diseases, thereby improving patient outcomes while maintaining workplace safety.

5.4.1. Common Symptoms of Occupational Skin Diseases

Occupational skin illnesses are a common problem in the majority of industries, impacting not only the wellbeing of employees but also the economic viability of firms. The most common symptom is dermatitis, which is skin inflammation characterized by redness, itching, and scaling. Contact dermatitis can be categorized into irritant and allergic types, with the latter typically developing through contact with hazardous substances , such as chemicals, metals, or plant allergens. This condition is prone to chronic dermatological complications if left untreated. Industries construction, healthcare, and manufacturing subject workers to a high risk, enabling a better understanding of preventive measures and treatment options, thereby promoting a healthier work environment and reducing absenteeism. Itching, of the most common signs of occupational skin diseases. Employees also typically report mild to severe discomfort that severely impairs their daily activities. Itch may come with observable signs , such as rashes or dryness, leading to a cycle of scratching that exacerbates the condition and makes it susceptible to secondary infection. Extended exposure may also lead to systemic manifestations, and it is therefore crucial that employers be informed about the implications of skin health on the general well-being of their workers. Employing effective measures to minimize skin irritants and giving the workers a prompt medical checkup is essential in shielding the workers against experiencing the debilitating effects of the symptoms. Furthermore, severe occupational skin disease can manifest in blistering, dermatitis, or even skin malignancy in extreme situations. Such diseases can be caused by prolonged exposure to toxic substances, such as industrial chemicals, or by continuous mechanical rubbing. Hot weather and repetitive activity can also cause skin damage. One highly troublesome complaint reported among certain medical practitioners concerns vaccination side effects, such as the recent Singaporean findings of mild but noteworthy skin reactions to the Pfizer-BioNTech COVID-19 vaccine in people with a history of eczema or sensitive skin (Lim et al., 2021). This underscores the need to monitor all aspects of occupational skin health so that employers and employees can work together to minimize risk and achieve optimal health outcomes in the workplace.

5.4.2. Diagnostic Methods Used by Healthcare Professionals

Diagnostic methods used by clinicians in occupational skin disease are crucial to the detection and treatment of processes caused by workplace exposures. Diagnoses often begin with a patient history, which includes assessing the patient's occupational exposure to an allergen or irritant. This is followed by medical providers conducting complete physical examinations of the affected skin. Visual inspection, while rudimentary, can be supplemented by sophisticated techniques, such as dermatoscopy that allows close examination of skin lesions. Furthermore, physicians can recommend patch testing to identify specific allergens responsible for contact dermatitis, thereby facilitating targeted interventions and treatment protocols required for healing and preventing recurrence. Technological advances have also enhanced the diagnostic capabilities of healthcare professionals dealing with occupational skin diseases. Mobile health technologies and devices are of irreplaceable worth in aiding clinicians by permitting disease surveillance and monitoring patient outcomes efficiently. For instance, telemedicine enables dermatologists to share information and provide real-time consultations, which is particularly beneficial for clinicians in remote areas facing potential epidemics. Furthermore, electronic health record integration facilitates the organized collection of patient information, enabling greater monitoring of disease patterns and analysis of emerging trends associated with unique work environments. As specified, the creation of these tools enhances diagnosis and communication and cooperation among healthcare providers, ultimately contributing to a more holistic approach to the management of occupational dermatoses (Cesario et al., 2014). Education and training of the medical staff are also crucial in refining diagnostic methods for occupational skin disorders. Continuous professional development workshops can provide staff with fresh data on the latest dermatological assessment and treatment protocols. Involvement in multidisciplinary forums—where skin experts, allergists, and occupational health specialists convene—refines comprehension of complex cases. Moreover, healthcare professionals are also prompted to consider ethical aspects, particularly patient confidentiality and autonomy, in the case of diagnostic examinations, for instance, the process of obtaining consent for skin biopsies under some circumstances. Competent health professionals experienced in new diagnostic techniques can do much to stem the spread of occupational skin diseases and indirectly improve workplace health outcomes (Gostin, 1989) (Figure 5.10).

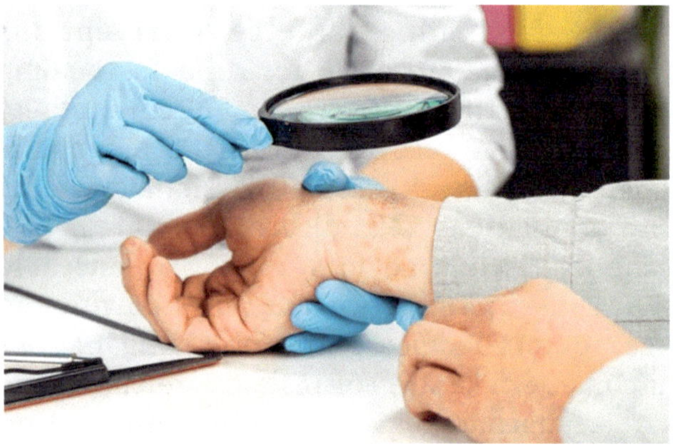

Figure 5.10. Healthcare professionals play identifying skin conditions that arise from workplace exposures.

Source: https://www.shutterstock.com/image-photo/dermatologist-wearing-gloves-examines-skin-600nw-1866052180.jpg.

5.4.3. Importance of Early Detection and Intervention

The significance of early diagnosis and intervention of occupational skin disease cannot be overemphasized. These diseases usually take years to develop, quietly progressing until they arrive at advanced stages, resulting in more extreme health problems for the afflicted. Providing measures for early detection, including regular skin checks and occupational education, encourages proactive risk-management strategies across various occupations. For instance, workers exposed to hazardous chemicals or constant workplace irritation can be significantly assisted by early detection of skin abnormalities. With this, employers can reduce the cost of such conditions not only on employees' health but also on overall workplace productivity. Early treatments, along with rigorous preventive measures, create a twofold safety net that has proven effective with respect to workplace health outcomes. Further, early intervention is likely to lead to more effective treatment regimes that minimize the risk of chronic skin disease. For instance, prompt measures like modification of work environments could greatly alleviate the severity and incidence of skin diseases such as dermatitis and psoriasis. By focusing on early intervention, health care professionals can develop individualized treatment plans based on specific risk factors and workplace exposures.

This customized approach maximizes recovery outcomes and reduces prolonged absenteeism by ensuring that employees receive appropriate care before complications develop. Early intervention is also less costly to employers and employees in the long term as it reduces the cost impact of treatments done in advanced stages and ongoing healthcare expenses for chronic skin conditions. In addition to ensuring individual health and workplace effectiveness, early diagnosis and intervention are also key in enhancing overall public health outcomes. When occupational skin diseases are identified and treated promptly, the spillover impact reaches the larger environment outside the workplace. Healthcare systems are better positioned to plan ahead and budget accordingly, ultimately resulting in population-level cost savings. By prioritizing early detection and intervention practices in workplaces, firms can cultivate a culture of health and safety that not only protects workers but also motivates the broader population to address preventable health issues. This visionary text aligns with public health objectives, such as reducing overall disease burden and improving quality of life, and it emphasizes the imperative to create systematic systems for early intervention in occupational dermatology situations (Fang et al., 2022; Bray et al., 2024).

Test Your Knowledge

1. What are the most common symptoms of occupational skin diseases?
2. Which occupational skin diseases commonly present with contact dermatitis?
3. What diagnostic tests are commonly used to identify occupational allergens causing skin diseases?

5.5. Prevention Strategies

Learning Outcome

1. Understand the utilization of personal protective equipment (PPE) in preventing occupational skin diseases.
2. Describe workplace safety protocols and training.
3. Explain the role of employers in preventing skin diseases.

Occupational dermatitis and skin cancer are of great concern to employees in most sectors. The right prevention methods must be implemented in a bid to guarantee that these risks are averted and employees' health is maintained. Enhancing worker training and education on potential hazards encountered in the workplace is a simple step that can help ensure this. Developing a culture of awareness gives employees the ability to identify irritants and allergens at an early stage, thereby reducing exposure.

Furthermore, organizations should accord skin protection the necessary attention through the provision of personal protective equipment (PPE), such as gloves and protective clothing, to suit the nature of work and associated hazards in their work environments. Providing workers with full information on the use and care of PPE is essential to maximizing its protective effect, thereby reducing incidents of work-related skin diseases. In conjunction with educational interventions, the implementation of engineering and administrative controls is essential to the overall prevention of occupational skin disease. Organizations use ventilation systems to reduce airborne irritants and accomplish design modifications to reduce skin exposure to harmful chemicals. Additionally, administrative measures establishing exposure limits and staggering job assignments can reduce the frequency and duration of skin contact. Routine observation of work environments is also paramount for detecting emerging risks and ensuring compliance with safety laws. Establishing an environment with inherently minimized risk factors enables organizations to reduce the incidence of serious skin disease among workers, thereby improving their health and productivity.

Early diagnosis and pioneering biomarker studies play a central role in preventive strategies for occupational skin disease. Prompt identification of risk factors and symptoms will lead to early intervention and control. Non-invasive procedures, including tape stripping of the stratum corneum, provide valuable methods for assessing skin health and evaluating the effectiveness of preventive measures. Advances in biomarker science illustrate the applicability of such testing in assessing subtleties in the skin's barrier function resulting from occupational exposure. By integrating these biologic markers into occupational health assessments in a systematic way, employers can provide targeted interventions and encourage healthier workplaces that, in the long term, will reduce the prevalence of occupational skin disease.

5.5.1. Personal Protective Equipment (PPE)

Personal protective equipment (PPE) use is vital to preventing occupational skin diseases, which have become increasingly prevalent in most workplaces in recent years. Properly fitted and well-designed PPE masks, gowns, and gloves, is a vital barrier against noxious substances that can lead to skin irritation or contact dermatitis. Because most jobs, particularly those in manufacturing and healthcare, expose workers to sensitizers and irritants, proper use of PPE is paramount. Utilization of PPE, strategically coupled with the prevention of direct contact of skin with harmful chemicals, not only protects the skin from contact with dangerous chemicals but also prevents long-term health consequences attributable to cumulative exposure. Therefore, organizations must place strong emphasis on PPE training to ensure that workers are informed about the importance and proper use of protective equipment to prevent skin diseases in the workplace. Furthermore, current guidelines point out the importance of PPE in managing some conditions , such as hand eczema in workers. Evidence indicates that hand eczema, a common inflammatory skin condition, requires ongoing education for healthcare practitioners on its management. As highlighted in the guidelines developed by the European Society of Contact Dermatitis, familiarization with measures for prevention in the use of PPE can be the difference between life and death for those who are affected (Jacob et al., 2021). Adding training in PPE to the overall curriculum of occupational health can enhance awareness and adherence among employees. This program not only improves workers' health but also reduces the economic burden of treatment and the productivity losses associated with skin diseases. Therefore, an integrated implementation strategy for PPE can lead to a remarkable decline in occupational skin disease incidence. Additionally, the dynamic process of occupational health necessitates continuous updating of PPE guidelines in response to emerging evidence and guidelines. The 2021 European Resuscitation Council Guidelines emphasize the need for evidence-based practice in various occupational environments, including the didactic role of PPE for handling emergencies (Gavin et al., 2021). As industries learn to address emerging challenges such as technological advancement and new chemicals, it is critical that responses through PPE are both pertinent and effective. There must be periodic training and testing intervals to foster compliance and effectiveness in preventing skin illnesses. Such an active employment of PPE, aside from protecting worker health, also comes a long way towards fostering a culture of safety and awareness in employers. Employers can also further guarantee their employees' safety against the ever-present threat of occupational skin illness by embracing and maintaining the practice of PPE (Figure 5.11).

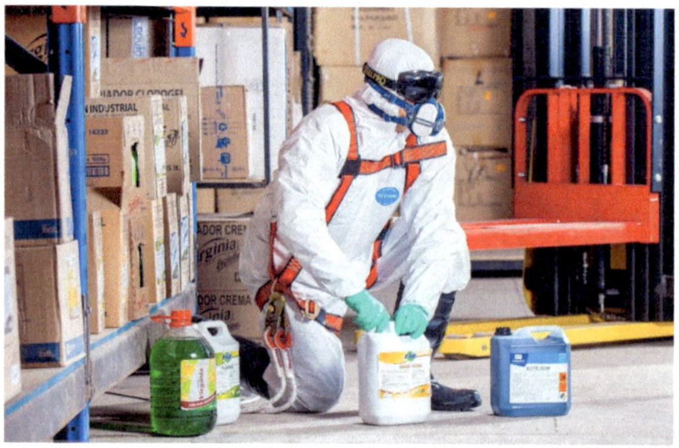

Figure 5.11. The use of personal protective equipment (PPE) is crucial for preventing occupational skin diseases.

Source: https://www.hsestudyguide.com/wp-content/uploads/2024/02/pexels-photo-209230-1.jpeg.

5.5.2. Workplace Safety Protocols and Training

Poor workplace safety procedures significantly contribute to the prevention of occupational skin diseases resulting from prolonged exposure to toxic substances or conditions. To prevent such exposures, organizations must implement comprehensive training sessions that familiarize employees with potential skin hazards, appropriate personal protective equipment (PPE), and teach safe handling practices. Effective training sessions should be scheduled to cultivate an awareness of specific skin conditions specific to certain work environments, including dermatitis, allergic contact dermatitis, and infections. Such training helps staff recognize early symptoms and encourages prompt reporting to their managers, thereby decreasing the incidence of these conditions. In addition, the workplaces can be supported by periodic safety audits and health examinations to ensure adherence to the established protocols, such that changes and improvements in the organization's safety culture can be addressed if necessary (Fang et al., 2022).

The application of advanced technology in workplace safety training can improve workers' knowledge and compliance regarding skin health. Wearable devices and Internet of Things worker solutions are valuable tools that monitor constantly changing environmental conditions and personal exposure levels, providing real-time information that enables immediate responses to potential hazards. For instance, health wearables designed to track sun exposure can alert outdoor workers to apply sunscreen or seek shade, thereby significantly reducing the risk of skin cancer from UV radiation. Moreover, predictive analytics can help organizations identify trends in skin health issues, enabling preventive measures to mitigate risks before they reach dangerous levels. Integrating such technologies into organizational occupational safety strategies ensures that employees are equipped with the latest knowledge and resources necessary to protect their skin health, thereby fostering a safety culture (Patel et al., 2021). Beyond training and technology implementation, a positive workplace culture is essential for enforcing safety measures and minimizing occupational skin disease. It requires creating an environment with open lines of communication between workers and the company, so that people feel free to report health issues and incidents without fear of retaliation. Management should actively engage in sharing skin health programs by releasing products, such as skincare products, educational materials, and dermatology consultation access. By maintaining employee well-being, organizations create a culture of prevention and care that translates into improved overall workplace satisfaction. Moreover, participation in health and well-being programs can yield better morale and productivity among employees, as an example to show that investment in health and safety is good for employers and employees in the long run (Patel et al., 2021) (Figure 5.12).

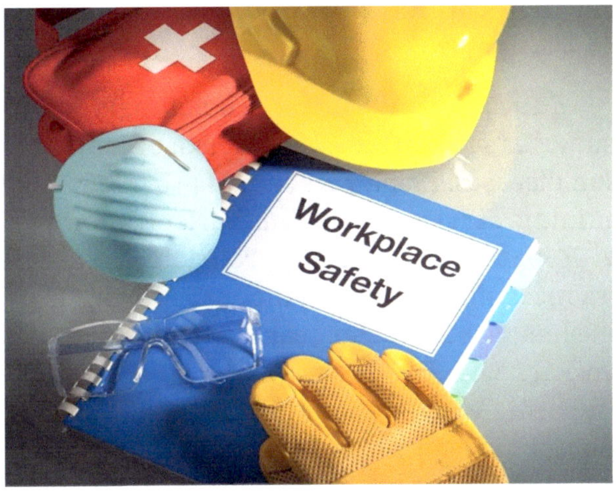

Figure 5.12. Effective workplace safety protocols are crucial in preventing occupational skin diseases.

Source: https://d8it4huxumps7.cloudfront.net/uploads/images/65fac27c5c471_2.jpg?d=2000x2000.

5.5.3. Role of Employers in Preventing Skin Diseases

The employers have a critical role to play in ensuring the prevention of occupational skin disorders through fostering a work culture where skin care is a priority. This involves proper risk analysis and compliance of protective procedures based on work environments. Employers can identify potential skin irritants and allergens in the workplace by collaborating with occupational health professionals. For instance, they may recommend low-irritancy products and personal protective equipment (PPE) with low sensitization potential so that employees may be safeguarded against adverse exposure. Secondly, promoting skin creams as an active barrier can substantially reduce the risk of dermatitis, demonstrating an employer's concern for employees. This preventive measure not only reduces the incidence of skin diseases but also enhances morale and productivity across the workplace, illustrating how preventive health measures can be of dual value for employees and the company in the long term (Filon et al., 2025).

Education is also a crucial part of an employer's role in the prevention of occupational skin diseases. Employers should provide regular training sessions that familiarize employees with potential risks, appropriate skin-care practices, and the importance of reporting signs of skin disease at an early stage. Educating workers with better knowledge is a means of preparing workers with information regarding the risks they are likely to encounter as well as encouraging them to apply protective measures on their own. Providing regular explanations of the importance of maintaining skin integrity to employees also demonstrates employers' commitment to employee health. Integration of health education campaigns can also help demystify skin diseases, making employees more likely to report early for intervention when symptoms appear. Therefore, an employer's investment in education can promote a proactive health culture that reduces the incidence of occupational skin diseases and promotes long-term workforce sustainability (Marcinkiewicz et al., 2024). Monitoring and surveillance of skin conditions are the most important parts of an employer's function in the prevention of occupational skin disease. By adopting regular medical check-ups and routine medical examinations, the employers are able to detect workers at risk early on and render early treatment and diagnosis a possibility. Occupational health services must conduct regular screenings to identify signs of irritant contact dermatitis and other conditions among workers. By taking this step, employers can tailor their preventive measures to address an employee's specific concerns and risk factors. Furthermore, by making the reporting of skin issues easy for workers, there is an opportunity for timely intervention and appropriate guidance. This constant commitment not only highlights the responsibility of employers to maintain a healthy working environment but also strengthens a healthy culture that respects preventive care and early intervention, and ultimately leads to a healthier workforce (Filon et al., 2025).

Test Your Knowledge

1. What types of personal protective equipment (PPE) are commonly used to prevent occupational skin diseases?
2. What workplace safety protocols can help minimize the occurrence of occupational skin diseases?

5.6. Treatment Options

Learning Outcome

1. Understand topical treatments and medications.
2. Discuss systemic treatments for severe cases.
3. Explain the importance of follow-up care and management.

The therapies for occupational skin diseases vary significantly depending on the specific condition and case severity. The treatments in most instances include pharmacological interventions, lifestyle modifications, and protective measures to reduce exposure to irritants. Dermatological therapy, for instance, may include topical corticosteroids to reduce inflammation and pruritus. Systemic medications, such as immunosuppressives, may be employed for severe conditions to manage chronic cases. In addition, protective barriers such as gloves and masks are recommended for patients handling hazardous substances to minimize exposure through skin contact. Individualized treatment protocols are also requiredgiven that , given that the effectiveness of such interventions may vary among patients based on occupational exposure risk and personal medical history, necessitating a tailored approach to manage symptoms effectively. In conditions contact dermatitis and eczema, preventing exposure to irritants and allergens can significantly influence treatment outcomes. This may be in the form of adjustments to workplace settings and processes, including improved ventilation and the use of less toxic chemicals. Education on skin care practices following contact with irritants can also facilitate healing and prevent relapse. In addition, it should be ensured that patients are motivated to attend regular follow-up visits to monitor their skin condition. Empirical evidence shows that active changes in lifestyle and the environment result in a significant decline in symptoms and frequency of flare-ups. In general, effective control of occupational skin diseases depends on a multifaceted approach that integrates medical care with practical lifestyle modifications to ensure long-term skin health. New forms of therapy for occupational dermatitis are emerging; therefore, it is essential that the development of therapeutic options for these diseases continue unabated. Modalities , such as laser therapy and phototherapy are being evaluated for efficacy in managing occupational exposure-related chronic skin diseases. The genetic factors underlying these diseases are also being studied, which may lead to more targeted therapies in the future. As a component of this dynamic environment, clinicians have to pay special attention to the patient's individual situation the work context and existing illness conditions, when issuing a treatment protocol. Significant importance should also be given to optimizing patient education, which enables individuals to understand their conditions and the range of available treatment modalities. By encouraging well-informed decisions, patient compliance will increase, and, consequently, better health outcomes in occupational skin disease management will be achieved.

5.6.1. Topical Therapies and Medicines

Management of occupational skin diseases typically involves topical medications and treatments, which can provide localized relief for a variety of inflammatory skin diseases that present after occupational exposure. Topical corticosteroids have long been established as a first-line treatment for these diseases. Their capacity to dampen inflammation and provide symptomatic relief makes them a key component of the treatment regimen. Even so, systemic and cutaneous adverse effects must be considered, as they can lead to problems in chronic treatment. A consensus among professionals has highlighted the need for clinicians to weigh the effectiveness of topical corticosteroids against the potential medical-legal risks of their prescription (Burshtein et al.,

2025). Accordingly, therapy with a holistic strategy must encompass patient education on proper use and the potential for side effects to maximize therapeutic benefit. Beyond corticosteroids, recent advances in topical therapy have provided clinicians with alternatives for managing occupational skin disorders. New non-steroidal drugs , such as difamilast and delgocitinib have emerged in meta-analysis and network meta-analysis of their efficacy and safety. These medications have been shown to improve Eczema Area and Severity Index (EASI) and Investigator Global Assessment (IGA) scores in conditions such as atopic dermatitis, which is prevalent in workplaces. Investigations have found that difamilast, for example, has an acceptable safety margin, lower rates of acne than other treatments, and a favorable profile (Murota et al., 2025). Such developments suggest that the landscape of topical treatment of occupational dermatoses is evolving as more lines of therapy can be properly used. Moreover, the utilization of targeted topical treatments foreshadows the move toward personalized treatment regimens in the management of occupational dermatoses. Specifically for individual inflammatory pathways, these newer treatments aim to maximize patient outcomes without increasing the risk of side effects typically associated with conventional corticosteroids. Recommendations from recent systematic reviews highlight the importance of assessing efficacy and safety when selecting appropriate topical therapy (Murota et al., 2025). Since occupational dermatoses are highly individualized among patients due to diverse exposures and genetic determinants, practitioners will require advanced knowledge of these treatments. This will not only increase patient compliance but also pave the way for better long-term care of occupational dermatoses and hence decrease the burden on affected populations (Figure 5.13).

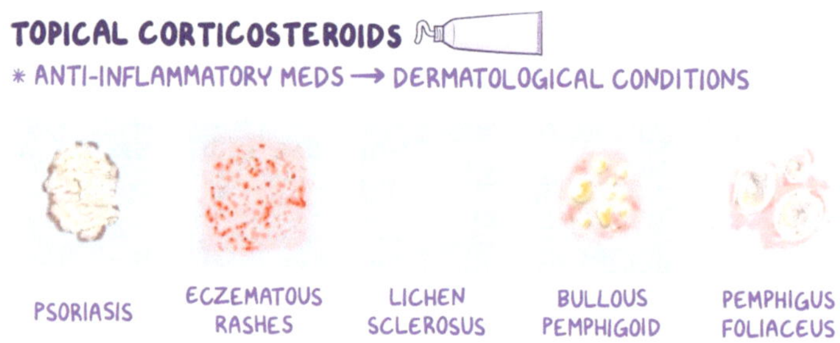

Figure 5.13. Topical corticosteroids are a common and effective first-line treatment for various occupational skin diseases.

Source: https://d16qt3wv6xm098.cloudfront.net/TP7ORpeXTk_eFa6O30_wcTEMQ36wKX-P/_.jpg.

5.6.2. Systemic Treatments for Severe Cases

Systemic treatments for serious occupational dermatoses are necessary to manage conditions that significantly impair the person's quality of life and work ability. Systemic treatments are particularly needed for patients with diseases , such as atopic dermatitis and scleroderma, in whom local treatments may prove to be inadequate. Systemic treatments comprise a broad spectrum of pharmacological agents, including biologics and immunosuppressants, which target the pathologic inflammatory pathways. For instance, lebrikizumab, an innovative biologic, demonstrated therapeutic efficacy comparable to established therapies such as dupilumab in the management of moderate-to-severe atopic dermatitis, improving patients' symptomatic relief and functional ability in occupational tasks (Omali et al., 2024). Individualized systemic treatment regimens not only alleviate symptoms but also reduce disease flares triggered by occupational exposure, thereby maximizing work performance and quality of life. Scleroderma, a chronic disease with skin thickening and multi-organ complications, is particularly challenging in the workplace, particularly for those whose work is in the hands (Omali et al., 2024). Scleroderma systemic therapy aims to slow the disease's progression and its adverse effects on daily functioning, particularly for those whose work entails fine motor skills. Practical adaptations of the working environment, alongside systemic therapy, help patients to remain productive and reduce the psychological burden accompanying chronic disease.

The use of therapeutic methods, along with ergonomic adjustments, can prolong a patient's working years and therefore supports the need to incorporate medical and occupational health interventions in the management of severe systemic skin diseases. Supporting pharmacologic therapy, regular monitoring, and care are integral parts of a comprehensive treatment regimen in workers with serious occupational dermatoses. Regular assessment of therapy efficacy, side effects, and functional status enables appropriate decisions about therapy adjustments. Clinical studies have found that patients who respond well to systemic treatments experience substantial quality-of-life improvements, including alleviation of the physical limitations their diseases impose (Jonathan et al., 2024). Also, multidisciplinary collaboration among occupational health professionals, employers, and dermatologists is essential to creating a healthy workplace and improving employee productivity and well-being. This coordinated management of serious cases both enhances patient outcomes and pays dividends for organizations by maintaining a healthier workforce and ultimately reducing economic costs due to absenteeism and lost work capacity (Figure 5.14).

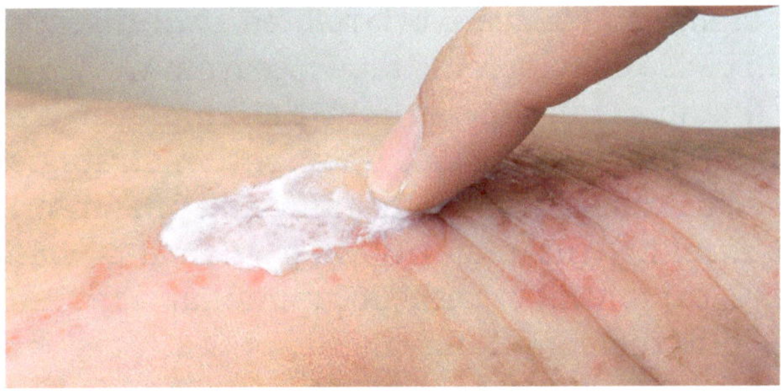

Figure 5.14. Immunosuppressants are used to treat occupational skin diseases.

Source: https://amperna.com/cdn/shop/articles/AMPERNA-immunosuppressants_49cd80c6-a1c3-4f68-8a14-201b1f9f15f4.jpg?v=1738196111.

5.6.3. Importance of Follow-Up Care and Management

In occupational skin disease care, follow-up is as essential as it can be. Follow-up appointments enable treatment physicians to monitor the progress of affected individuals, assess the effectiveness of treatment regimens, and address emerging symptoms. Through such aggressive monitoring, complications that are most likely to be prevented as conditions , such as contact dermatitis or eczema, typical of workplace exposures, have a running start at developing full-blown problems. Such surveillance is especially needed in high-risk skin-disease occupations, where constant observation and adjustments to protective protocols can effectively minimize symptoms and improve employees' lives. With open communication between patients and health care providers during follow-up visits, a more tailored treatment regimen may be devised, thereby maximizing long-term patient outcomes. Apart from this, structured follow-up programs have been found to provide occupational stability advantages in other respects. For instance, among metal workers, those enrolled in a comprehensive follow-up care program experienced fewer job losses due to work-related skin conditions. This is significant since work-related skin diseases can cause considerable time loss from work and a financial burden on both the employer and the employee. Through intervention strategies such as skin protection training and one-on-one counseling, the majority of participants were able to continue with occupational activities despite the conditions. Evidence indicates that job retention not only supports economic self-sufficiency among workers but also improves psychological well-being, underscoring the value of follow-up care (Wilke et al., 2018). Moreover, follow-up care is instrumental for educating patients on effective self-management techniques for their skin disease. Through ongoing education and support, patients are better able to recognize early warning signs of deteriorating conditions and implement protective practices tailored to their occupational environments. This allows for greater compliance with suggested protective practices, such as donning gloves or barrier creams on a regular basis. In addition, regularly evaluating disease severity encourages collaboration between patients and their treatment providers, allowing treatment plans to be adjusted as needed. As evidenced by increased patient satisfaction and perceived control of disease in ongoing programs, emphasis on follow-up care and management in occupational environments eventually leads to long-term reduction of both incidence and severity of occupational skin diseases (Wilke et al., 2018).

Test Your Knowledge

1. What are the first-line topical treatments commonly used for occupational irritant and allergic contact dermatitis?
2. When are systemic treatments indicated in occupational skin diseases?

SUMMARY

In summary, occupational skin diseases are significant health hazards across various industries and workplaces. The state of disorders among employees depends on numerous factors, from environmental contact and work habits to individual susceptibility. Such a multifactorial etiology underscores the need for effective preventive strategies and sound management practices to prevent employee exposure to potential harm. The link between workplace exposure and the development of skin disorders highlights the need for regular education and training in these areas to alert workers and employers to risks and to maximize techniques for reducing exposure. A comprehensive occupational health strategy not only maintains workers' safety but also supports overall productivity and employee morale. Moreover, it is essential to understand the demographic determinants of occupational dermatoses so that intervention campaigns can be suitably tailored. For instance, ethnicity plays a role in the perception of such diseases, as has been witnessed in observations that document unequal occurrences of chronic illnesses in various ethnic groups within the work environment. Evidence suggests that UK South Asians, for example, are likely to have greater proportions of limiting long-term illness compared to other groups because of occupational hazards and the availability of preventive care (Clay et al., 2004). Interventions that work effectively in occupational health must account for such inequalities to ensure inclusivity, cultural appropriateness, and responsiveness to the specific needs of diverse worker groups. It is pivotal in providing equal health outcomes across various occupational groups. Ultimately, policy formulation and enforcement in the workplace are paramount to addressing occupational skin diseases. As the evidence suggests, preventive measures extensive surveillance, risk assessment, and the establishment of safety standards can significantly reduce cases of these diseases. Furthermore, fostering a work culture of skin health and wellbeing, for instance through workshops and health promotion activities, is essential for sensitizing employees (Atmaca et al., 2016). Training programs should focus on educating employees about protective equipment, skincare procedures, and symptom reporting. As businesses do this, they not only protect their employees but also contribute to having a healthier workforce that ultimately benefits society as a whole.

Occupational skin disorders are a serious public health concern, particularly in workplaces where workers are continuously exposed to toxic chemicals. Dominant themes highlight that occupational skin disorders do not only occur as a direct consequence of exposure to irritants and allergens but also through organizational problems within the workplace. For instance, the prevalence of dermatological issues across demographic and ethnic groups may vary and warrant scrutiny. Specifically, UK South Asians, while being underrepresented in hazardous occupations, have greater proportions of limiting long-term illness compared to other populations, and this affects their workplace participation and state of health (Clay et al., 2004). This kind of observation underscores the need for targeted health and safety interventions to address the unique needs of these workers and improve their overall occupational well-being. Furthermore, the economic impacts of occupational skin disease are substantial to both employers and employees. Skin disease can lead to higher absenteeism, lower job satisfaction, and increased healthcare costs, all of which can undermine organizational effectiveness. Rhetoric in the literature emphasizes successful workplace safety programs that meet regulatory standards while also promoting a prevention and awareness culture among employees. Systematic safety and health activities must cover a risk assessment of the work environment, including exposure to chemicals and physical agents, as well as ergonomic factors (Pouliakas, K.,

& Theodossiou, I., 2010). Prioritizing workers' health is not only an ethical imperative; it is also a strategic way to reduce the significant social and economic burden of occupational skin disease. Lastly, future research directions should focus on enhancing monitoring and data collection on occupational skin disorders among oppressed communities. The evidence here indicates a need for improved methodology capable of measuring a wide range of occupational safety and health (OSH) indicators, including environmental and individual determinants of skin disease. Through detailed analysis of existing data and by stimulating interdisciplinary alliances, stakeholders can identify knowledge gaps and develop focused interventions for at-risk groups (Pouliakas, K., & Theodossiou, I., 2010). Project schemes, such as occupational health promotion workshops designed especially for ethnic minorities, can be a useful resource in managing occupational dermatitis hazards, thus leading to healthy workplaces in different sectors (Clay et al., 2004).

KEY TERMS FROM THIS CHAPTER

- Allergic contact dermatitis (ACD)
- Allergic reactions
- Atopic dermatitis
- Autoimmune correlations
- Biological agents
- Causative agents
- Community-level engagement
- Contact dermatitis
- COVID-19 pandemic
- Critical health
- Dermatological infections
- Dermatoses
- Disease patterns
- Eczema Area and Severity Index (EASI)
- Exposure risks
- Health care resources
- Health care sector,
- Healthcare providers

CRITICAL THINKING QUESTIONS

1. **Which of the following is the most common type of occupational skin disease?**
   a. Psoriasis
   b. Occupational contact dermatitis
   c. Skin cancer
   d. Acne
2. **Which of the following is a primary cause of occupational skin diseases?**
   a. Excessive sun exposure only
   b. Genetic predisposition only
   c. Exposure to irritants and allergens at the workplace
   d. Poor diet
3. **Which group of workers is most at risk for occupational skin diseases?**
   a. Office workers with no contact with chemicals
   b. Construction workers, hairdressers, and healthcare workers
   c. Software developers
   d. Teachers
4. **What is a common symptom of occupational skin diseases , such as contact dermatitis?**
   a. Itching, redness, and scaling of the skin
   b. Blurred vision
   c. Hair loss
   d. Muscle weakness
5. **Which of the following is an effective prevention strategy for occupational skin diseases?**
   a. Regular use of sunscreen only
   b. Avoiding all physical activity at work
   c. Taking antibiotics daily
   d. Using personal protective equipment (PPE) like gloves and barrier creams

Short Answer Questions

1. What are the main types of occupational skin diseases commonly seen in the workplace?
2. What are the primary causes and risk factors associated with occupational skin diseases?
3. Which worker populations are at higher risk of developing occupational skin diseases?
4. What are common symptoms indicating the presence of an occupational skin disease?
5. What prevention strategies are effective in reducing the incidence of occupational skin diseases?
6. What are typical topical treatments used for occupational skin diseases?
7. When are systemic treatments indicated for occupational skin diseases, and what options are available?
8. Why is early diagnosis and ongoing management important in occupational skin diseases?

Answer to Critical Thinking Questions

1. (b); 2. (c); 3. (b); 4. (a); 5. (d)

REFERENCES

1. Aboulmira, A., Hrimech, H., & Lachgar, M. (2024). Skin Diseases Classification with Machine Learning and Deep Learning Techniques: A Systematic Review. *International Journal of Advanced Computer Science and Applications, 15*(10). https://doi.org/10.14569/ijacsa.2024.01510118Abuzreda, A. (2025). Comprehensive administrative and engineering strategies for radiation protection and occupational health safety. *Clinical and Medical Engineering Live*. https://www.semanticscholar.org/paper/c8b269bbced6dc1a6b9d33ee95f5e76b310a01cc (accessed on 21st July 2025).
2. Al-Delaimy, W. K., Larsen, C. W., & Pezzoli, K. (2014). Differences in health symptoms among residents living near illegal dump sites in Los Laureles Canyon, Tijuana, Mexico: A cross-sectional survey. https://core.ac.uk/download/323065370.pdf (accessed on 21st July 2025).
3. Aledani, E. M., Gurramkonda, J., Chaudhri, S. I., Amin, A., Panjiyar, B., Al-taie, D. S., & Nath, T. S. (2024). COVID-19-related risk factors for developing occupational contact dermatitis along with its incidence, prevention, and management: A systematic review. *Cureus, 16*. https://www.semanticscholar.org/paper/2de2de4b51c729a81240f9b2e0a75bed7ee84d4a (accessed on 21st July 2025).
4. Ali, H., Khan, E., & Ilahi, I. (2019). Environmental chemistry and ecotoxicology of hazardous heavy metals: Environmental persistence, toxicity, and bioaccumulation. *Journal of Chemistry, 2019*, 1–14. https://doi.org/10.1155/2019/6730305 (accessed on 21st July 2025).
5. Atmaca, M., Fineberg, N. A., Fontenelle, L. F., Grant, J. E., et al. (2016). The classification of obsessive–compulsive and related disorders in the ICD-11. https://core.ac.uk/download/213085588.pdf (accessed on 21st July 2025).
6. Balla, M. P., Marsico, C., Marsico, S., Massoni, F., et al. (2017). Work-related allergic rhinitis: A contemporary review of the literature. https://core.ac.uk/download/154947305.pdf (accessed on 21st July 2025).
7. Bizel, G., Einstein, A., Jaunjare, A. G., & Jagannathan, S. (2024). Machine learning study: Identification of skin diseases for various skin types using image classification. *Journal of Big Data and Artificial Intelligence*. https://www.semanticscholar.org/paper/9f429abb5a47a5b73c57ad635fc66d3f41b28f43 (accessed on 21st July 2025).
8. Bray, F., Laversanne, M., Sung, H., Ferlay, J., Siegel, R. L., Soerjomataram, I., & Jemal, A. (2024). Global cancer statistics 2022: GLOBOCAN estimates of incidence and mortality worldwide for 36 cancers in 185 countries. *CA: A Cancer Journal for Clinicians, 74*, 229–263. https://doi.org/10.3322/caac.21834 (accessed on 21st July 2025).
9. Burak, I. I., & Cherkasova, O. A. (2013). Labor safety. https://core.ac.uk/download/53873565.pdf (accessed on 21st July 2025).
10. Burshtein, J., Chovatiya, R., Golant, A., Zakria, D., Shah, M., Lio, P., & Lebwohl, M. (2025). Risks of topical corticosteroid therapy and role for advanced targeted topical treatments for inflammatory skin diseases: An expert consensus panel. *Dermatology Online Journal, 31*(1). https://www.semanticscholar.org/paper/1b85d15cca70f521fc4848c792b1385e1645030f (accessed on 21st July 2025).
11. Cesario, M., Luz, S., & Masoodian, M. (2014). Disease surveillance and patient care in remote regions: An exploratory study of collaboration among healthcare professionals in Amazonia. https://core.ac.uk/download/29202884.pdf (accessed on 21st July 2025).

12. Clay, D., Davies, R., Elias, P., Gumber, A., et al. (2004). Review of the occupational health and safety of Britain's ethnic minorities. https://core.ac.uk/download/105299.pdf (accessed on 21st July 2025).

13. Crivellaro, M., Malipiero, G., Maculan, P., Senna, G., Passalacqua, G., & Maestrelli, P. (2020). Severe asthma due to occupational exposure to Guar Gum: Is lipid transfer protein involved? *Occupational and Environmental Medicine, 77*, 427–427. https://www.semanticscholar.org/paper/468db9f7aaeab45352ff1b1ba86bf0c0bcb28323 (accessed on 21st July 2025).

14. De Luca, A., Di Ninno, F., Ferretti, F., Marani, G., et al. (2017). Screening for tuberculosis in health care workers: Experience in an Italian teaching hospital. https://core.ac.uk/download/84928372.pdf (accessed on 21st July 2025).

15. Drozdowska, A., Drozdowski, P., Jaworski, A., Bula, D., Adamczyk, D., & Reich, A. (2023). The novel questionnaire assessing occupational exposure to the risk factors of contact allergy among health professionals. *Advances in Dermatology and Allergology/Postępy Dermatologii i Alergologii, 40*, 291–297. https://www.semanticscholar.org/paper/a5e52ccdc1fbe8458bd1c4004b3caf43703a40f4 (accessed on 21st July 2025).

16. Dvornikov, A., Gusev, E. I., Martynov, M., Lashch, N., Gaydina, T., Chukanova, A. S., & Boyko, A. (2024). Autoimmune skin diseases in multiple sclerosis: Comorbidity issues and the impact of pathogenetic therapy. *Annals of the Russian Academy of Medical Sciences*. https://www.semanticscholar.org/paper/32fb55976fbed3a537f8e590e78d02330f505430 (accessed on 21st July 2025).

17. Ferronato, N., & Torretta, V. (2019). Waste mismanagement in developing countries: A review of global issues. *International Journal of Environmental Research and Public Health, 16*, 1060–1060. https://doi.org/10.3390/ijerph16061060 (accessed on 21st July 2025).

18. Gauci, M., & Vella, N. (1997). Occupational screening. https://core.ac.uk/download/46601749.pdf (accessed on 21st July 2025).

19. Gostin, L. (1989). Hospitals, health care professionals, and AIDS: The right to know the health status of professionals and patients. https://core.ac.uk/download/56357585.pdf (accessed on 21st July 2025).

20. Holness, D., Kudla, I., DeKoven, J., & Skotnicki, S. (2020). The utility of an occupational contact dermatitis patch test database in the analysis of workplace prevention activities in Toronto, Canada. *Annals of Work Exposures and Health*. https://www.semanticscholar.org/paper/ffb019eb314775119878f10ba6114b41d11ba4f4 (accessed on 21st July 2025).

21. Karpova, O., Filimonov, S. N., & Semenikhin, V. A. (2022). Industrial ecology and skin diseases. *Russian Journal of Occupational Health and Industrial Ecology*. https://www.semanticscholar.org/paper/35f962f50b139c25e54e379a0470b93af925110d (accessed on 21st July 2025).

22. Kezic, S., de Boer, F. D., & van der Molen, H. F. (2024). O-129 Non-invasive biomarkers for early detection and prevention of work-related skin diseases. *Occupational Medicine*. https://www.semanticscholar.org/paper/1ad7f96597079fe91231e679abe1c14934b69103 (accessed on 21st July 2025).

23. Kim, D., Kim, A., Kim, H., Lee, S., Seo, B., Suh, H., Sim, C., et al. (2022). Nickel dust-induced occupational contact dermatitis by welding and grinding work in shipyard workers: A report of nine cases. *Annals of Occupational and Environmental Medicine, 34*. https://www.

semanticscholar.org/paper/499b6745bc45e616d8255775436e8c168bbb3288 (accessed on 21st July 2025).

24. Larese Filon, F., & Rui, F. (2025). [Occupational allergic dermatitis: The role of the occupational physician in prevention]. *Giornale Italiano di Medicina del Lavoro ed Ergonomia*. https://www.semanticscholar.org/paper/5e2765ea994f137ef63fafb3449a9b0236069c79 (accessed on 21st July 2025).

25. Lim, S. M., Chan, H. C., Santosa, A., Quek, S. C., Liu, E. H. C., & Somani, J. (2021). Safety and side effect profile of Pfizer-BioNTech COVID-19 vaccination among healthcare workers: A tertiary hospital experience in Singapore. *Annals of the Academy of Medicine Singapore, 50*, 703–711. https://doi.org/10.47102/annals-acadmedsg.2021160 (accessed on 21st July 2025).

26. Marcinkiewicz, A., Walusiak-Skorupa, J., Wdówik, P., Zarębska-Michaluk, D., Inglot, M., Władysiuk, M., Prycel, T., et al. (2024). [Guidance for the occupational medicine service regarding the prevention of hepatitis C and HIV infection in Poland]. *Medycyna Pracy*. https://www.semanticscholar.org/paper/52bfcab01f5431674075ad1bceea6de7c7dfc0ae (accessed on 21st July 2025).

27. Montero-Odasso, M., van der Velde, N., Martin, F. C., Petrović, M., Tan, M. P., Ryg, J., Aguilar-Navarro, S. G., et al. (2022). World guidelines for falls prevention and management for older adults: A global initiative. *Age and Ageing, 51*. https://doi.org/10.1093/ageing/afac205 (accessed on 21st July 2025).

28. Mourad, R. A. H. (2022). Impact of climate change on occupational health and its possible preventive strategies (Review article). *Egyptian Journal of Occupational Medicine*. https://www.semanticscholar.org/paper/1e8478f3effdd17b6afda2720533c7ba66825b42 (accessed on 21st July 2025).

29. Murota, H., Nakahara, T., Wang, X., Matsukawa, M., Takeda, H., Kondo, T., & Yamato, K. (2025). Systematic literature review and network meta-analysis of clinical efficacy and safety of topical treatments for patients with atopic dermatitis. *Dermatology and Therapy, 15*, 1045–1062. https://www.semanticscholar.org/paper/f10b2f4661efda21a59f6de9f3e47ddb69bf5688 (accessed on 21st July 2025).

30. Office of Publication Services, Boston University Medical Center. (1989). *Progress*. https://core.ac.uk/download/142070617.pdf (accessed on 21st July 2025).

31. Omali, A., Wifaq, K., Tahri, L., Youabd, S., & El Kholti, A. (2024). O-226 Systemic scleroderma and occupational impacts: A case report. *Occupational Medicine*. https://www.semanticscholar.org/paper/0b78b74a6e0d63a13a6729b60cb936e785f24edc (accessed on 21st July 2025).

32. Patel, V., Chesmore, A., Legner, C., & Pandey, S. (2021). Trends in workplace wearable technologies and connected-worker solutions for next-generation occupational safety, health, and productivity. *Advanced Intelligent Systems, 4*. https://doi.org/10.1002/aisy.202100099 (accessed on 21st July 2025).

33. Perkins, G. D., Gräsner, J. T., Semeraro, F., Olasveengen, T. M., Soar, J., Lott, C., Van de Voorde, P., et al. (2021). European Resuscitation Council guidelines 2021: Executive summary. *Resuscitation, 161*, 1–60. https://doi.org/10.1016/j.resuscitation.2021.02.003 (accessed on 21st July 2025).

34. Pouliakas, K., & Theodossiou, I. (2010). An inquiry into the theory, causes and consequences of monitoring indicators of health and safety at work. https://core.ac.uk/download/177141.pdf (accessed on 21st July 2025).

35. Ruettermann, M., Hermann, R. M., Khatib-Chahidi, K., & Werker, P. M. N. (2021). Dupuytren's disease—Etiology and treatment. *Deutsches Ärzteblatt International*. https://doi.org/10.3238/arztebl.m2021.0325 (accessed on 21st July 2025).

36. Shakik, S., Arrandale, V. H., Holness, D. L., MacLeod, J., McLeod, C., Peter, A., & Demers, P. A. (2019). Dermatitis among workers in Ontario: Results from the Occupational Disease Surveillance System. *Occupational and Environmental Medicine, 76*, 625–631. https://doi.org/10.1136/oemed-2018-105667 (accessed on 21st July 2025).

37. Siegel, R. L., Miller, K. D., Fuchs, H. E., & Jemal, A. (2021). Cancer statistics, 2021. *CA: A Cancer Journal for Clinicians, 71*, 7–33. https://doi.org/10.3322/caac.21654 (accessed on 21st July 2025).

38. Silverberg, J. I., Bieber, T., Paller, A. S., Beck, L. A., Kamata, M., Puig, L., Wiseman, M., et al. (2024). Efficacy comparison of targeted systemic monotherapies including lebrikizumab for moderate-to-severe atopic dermatitis: A network meta-analysis. *SKIN: The Journal of Cutaneous Medicine*. https://www.semanticscholar.org/paper/0e5e1acc9885d2aef297dad0425de31ba684b7a3 (accessed on 21st July 2025).

39. Thyssen, J. P., Schuttelaar, M. L. A., Alfonso, J. H., Andersen, K. E., Angelova-Fischer, I., Arents, B. W. M., Bauer, A., et al. (2021). Guidelines for diagnosis, prevention, and treatment of hand eczema. *Contact Dermatitis, 86*, 357–378. https://doi.org/10.1111/cod.14035 (accessed on 21st July 2025).

40. Wilke, A., Gediga, G., Goergens, A., Hansen, A., Hübner, A., John, S. M., Nordheider, K., et al. (2018). Interdisciplinary and multiprofessional outpatient secondary individual prevention of work-related skin diseases in the metalworking industry: 1-year follow-up of a patient cohort. *BMC Dermatology, 18*. https://doi.org/10.1186/s12895-018-0080-2 (accessed on 21st July 2025).

41. Yalamanchi, V., Vadlamani, S., & Vennam, S. (2022). Occupational health problems and major risk factor profile of non-communicable diseases among workers in the aquaculture industry in Visakhapatnam. *Journal of Family Medicine and Primary Care, 11*, 3071–3076. https://www.semanticscholar.org/paper/1a8c1e9d29da8ac258420ca8c684659b95da8b49 (accessed on 21st July 2025).

42. Zota, A. R., & Shamasunder, B. (2017). The environmental injustice of beauty: Framing chemical exposures from beauty products as a health disparities concern. *American Journal of Obstetrics and Gynecology, 217*, 418.e1–418.e6. https://doi.org/10.1016/j.ajog.2017.07.020 (accessed on 21st July 2025).

43. Zuo, R. L., Liu, T., & Zhang, W. (2025). [A case report of acute poisoning caused by skin contact with cyanamide]. *Zhonghua Lao Dong Wei Sheng Zhi Ye Bing Za Zhi = Zhonghua Laodong Weisheng Zhiyebing Zazhi = Chinese Journal of Industrial Hygiene and Occupational Diseases, 43*(4), 302–304. https://www.semanticscholar.org/paper/4d849002fa75b0efa5e81ed589dbb1377ccfb9d2 (accessed on 21st July 2025).

DRUG REACTIONS AND ADVERSE CUTANEOUS DRUG ERUPTIONS

6

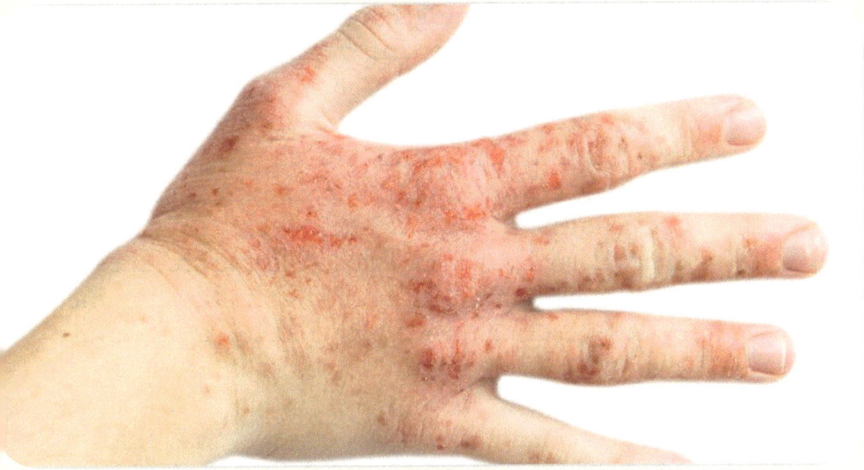

LEARNING OBJECTIVES

After studying this chapter, you will be able to:

1. Understand the mechanisms of drug reactions
2. Classify adverse cutaneous drug eruptions
3. Describe common drugs associated with cutaneous reactions
4. Focus on the diagnosis of adverse cutaneous drug eruptions
5. Explain how to manage drug reactions
6. Discuss how to prevent adverse drug reactions

Introduction

Understanding drug reactions is of great importance to dermatology, particularly in the study of cutaneous drug eruptions. Drug reactions are multidimensional interactions between pharmacologic agents and individual patients' responses, resulting in various dermatological presentations. Adverse drug reactions vary from mild and self-limiting cutaneous irritation to serious and potentially life-threatening conditions , such as Stevens-Johnson syndrome and toxic epidermal necrolysis. Assessing such reactions requires deep insight into the mechanisms involved, which are likely immune-mediated cascades that trigger inflammation and cell injury in the skin. Identification of the nature and severity of cutaneous reactions is most important to enable dermatologists to institute appropriate management, especially maximizing patient safety and preventing therapy interruptions. Among the wide range of drugs with the potential to cause cutaneous adverse reactions, those used for oncological therapies, for example, immune checkpoint inhibitors, have emerged as significant due to their unique mechanisms of action. Especially those targeting the programmed death cell protein 1 (PD-1) and PD-L1 are increasingly used in cancer therapy. While these represent an improvement in oncological therapy by enhancing anti-tumor immunity, they also introduce a new set of immune-related adverse events (irAEs) that primarily affect the skin. The skin findings range from maculopapular rashes to more severe forms , such as lichenoid dermatitis and dermatomyositis, hence complicating the clinical handling of cancer patients. Early diagnosis and proper management of these cutaneous responses are important in maintaining a balance between the effectiveness of cancer treatment and preventing the danger of serious cutaneous adverse effects (Bhardwaj et al., 2022).

In addition, the alimentary tract drug reactions unveil another dimension of drug-induced dermatological complications. A review of the surveillance reports of the Italian Group for Epidemiologic Research in Dermatology shows that cutaneous adverse reactions to the drugs, while present, are not very common and usually well-tolerated. The most frequent reactions, such as urticaria, angioedema, and exanthema, account for approximately 70% of cases. Besides, a reassuring image is encountered concerning antiulcer and antiemetic drugs, which appear to induce fewer cutaneous adverse reactions compared to other categories of drugs. This fact emphasizes the importance of systematized monitoring and reporting of drug reactions to alimentary drugs, as identification of dermatologic signs can lead to more appropriate patient care and more comprehensive information on drug safety (Epidemiologici GIS in Dermatologia, 1996).

Definition of Drug Reactions

Drug reactions are a broad range of undesirable effects that may arise as a consequence of drug administration. They can be divided primarily into adverse drug reactions (ADRs) and drug allergies, both with various pathophysiological mechanisms. ADRs are likely to be non-immune-mediated and can occur in any individual under the appropriate conditions, depending on factors like dose and vulnerability of the individual. For instance, typical presentations include gastrointestinal distress or cutaneous manifestations, such as rashes or pruritus. These latter presentations have both dermatological and non-dermatological etiologies and tend to complicate diagnosis and treatment. Recognition of such reactions is important in dermatology, where consequences for patient quality of life can be extensive and where cause-specific diagnostic work-up and therapeutic modalities are required. One of the most significant characteristics of drug reactions is the presence of hypersensitivity reactions, wherein the immune system mistakenly targets a drug as harmful. This type of reaction ranges from cutaneous manifestations that are mild, such as urticaria, to severe manifestations like Stevens-Johnson syndrome or toxic epidermal necrolysis. These severe manifestations are of significant concern in dermatology due to their potential to produce high morbidity and mortality. The challenge is not only to monitor the signs and symptoms but also to be capable of distinguishing between idiosyncratic reactions that may be linked to genetic factors and predictable reactions that are dose-dependent. Interestingly, with the advent of novel therapeutic modalities, including biologics and targeted drugs, there has been increased recognition of new cutaneous adverse drug eruption patterns that require greater attention and research from clinicians. The awareness of drug reactions extends beyond facile definition; it entails meticulous regard for their broad array of presentations, such as pruritus, experienced by a vast majority of individuals on medication. Population studies estimate chronic pruritus occurs in 7% of the general population, increasing further in specific patient groups, such as individuals with dermatologic disorders or on long-term therapy. Moreover, pruritus can also arise as a side effect of medication, complicating treatment effectiveness and necessitating multidisciplinary treatment approaches. Recognizing and managing dermatological adverse effects is essential to preserve a patient's quality of life and avoid deleterious acclimatization to necessary therapy. Hence, an interdisciplinary step, emphasized in recommendations those formulated by specialists in chronic pruritus, is vital to resolving complex drug issues in dermatology, ultimately affecting therapeutic guidelines and patient care (Figure 6.1).

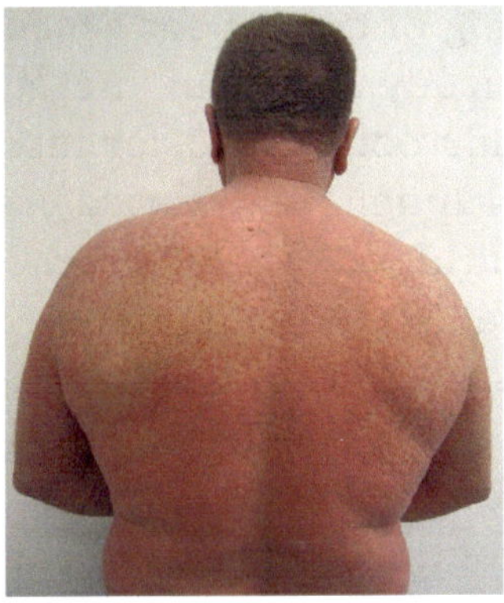

Figure 6.1. A rash due to a drug reaction.

Source: https://upload.wikimedia.org/wikipedia/commons/thumb/0/06/Drugreaction.jpg/800px-Drugreaction.jpg.

Importance of Understanding Drug Reactions in Dermatology

The value of learning to recognize drug reactions in dermatology cannot be overstated, as these reactions often represent the first clinical manifestation of toxic events after pharmacological interventions. Cutaneous drug adverse reactions (CADRs) are a group of dermatologic manifestations that evolve with systemic drug exposure, and therefore, proper detection and management are essential for maintaining the best patient outcomes. The literature indicates that as many as 10% of patients referred to the hospital are subjected to CADRs, highlighting their prevalence and the need for greater awareness among doctors. Identification of the causative agent is necessary to formulate the treatment regimen, and this is generally achieved by discontinuing the offending drug. By gaining a deeper understanding of the mechanisms and triggers of CADRs, dermatologists can significantly improve patient outcomes and reduce complications from unrecognized or inadequately managed drug eruptions (Sutaria et al., 2024). In addition, the study of drug reactions provides valuable information about the interface between pharmacology and immunology. Conditions , such as fixed-drug eruptions (FDE) are the prototype immune-mediated responses that produce cutaneous manifestations in the area of drug exposure. Data from case reports, such as the case report of a 51-year-old man who developed FDE after administration of cefadroxil, give us insight into the immunological process underlying conditions, such as the contribution of CD8+ memory T cells and cytokine release. Its comprehension not only facilitates early diagnosis and treatment but also supports foundational understanding that can be applied to the formulation of preventive interventions. Hence, recognition of the patterns and potential risks of different drug classes enhances clinicians' ability to predict and prevent adverse reactions before they become serious health threats (Agrawal et al., 2024). In addition, the added complexity of polypharmacy pharmacological regimens imposed in elderly patients or those with multiple comorbidities heightens the need for in-depth knowledge of drug reactions in dermatology. The complexity of these patients in general requires awareness of the drug interactions and potential cumulative adverse drug effects, the presentation of which is often cutaneous. By employing overall strategies that include patient education and close observation, practitioners can minimize the risk of cutaneous drug eruptions. A thorough knowledge of drug reactions not only informs safer prescribing but also promotes an active approach in dermatology that emphasizes vigilant monitoring and timely interventions. Thus, the requirement to be informed regarding drug reactions involves not only reactive therapy but also the promotion of a proactive, well-educated model of healthcare (Sutaria et al., 2024).

Overview of Common Types of Drug Reactions

It is crucial to learn the various types of drug reactions in dermatology, particularly with the prevalence of cutaneous drug eruptions. Drug reactions can be broadly categorized into two types: allergic and non-allergic reactions. Allergic reactions occur when the immune system falsely identifies a drug as a threatening substance, which causes an exaggerated reaction. The presentations are usually manifested as urticaria, angioedema, and anaphylaxis. On the other hand, non-allergic drug reactions are typically mediated by idiosyncratic reactions, dose-related toxicity, or pharmacologic effects and may vary greatly from person to person. The differential diagnosis between these two types is paramount to accurate diagnosis and treatment of drug-induced skin eruptions that have a major impact on clinical practice.

Among the common presentations of allergic drug reactions, cutaneous involvement is especially prevalent, often presenting as maculopapular eruptions. These eruptions can be of mild to severe degrees, with the potential of advancing to more dangerous conditions like Stevens-Johnson syndrome or toxic epidermal necrolysis. Reactions usually precipitated by common drugs include antibiotics and anticonvulsants, further emphasizing the need for clinicians to exercise due care in monitoring patients being subjected to these drugs. Causative drug identification is necessary in order to avoid the recurrence of the condition and to treat the symptoms. In certain cases, desensitization protocols must be implemented, underscoring the complexity of managing drug allergies in dermatologic practice. Non-allergic drug reactions, while often less emergently problematic than their allergic equivalents, remain pertinent in the dermatologic context due to their frequency and multidisciplinary presentation. These reactions are most commonly the result of the drug's pharmacologic action or incidental toxic exposure from cumulative dosing. Recognition of such reactions could require an in-depth understanding of the patient's medical history and pharmacodynamics of the administered drugs. Antimicrobial drugs, for instance, might cause skin eruptions with varied presentations, thereby requiring tailored approaches to treating skin health and underlying issues. As the field continues to advance, the creation of new therapeutic drugs requires ongoing education regarding potential drug reactions in order to provide the optimal situation in patients and to continually improve dermatological treatment.

6.1. Mechanisms of Drug Reactions

Learning Outcome

1. Understand pharmacological mechanisms for adverse cutaneous drug reactions (ACDRs).
2. Discus about immunological mechanisms in understanding drug reactions and adverse cutaneous drug eruptions.
3. Deal with genetic predisposition to drug reactions.

The multifactorial complexity of drug reactions, particularly dermatological reactions, stems from the interplay between drug action and the individual's immune system. Drug reactions can be classified generally into immediate hypersensitivity reactions, which occur within minutes to hours after exposure, and delayed-type hypersensitivity reactions that occur after days. The immediate reactions are likely to include the activation of IgE antibodies and mast cells to shed inflammatory mediators , such as histamine, while delayed-type reactions are largely mediated by T-lymphocytes and may lead to a range of cutaneous eruptions. Understanding these mechanisms is important for dermatologists to diagnose and distinguish benign from life-threatening illnesses, because eruptions can be precursors to severe outcomes such as Stevens–Johnson syndrome or toxic epidermal necrolysis. Identification of such cues may be helpful in successful management (Yan et al., 2025). Cutaneous drug eruptions also exhibit diverse morphological features and distinctive properties that may aid clinical diagnosis. The typical presentations include morbilliform eruptions, urticaria, and fixed drug eruptions, each representing distinct underlying mechanisms. Morbilliform rashes, for instance, are likely to appear as erythematous papules and macules and usually represent minor drug reactions. Urticaria is characterized by wheals and is primarily due to mast cell degranulation. Differences in presentation indicate the need for thorough knowledge of drug characteristics and patient susceptibility, including genetic influences that may affect drug metabolism and immune function. Differences are pivotal to establishing an effective management plan and optimal patient care (Abhinesh et al., 2024).

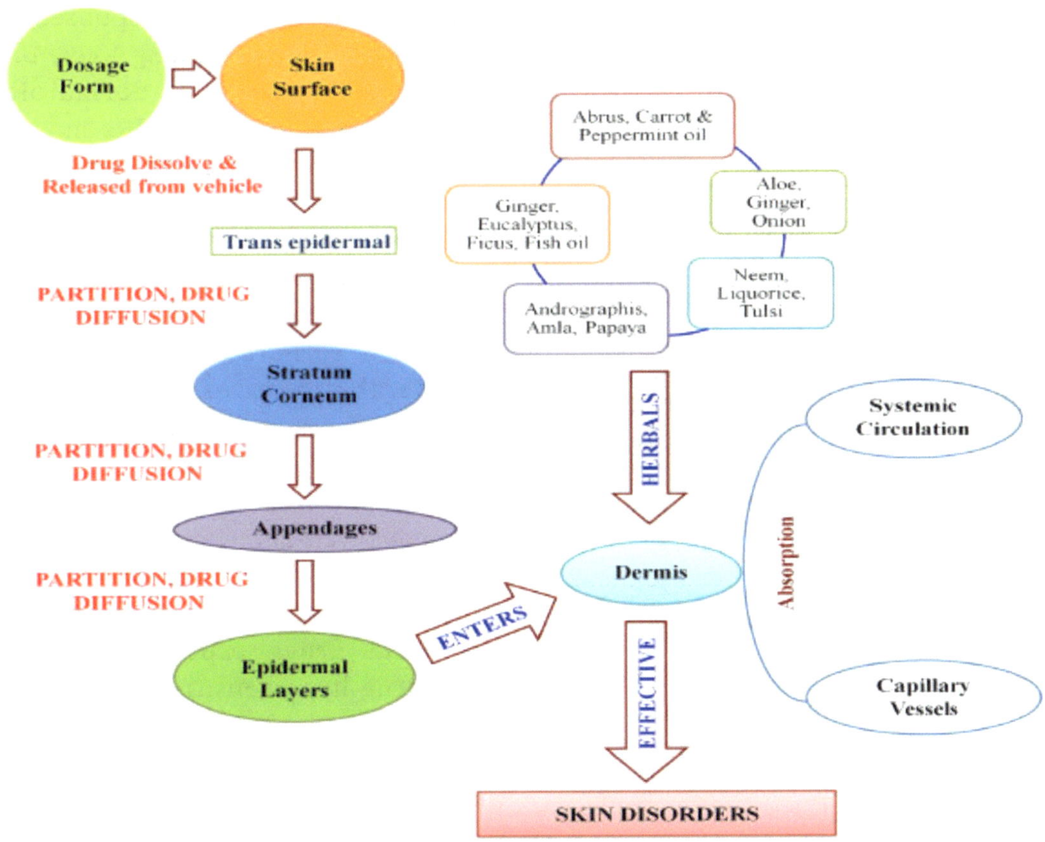

Figure 6.2. Mechanism of drug absorption through skin.

Source: https://www.researchgate.net/profile/Ashima-Ahuja/publication/342369212/figure/fig2/AS:923366160617472@1597159056334/Fig-2-Mechanism-of-drug-absorption-through-Skin.jpg.

Detection and categorization of the causative agents in drug reactions require proper evaluation and clinical judgment. Recognition of the causative drugs observed with extreme cutaneous reactions serves clinicians in performing risk stratification in patients with drug-induced adverse effects. First-line investigations should focus on taking a careful history, including medication exposure, demographic factors, and clinical presentation.

A study of 130 patients found that the most frequently implicated drugs were associated with a range of events, from maculopapular rashes to exfoliative dermatitis. Owing to diverse presentations and pathogenic mechanisms, identifying the drugs most commonly inducing these reactions is necessary for dermatologists and can significantly improve patient safety in prescribing (Abhinesh et al., 2024) (Figure 6.2).

6.1.1. Pharmacological Mechanisms

Pharmacological pathways of cutaneous drug adverse reactions (ACDRs) are central to understanding how drugs can trigger harm to the skin. These reactions can be idiosyncratic or dose-dependent, often resulting from complex interactions between the drug, the immune system, and the individual's genetic predisposition. Certain drugs cause immune responses that manifest as various dermatoses, ranging from benign rashes to potentially life-threatening syndromes such as Stevens-Johnson syndrome.

The division of these reactions is normally predicated upon their timing, clinical presentation, and pharmacological profile of the offending drug. Furthermore, a deeper understanding of the pharmacokinetics and pharmacodynamics of these drugs can help clinicians predict which patients are more susceptible to such reactions, enabling more individualized therapy regimens and enhancing patient safety in dermatology, as highlighted by recent advances in methods for skin lesion evaluation (Ban et al., 2024). It is observed from studies that drug classes like antibiotics and non-steroidal anti-inflammatory drugs are most frequently involved in ACDRs. Cutaneous drug adverse reactions have been investigated to determine that the most commonly presenting clinical condition is an erythematous maculopapular rash, with more severe forms like bullous exfoliative eruptions being evident in less frequent instances. Pharmacological processes, such as interactions between metabolites and skin immune cells, are vital when evaluating drug-related adverse effects. For instance, the metabolism of certain drugs can yield reactive intermediates that modify proteins and trigger cascading inflammatory responses, leading to skin lesions. Understanding these biochemical principles can assist dermatologists in diagnosing and treating ACDRs and underscores the importance of integrating pharmacological knowledge into clinical practice (Panigrahy et al., 2024). Also, therapy of ACDRs demands thorough knowledge of the causative drug's pharmacological properties. Drug withdrawal remains a cornerstone of management and considerably reduces the violence and the duration of reaction. After withdrawal of the causative drug, improvement usually occurs, which emphasizes the interconnection between cutaneous well-being and pharmacologic effect. Reporting of ACDRs emphasizes the need for close observation of patients on possibly hazardous drugs, especially in the event of prior drug hypersensitivity. In line with more individualized therapy in dermatology, the inclusion of robust pharmacologic categorization and patient history would be required to prevent ACDRs. This approach, besides aiming to enhance therapeutic outcomes, reduces healthcare burdens associated with coping with negative reactions (Ban et al., 2024) (Figure 6.3).

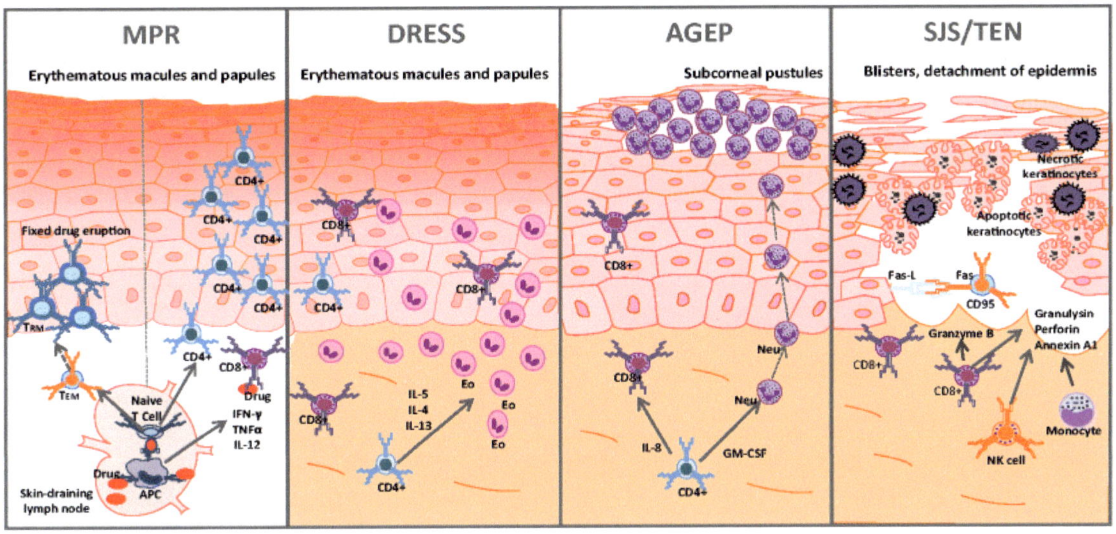

Figure 6.3. Pathophysiological mechanisms underlying adverse cutaneous drug reactions.

Source: https://www.researchgate.net/profile/Lars-French/publication/283687230/figure/fig2/AS:960060809310211@1605907742423/Pathophysiological-mechanisms-underlying-adverse-cutaneous-drug-reactions-Maculopapular.gif.

6.1.2. Immunological Mechanisms

Immunological events have a marked impact on drug reactions and cutaneous drug eruptions, particularly those occurring as localized fixed-drug eruptions (FDE). Presenting as a recurrence of lichenoid eruptions at specific locations on the skin after repeated exposure to the causative agent, FDE represents a classic illustration of the adaptive immune system's memory response. A relevant example is a 51-year-old patient with blisters and brown-black macules after cefadroxil, a first-generation cephalosporin. In this case, the patient's immune system mounted an immediate reaction mediated by CD8+ memory T cells, which recognize the drug as foreign and induce inflammation at the site of contact. The study of such cases helps to understand the pathogenesis of FDE and supports the role of the immunological response in the etiology of drug-induced dermatological disorders (Agrawal et al., 2024). Other than localized forms like FDE, there may be more serious cutaneous adverse drug reactions (CADRs), which are likely to be accompanied by systemic manifestations and may be life-threatening in nature. Mechanistically, these life-threatening cutaneous eruptions, such as Stevens-Johnson syndrome (SJS) and drug reaction with eosinophilia and systemic symptoms (DRESS), tend to be T-cell mediated. Drug-specific activation of T cells can cause extensive apoptosis of keratinocytes, akin to a burn-like phenomenon on the skin. Identification of the immunological pathways responsible for these adverse effects enables clinicians to identify at-risk patients and treat these potentially fatal conditions with proper urgency. Differential diagnosis of CADRs from infection, which may mimic one another, is yet another confounding factor in dermatological assessments (Morgillo et al., 2022). Knowledge of the immunological pathways underlying drug-induced cutaneous reactions is important for both prevention and effective intervention. Because some drugs have a tendency to initiate severe cutaneous reactions, the doctor should be well conversant with the toxicological profiles of such drugs. Increased knowledge of drug-drug interactions and their immunogenicity allows clinicians to closely monitor patients and mitigate the risks posed by certain treatments. Furthermore, the role of cytokines and immune mediators in the pathogenesis of cutaneous eruptions makes personalized medicine valuable in dermatology, where treatment regimens can be tailored based on individual immunological responses. Such a strategic approach can lead to improved patient outcomes and safer therapeutic practices while managing adverse drug reactions (Morgillo et al., 2022) (Figure 6.4).

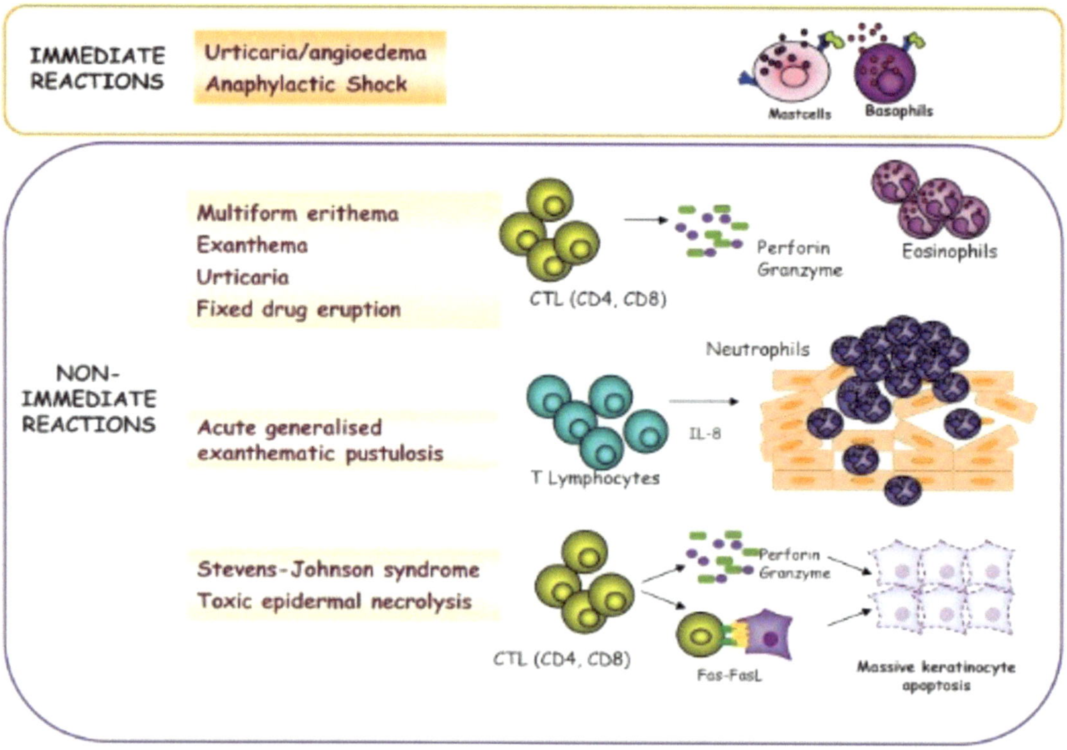

Figure 6.4. Immunological mechanism in immediate and non-immediate reactions to drugs.

Source: https://www.researchgate.net/publication/230798896/figure/fig2/AS:202539669692419@1425300628794/Immunological-mechanism-in-immediate-and-non-immediate-reactions-to-drugs.png.

6.1.3. Genetic Predisposition to Drug Reactions

The phenomenon of genetic susceptibility significantly influences drug reaction risk and severity, particularly that of cutaneous adverse drug reactions (CADRs). A single gene variant, especially drug-metabolizing enzymes and immune-related gene polymorphisms, may lead to altered pharmacokinetics and pharmacodynamics of drugs. For instance, some people with specific genetic markers may metabolize drugs more rapidly or more slowly than the general population, resulting in suboptimal therapeutic effects or enhanced toxicities, for example, poor skin reactions. It is important to recognize this genetic diversity because it provides a basis for individualized therapy, in which treatment modalities can be tailored to an individual's genetic makeup to avoid drug reactions and enhance patient safety in clinical practice. The genetic environment that determines drug reactions also includes the HLA (human leukocyte antigen) system, which plays a critical role in drug-induced immune responses. Certain HLA alleles have been strongly associated with specific drug-induced cutaneous reactions. An example is patients with the HLA-B*15:02 allele, who are at considerable risk of developing Stevens-Johnson syndrome when exposed to carbamazepine, a common anticonvulsant. The association has emphasized the utility of genetic screening in the detection of susceptible populations, particularly for high-risk drugs. As drug reactions remain a high-priority issue in dermatology, incorporating genetic testing into clinical practice can help dermatologists prescribe safe and effective medications, enhance overall patient care, and mitigate the healthcare burden of drug-induced adverse reactions (Panigrahy et al., 2024). Last but not least, the interplay between genomics and the environment cannot be overlooked when dealing with drug reactions. While genetic susceptibility provides the background for potential harmful effects, additive environmental factors, such as drug interactions and general state of health, can initiate these reactions. For instance, polypharmacy patients are often at increased risk for CADRs, particularly if they are genetically predisposed to certain drugs. This multidimensional interaction underscores the need for an integrated approach that combines genetic and environmental assessments to accurately predict and prevent major cutaneous drug eruptions. With continued advances in pharmacogenomics, the path is set for a more robust rationale for these complex interactions, enabling improved management strategies in dermatology (Sutaria et al., 2024).

Test Your Knowledge

1. What are the pharmacological mechanisms behind adverse drug reactions (ADRs)?
2. How do immunological mechanisms contribute to drug hypersensitivity reactions?

6.2. Classification of Adverse Cutaneous Drug Eruptions

Learning Outcome

1. Understand exanthematous drug eruptions.
2. Discuss urticarial drug eruptions.
3. Focus on severe cutaneous adverse reactions (SCARs).

Cutaneous drug eruptions are heterogeneous and can be classified based on clinical presentation and underlying mechanisms. The two broad categories are exanthematous drug eruptions, typically presenting as measles-like, widespread rashes, and urticarial drug reactions, which consist of raised welts or hives. Another significant classification is fixed drug eruptions, which are fixed and recur at the same site upon reexposure to the offending agent. Drug hypersensitivity syndromes, though less common, are serious systemic reactions involving fever, lymphadenopathy, and multiorgan involvement and necessitate immediate medical therapy. This grouping facilitates dermatologists in diagnosing and managing cutaneous reactions by associating the symptoms with the corresponding drug classes and mechanisms, and eventually enhances patient safety and treatment results. The spectrum of cutaneous drug eruptions that are adverse in nature typically involves the immune system, which is critical to their causation. Drug eruptions can be immunological, in which the body recognizes the drug or its metabolite as foreign and mounts an inflammatory response. This occurs with the administration of immunomodulatory drugs such as pembrolizumab, in which several patients developed cutaneous side effects, including macular papular eruptions and pruritus. Notably, such drug-induced skin eruptions can also be associated with positive treatment responses in patients with melanoma, suggesting that immune activation may benefit the overall therapeutic response. Such information underscores the importance of understanding the immunological mechanisms of drug eruptions, as this can inform methods to predict patient responses to certain treatments, guiding clinical decisions. Photosensitivity is another crucial factor in the categorization of cutaneous drug eruptions, where some drugs initiate skin reactions after exposure to light. Phototoxicity and photoallergy exhibit distinct pathogenetic mechanisms that affect not only the clinical management of drug reactions but also the choice of treatment drugs. Many drugs—across antimicrobials, NSAIDs, and chemotherapeutic agents—have been implicated in photosensitivity reactions, and this emphasizes the need for vigilance among clinicians. Understanding the specific mechanisms of photosensitivity can prevent undesirable effects by choosing another drug or taking preventive measures, such as using sunscreen. Thorough knowledge of the categorization of cutaneous drug eruptions, such as photosensitivity, equips dermatologists with the correct tools to evaluate, manage, and even avoid these reactions in practice, ultimately enhancing patient quality of life and treatment compliance.

6.2.1. Exanthematous Drug Eruptions

Exanthematous drug eruptions represent a significant category of cutaneous adverse reactions, appearing predominantly as morbilliform rashes made up of erythematous macules and papules. Drug eruptions can represent a diagnostic dilemma since they can mimic most infectious diseases and other skin conditions. The importance of accurate diagnosis of exanthematous drug eruptions lies not only in the need for prompt treatment but also in the need to differentiate between low-risk and high-risk reactions. While the majority of cases can be attributed to benign causes, for example, common pharmacologic agents, a fraction of them may herald serious conditions, such as Stevens-Johnson syndrome or toxic epidermal necrolysis. Thus, understanding the entire clinical picture is essential for dermatologists to effectively treat these patients and achieve the best possible health outcomes when faced with potentially fatal complications. In dermatology, therapy of exanthematous drug reactions needs to be multi-dimensional, addressing both patient education and vigilant monitoring. Doctors must be adept at identifying the clinical features that can distinguish severe drug eruptions from the benign types. For instance, some details, such as the spread, direction, and accompanying symptoms of the eruption, may provide valuable clues regarding the etiology. The identification of the potential causative agents is also vital in treatment decisions, ranging from drug cessation to initiation of supportive measures. The clinical algorithm developed to diagnose the various presentations of morbilliform rashes remains an excellent tool for clinicians. This systematic approach would help distinguish high-risk conditions, ultimately improving patient outcomes in the management of drug-related adverse reactions (Yan et al., 2025).

Further research on the epidemiology and pathophysiology of exanthematous drug eruptions is needed to advance knowledge in this area of dermatology. Understanding the varied stimuli that elicit such eruptions not only facilitates better preventive strategies but also enhances clinical practice by reducing diagnostic specificity. It also validates the merits of personalized medicine in dermatologic care, as it recognizes that the same patients will respond differently to identical medications. As described in the literature, a scrupulous examination of cutaneous drug reactions enables clinicians to develop individualized management strategies that balance efficacy and safety (Wützner, 2020). It is therefore vital to create awareness and education regarding exanthematous drug eruptions among clinicians because this can result in a decrease in morbidity as well as an increased exploration of drug interaction and side effects in clinical practice (Figure 6.5).

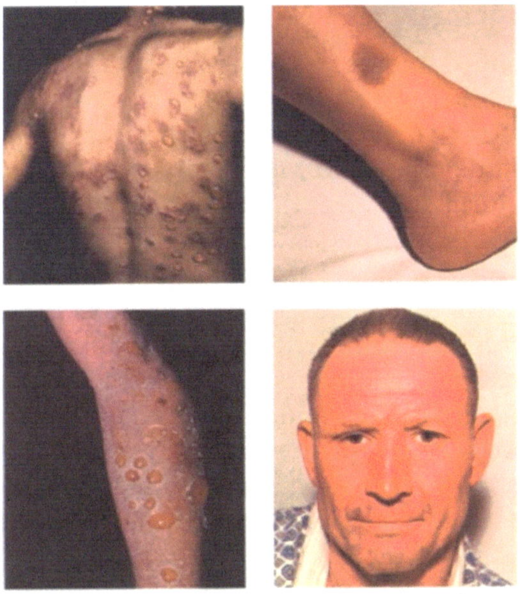

Figure 6.5. Drug eruptions. (A) Bullous dermatitis medicamentosa caused by sulfathiazole. (B) Fixed drug eruption caused by phenolphtalein. (C) Bullous erythema multiforme. (D) Diffuse photosensitivity reaction.

Source: https://upload.wikimedia.org/wikipedia/commons/3/3d/Drug_eruptions.jpg.

6.2.2. Urticarial Drug Eruptions

Urticarial drug eruptions are a significant subgroup of skin drug reactions characterized by the acute development of itchy wheals (hives) on the skin. These eruptions can result from a number of drugs, including antibiotics, nonsteroidal anti-inflammatory drugs, and certain biologics. When presenting with an urticarial reaction, it is essential that clinicians perform a detailed inquiry into their drug history and identify the probable offenders. The pathophysiological process in such eruptions is most often immunologically driven, with mast cell and basophil activation playing a central role, leading to the release of histamine and other inflammatory mediators. Urticarial drug eruptions need early diagnosis because they can occur very suddenly, even within hours of medication. Physicians need to distinguish urticarial reactions from other cutaneous manifestations, such as angioedema or maculopapular eruptions, to provide appropriate therapy and prevent complications. The management of urticarial drug eruptions is largely the immediate cessation of the offending agent, along with symptomatic relief. Antihistamines are the cornerstone of therapy, which optimally relieves pruritus and reduces wheal formation. In acute reactions, systemic corticosteroids may be necessary to control inflammation and prevent worsening. Moreover, educating the patient about their specific drug allergy is important for preventing recurrences. The potential for cross-reactivity between some classes of drugs necessitates careful avoidance and consideration of similar drugs. Due to the nature of some urticarial eruptions to progress to more severe reactions, for example, anaphylaxis, special follow-up and monitoring are indicated in the management of such patients. Understanding the nuances of drug-induced urticarial eruptions can significantly enhance patient care and induce more prudent prescribing. Study acknowledges the importance for dermatologists and physicians to become familiar with the range of cutaneous drug reactions, such as urticarial eruptions, in a way that they can provide more effective diagnostic and therapeutic strategies. Approximately 2% of all skin adverse reactions are serious, but most are benign in etiology (Abhinesh et al., 2024). This necessitates clinicians to refine their skills in differentiating differences in forms of drug eruption. Furthermore, extensive research, such as that evaluating drug-related skin reactions, contributes to identifying common drug perpetrators and their corresponding clinical morphologies, thereby enhancing patient safety (Yan et al., 2025). As technology continues to evolve, new research will definitely play an essential role in evaluating and expanding the understanding and management of drug reactions, guiding the direction of dermatological practices in the management of urticarial eruptions and other cutaneous adverse reactions (Figure 6.6).

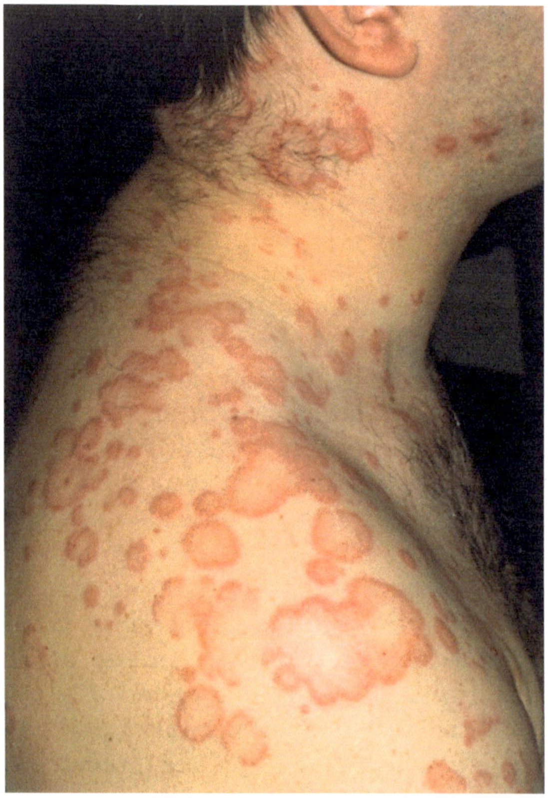

Figure 6.6. Urticarial drug eruptions represent a significant subset of cutaneous drug reactions.

Source: https://www.clinicaladvisor.com/wp-content/uploads/sites/11/2018/12/urticaria0310_wheals_90990.jpg.

6.2.3. Severe cutaneous Adverse Reactions (SCARs)

Treatment of severe cutaneous adverse reactions (SCARs) is a vexing problem for dermatology and pharmacology. SCARs, which include Stevens-Johnson syndrome (SJS) and toxic epidermal necrolysis (TEN) among others, are characterized by massive separation of the skin and mucous membranes and commonly lead to serious morbidity or mortality. SCARs are drug-induced and are most commonly associated with antibiotics, anticonvulsants, and non-steroidal anti-inflammatory drugs (NSAIDs). Early detection of SCAR signs is crucial for prompt intervention, as delays in treatment play a major role in worsening patient outcomes. Management should also be multidisciplinary, involving dermatologists, allergists, and systemic physicians, to allow the maximum options for management that prevent long-term sequelae, thereby improving quality of life in these patients. Scientific studies have shown the complex immunological mechanisms in SCARs that make them difficult to treat. In the case of immune checkpoint inhibitors (ICIs), for instance, cutaneous immune-related adverse events (IrAEs) become increasingly known in oncology. They present with heterogeneity in terms of presentation, severity, and response to treatment. In a phase IV real-world analysis on the basis of the Melskintox database, multiple types of cutaneous IrAEs were presented in melanoma-treated patients. Importantly, the study categorizes drug eruptions and inflammatory dermatoses, noting that such responses can significantly impede existing cancer therapies. Additionally, severe delayed reactions are not uncommon, underscoring the importance of close follow-up and early dermatologic evaluation, as timely intervention can prevent potentially lethal complications in patients undergoing immunotherapy (L'Orphelin et al., 2023). The prognostic value of SCARs runs deep, according to a retrospective study that focused on severe blistering skin eruptions caused by ICIs. Though the occurrence of the life-threatening adverse effects is uncommon, the effect can prove to be fatal, with the study having reported a whopping 25% mortality among affected patients. Findings indicated difficulty in early diagnosis, revealing that the majority of cases of epidermal necrolysis were misdiagnosed, thus complicating management. The study reinforced a homogeneous clinical presentation, with a median onset of 52 days from the time treatment was started, pointing to the importance of early symptom recognition in order to provide timely treatment interventions. Enhanced awareness and research into the pathophysiology and management of SCARs in dermatology, and indeed across a broader spectrum, are needed, given their high mortality and morbidity in patients (Oro et al., 2022) (Figure 6.7).

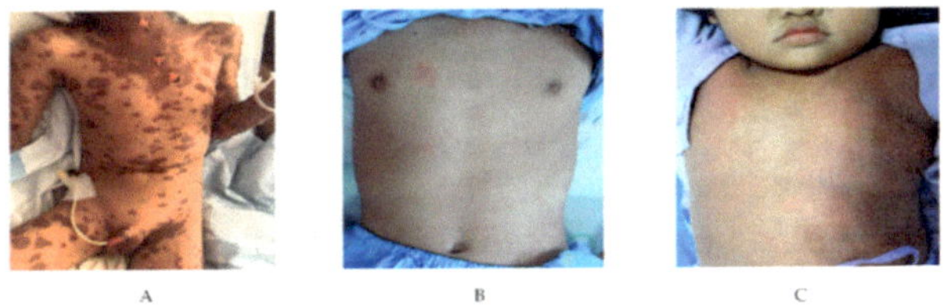

Figure 6.7. Severe cutaneous adverse drug reactions. (A) indicates Stevens–Johnson syndrome (SJS)/toxic Epidermal necrolysis (TEN), (B) indicates drug reaction with eosinophilia and systemic symptoms (DRESS) and (C) indicates acute generalized exanthematous pustulosis (AGEP).

Source: https://www.mdpi.com/pharmaceuticals/pharmaceuticals-14-01077/article_deploy/html/images/pharmaceuticals-14-01077-g002-550.jpg.

Test Your Knowledge

1. What are the typical clinical features of exanthematous (morbilliform) drug eruptions?
2. How do urticarial drug eruptions differ from exanthematous eruptions in onset and appearance?

6.3. Common Drugs Associated with Cutaneous Reactions

Learning Outcome

1. Understand antibiotics and their cutaneous effects.
2 .Describe anticonvulsants and skin reactions.
3. Discuss non-steroidal anti-inflammatory drugs (NSAIDs).

The drugs that cause cutaneous reactions are numerous, making pharmacotherapy difficult for patients. Of the numerous drugs that cause this, nonsteroidal anti-inflammatory drugs (NSAIDs) are among the most frequent causative agents of eruptions on the skin, including urticaria and fixed drug eruption. Pathophysiology of such reactions is normally through hypersensitivity mechanisms, where the immune system mistakenly identifies such drugs as harmful substances. Thus, patients can develop symptoms ranging from a mild rash to a severe illness such as Stevens-Johnson syndrome. This is a stark indication of the importance of dermatological monitoring of patients who receive NSAIDs, as early identification and treatment can decrease complications. In other common drugs , such as antibiotics, namely penicillins and sulfonamides, the incidence of cutaneous adverse reactions is also high. These instances indicate the need for health care practitioners to be aware of the cutaneous effects associated with commonly used drugs. The hallucinogenic and psychedelic drugs are now increasingly popular not only because of their therapeutic potential but also because of their less-well-published cutaneous side effects. A critical review of all studies linking these drugs to dermatologic reactions revealed a striking incidence of adverse eruptions. Cannabis, for instance, was implicated in several hypersensitivity responses, including type I hypersensitivity, most often caused by cutaneous contact. It is reported that patients may form vesicular contact dermatitis or erythema multiforme-like reactions with the systemic ingestion of such drugs. Similarly, MDMA has been associated with varied cutaneous presentations, while ketamine and psilocybin also explain a variety of dermatological responses. This fresh information points toward carrying out additional research on the cutaneous reactions of hallucinogens and psychedelics because clinicians must remain current with these potential interactions in order to effectively treat patients (Rahman et al., 2024). For drugs targeted, such as enfortumab vedotin, have emerged as effective therapies for complex malignancies but also created cutaneous side effects. Enfortumab vedotin, a drug-antibody conjugate, has been known to induce toxic erythema after its interaction with nectin-4 present on the skin. Painless, erythematous plaques limited to the trunk and extremities can occur in treated patients and show histopathologic findings of interface dermatitis. This presents a two-edged sword: clinicians are challenged to balance the effectiveness of treatment against the risk of cutaneous adverse events. Fortunately, most such cutaneous side effects are manageable. Their management is successful by measures generally in the form of topical corticosteroids, allowing therapy to go on without drug withdrawal. By documenting such reactions, the dermatological community can enhance its expertise and preparedness to address the cutaneous ramifications of evolving cancer treatments (Casale et al., 2024).

6.3.1. Antibiotics and Their Cutaneous Effects

The use of antibiotics in clinical practice is impossible without them; however, their application is often accompanied by cutaneous adverse drug reactions (CADRs) that can range from an insignificant rash to severe skin disease. Among the various CADR categories, antibiotics fall among the leading CADR causes and accounted for 42.15% of the reactions documented in a recent study (Panigrahy et al., 2024). The most common clinical presentation reported was an erythematous maculopapular rash, which typically appears within days of initiation of drug therapy and is a manifestation of hypersensitivity. Although most patients develop mild reactions, fulminant presentations , such as Stevens-Johnson syndrome and toxic epidermal necrolysis can occur and necessitate immediate medical intervention. This association highlights the importance of vigilant monitoring for cutaneous manifestations in patients on antibiotics. Aside from that, properties of cutaneous effects of antibiotics all converge at the condition, fixed drug eruption (FDE), a unique type of CADR. In FDE, re-exposure to the offending agent leads to recurrent lesions on the skin at a single site, and such an offender in the majority of cases is an antibiotic, such as co-trimoxazole, one of the most frequent culprit drugs (McClatchy et al., 2022). The lesions are typically well-defined erythematous plaques that can progress to produce blisters or erosions. Awareness of the pathophysiology of FDE, such as T-cell mediated immunity, can aid in discriminating it from other dermatoses and, therefore, ensure appropriate management. In view of the fact that antibiotics are commonly implicated in such cutaneous reactions, increased vigilance by treating physicians to detect at-risk patients is necessary to prevent re-exposure to these drugs. Effective management of CADR secondary to antibiotic treatment is dependent on a prompt diagnosis and immediate withdrawal of the offending drug. An earlier retrospective analysis found that, in 76% of identified cases, the offending antibiotic was withdrawn, and 52% of patients recovered (Panigrahy et al., 2024). The statistic indicates that prompt diagnosis and intervention could significantly reduce the duration and severity of cutaneous reactions. In addition, clinicians should be alert for first-time presentation of drug-induced skin eruptions as well as for repeated reactions when the patient is re-exposed to antibiotic drugs. Avoiding misunderstandings through effective communication with the patient about possible skin reactions and making them aware of the need to report symptoms is an important measure. By encouraging proactive and well-informed management of cutaneous antibiotic effects, dermatologists can significantly mitigate adverse outcomes and enhance patient safety in therapeutic practice (Figure 6.8).

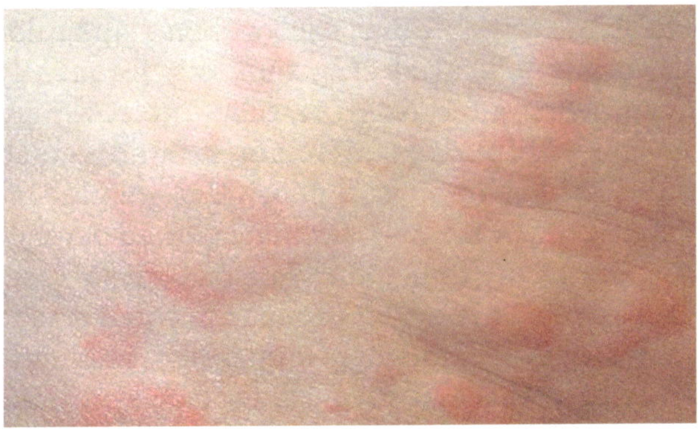

Figure 6.8. Cutaneous adverse reactions to antibiotics.

Source: https://www.summitdermatology.com/wp-content/uploads/2018/03/urticaria1.jpg.

6.3.2. Anticonvulsants and Skin Reactions

Anticonvulsants are widely used to treat seizure disorders but are also well known for their propensity to induce numerous cutaneous reactions. Of these, aromatic amine anticonvulsants, including carbamazepine and phenytoin, are particularly well known to induce skin eruptions. The reactions can range as mildly as exanthematous drug eruptions, which are usually supported by maculopapular rashes, or as severe as Stevens-Johnson syndrome and toxic epidermal necrolysis. The frequency of these cutaneous side effects has been surprising, with reports of up to 100 severe cutaneous reactions per 1000 new users of these medicines. These facts emphasize the need for greater alertness among clinicians initiating therapy with these anticonvulsants, who should pay closer attention to dermatologic side effects. The association between certain anticonvulsants and cutaneous adverse reactions is further supported by case reports in which skin eruptions occurred shortly after therapy initiation. An example involves a reported case of a 12-year-old male patient who developed widespread maculopapular eruptions upon administration of phenytoin for neurocysticercosis, indicative of the drug's tendency to cause hypersensitivity reactions (Hu et al., 2020). With discontinuation of the offending drugs, the patient's symptoms also showed considerable improvement, underscoring the importance of early detection and timely treatment. Interestingly, such occurrences reflect a broader trend in dermatologic pharmacology, where early detection of drug eruptions can have a profound effect on patient care. Therefore, vigilant observation for cutaneous reaction is in order for prescribing clinicians, and an attenuating balance between therapeutic advantage and avoidable harm is again highlighted. Also, the dermatological impact of anticonvulsants extends beyond acute cutaneous reactions to include long-term effects on patient quality of life. The skin eruptions can lead to emotional distress, withdrawal from society, and poor compliance with drug regimens, ultimately compromising overall seizure disorder control. The composite effect is one healthcare providers must consider, as they weigh the complexities of treatment against the risk of side reactions. For example, the case of a 72-year-old man patient with erythema multiforme-like rash after the administration of tamsulosin highlights the duration of drug reactions in patients with comorbidities (Hu et al., 2020). Precautions to educate and closely observe patients for side effects can facilitate early interventions, thereby promoting an excellent healthcare experience among patients with epilepsy and other conditions requiring anticonvulsant therapy (Figure 6.9).

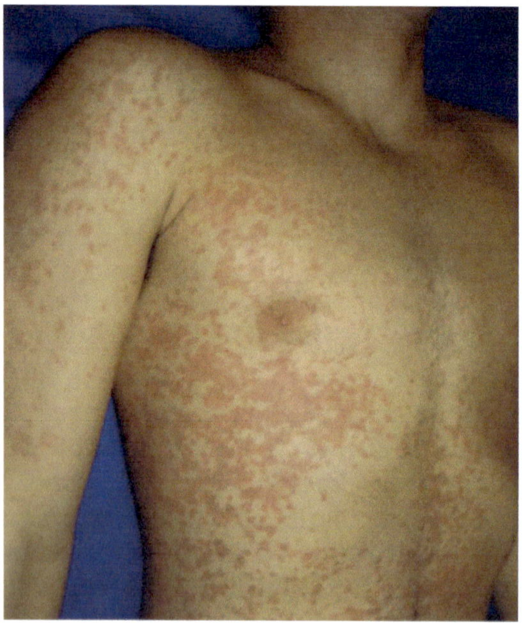

Figure 6.9. Anticonvulsants to induce various cutaneous reactions.

Source: https://i0.wp.com/obgynkey.com/wp-content/uploads/2019/01/m_zaoutis2_ch63_f001-1.png.?w=960.

6.3.3. Non-Steroidal Anti-Inflammatory Drugs (NSAIDs)

Non-steroidal anti-inflammatory drugs (NSAIDs) are a class of drugs that are widely prescribed for their analgesic and anti-inflammatory effects. They are widely used in rheumatoid arthritis, musculoskeletal pain, and inflammatory disorders. Besides their clinical use, NSAIDs have been associated with a range of adverse drug reactions (ADRs), particularly cutaneous eruptions. A significant subset of cutaneous drug reactions is causally related to NSAIDs and is thus an area of priority in dermatological practice. With patients being centered for treatment by physicians, awareness of the associations of NSAID use and cutaneous adverse events is essential. Vigilance in detecting such reactions enables better patient outcomes through earlier diagnosis and optimal management. Furthermore, the dynamic nature of patient-drug interactions in various populations necessitates that clinicians remain educated on the potential cutaneous effects of NSAIDs at all times. The evolving drug profile and new NSAIDs have also been behind changing patterns of adverse cutaneous reactions. According to recent literature, fixed drug eruptions (FDE) are also one of the most common manifestations of NSAID-induced cutaneous adverse drug reactions and account for a major majority of the cases in dermatological practices. In addition to FDE, other eruptions, such as maculopapular rashes and urticarial eruptions, are frequently encountered after NSAID intake. Interestingly, the age group most affected is middle-aged adults, which implies a specific demographic vulnerability that may be investigated further for genetic or environmental factors in drug reactions. These results underscore the importance of thorough clinical assessments to identify the cause of cutaneous eruptions resulting from NSAIDs, ultimately optimizing the effectiveness of treatment protocols (Gupta et al., 2021). Mechanism identification of NSAID-induced cutaneous drug reactions is crucial in order to prevent and successfully manage them. Pathophysiology of the reaction is generally multifactorial in nature, with complex interactions between drug chemical structure and the immune system of the host, manifesting as various clinical conditions. Delays or misdiagnoses can lead to catastrophic complications, which underscore the importance of thorough patient history and clinical examination in dermatology (Abhinesh et al., 2024). Implementation of an efficient ADR report system and surveillance can reduce resource utilization and improve drug safety practices. Interdisciplinary dialogue between dermatologists, allergists, and pharmacologists can enable healthcare workers to formulate practical methods to decrease the frequency and intensity of NSAID-induced dermatitis. Overall, heightened vigilance and ongoing research in this field are still required to minimize risks and maximize patient outcomes in dermatology (Figure 6.10).

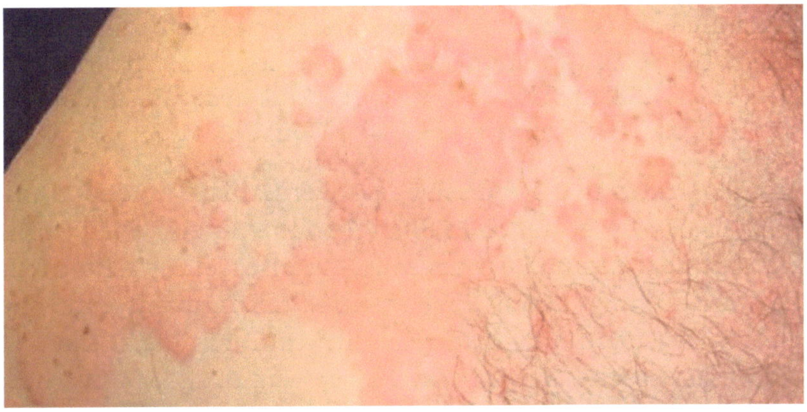

Figure 6.10. Urticaria (hives) is caused by non-steroidal anti-inflammatory drugs (NSAIDs).

Test Your Knowledge

1. Which types of cutaneous reactions are commonly caused by antibiotics?
2. What severe cutaneous adverse reactions are associated with anticonvulsants , such as carbamazepine and lamotrigine?
3. What types of skin reactions can be triggered by non-steroidal anti-inflammatory drugs (NSAIDs)?

6.4. Diagnosis of Adverse Cutaneous Drug Eruptions

Learning Outcome

1. Discuss clinical evaluation and history taking for diagnosing drug reactions and adverse cutaneous drug eruptions.
2. Describe patch testing and its role.
3. Understand laboratory tests and imaging studies.

Diagnosis of cutaneous drug eruptions (ACDEs) is a job demanding a thorough understanding of clinical presentation as well as the pathologic mechanisms involved. A credible diagnosis largely hinges on the detection of typical clinical patterns in different drug reactions. While established medical science has a rudimentary understanding of the biology involved, doctors must build on this knowledge using clinical classification schemes to improve diagnostic accuracy. For example, common conditions such as maculopapular exanthema and fixed drug eruptions can often be diagnosed by their characteristic appearance but may present differently from patient to patient. Awareness of these patterns not only helps with early diagnosis but also influences treatment modalities to a large extent, as early recognition of the offending drug is of utmost importance in avoiding adverse drug reactions (Malhotra et al., 2021). In addition to clinical observation, clinical assessment scales are required to establish the drug's causality and the severity of skin eruptions. One of these scales is the Naranjo Probability Scale, which clinicians can use to attribute symptoms to drugs in a stepwise fashion. It helps establish a causal relationship through patient history, treatment duration, and symptom resolution. Equally, Hartwig and Siegel's scale gives a powerful means of measuring the severity of adverse drug reactions as mild, moderate, or severe. Statistical results, for example, incidence rates in studies, place the importance of formalized measurements in evidence. For instance, a certain study conducted in India observed a 0.09% frequency of cutaneous adverse drug reactions, out of which fixed drug eruptions accounted for the majority (Malhotra et al., 2021). The figures state that accurate diagnosis and classification are the cornerstone to understanding and managing ACDEs.

The global epidemiological trend of cutaneous adverse drug reactions makes the diagnostic process even harder. As shown by evidence in Shanghai, the heterogeneity of response and drugs involved is a dilemma that health practitioners must tread carefully. The occurrence of S-CADRs, as shown by the study, is alarming: about 22% of cases fall into this category, underscoring the imperative need for early detection and management. Antimicrobials, the largest drug category involved in these reactions, show the danger posed by certain drugs and the necessity of a rigorous monitoring scheme. Knowing the frequency of CADRs by demographic group, like age and sex, is essential to the planning of specific preventive strategies and treatment regimens, which not only cut down on the incidence of such reactions but also enhance overall patient safety and management (Figure 6.11).

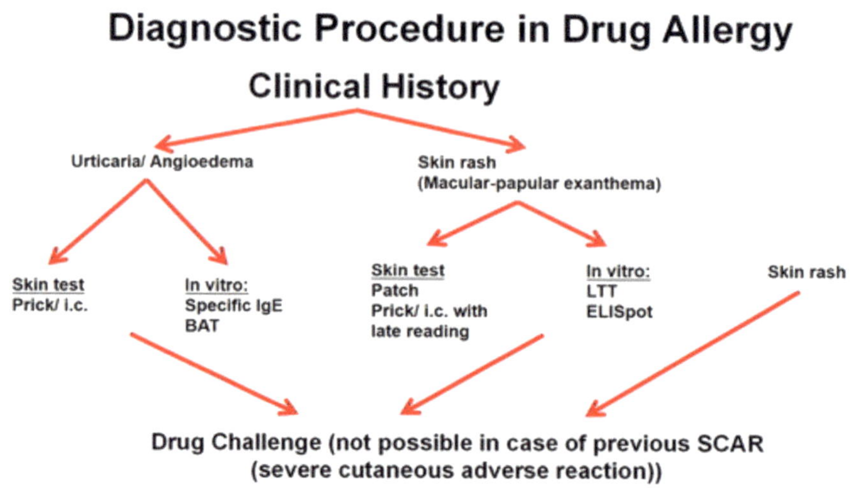

Figure 6.11. Diagnostic procedure in drug allergy.

Source: https://www.tandfonline.com/cms/asset/8c8c6c73-0aa7-498d-90cb-4127ea3608df/icot_a_1319379_f0005_c.jpg.

6.4.1. Clinical Evaluation and History Taking

In dermatology, clinical examination and history taking are the keys to the diagnosis of cutaneous adverse drug eruptions and drug reactions. A good history can yield important details about recent drug intake, past allergies, and any comorbid diseases that could increase the risk of adverse effects.

Most importantly, in cutaneous adverse drug reactions (CADR), the identification of the timing and type of symptom occurrence in relation to drug exposure is of utmost importance. Studies have shown a significant correlation between certain pharmacological drugs, specifically antibiotics, and CADR presentation. For instance, among 272 reported CADR cases, most were due to antibiotics, highlighting the importance of seeking potential offenders through a detailed medical history (Panigrahy et al., 2024). A patient's medication history is critical for obtaining key information that can guide clinicians in identifying likely offending agents in cutaneous manifestations. Clinical assessment is not limited to historical data; it also includes proper physical examination. When evaluating patients for skin drug reactions, dermatologists must use a systematic approach to assess the rash's distribution and morphology. Each presentation, such as maculopapular eruptions, urticaria, or serious conditions such as Stevens-Johnson syndrome, requires keen observation skills for appropriate categorization. These tests not only help determine the offending drug but also help clinicians determine the severity of the response. A study found that, among CADR cases, timely detection and withdrawal of the offending agent were key to improving patient outcomes, and over half of patients improved after drug withdrawal (Panigrahy et al., 2024). Thus, a detailed assessment is important for the appropriate management of such complex cases of drug-induced skin conditions. Moreover, advances in the understanding of the related immunologic mechanisms have improved clinical evaluation in the management of adverse drug reactions. Certain immune indicators, including interleukin-21 (IL-21), have also been of interest for their potential roles in the pathogenesis of drug eruptions. Research has demonstrated that higher IL-21 levels are associated with the severity of erythema multiforme and Stevens-Johnson syndrome, and this finding has opened a new door for prognostic assessment in CADR cases. By incorporating such biochemical studies into clinical examinations, dermatologists can better refine their evaluation and stratify patient risk. Therefore, this combined practice of patient history and clinical evaluation allows dermatologists not only to diagnose and manage drug reactions but also to undertake preventive measures to prevent complications of adverse drug reactions.

6.4.2. Patch Testing and Its Role

Patch testing is a significant diagnostic tool in dermatology for the diagnosis of contact allergies secondary to drugs and other chemicals. Patch testing is a technique in which small amounts of allergens are placed under occlusion on the skin to allow clinicians to evaluate allergic reactions over time. Patch testing is very significant in drug reactions to distinguish a true allergic reaction from an irritant reaction. Such discrimination is equally vital for providing appropriate treatment regimens, since incorrect diagnosis can lead to improper treatment and exacerbation of patient conditions. By accurately identifying the specific allergens that provoke it, dermatologists can advise patients on potential risk factors in their drug regimens and implement preventive measures to avoid further cutaneous drug eruptions. One of the applications of patch testing is its value in diagnosing conditions such as symmetrical drug-related intertriginous and flexural exanthema (SDRIFE), an allergic condition usually linked to systemic drugs. More recent studies have found that patch testing is useful in diagnosing SDRIFE, particularly when routine laboratory investigations yield negative results. For instance, two cases of SDRIFE-like eruptions following COVID-19 vaccination illustrate the importance of patch testing in distinguishing vaccine-related skin reactions from other adverse drug reactions. Despite the complexities of these eruptions' pathogenesis, effective patch testing protocols enabled dermatologists to validate vaccine involvement, which in turn informed clinical decision-making and provided patient-specific care (Lahouel et al.,

2022). Moreover, patient safety and health are the therapeutic benefits of patch testing for drug allergy. Effective determination of an allergen allows one to develop alternative treatment plans, hence preventing potential future allergic responses to a specific drug. Effective patient education about identified allergens also helps individuals advocate for themselves when they are prescribed medications in the future.

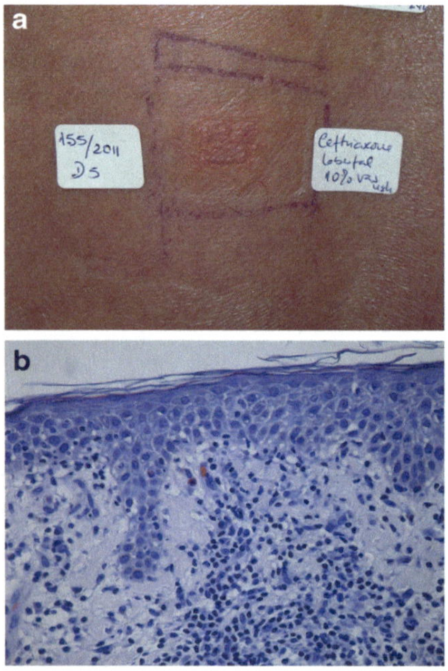

Figure 6.12. A positive patch test reaction to ceftriaxone at 10% pet, manipulated from the powder of the intravenous drug, was observed at day 3 in a case of maculopapular exanthema. b Histopathology of the patch test (H&E) showing a dermal perivascular infiltrate of mononuclear cells and eosinophils, vacuolar degeneration of the basal layer, and lymphocyte exocytosis.

Source: https://www.researchgate.net/publication/330739876/figure/fig3/AS:963442898911281@1606714095680/a-Positive-patch-test-reaction-to-ceftriaxone-at-10-pet-manipulated-from-the-powder-of.png.

In the broader context of dermatology, patch testing enhances understanding of drug hypersensitivity and raises awareness among patients and healthcare providers of the potential consequences of allergic reactions. With the continuous advances in the field of dermatology, the implementation of patch testing innovations is essential to improve patient outcomes in the context of drug and cutaneous adverse drug reactions (Montinari et al., 2020) (Figure 6.12).

6.4.3. Laboratory Tests and Imaging Studies

In dermatology, imaging studies and laboratory tests are vital diagnostic tools for identifying adverse cutaneous drug reactions (ACDRs). The tests not only determine the exact drug that caused a patient's eruption of the skin but also eliminate other forms of dermatological conditions that can be drug reaction mimics. An example is the skin biopsy that will present histopathological proof of ACDRs in the form of unique patterns, like focus on interface dermatitis or peri-vascular infiltrates. Accurate diagnosis can be ascertained by a multi-dimensional process, where patient history and laboratory reports are merged because the intricacies involved in drug interactions require thorough investigation (cited in (Abhinesh et al., 2024). This is important because timely treatment greatly reduces the risk of life-threatening complications from these reactions. Imaging studies are also engaged in examining severe adverse cutaneous drug reactions, particularly when agents are suspected to engage the system. Methods , such as ultrasonography may be employed to measure edema within the soft tissues or to detect alterations deeper within the skin that are not visible in the epidermis. Moreover, imaging could be used to track the progression of drug eruptions, especially when reactions are severe or have caused secondary infections. The integration of laboratory examinations with imaging can give a more comprehensive insight into the status of the patients, thereby allowing effective clinical decisions and management interventions (cited in (Aditi et al., 2024). Lastly, these technologies enable health care providers to react in a timely manner and improve patient outcomes in the course of acute drug reaction attacks. In spite of their importance, the value of laboratory tests and imaging techniques in ACDR diagnosis is marred by several limitations. The variations in the clinical manifestations of drug eruptions often overlap with those of other dermatological conditions, making interpretation challenging. Moreover, the lack of definitive laboratory tests means that physicians often rely on clinical judgment and contextual knowledge to provide accurate diagnoses. As found through research, awareness of the most common etiological agents, as well as ACDR's clinical presentation, can overcome most such limitations (cited in Abhinesh et al., 2024). Heightened sensitivity, coupled with systematic documentation and careful observation of skin reactions, can improve diagnostic precision and protect patients in the management of drug reactions, underscoring the need for ongoing education in this area (Figure 6.13).

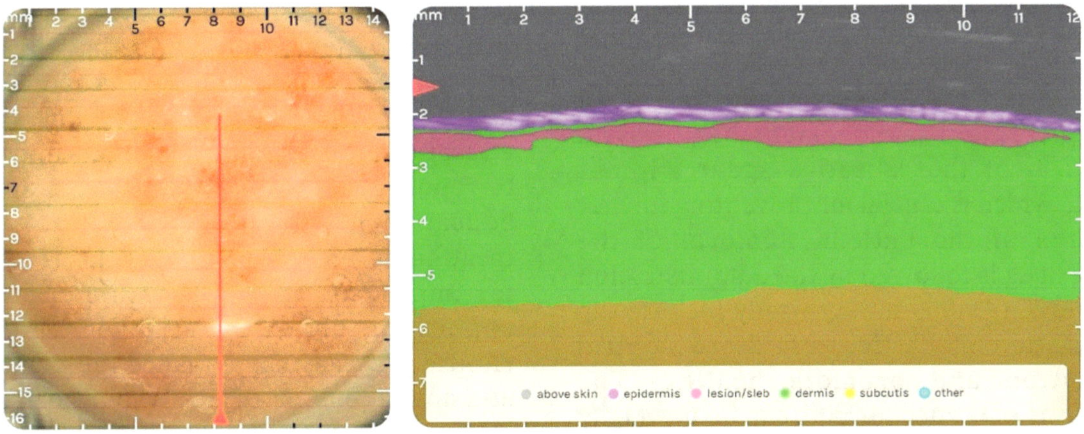

Figure 6.13. Optical (left) and ultrasound image (right) of the lesion: The subepidermal low-echogenic band (SLEB) can be seen on the ultrasound image colored in pink, between the epidermis and dermis.

Source: https://www.mdpi.com/diagnostics/diagnostics-14-00575/article_deploy/html/images/diagnostics-14-00575-g004.png.

Test Your Knowledge

1. Why is a detailed clinical history essential in diagnosing cutaneous drug eruptions?
2. How does physical examination assist in the diagnosis of drug-induced skin reactions?
3. What is the role of patch testing in the evaluation of cutaneous drug reactions?

6.5. Management of Drug Reactions

Learning Outcome

1. Understand immediate management of adverse cutaneous drug eruptions.
2. Focus on long-term management and follow-up.
3. Explain the role of dermatologists in managing drug reactions.

Management of drug reactions, particularly severe cutaneous adverse drug reactions (SCADRs), must follow a methodical approach to achieve therapeutic success and to protect the patient. Initial management begins with the removal of the causative agent without hesitation, which is crucial for preventing further aggravation of the patient. Removal of the offending drug is followed by the administration of the following steps that typically include the administration of corticosteroids to control inflammation and promote healing. The effectiveness of corticosteroids can be markedly improved if used in combination with other immunomodulatory drugs , such as cyclosporine. Research indicates that the treatment not only reduces the interval to disease worsening but also improves patient prognosis, underscoring the importance of individualized therapeutic interventions in SCADR (Patel et al., 2023). Thus, there is a need for a multidisciplinary team of clinicians and dermatologists to provide the best treatment for patients. For cases that involve epidermal growth factor receptor (EGFR) inhibitors, reactions to drugs are particularly complex due to the increased frequency of cutaneous toxicities. These responses, ranging from acneiform eruptions to their more severe mucocutaneous counterparts, can substantially affect a patient's quality of life and the success of oncologic interventions. More than merely treating the signs, successful management involves thorough evaluation and continued dermatologic follow-up. Multidisciplinary therapy by oncologists and dermatologists improves treatment adherence and enables long-term use of EGFR inhibitors, even in patients who may have initially required dose reductions due to side effects. A research showed that multidisciplinary treatment was effective in the resumption of therapy for almost all patients with a history of drug-induced cutaneous reactions, thus emphasizing the significance of specialized management guidelines for this condition (Gisondi et al., 2021). As knowledge of drug reactions improves, so too must our vigilance as healthcare workers in observing how patients respond to medications. Effective management of drug reactions is not only reactive but also includes preventive strategies, such as patient education on potential side effects and the need to report any unusual skin lesions. Continuing education for medical professionals on new treatments and associated risks is important for improving patient outcomes. Second, the application of patient-reported outcomes in clinical practice may enhance the identification and management of adverse drug reactions, along with a multidisciplinary response to patient safety. Lastly, communication between dermatologists, oncologists, and general practitioners is on the leading edge of planning the overall management plan, encouraging both clinical practice and patient care in drug-induced dermatologic diseases.

6.5.1. Immediate Management Measures

The cutaneous drug eruptions' emergency management needs a multi-dimensional approach, beginning with the immediate identification and discontinuation of the offending drug. Once rashes or urticaria are detected, doctors must immediately inquire about recent drug intake to identify the suspected offenders. Discontinuation of the drug is immediately necessary since continued use would aggravate the reaction and deteriorate the patient's health. Besides withdrawal of the offending substance, supportive treatment, including antihistamines and topical corticosteroids, plays a pivotal role in the relief of symptoms. In addition to relieving eruption discomfort, these measures prevent secondary progression to more severe cutaneous drug eruptions that may affect overall patient quality of life.

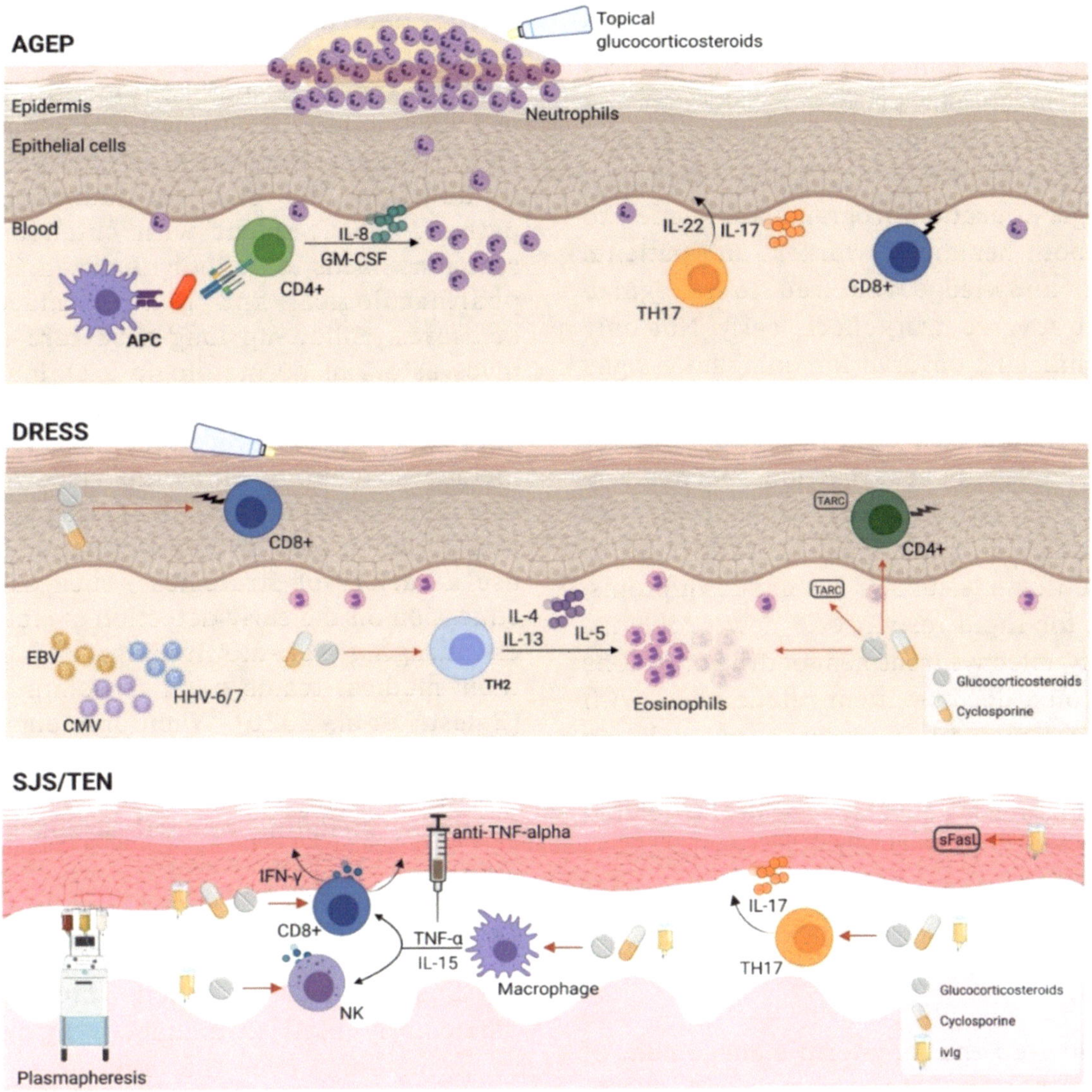

Figure 6.14. Mechanisms and pharmacological management for T-cell-mediated reactions.

Source: https://www.frontiersin.org/files/Articles/923991/fmed-09-923991-HTML/image_m/fmed-09-923991-g002.jpg

Where the reaction is likewise severe, such as in Stevens-Johnson syndrome or toxic epidermal necrolysis, rapid intervention is likewise crucial. Hospital admission may be necessary to provide supportive therapy, such as fluid resuscitation and relief of pain. Systemic corticosteroid injection or immunosuppressive therapy may also be needed in these cases to control inflammation and regulate immune responses. Serious observation in a critical care setting enables an aggressive approach to the treatment of dermatologic manifestations, while concurrently providing care for concomitant systemic effects. Significantly, familiarity with procedures for identifying important drug reactions ensures that health practitioners respond adequately and effectively, provided that this requires a well-defined management policy based on current knowledge. Education programs are needed to educate both healthcare workers and patients with the knowledge required to recognize and treat adverse drug effects early. Not only should clinicians observe for immediate signs and symptoms upon initiation of medication, but they should also educate patients about the risk of delayed-onset reactions, particularly with monoclonal antibody drugs (Paganini et al., 2025). Patients must be cautioned to report new skin lesions or systemic symptoms, allowing for rapid response to new problems. Ultimately, effective treatment of drug eruptions is based on a doctor-patient relationship, with effective communication serving as a foundation for promoting beneficial treatment results without aggravating adverse drug events related to pharmacotherapy (Kherallah et al., 2025) (Figure 6.14).

6.5.2. Long-Term Management and Follow-Up

Good follow-up and long-term management of patients in the event of drug reaction and adverse cutaneous drug eruption-susceptible patients are important in the practice of dermatology, given the rising number of such incidents. The need for ongoing observation is that one must monitor not only the temporary effect of drug treatment but also the risk for long-term or recurrent reactions that may be manifested. Prompt detection and intervention are crucial since cutaneous drug reactions can manifest in multiple ways, from maculopapular eruptions to more severe complications , such as Stevens-Johnson Syndrome (Rahman et al., 2020). Patient history and drug reactions should be monitored by clinicians to enable timely modification of therapy upon the occurrence of adverse effects. In addition, establishing an open forum for patient experience may help identify patterns in drug reactions to inform future management and provide a framework for integrated care. In addition, the plan for management of patients who present with cutaneous drug reactions needs to be individualized, including pharmacological and non-pharmacological measures. Follow-up long-term care typically involves serial dermatologic examinations to reassess skin status, particularly if patients have experienced severe reactions. This could include scheduling follow-up visits at cycles coincident with the cycles of drug treatment and potential side effects. Dermatologists can use a variety of strategies , such as patient education on the early detection of side effects, encouraging self-monitoring, and keeping their medical teams open to communication (Balestri et al., 2020). When problematic drug eruptions are encountered, better outcomes can be achieved with a multidisciplinary team response, including referral to specialists in areas such as rheumatology or immunology, to address concurrent disease and to consider the benefits and risks of continued therapy.

Lastly, personalized medicine is particularly used to manage drug reactions in dermatology over the long term. Tailored treatment regimens to an individual patient's unique genetic, environmental, and lifestyle factors can maximize therapeutic benefit while reducing risk. Emerging investigations into the mechanisms of drug-induced adverse effects have the potential to uncover biomarkers that predict susceptibility to specific drug-induced skin eruptions (Rahman et al., 2020). This could significantly change follow-up treatment by enabling clinicians to preselect safer drugs earlier, based on a patient's profile. Additionally, as therapeutic models evolve, the incorporation of biological agents into long-term therapeutic protocols has become a standard component of the management of hard-to-treat drug-induced skin eruptions. Constant monitoring of treatment efficacy and side effects is vital to ensure effective and safe long-term management for patients.

6.5.3. Dermatologists' Role in Drug Reactions Management

Management of drug reactions, particularly cutaneous adverse drug reactions (CADRs), is a vital area in dermatology that requires the skilled hand of dermatologists. Drug reactions could be as insignificant as a slight rash or as severe as a debilitating condition, so it involves a high-level understanding of drug interactions and patient reactions. Dermatologists play a critical role in identifying and diagnosing such drug reactions, as they may present in various forms that resemble other dermatological conditions. Their expertise enables them to effectively distinguish CADRs from other skin diseases. In addition, this differentiation is critical to implementing appropriate management approaches, as misdiagnosis will lead to inappropriate management and deterioration of the patient's condition. By using advanced diagnostic facilities and techniques, dermatologists significantly contribute to optimizing patient outcomes in cases of potentially disabling drug reactions. In addition to accurate diagnosis, dermatologists are responsible for coordinating CADR treatment through a combination of causative agent withdrawal and supportive therapy. Causative drug withdrawal is at times the foundation of treatment, as per the literature that addresses CADR management, such as from antibiotic or anticonvulsant therapy (Sutaria et al., 2024). In addition, they may use therapies to reduce symptoms of the reactions, such as corticosteroids or antihistamines, based on eruption severity and type. Effective management may require dermatologists to collaborate with other healthcare providers to provide comprehensive care. This interprofessional approach not only enhances the management of adverse reactions but also provides a setting for educating other clinicians about the complexities of drug reactions and their dermatological manifestations. Moreover, the integration of digital software and applications into CADR management is an important advancement in dermatologic practice.

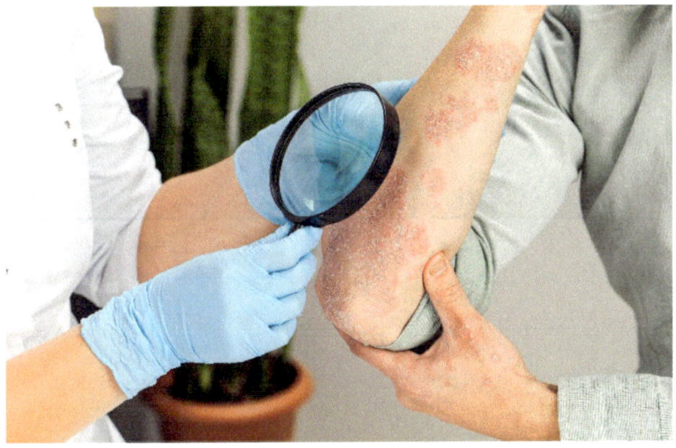

Figure 6.15. Dermatologists play a crucial role in the diagnosis and management of drug reactions, particularly cutaneous adverse drug reactions (CADRs).

Source: https://images.squarespace-cdn.com/content/v1/6201a35299bac77b09db4ba3/08d5b040-2dbb-41b9-842e-1997e58e191e/bigstock-A-Dermatologist-Wearing-Gloves-399579221.jpg.

Current studies have shown that online applications can effectively augment the knowledge of non-dermatology practitioners in the detection and treatment of CADRs (Chaisriya et al., 2024). The applications are employed to enhance awareness of potential drug reactions, thereby enabling faster and more accurate diagnoses. Dermatologists can use such technological innovation to augment peer education, particularly among non-experts, thereby expanding their purview beyond direct patient care. By way of digital training and resource development, dermatologists can facilitate the coordination of a multidisciplinary intervention that better empowers all healthcare professionals to manage drug reactions, with emphasis on their integral role in ensuring safe therapeutic practice in healthcare facilities (Figure 6.15).

Test Your Knowledge

1. What are the key immediate steps in managing a suspected cutaneous drug reaction?
2. What role do dermatologists play in the management of drug-induced skin reactions?
3. Why is follow-up care important in patients who have experienced a drug reaction?

6.6. Prevention of Adverse Drug Reactions

Learning Outcome

1. Explain the importance of patient education.
2. Understand the strategies for minimizing risk.
3. Discuss the role of pharmacovigilance in prevention.

Prevention of drug adverse reactions (ADRs) is an important consideration for dermatology, especially due to the expanding list of drugs that exist as treatment options. Prevention is successful when based on a thorough understanding of the patient's history, interactions among medications, and the known risk factors inherent to particular drugs. A key method for reducing ADRs is to use comprehensive screening procedures before initiating any treatment regimen. For instance, dermatologists should screen patients for potential allergy, pre-existing conditions, and other drugs patients are taking. By identifying candidates at high risk, practitioners are able to plan treatment regimens that exclude the risk of cutaneous adverse eruptions, and hence protect the health and well-being of patients." Dermatologists must inform patients about the potential side effects of prescribed medications in an effective manner, emphasizing the importance of early reporting of adverse reactions. Engaging patients in their own care not only empowers them but also enhances adherence to treatment regimens and reduces the risk of complications. In addition, regular follow-ups enable effective monitoring of patients, particularly those receiving high-risk regimens, such as immunosuppressive immunomodulators. For example, patients undergoing treatment for infections exacerbated by COVID-19 must be carefully monitored and educated about signs to watch for, as drug-to-drug interactions or changes in health status can cause serious cutaneous reactions (Seirafianpour et al., 2020).

Additionally, the use of advanced pharmacogenomic testing is a promising approach to reducing ADRs. By identifying genetic variants that affect drug metabolism, dermatologists can tailor treatment regimens to patient profiles. Such a personalized treatment regimen could significantly decrease the incidence of adverse effects caused by drugs like taxanes, which are typically associated with dermatotoxicities. Knowledge of genetic susceptibility enables clinicians to make informed decisions about drug selection and dosing regimens, thereby maximizing patient outcomes. Implementation of these preventive measures not only addresses the existing issue of drug reactions but also opens new avenues toward safer, more effective therapeutic options in dermatology (Sibaud et al., 2016).

6.6.1. Patient Education's Importance

Patient education is the key to effective dermatologic practice. Educating patients about medications, the potential for drug reactions, and the recognition of cutaneous adverse drug reactions can empower practitioners to help patients take control of their treatment. Patient education about the manifestations of cutaneous adverse drug reactions (CADRs) is relevant as early detection can help in early treatment and reduce complications. The harmless rashes or the more dangerous Stevens-Johnson syndrome that CADRs can resemble underscore the need for well-educated patients who can identify warning signs early. Greater awareness is causally linked to improved patient outcomes, thereby highlighting education as a step toward reducing the costs of preventable drug reactions to society and the economy (Sutaria et al., 2024). Moreover, patient education enhances effective communication between healthcare providers and patients, fostering a partnership that optimizes therapeutic outcomes. Knowing the possible side effects of drugs, patients can realistically discuss with the health team changing treatments or alternative modes of therapy. A high percentage of CADRs is brought about by easily identifiable causes, that is, drug interactions or incorrect dosing, according to research. By resolving these concerns through education, clinicians can reduce the prevalence of CADRs and enhance safer drug practices. Informed decision-making is also emphasized, with patients informed about treatment plans more likely to be compliant, ultimately producing improved overall health outcomes (Panigrahy et al., 2024). In addition to initiating compliance and reducing drug reactions, patient education also plays an important role in promoting a culture of safety within the healthcare system. Once patients are informed about their medication, they can help ensure safety by reporting any unintended side effects they may have experienced or by questioning inconsistencies in their treatment plan. This forward-looking approach not only benefits individual patients but also enhances the overall body of knowledge on medication safety. To the extent that cutaneous drug reactions remain a significant public health problem, integration of robust patient education programs into dermatologic practice is imperative. With appropriate educational tools and resources, patients are better able to manage their treatments and their complexities, leading to improved control of CADRs and greater confidence in the healthcare system (Sutaria et al., 2024).

6.6.2. Strategies for Minimizing Risk

Effective management of drug reactions and cutaneous adverse drug eruptions requires the implementation of risk-reducing, holistic strategies. Foremost among these measures is identification and knowledge of high-risk patients, particularly those who are elderly or have polypharmacy, since they are most prone to experiencing cutaneous adverse drug reactions (CADRs) (Sutaria et al., 2024). Health care providers need to conduct intensive pre-treatment assessments, such as thorough medication histories and allergy profiles, to identify those at greatest risk. Patient education is also an important aspect of risk reduction, with patients being required to inform health care providers when any abnormal skin changes are first noticed. Adopting stringent monitoring protocols, particularly during the launch of new drugs, can also facilitate early identification of adverse reactions, thereby limiting the severity and duration of cutaneous eruptions. Another important approach to the reduction of risk in instances of adverse drug reactions (ADRs) is the utilization of pharmacogenetic testing. Pharmacogenetic tests can identify genetic markers that may increase the risk of serious side effects, particularly with drugs that cause dermatologic effects. For instance, understanding how HLA alleles are used to predict adverse drug reactions can render prescribing more evidence-based, particularly in those at risk of severe reactions like Stevens-Johnson syndrome (SJS) or toxic epidermal necrolysis (TEN) (Palafox et al., 2024). By selecting medications that take genetic profile and medical history into consideration, healthcare professionals can substantially reduce the incidence of adverse skin events. Educational programs for both patients and healthcare professionals on pharmacogenomics are necessary to support more individualized treatment practices, ultimately improving patient safety. Finally, ongoing professional development and training for healthcare professionals are required to keep up-to-date with the most recent research into cutaneous adverse drug reactions. Because dermatological conditions related to drug reactions can evolve with new medications, providers must be informed about new recommendations and evidence. Regular workshops, group discussions, and access to current literature can help providers identify and treat drug eruptions more effectively. Creating a culture of reporting and adverse-effect analysis in health care systems can also increase awareness and control of treatment, leading to improved patient outcomes. All these steps offer assurances that healthcare practitioners are adequately trained to handle the complexities of drug interactions and therefore safer prescribing and ultimately reduced risk of CADRs.

6.6.3. Pharmacovigilance Role in Prevention

Pharmacovigilance plays an essential role in preventing drug reactions and cutaneous adverse drug eruptions, particularly in dermatology. Pharmacovigilance aims to find new safety issues and improve the safety profiles of drugs through the systematic monitoring, reporting, and assessment of adverse drug reactions (ADR). This method is crucial for identifying the risk factors associated with some drugs allopurinol, which has been associated with severe cutaneous adverse reactions (SCARs), such as Stevens-Johnson syndrome and toxic epidermal necrolysis. Continuous surveillance enables the clinician to provide informed advice when prescribing dermatological therapy and supports early detection of potential adverse effects, ultimately leading to improved patient safety and optimal therapeutic outcomes. The general purpose of pharmacovigilance is to reduce risks of drug use, affirming the value of vigilant monitoring in dermatology. Effective pharmacovigilance not only helps identify adverse cutaneous drug eruptions but also enables the implementation of risk-minimization measures. Drug safety organizations are likely to use data from pharmacovigilance systems to develop recommendations and guidelines on drug use to enhance safety profiles. For instance, studies with medications like allopurinol demonstrate the necessity for close monitoring, especially in populations at high risk like the elderly, who are at a higher risk for severe cutaneous ADRs. The information obtained from databases of reports enables clinicians to make better-informed decisions, modify medication regimens, and potentially reduce the incidence of serious cutaneous adverse reactions. Besides, patient education participation in signs and symptoms of ADRs is important in encouraging active healthcare behavior, whereby patients report voluntarily any drug-related adverse effects in a timely manner. Finally, coordination among clinicians, pharmacists, and regulatory agencies within the pharmacovigilance system strengthens communication channels and promotes a safety culture in dermatology. Collaboration among such stakeholders facilitates the timely release of findings from pharmacovigilance activities, for instance, alerts on serious skin reactions associated with some drugs. Such information is essential for updating clinical guidelines and for sensitizing prescribers to safer practice, thereby minimizing the incidence of ADRs. With technology, real-time monitoring and reporting are also possible through electronic health platforms, which can revolutionize pharmacovigilance practice. With the active participation of healthcare providers and patients in the pharmacovigilance process, the dermatologic community can unite and be positioned to prevent adverse drug reactions and ensure safe administration of therapies, thereby advancing the overall objective of improved patient care (Figure 6.16).

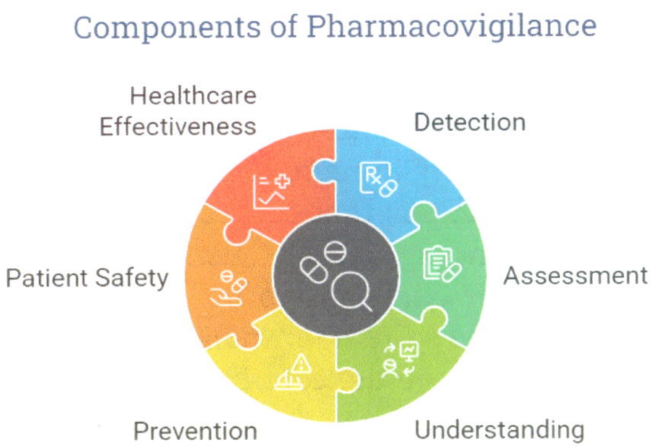

Figure 6.16. Components of pharmacovigilance.

Source: https://pharmuni.com/wp-content/uploads/2025/02/Definition-of-Pharmacovigilance-visual-selection.png.

Test Your Knowledge

1. Why is patient education critical in preventing adverse drug reactions?
2. What strategies can healthcare providers use to minimize the risk of ADRs
3. What is the role of pharmacovigilance in preventing adverse drug reactions?

SUMMARY

In concluding the analysis of drug reactions and cutaneous adverse drug reactions (CADRs) in dermatology, the incidents are increasingly evident to be a significant, though preventable, health issue in clinical practice. The findings of various studies suggest a range of CADRs, with common presentations including erythematous maculopapular rashes and severe presentations such as Stevens-Johnson Syndrome and toxic epidermal necrolysis. As indicated by studies, most patients indicated improvement after offending drugs were discontinued, early detection and withdrawal of offending drugs are critical in reversing the impacts of CADRs on patient health (Panigrahy et al., 2024). Lastly, enhanced awareness among health professionals of the detection and treatment of such reactions can significantly impact patient outcomes and reduce the burden on health systems. Secondly, epidemiological knowledge of CADRs underscores the necessity of collecting data systematically to inform best practices in dermato-care. For instance, studies aimed at cohorts from different geographical locations, particularly in regions where HIV and other systemic diseases are prevalent, unveil complexity in drug reactions that can be addressed with subtle strategies (Blank et al., 2024). The identification of offending agents, such as antibiotics and some antiretroviral medications, provides a critical basis for clinicians to be alert and consider alternative therapies when prescribing. By establishing an active system for monitoring adverse drug reactions, healthcare systems are better positioned to manage the delicate balance between dermatological well-being and pharmacotherapy. In the future, the continued implementation of robust pharmacovigilance programs and educational interventions is required to address the challenges at the interface posed by CADRs. Such programs facilitate not only reporting and analysis of adverse effects but also clinician sensitization and patient education about potential cutaneous side effects. The integration of multidisciplinary approaches, combining the strengths of dermatology, pharmacology, and public health, will continue to enhance our understanding of adverse drug events and improve the safety profile of medication therapy. Last but not least, continued research and interdisciplinarity will play a vital role in advancing the prevention and management of drug reactions and CADRs, ultimately improving patient care worldwide.

In dermatology, drug eruptions and adverse cutaneous drug reactions are crucial to understand in order to treat the patient appropriately. These adverse cutaneous drug eruptions manifest as various dermatological conditions, which cause severe morbidity on the patient's quality of life. It is essential to categorize these eruptions according to clinical presentation and pathogenic mechanisms. For example, some reactions occur as soon as after exposure to drugs, while others take weeks or months to become evident, hence making diagnosis and management more difficult. The identification of such patterns enables clinicians to more accurately predict potential reactions, allowing timely interventions and improved patient outcomes. Furthermore, obtaining a detailed history of drug use, such as the onset and duration of symptoms, is critical in determining the causative drugs responsible for such adverse reactions. Yet another significant component of drug reaction adverse research is the application of pharmacogenomics, which helps tailor treatment by employing patients' individual genetic profiling. Genetic variables influence how patients process medications, thereby modifying drug efficacy and safety profiles. Identification of these factors can guide dermatologists to select safer treatments to avoid cutaneous eruptions. Additionally, ongoing research is crucial for identifying accurate genetic markers associated with increased sensitivity to certain drugs. Using such information, healthcare practitioners can implement more personalized therapeutic interventions that not only increase therapeutic efficacy but also minimize skin reactions and enhance patient satisfaction and medication adherence. Furthermore, treatment options continue to evolve, with the incorporation of natural products and their therapeutic applications in dermatology. As further illustrated by recent studies, natural-derived drugs possess anti-inflammatory, antioxidant, and antimicrobial activities and therefore may serve as alternatives for the treatment of numerous skin ailments, including drug-induced conditions. Combining these natural substances with modern medicines might yield synergistic effects, enhancing overall treatment efficacy and reducing side effects (Zaid et al., 2022). However, promising as these options appear, additional clinical trials are necessary to confirm their safety and efficacy. Continuing our understanding of these treatments will not only enhance dermatological practice but also provide patients with safe, tolerable options for treating drug reactions and skin eruptions (Kilburn et al., 2023).

KEY TERMS FROM THIS CHAPTER

- Adverse drug reactions (ADRs)
- Anticonvulsants
- Cancer therapy
- CD8+ memory T
- Cutaneous drug adverse reactions (CADRs)
- Cutaneous toxicities
- Dermatological reactions
- Dermatomyositis
- Drug allergies
- Angioedema
- Anti-tumor immunity
- Catastrophic complications
- Cutaneous adverse effects
- Cutaneous drug eruptions
- Cytokines
- Dermatological treatment
- Diagnostic specificity
- Drug eruptions

CRITICAL THINKING QUESTIONS

1. **Which of the following best describes a Type IV hypersensitivity reaction involved in adverse cutaneous drug eruptions?**
   a. Immediate IgE-mediated reaction causing anaphylaxis
   b. Cytotoxic reaction involving antibody-dependent cell lysis
   c. Immune complex deposition in tissues, causing inflammation
   d. T-cell-mediated delayed hypersensitivity reaction
2. **Which drug class is most commonly associated with Stevens-Johnson Syndrome (SJS) and Toxic Epidermal Necrolysis (TEN)?**
   a. Beta-blockers
   b. NSAIDs
   c. Sulfonamides
   d. Antacids
3. **A patient develops a widespread erythematous maculopapular rash 7 days after starting ampicillin. There are no systemic symptoms. What is the most likely diagnosis?**
   a. Morbilliform (exanthematous) drug eruption
   b. Urticaria
   c. Fixed drug eruption
   d. Drug-induced lupus
4. **What is the first step in the management of a suspected drug-induced cutaneous reaction?**
   a. Administer corticosteroids
   b. Prescribe antihistamines
   c. Perform a skin biopsy
   d. Discontinue the suspected drug immediately
5. **Which of the following is a key strategy in preventing serious adverse cutaneous drug reactions in high-risk patients?**
   a. Routine antibiotic prophylaxis
   b. Patch testing for all medications
   c. Pharmacogenetic screening
   d. Starting multiple drugs simultaneously

Short Answer Questions

1. What are the main immunological mechanisms underlying adverse cutaneous drug eruptions (ACDEs)?
2. What are the most common clinical types of adverse cutaneous drug eruptions?
3. Which drugs are most commonly associated with serious cutaneous adverse drug reactions (SCARs).
4. How is an adverse cutaneous drug eruption diagnosed?

Answer to Critical Thinking Questions

1. (d); 2. (c); 3. (a); 4. (d); 5. (c)

REFERENCES

1. N, A., Salam, A., Gp, R., & Challa, T. (2024). Unraveling the tapestry of adverse cutaneous drug reactions: A clinico-epidemiological study. *IP Indian Journal of Clinical and Experimental Dermatology, 10*(2), 176–181. https://doi.org/10.18231/j.ijced.2024.032Agrawal, P., Kunkulol, R., & Ghodke, K. D. (2024). Eruptions in focus: Cefadroxil and the uncommon realm of fixed-drug reactions: A case report. *International Journal of Basic & Clinical Pharmacology*. https://www.semanticscholar.org/paper/5cca99d655f9481b3602aef7d7a3f9050468eb23 (accessed on 21st July 2025).
2. Algazi, A., Daud, A., Gubens, M., Lin, L., et al. (2015). Pembrolizumab cutaneous adverse events and their association with disease progression. https://core.ac.uk/download/573402193.pdf (accessed on 21st July 2025).
3. Balestri, R., Magnano, M., Girardelli, C. R., Bortolotti, R., & Rech, G. (2020). Long-term safety of combined biological therapy in a patient affected by arthropathic psoriasis and atopic dermatitis. *Dermatologic Therapy, 33*. https://www.semanticscholar.org/paper/6790476d5d7a0e604c08822f8d430b8fea5407e8 (accessed on 21st July 2025).
4. Ban, E. G., Lechsner, P., Dho-Nagy, E. A., Balan, M. A., Major-Szakács, I., Brassai, A., Simon-Szabó, Z., et al. (2024). Novel strategy in the detection of adverse cutaneous drug reactions: A case series study. *Diagnostics, 14*. https://www.semanticscholar.org/paper/c08e6c21779f7240bc929b832ee56cbe905ea2d6 (accessed on 21st July 2025).
5. Bhardwaj, M., Chiu, M. N., & Sah, S. P. (2022). Adverse cutaneous toxicities by PD-1/PD-L1 immune checkpoint inhibitors: Pathogenesis, treatment, and surveillance. *Cutaneous and Ocular Toxicology, 41*, 73–90. https://www.semanticscholar.org/paper/7f50b0da12fc3af1706470793127fc5f587f69a1 (accessed on 21st July 2025).
6. Blank, S., Recke, A., Konyana, S. P. P., Teixeira, N., Pirjol, L., Thwala, B., Nkoyane, W., et al. (2024). Spectrum of offending drugs and cutaneous adverse drug reactions requiring hospitalization in a tertiary South African hospital in TB/HIV endemic setting. *Frontiers in Allergy, 5*. https://www.semanticscholar.org/paper/1e1f9eb13f5006827e0568ce1fc048d36f2c4ed5 (accessed on 21st July 2025).
7. Casale, F., Roth, G., Wan, K., & Saab-Chalhoub, M. W. (2024). Enfortumab vedotin drug eruption: Cutaneous adverse events and histopathologic findings. *The American Journal of Dermatopathology, 46*, 538–541. https://www.semanticscholar.org/paper/e65fe985828b46b03b843c9ecc5aa671edb6d938 (accessed on 21st July 2025).
8. Chaisriya, K., Tawanwongsri, W., Mettarikanon, D., Ameentranon, N., Eden, C., Inthongpan, M., & Sindhusen, S. (2024). Web application for assisting non-dermatology physicians in learning and managing patients with common cutaneous adverse drug reactions: A multicenter randomized controlled trial. *Annals of Medicine, 56*. https://www.semanticscholar.org/paper/7bdcac10be5721a0f8b37aa1020d6a7635d1eaf7 (accessed on 21st July 2025).
9. Gisondi, P., Geat, D., Mattiucci, A., Lombardo, F., Santo, A., & Girolomoni, G. (2021). Incidence of adverse cutaneous reactions to epidermal growth factor receptor inhibitors in patients with non-small-cell lung cancer. *Dermatology, 237*, 929–933. https://www.semanticscholar.org/paper/fe0ea72b5a03baea914f1083a75159e7230b01a5 (accessed on 21st July 2025).

10. Gruppo Italiano Studi Epidemiologici in Dermatologia (1996). Cutaneous reactions to alimentary tract medications: Results of a seven-year surveillance program and review of the literature. *Dermatology, 193*(1), 11–16. https://www.semanticscholar.org/paper/59764da28de1b8fd45406e78450700b567414a49 (accessed on 21st July 2025).

11. Gupta, D., Gairola, B., Kumar, B., Bharath, M., & Ansari, M. S. (2021). A study and evaluation of cutaneous adverse drug reaction in the patients attending dermatology department of tertiary care teaching hospital in Eastern Uttar Pradesh. *International Journal of Basic and Clinical Pharmacology, 10*, 664. https://www.semanticscholar.org/paper/8f30feba7ac899066b37215345e8c1c832222e68 (accessed on 21st July 2025).

12. Hu, L., Dong, J., & Zhang, S. (2020). Tamsulosin-associated erythema multiforme-like eruption. *American Journal of Therapeutics*. https://www.semanticscholar.org/paper/7f92ec54c5ea0c69ef7664fc5b68f625b8f7eba3 (accessed on 21st July 2025).

13. Kherallah, K., Ahmad, I., Bandara, A., Kattoula, J., Rodriguez, I., & Worswick, S. (2025). Adverse cutaneous reactions to monoclonal antibodies: Stevens-Johnson syndrome, toxic epidermal necrolysis, erythema multiforme, and fixed drug eruption–A systematic review. *Biomedicine Hub, 10*, 105–115. https://www.semanticscholar.org/paper/ae800c3fe623da2ffa79dcd1b9a87172ef3f55a7 (accessed on 21st July 2025).

14. Kilburn, L., Khuong-Quang, D. A., Hansford, J. R., Landi, D., van der Lugt, J., Leary, S., Hernáiz Driever, P., et al. (2023). The type II RAF inhibitor tovorafenib in relapsed/refractory pediatric low-grade glioma: The phase 2 FIREFLY-1 trial. *Nature Medicine, 30*, 207–217. https://doi.org/10.1038/s41591-023-02668-y (accessed on 21st July 2025).

15. L'Orphelin, J. M., Cassecuel, J., Kandolf, L., Harwood, C. A., Tookey, P. M., Junejo, M. H., Hogan, S., et al. (2023). Cutaneous manifestations induced by check point inhibitors in 120 melanoma patients—The European MelSkinTox study. *Journal of the European Academy of Dermatology and Venereology, 37*, 1606–1615. https://doi.org/10.1111/jdv.19112 (accessed on 21st July 2025).

16. Lahouel, I., Ben Salah, N., Ben Fadhel, N., Chahed, F., Ouni, N. E. I., Belhadjali, H., Aouam, K., et al. (2022). Symmetrical drug-related intertriginous and flexural exanthema-like eruption after COVID-19 vaccine. *Journal of the European Academy of Dermatology and Venereology, 36*. https://doi.org/10.1111/jdv.18108 (accessed on 21st July 2025).

17. Malhotra, S., Kaur, B., & Kaur, I. (2021). A prospective study of clinical spectrum of cutaneous adverse drug reactions and their incidence in Indian population. *IP Indian Journal of Clinical and Experimental Dermatology*. https://www.semanticscholar.org/paper/91052bad37b90d1d9947683830a3ed5dd1595b31 (accessed on 21st July 2025).

18. McClatchy, J., Yap, T., Nirenberg, A., & Scardamaglia, L. (2022). Fixed drug eruptions–The common and novel culprits since 2000. *JDDG: Journal der Deutschen Dermatologischen Gesellschaft, 20*. https://www.semanticscholar.org/paper/0761a5703628f300b9370b08d8594843a5d90ebb (accessed on 21st July 2025).

19. Mohd Zaid, N. A., Sekar, M., Bonam, S. R., Gan, S. H., Lum, P. T., Begum, M. Y., Mat Rani, N. N. I., et al. (2022). Promising natural products in new drug design, development, and therapy for skin disorders: An overview of scientific evidence and understanding their mechanism of action. *Drug Design Development and Therapy, 16*, 23–66. https://doi.org/10.2147/dddt.s326332 (accessed on 21st July 2025).

20. Montinari, M., Atzori, L., Valdevit, S., & Rongioletti, F. (2020). Erythema annulare centrifugum with anosmia and ageusia in a SARS-CoV-2 exposed patient successfully treated with doxycycline. *International Journal of Dermatology, 60*, 384–386. https://doi.org/10.1111/ijd.15356 (accessed on 21st July 2025).

21. Moretta, A., Scieuzo, C., Petrone, A. M., Salvia, R., Manniello, M. D., Franco, A., Lucchetti, D., et al. (2021). Antimicrobial peptides: A new hope in biomedical and pharmaceutical fields. *Frontiers in Cellular and Infection Microbiology, 11*. https://doi.org/10.3389/fcimb.2021.668632 (accessed on 21st July 2025).

22. Morgillo, A., Marovino, E., Mazzarella, M., Barbagiovanni, V., & Randazzo, M. F. (2022). Severe cutaneous adverse drug reactions: From causes to mechanisms. *Qeios*. https://www.semanticscholar.org/paper/b92f8b4f36cea20e0c7da0861f52b70ea0571b6d (accessed on 21st July 2025).

23. Morsy, H., Ibrahim, F., Negm, D., Mwafey, I., & Hanna, M. (2023). Serum interleukin-21 level in patients with severe adverse cutaneous drug reactions and correlation with disease severity. *Journal of Current Medical Research and Practice, 8*, 12–16. https://www.semanticscholar.org/paper/9a0b8b7cecbb65f00d686da649f9e2b9f876e5b7 (accessed on 21st July 2025).

24. Fang, Wei-Cheng1; Chou, Pei-Chien5; Chiu, Li-Wen1; Ke, Chiao-Li2,4; Cheng, Shih-Tsung1,3. Dermoscopy as a Diagnostic and Monitoring Tool for Recurrent Extramammary Paget's Disease. Indian Journal of Dermatology 67(6):p 819-820, Nov–Dec 2022. | DOI: 10.4103/ijd.ijd_771_22 (accessed on 21st July 2025).

25. Oro, S., Milpied, B., Badrignans, M., Carrera, C., Elshot, Y. S., Bensaïd, B., Segura, S., et al. (2022). Severe blistering eruptions induced by immune checkpoint inhibitors: A multicenter international study of 32 cases. *Melanoma Research, 32*, 205–210. https://doi.org/10.1097/cmr.0000000000000819 (accessed on 21st July 2025).

26. Paganini, C., Mortato, E., Tofani, L., Belcastro, A., Talamonti, M., Di Raimondo, C., Bianchi, L., et al. (2025). Rosacea-like eruptions associated with upadacitinib in atopic dermatitis: Two case reports and management strategies. *Dermatology Reports*. https://www.semanticscholar.org/paper/93be00efa139af3a5e9322c34b48120c3612293d (accessed on 21st July 2025).

27. Palafox-Romo, R., & Méndez-Flores, S. (2024). Cutaneous adverse drug reactions to antiseizure medications. *Journal of Epilepsy Research, 14*, 53–58. https://www.semanticscholar.org/paper/f8ecfcbb7506836fc41cb4225b07f69c10760199 (accessed on 21st July 2025).

28. Pandhi, D., & De, D. (2020). Use of immunosuppressants/immunomodulators in autoimmune/inflammatory dermatologic diseases during COVID-19 pandemic—General recommendation based on available evidence. *Indian Dermatology Online Journal, 11*, 526–526. https://doi.org/10.4103/idoj.idoj_414_20 (accessed on 21st July 2025).

29. Panigrahy, A., Begum, A., Pingali, U., Padmaja, M., & Sajeev, A. (2024). Evaluation of cutaneous adverse drug reactions in a tertiary care hospital in southern India: A retrospective analysis. *Asian Journal of Pharmaceutical and Clinical Research*. https://www.semanticscholar.org/paper/7dca3435b93f2363be4c8316a8020f7fcff22956 (accessed on 21st July 2025).

30. Patel, L., Shah, S. P., Jangid, N., Desai, C., & Shah, B. (2023). Effectiveness of corticosteroids alone versus corticosteroids and cyclosporine in the management of patients with severe cutaneous drug reaction. *Journal of Clinical and Diagnostic Research*. https://www.semanticscholar.org/paper/fe202c85e0a9a0d9c47bcfa6d12b4b227664bb44 (accessed on 21st July 2025).

31. Patil, A. B., Rajashekhar, N., & Sushma, A. (2024). Cutaneous adverse drug reactions: Clinical pattern and causative agents in a tertiary care center in central Karnataka. *International Journal of Scientific Research*. https://www.semanticscholar.org/paper/17e106e06b6f8cc6049d5435dc3d80a7bf895dd5 (accessed on 21st July 2025).

32. Pfützner, W. (2020). Cutaneous adverse drug reactions. *Pediatric Dermatology*. https://www.semanticscholar.org/paper/89f5a69c35ae5d70427b4038af56be99965f9a5d (accessed on 21st July 2025).

33. Rahman, M., Khan, A., Chandra, P., Sharmin, L., Rahman, F., & Jamil, A. (2020). Cutaneous drug reactions in children attending a tertiary care hospital. *Taj: Journal of Teachers Association, 33*, 56–62. https://www.semanticscholar.org/paper/f0a6d5f722627c76e6e3037cfd11b090209caf58 (accessed on 21st July 2025).

34. Rahman, S. M., Salem, Y., & Hussain, A. (2024). Trips through the skin: Reviewing cutaneous drug reactions to psychedelics and hallucinogens. *Dermatitis: Contact, Atopic, Occupational, Drug*. https://www.semanticscholar.org/paper/80939c30ae4c0da8b28c2726b5dd2f7319f98269 (accessed on 21st July 2025).

35. Ravishankar, M., & Rakshith, N. (2015). Phenytoin/albendazole induced exanthematous eruptions: A case report. *International Journal of Basic and Clinical Pharmacology, 4*, 586–589. https://www.semanticscholar.org/paper/419e0e60e5caeb66982fdfda5ed2b946215acdb1 (accessed on 21st July 2025).

36. Scavone, C., Di Mauro, C., Ruggiero, R., Bernardi, F. F., Trama, U., Aiezza, M. L., Rafaniello, C., et al. (2019). Severe cutaneous adverse drug reactions associated with allopurinol: An analysis of spontaneous reporting system in Southern Italy. *Drugs – Real World Outcomes, 7*, 41–51. https://doi.org/10.1007/s40801-019-00174-7 (accessed on 21st July 2025).

37. Seirafianpour, F., Sodagar, S., Pour Mohammad, A., Panahi, P., Mozafarpoor, S., Almasi, S., & Goodarzi, A. (2020). Cutaneous manifestations and considerations in COVID-19 pandemic: A systematic review. *Dermatologic Therapy, 33*. https://doi.org/10.1111/dth.13986 (accessed on 21st July 2025).

38. Sibaud, V., LeBoeuf, N. R., Roché, H., Belum, V. R., Gladieff, L., Deslandres, M., Montastruc, M., et al. (2016). Dermatological adverse events with taxane chemotherapy. *European Journal of Dermatology, 26*, 427–443. https://doi.org/10.1684/ejd.2016.2833 (accessed on 21st July 2025).

39. Sutaria, A., Rawlani, S., & Sutaria, A. (2024). Causes and management of cutaneous adverse drug reactions: A comprehensive review. *Cureus, 16*. https://www.semanticscholar.org/paper/bc42031e280b8bfbcc8c52c4556e0db97fb35a83 (accessed on 21st July 2025).

40. Weißhaar, E., Szepietowski, J. C., Dalgard, F., Garcovich, S., Gieler, U., Giménez-Arnau, A. M., Lambert, J., et al. (2019). European S2k guideline on chronic pruritus. *Acta Dermato Venereologica, 99*, 469–506. https://doi.org/10.2340/00015555-3164 (accessed on 21st July 2025).

41. Yan, A., Madigan, L., Korman, A. M., Shearer, S., Dulmage, B., Patel, T., Milani-Nejad, N., et al. (2025). Morbilliform eruptions: Differentiating low-risk drug eruptions, severe cutaneous adverse reactions, viral eruptions, and acute graft-versus-host disease. *American Journal of Clinical Dermatology, 26*, 379–393. https://www.semanticscholar.org/paper/dfd7f752ed7d1c39026ecb01eb93a1c150121280 (accessed on 21st July 2025).

COSMETIC DERMATOLOGY AND AESTHETIC PROCEDURES

7

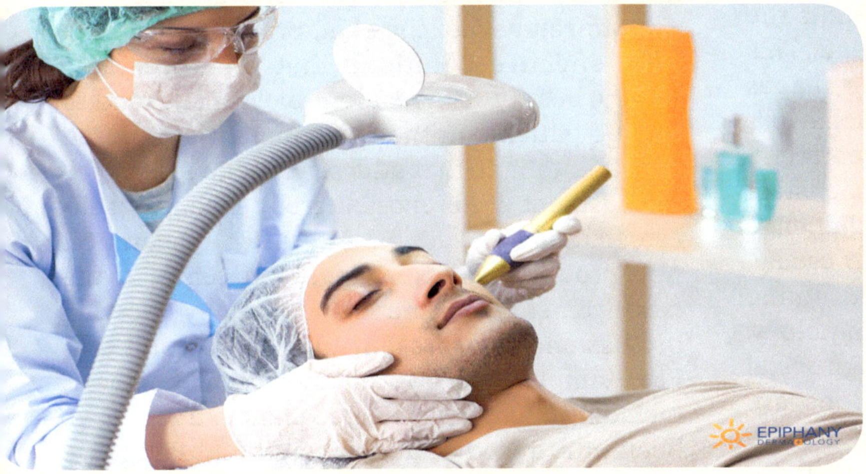

LEARNING OBJECTIVES

After studying this chapter, you will be able to:

1. Understand the historical background of cosmetic dermatology
2. Describe common cosmetic dermatology procedures
3. Differentiate between non-invasive and invasive procedures
4. Explain the role of technology in cosmetic dermatology
5. Discuss the intersection of ethical considerations and cosmetic dermatology
6. Focus on the future of cosmetic dermatology

Introduction

The cosmetic dermatology market has witnessed unprecedented growth in recent years, driven primarily by cultural expectations of beauty and the increasing accessibility of advanced aesthetic treatments. At the heart of this shift is the ubiquitous influence of social media, which is not just a source of communication but also an influential source of information and inspiration regarding skin care and aesthetic development. For the majority of the population, social media platforms , such as Instagram and Snapchat have become arenas for procuring and debating cosmetic dermatologic options. This shift underscores the dual role of social media: it, on the one hand, increases awareness of skin conditions and aesthetic treatments, but, on the other hand, provides a wealth of information, much of which may lack medical accreditation. Hence, the overlap between social media and cosmetic dermatology raises critical issues regarding the consumption of information and subsequent personal health decision-making, particularly among young people (Alsatti et al., 2023). Recent research identifies that social media's effect on people's decision-making process regarding cosmetic procedures is particularly significant in some population segments, such as teenagers and young adults. In a comprehensive study conducted in Jeddah, Saudi Arabia, nearly half of respondents reported seeking aesthetic treatments, with social media as a primary source of information about these treatments. The research identified not just high use of face filters on platforms like Snapchat, but also a great deal of association between one's demographic characteristics, like gender and age, and the intention to receive aesthetic enhancements. This trend shows how social media not only shapes perceptions of beauty but also specific behaviors related to seeking dermatological treatment. As healthcare professionals remain the most credible source of information, the challenge is how to integrate expert advice with casual, largely unproven advice disseminated online (Joshi et al., 2022). In cosmetic dermatology, online information dissemination through social media is immediate. The repercussions are double-edged: although such social networks provide valuable knowledge and promote group forums for skin care, they also pose risks to the dissemination of misinformation. Unverified posts and recommendations can misdirect users to potentially unsafe decisions in dermatological interventions. While the beauty market increasingly uses social media to sell products, particularly to young women with skin problems, the dual nature of these platforms warrants critical examination. Social media influence is changing the progression of dermatologic consultations into an add-on to the usual recommendation from dermatologists. Therefore, maintaining a balance between embracing the benefits of social media and maintaining a core of reliable medical advice is essential for facilitating well-informed decision-making regarding cosmetic dermatology and aesthetic treatments (Alsatti et al., 2023).

Definition of Cosmetic Dermatology

Cosmetic dermatology is an offshoot of dermatology that focuses on treatments to primarily enhance the external appearance of the skin through a variety of non-invasive and minimally invasive procedures. Cosmetic dermatology is intended to treat a range of concerns, including aging, uneven skin tone, acne scarring, and textural irregularities. With techniques such as chemical peels, laser therapy, fillers, and injectables, cosmetic dermatology aims to rejuvenate the skin, providing patients with effective solutions that enhance their natural beauty. As a result, professionals tend to engage patients in the development of tailored treatment plans that address unique skin types and aesthetic preferences, thereby enhancing self-esteem and satisfaction with their appearance. New products and technologies are central to the advancement of cosmetic dermatology, allowing professionals to present innovative solutions. For example, recent advances in cosmetic fibers, including microencapsulated plant extracts, have been introduced as a novel method to improve skin hydration and reduce the appearance of cellulite during physical exercise (Özlem et al., 2024). These technologies not only provide functional outcomes but also enhance the overall patient experience by integrating everyday wear with therapeutic benefits. In addition, ongoing advances in injectable and laser technologies enable greater precision and efficacy, resulting in minimal downtime and more predictable outcomes for patients seeking aesthetic enhancement. In addition to esthetic enhancement, the role of cosmetic dermatology overlaps with that of medical dermatology, namely, the diagnosis and treatment of skin disease. For instance, preoperative imaging techniques like ultrasound have been recognized to have a significant role in surgical planning in disorders , such as melanoma and non-melanoma skin cancers. By quantifying lesion severity and local extent, these methods assist dermatologists in selecting appropriate treatment options and optimizing patient outcomes (Cri Dșan et al., 2024). This integration of cosmetic and medical specialties underscores the whole-person focus of contemporary dermatology and points to its commitment not only to aesthetically enhancing features but also to improving overall skin health (Figure 7.1).

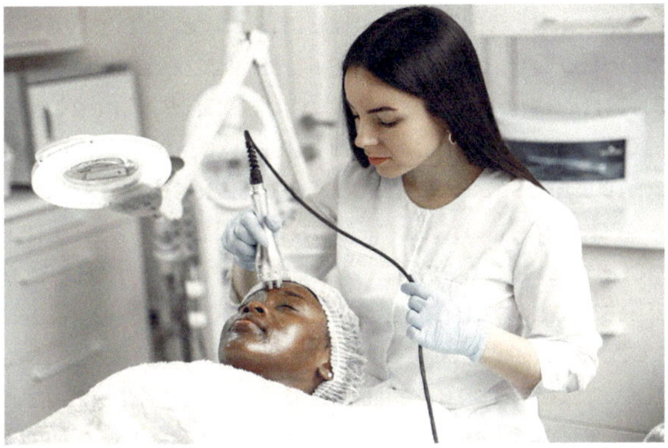

Figure 7.1. Illustration of cosmetic dermatology.

Source: https://aptinjectiontraining.com/wp-content/uploads/2022/06/Featured.jpg.

Importance of Aesthetic Procedures in Modern Society

Now, cosmetic treatments have transcended the limits of luxury and have become inseparable from self-preservation and self-expression. Individuals opt for cosmetic enhancement increasingly, which once more demonstrates the intense relationship between appearance and psyche. Aesthetic treatments range from simple treatments like Botox to extensive surgery, making a larger population accessible to achieve the desired appearance.

Aesthetic concern is not vanity, it is a sign of human beings' need to participate with confidence in social as well as working environments. As society continues to promote youthfulness and beauty, the role of dermatological aesthetics is crucial to fostering a sense of belonging and acceptance across all segments of society. Furthermore, advancements in cosmetic dermatology have massively expanded the scope of aesthetic treatments, making them safer and more feasible than ever before. Technologies adipose-derived stem cell (ADSC)-based treatments exemplify how science and aesthetics converge and how innovative techniques can enable both therapeutic and cosmetic effects. ADSC-exosomes (ADSC-exos) enhance tissue regeneration and repair, offering patients revolutionary treatments for both aesthetic conditions and skin health (Papadopoulos et al., 2024). All of these points to a very significant trend in aesthetics: more and more patients are opting for treatments that enhance not only appearance but also overall skin health and vitality, embracing a multifaceted definition of beauty. Therefore, cosmetic dermatology also keeps up with the times, continually responding to and adjusting to the increasingly complex beauty standards of today. Moreover, the social significance of aesthetic treatments extends beyond individual enhancement; they entail broader discussions about cultural mandates and the democratization of beauty. Growing popularity has also prompted discussions about body positivity and individual autonomy regarding appearance. When people engage in aesthetic enhancements, they are likely to violate conventional beauty norms, producing variations among cultures and groups. This movement tends to drive the concept of beauty toward greater inclusivity, guided by personal tastes rather than societal pressures. Besides, as the cosmetics industry keeps expanding, it promotes economic growth, with various employment opportunities and is spurred by constant research into the new uses of some of the materials and those in the Fungi kingdom because they are primarily studied for their characteristics in cosmetic treatment and application (Corbu et al., 2023). Thus, the worth of aesthetic treatments in our modern world is multifaceted, intersecting individual wants with broader economic and cultural agendas.

7.1. Historical Background

Learning Outcome

1. Understand the evolution of cosmetic dermatology practices.
2. Discuss key milestones in aesthetic procedures.
3. Focus on cultural influences on beauty standards.

The historical evolution of cosmetic dermatology cannot be separated from cultural perceptions of beauty, health, and social status. All the ancient civilizations, including the Egyptians, Greeks, and Romans, employed natural preparations heavily, such as oils, plants, and minerals, for improving and protecting the skin. The use of kohl, a powder made from lead sulfide, is an outstanding example of their early efforts to beautify the eyes and protect them from the sun's glare. In the Middle Ages, cosmetic practices waxed and waned with shifting moral standards, but a taste for aesthetic treatments returned to favor during the Renaissance. Changes in societal expectations, as well as advances in materials and techniques, ultimately set the stage for cosmetic dermatology in modern times. The history of these ancient practices demonstrates how beauty and utility have shaped dermatologic progress over the ages, culminating in the sophisticated procedures of today. The 20th century marked a watershed for cosmetic dermatology, spurred by advances in technology and a new consumer culture celebrating the appearance of youth. Newly developed surgical techniques, as well as the introduction of less invasive procedures such as Botox and dermal fillers, contributed substantially to a cultural shift in the conception of aesthetic enhancement. Physicians began to expand the scope of dermatology, recognizing that physical beauty and mental well-being are inextricably linked. Above all, growing concern about body dysmorphic disorder accompanied the popularity of cosmetic surgery; it has prompted practitioners to consider ethical concerns when deciding whether to operate on patients, with special regard for the safety of patients and informed decision-making. Since it has been found that with an increased number and popularity of cosmetic surgery and procedures, more patients are likely to approach clinicians from proximate specialties with body dysmorphic disorder. Because ethical, safety, and legal concerns are involved in aesthetic treatments for such patients, accurate identification and appropriate treatment selection are required (Susan et al., 2017). In recent times, there has been a discernible trend toward more natural and holistic principles of cosmetic dermatology. There has been heightened public awareness of the potential adverse effects of certain cosmetic ingredients, and consumers have turned to safer alternatives, thereby increasing the use of natural extracts in products. For example, skin-whitening treatments, hitherto governed by conventional synthetic compounds, are increasingly subject to health legislation and ethical concerns. Recent research has highlighted the risks of conventional depigmenting agents such as hydroquinone, necessitating a reevaluation of such applications (Burger et al., 2016). At the same time, research into natural plant extracts as potential alternatives holds promise, and there is a trend towards more sustainable and healthy alternatives in the cosmetic industry. This development is not merely a reflection of changes in consumer trends but also a profound impact on dermatologic practice, underscoring the importance of patient education and regulatory oversight of cosmetic procedures.

7.1.1. Evolving Practice of Cosmetic Dermatology

The evolution of practices in cosmetic dermatology has largely been influenced by technology and changes in societal values toward beauty. Historically, treatments were limited to invasive procedures and basic surface applications for enhancing beauty. The past decades have, however, seen a revolutionary change, primarily as a result of technology that allows for non-invasive and minimally invasive procedures. Such technological improvements high-tech laser technologies and the manufacturing of a variety of aesthetic products, have expanded the scope and functionality of cosmetic dermatology treatments. Therefore, physicians can now offer sophisticated treatments that address multifaceted aesthetic concerns and enhance patient satisfaction through specialized consultations that integrate medical science with artistic reasoning (Haykal et al., 2023). This integration of technology and beauty has significantly affected the patient experience, enabling more personalized and effective outcomes in cosmetic dermatology. Social media has played a particularly significant role in raising awareness about cosmetic dermatology, further propelling its evolution. With platforms Instagram and TikTok serving as centers of beauty trends, people's perceptions of cosmetic procedures have undergone a complete revolution. This democratization of beauty has broadened access for a larger population to explore and study aesthetic treatments, transforming the patient demographics receiving such treatments in a radical way. Younger people, who in most instances are pushed by social media trends, are now explicitly seeking treatments that were previously obtained primarily by older patients (Hogan et al., 2021). Data shared on the internet not only sensitizes but also raises realistic hopes regarding outcomes, thereby contributing to increased patient autonomy and decision-making in cosmetic dermatology. Practitioners must therefore be attuned to such shifts in patient behavior and expectations and adapt their practices accordingly. Concurrent with technological and cultural transitions, the phenomenon of prejuvenation has evolved as a watershed in cosmetic dermatology practice. This term, which has been used to denote preventive treatments intended to maintain a youthful appearance before signs of ageing appear, indicates a significant shift in both patient and practitioner attitudes toward aesthetic treatment. The emphasis on early intervention, such as neurotoxins and dermal fillers, reflects rising awareness of the ageing processes and the skin's biology of health (Hogan et al., 2021). As younger generations learn about the benefits of early intervention, the practice of cosmetic dermatology will experience increasing demand for such preventive approaches. Not only does this transformation indicate the evolving character of cosmetic dermatology, but it also highlights the need to remain constantly educated and adaptable in the discipline to cater to a changing patient population (Figure 7.2).

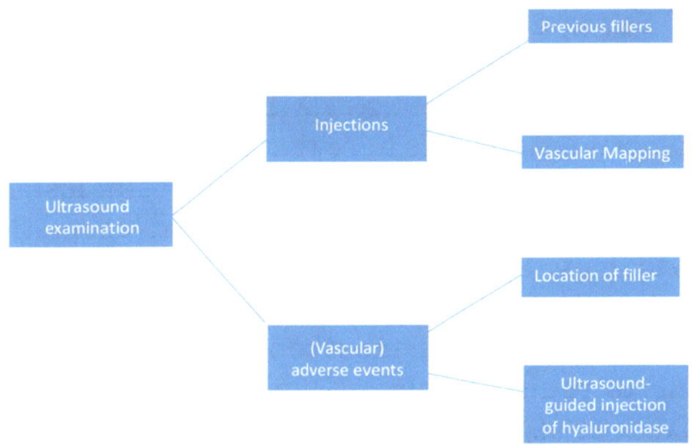

Figure 7.2. Flow chart describing the potential uses of US in cosmetic dermatology.

Source: https://www.researchgate.net/publication/365390626/figure/fig1/AS:11431281180583374@1691642435113/Flow-chart-describing-the-potential-uses-of-US-in-cosmetic-dermatology.png.

7.1.2. Key Milestones in Aesthetic Procedures

The history of aesthetic treatments has seen several milestone events that have profoundly transformed the field of cosmetic dermatology. One important step has been the development of minimally invasive techniques, which have gained prominence for their ability to deliver good outcomes without prolonged recovery or increased risk. Techniques such as Botox injections and fillers became feasible, enabling subtle facial modification without major surgery. Such technologies not only responded to increased patient demand for non-invasive options but also revolutionized cosmetic ideals and patient expectations in dermatology. The trend towards less invasive techniques reflects a patient-centered approach, with efficacy and safety as primary priorities in aesthetic treatments, fundamentally changing the manner in which dermatologists practice cosmetic medicine. Another milestone in aesthetic procedures is the advent of High-Intensity Focused Ultrasound (HIFU) as a non-invasive treatment for conditions , such as Basal Cell Carcinoma (BCC). Traditional surgical interventions for BCC, while effective, used to have cosmetic drawbacks, particularly in facial lesions. It is here that HIFU has made a significant breakthrough with successful lesion ablation accompanied by improved cosmetic outcomes. Studies have shown that patients undergoing HIFU experience minimal pain and rapid recovery, with most reporting satisfaction due to reduced scarring and effective healing (Calik et al., 2024). The successful inclusion of HIFU in BCC treatment protocols is a sign of a continued trend in aesthetic dermatology, where technology improves therapeutic outcomes and quality of life for patients, marking a new era in dermatologic oncology. Last but not least, the role of training and education in aesthetic treatments has been a key factor influencing their safety and effectiveness. Physicians are increasingly seeking specialty training in minimally invasive approaches to patient care delivery. The establishment of specialized dermatologic training programs for procedural techniques attests to the importance of extensive training in conducting aesthetic treatments. Moreover, peer-reviewed literature and clinical journal reviews have begun to examine and substantiate these methods, clarifying their efficacy and long-term outcomes (Meghe et al., 2024). As the field matures, continuous professional development among dermatologists will play an essential role in adopting the latest breakthroughs and ensuring that aesthetic treatments are performed safely and efficiently, thereby improving patient satisfaction and outcomes across aesthetic dermatology (Figure 7.3).

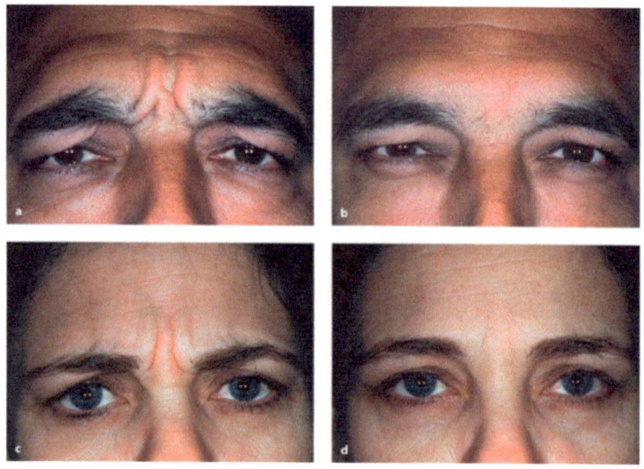

Figure 7.3. Relaxation of the frown lines in a woman and a man treated with Botox Cosmetic: before treatment and 4 weeks following treatment of the corrugator supercilii and procerus muscles.

Source: https://iamj.in/KAYA_CHIKITSA/images/upload/Cosmetic_Dermatology___Copy.pdf.

7.1.3. Cultural Influences on Beauty Standards

Cultural influences significantly shape the definition of beauty across the globe, shaping the perception of aesthetic value and preference in cosmetic dermatology. It is a historical trend that Western beauty standards have dominated the discourse on beauty, depicting predominantly Eurocentric features as the norm. However, the recent trend is toward embracing variable beauty standards across cultures. As noted by scholars, beauty standards are not culture-cross-compatible; what is considered beautiful in one culture may differ substantially in another. This has led to increased concern within the field of cosmetic dermatology that beauty interventions should adapt to and enhance ethnic features rather than blending them with Western standards, thereby fostering a pluralistic approach to aesthetic interventions (Arian et al., 2023). Moreover, the proliferation of social networking sites has exposed individuals to diverse standards of beauty, thereby promoting a high-level discussion of beauty tastes. In such instances, young adults are increasingly influenced by what they witness and hear online, creating demand for cosmetic procedures that align with these influences. Studies on attitudes towards cosmetic surgery among the college-aged population show an increasing interest often driven by the desire to improve one's appearance according to culture-dependent conceptions of beauty (Pearlman et al., 2022). With growing awareness and access, people are likely to seek cosmetic dermatological interventions that reflect their cultural orientation while simultaneously following global beauty trends. The dynamic between beauty ideals and cultural identity presents unique challenges and opportunities in the art of cosmetic dermatology. As practitioners navigate the nuances of varying aesthetic ideals, understanding patient motivation is critical. Increasingly, patients are being drawn to cosmetic surgery not simply to comply with Western standards but as a means of affirming their ethnic heritage. This cultural sensitivity compels clients to seek treatments that accentuate their features rather than conceal them in the name of standardized beauty. This shift assumes that cosmetic dermatology must evolve into a more culturally sensitive and inclusive practice, ultimately leading to better outcomes for individuals seeking to enhance their appearance while honoring their cultures (Arian et al., 2023).

Test Your Knowledge

1. How did cosmetic dermatology evolve from ancient beauty rituals to a specialized medical field?
2. What are the key milestones in aesthetic procedures?

7.2. Common Cosmetic Dermatology Procedures

Learning Outcome

1. Discuss Botox and its applications.
2. Understand dermal fillers and their uses.
3. Explain the use of chemical peels and skin resurfacing.

The specialty of cosmetic dermatology has evolved significantly, and numerous new procedures have been developed to treat a range of aesthetic concerns. Among the most in-demand treatments are non-surgical options such as Botox injections and dermal fillers, which offer a convenient choice for quick outcomes and minimal downtime. Botox is actually utilized to smooth out fine lines and wrinkles by temporarily paralyzing the muscles beneath, thereby alleviating the ruggedness on the skin surface. Similarly, dermal fillers provide fullness and volume to the lips and cheeks, say, to enhance facial contours. Besides the immediate cosmetic benefit, these treatments also positively affect individuals' self-esteem and overall contentment with themselves, an indication of the psychosocial impact that beauty treatments can exert on patients in addition to the physical improvement. In addition to injectables, lasers now occupy a niche in cosmetic dermatology as the treatment of choice for many skin conditions like pigmentation disorders, scarring, and photoaging. Laser resurfacing procedures use high-intensity light to target areas of the skin requiring treatment, ablate the outer layers, and stimulate collagen production. The healing process leads to flattening of the skin texture and reduction of imperfections. Fractional and ablative lasers are technologies that provide customized treatment, enabling dermatologists to tailor protocols to skin type and the patient's desired outcome. Introducing integrated skincare principles, including adjunct therapies, can further improve laser outcomes by reducing recovery time, underscoring the significance of holistic care in aesthetic clinics (Fabi et al., 2024). Care should be exercised in making the choice to undergo cosmetic dermatology procedures, particularly with patients' psychological conditions that may have an impact on patient satisfaction. According to research, patients with certain psychological profiles, such as high body dysmorphia or high expectations, are more prone to being at risk for dissatisfaction following aesthetic procedures (Toni et al., 2024). A thorough preoperative assessment, employing tools such as the Cosmetic Readiness Questionnaire (CRQ), would then identify such at-risk patients and provide them with appropriate advice and counseling before undergoing procedures. Acting proactively not only maintains patient health but also enhances the overall success rates of cosmetic dermatology procedures. Thus, it is important for practitioners and patients alike to understand the interplay between aesthetic desire and psychological preparedness in navigating the nuances of contemporary cosmetic procedures.

7.2.1. Botox and Its Uses

Botox is widely used in cosmetic dermatology because it effectively reduces facial wrinkles and fine lines. As a very purified form of botulinum toxin type A, Botox works by temporarily inhibiting the release of acetylcholine at the neuromuscular junction, inducing relaxation of the muscles of the regions it is administered to. Of the numerous applications of Botox, its cosmetic use has become incredibly fashionable, becoming the most widespread nonsurgical procedure in the world. With increasing demand, there is greater research into the various formulas employed, as clinicians seek to refine the safety and effectiveness of these treatments. Understanding the differences between products, such as onabotulinum toxin A, abobotulinum toxin A, and incobotulinum toxin A, is critical for clinicians in ensuring the maximum possible success with minimal risk associated with potency and immunogenicity (Fonfr Eía et al., 2018). Beyond cosmetic applications, Botox has been used extensively in medical interventions, reflecting its versatility. Originally used as a therapeutic agent, botulinum toxin A has come to be used to treat conditions such as chronic migraine and hyperhidrosis. Doctors utilize Botox injections to treat spasticity and dystonia, demonstrating the toxin's potential to treat so many various neurological ailments. Each new indication not only increases the therapeutic utility but also increases the number of clinicians approved to provide these injections safely. Nonetheless, the diversity of formulations obliges practitioners to understand the specific properties of Botox and its associated complications. Further study on pain control and other novel uses of Botox underscores its position as a multifaceted therapeutic agent for both aesthetics and medicine (Fonfr Eía et al., 2018). Botox incorporation into aesthetic dermatology is fraught with opportunities and challenges, and demands proper balance on the part of practitioners. With mounting demand for non-surgical facial rejuvenation, the industry faces significant challenges related to formulation differences, dosing, and patient safety. Since different formulations of Botox possess unique biochemical profiles, practitioners must undergo extensive training and have a strong understanding of clinical pharmacology to avoid complications, such as toxin spread. Additionally, there are patient education considerations regarding expectations and safety, particularly regarding immunogenicity and the need for touch-up treatments. Addressing these is crucial to the success of Botox administration in aesthetic treatments and ultimately to having patients and practitioners continue believing in the safety and efficacy of such life-altering injectable treatments (Samizadeh, S., & De Boulle, K., 2018) (Figure 7.4).

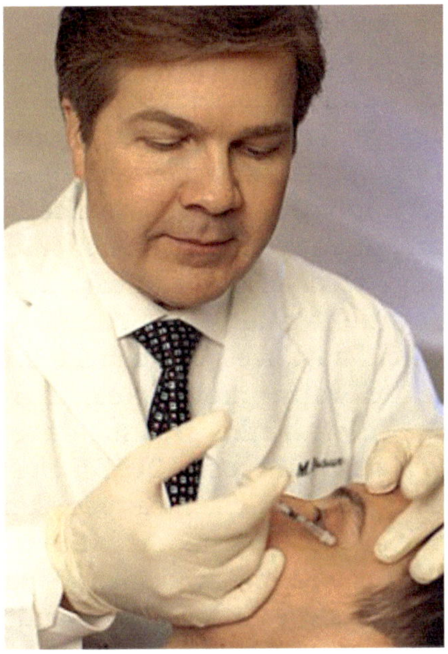

Figure 7.4. Botulinum toxin being injected in the human face.

Source: https://upload.wikimedia.org/wikipedia/commons/thumb/7/7f/Dr_Braun_Performs_a_Botox_Injection_%284035273577%29.jpg/250px-Dr_Braun_Performs_a_Botox_Injection_%284035273577%29.jpg.

7.2.2. Dermal Fillers and Their Uses

The use of dermal fillers revolutionized the cosmetic dermatology world by offering patients a new non-surgical way of addressing various aesthetic concerns, such as volume loss, wrinkles, and skin texture imperfections. Initially, in the 1980s, with the introduction of the first fillers, this field of aesthetic medicine expanded at a rapid rate, which has resulted in the current range of products formulated for particular indications. As highlighted by Dr. Pearlman et al., the innovation of HA fillers is a crucial step in this evolution, and the first FDA-approved HA filler was Restylane in 2003. This milestone occasion not only brought a new generation of filler technology but also provided worthwhile learning in patient protection and adverse effect management, which later shaped the existing standards of practice that govern the application of fillers (Schlesinger, 2023). Beyond simple cosmetic enhancement, the use of dermal fillers is also fraught with ethical issues, primarily concerning patient expectations and outcomes. Surprisingly, the imbalance of intentions and psychology among patients, mostly women, is able to influence their enjoyment of cosmetic treatments, sometimes leading to body dysmorphic disorders. As underscored by debates on ethical practice, dermatologists must navigate these complexities with finesse so that treatment regimens align with patients' actual needs while managing expectations (Keskinbora, K., & Kumbasar, E., 2023). This is an area of ethics that insists that dermatologists are not only skilled injectors but also empathetic practitioners who can manage the psychological dimensions embedded in cosmetic decisions. Finally, increased dermal fillers' popularity generated immense market growth, leading to the oversupply of products in the market. While this growth reflects strong competition and product development, it also necessarily breeds problems concerning standards and safety. According to Keskinbora, K., & Kumbasar, E. (2023), the use of Class 3 medical-grade material for injection is vital for minimizing complications such as tissue necrosis and infections caused by poorly performed procedures. Thus, practitioners must ensure that selected products meet safety standards to protect patients. As the field continues to advance, ongoing education and adherence to ethical medical practice will be crucial to upholding the integrity of aesthetic dermatology while promoting a positive patient experience and outcomes (Figure 7.5).

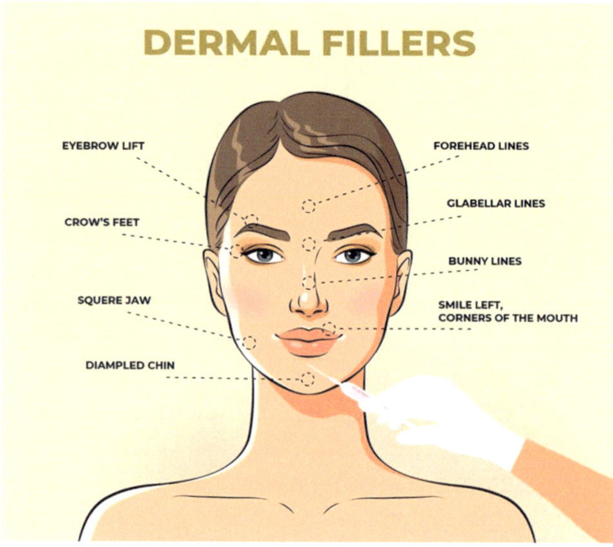

Figure 7.5. Dermal filler infographics.

Source: https://syraaesthetics.com/blog/wp-content/uploads/2023/11/Dermal-filler-Infographics-v2-1024x1024.jpg.

7.2.3. Chemical Peels and Skin Resurfacing

Cosmetic dermatology now encompasses various methods of skin resurfacing, and chemical peeling has emerged as a leading treatment. Chemical peeling involves applying chemical solutions to the skin, resulting in controlled exfoliation that reveals healthier, more refreshed-looking skin beneath. These treatments can correct several skin conditions, from acne scarring to fine wrinkles and pigmentation irregularities. The depth of peeling—superficial, medium, or deep—determines the extent of invasion into the skin and the recovery period. Chemical peels are therefore versatile tools that can both enhance the complexion and texture of the skin as well as treat mixed patient needs and wants. Such adaptability has rendered them a favorite in the field of cosmetic procedures, which increasingly seek treatments with reduced downtime and perceived results (Lipozen Jčić et al., 2010). In addition to chemical peels, skin resurfacing includes procedures such as lasers and dermabrasion. These treatments, such as chemical peels, aim to improve skin appearance by removing the outer layers, thereby promoting the growth of healthier skin. Laser resurfacing, indeed, has gained popularity due to its specificity and potential to target individual skin diseases, offering a tailored approach to cosmetic treatment. Moreover, technological innovations have led to nonablative resurfacing methods that induce healing through less invasive mechanisms than traditional approaches. Such advancements are emblematic of a growing tendency in cosmetic dermatology to prioritize clinical outcomes as much as patient safety and comfort. As the aesthetic field advances, clinicians increasingly integrate therapy modalities, combining chemical peels with other treatments to achieve optimal results (Ambrosio, 2018). Despite the numerous benefits of chemical peels and other resurfacing agents, it is important to introduce the treatments with the awareness of particular patient needs. Several factors, including skin type, condition, and personal aesthetic goals, play an important role in determining an ideal treatment approach. Hence, practitioners should prioritize thorough analyses and patient education before proceeding. Such emphasis on tailoring treatments not only optimizes results but also engenders patient trust and satisfaction. Given the ongoing increase in demand for aesthetic procedures, continuing education and training in aesthetic somatology are necessary. By closing the gap between dermatological science and aesthetic practice, professionals can assure patients safe, effective, and result-oriented skin treatments (Lipozen Jčić et al., 2010) (Figure 7.6).

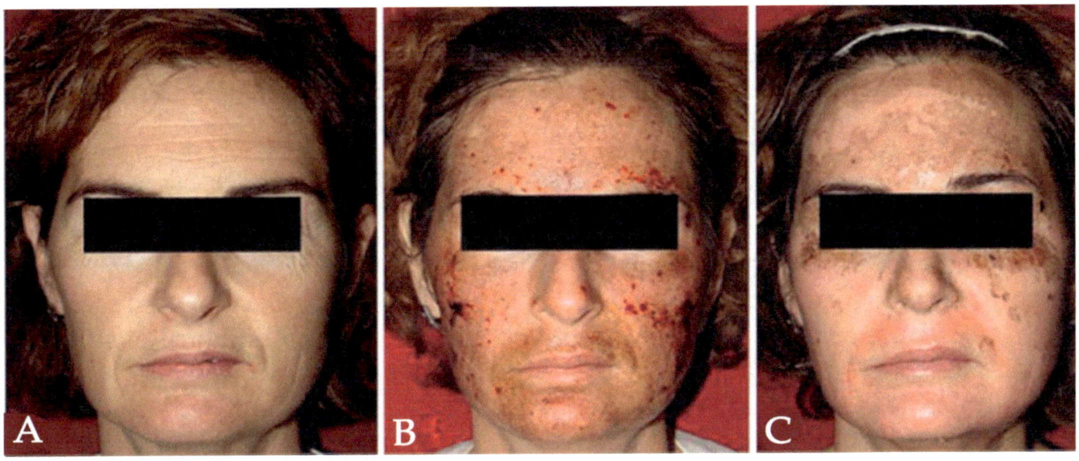

Figure 7.6. Various stages of before and after fractional resurfacing. a Before: Evident signs of skin laxness and wrinkles. Aspect b 2 days after and c 7 days after, with scabs almost gone.

Source: https://www.researchgate.net/profile/Mario-Trelles/publication/46125274/figure/fig2/AS:337031994593281@1457366097054/arious-stages-of-before-and-after-fractional-resurfacing-a-Before-Evident-signs-of-skin.png.

Test Your Knowledge

1. What are the primary medical and aesthetic applications of Botox, and how does it function at the muscular level?
2. How do dermal fillers differ in composition and use, and what factors determine the choice of filler for specific facial areas?
3. In what ways do chemical peels and other skin resurfacing techniques help improve skin texture and tone?

7.3. Non-Invasive versus Invasive Procedures

Learning Outcome

1. Explain the definition and examples of non-invasive procedures.
2. Understand the definition and examples of invasive procedures.
3. Describe risks and benefits associated with each type.

The choice between surgical and non-surgical treatment in cosmetic dermatology has a profound impact on patient satisfaction and outcome. Non-surgical treatments, such as chemical peels, microdermabrasion, and dermal fillers, have short downtime and low risk for complications. They are most often of interest to patients seeking improvement in appearance without the added stress that accompanies surgery. Secondly, numerous non-invasive procedures can be performed on an outpatient basis, allowing the patient to resume normal activity levels quickly. The development in technologies, for instance, in LED-RL therapy, is evidence of how the non-invasive approach can repair issues skin fibrosis in an optimal manner to promote healing and restrict scarring after surgical procedures (Heilman et al., 2019). This shift towards non-surgical treatments reflects a broader trend in patient demand, prioritizing convenience and safety alongside aesthetic considerations. Compared with this, surgical alternatives, such as facelifts and liposuction, tend to yield more pronounced results, often necessary for patients with significant skin laxity or fat gain. Surgical techniques are employed in these procedures to produce more dramatic alterations in a patient's facial appearance, suitable for individuals seeking a drastic change. While invasive procedures can yield long-term results, they carry inherent risks such as infection, scarring, and prolonged recovery periods. However, advances in surgical techniques and cosmetic procedures aim to mitigate these problems, making procedures more effective and safer. As noted through the example of skin cancer treatment, invasive procedures like excisional surgery remain essential for certain conditions, assuring removal of possibly harmful lesions (Löhr et al., 2017). Thus, understanding the implications and expected outcomes of each category is essential for both clients and practitioners. The choice between invasive and non-invasive treatments also requires careful consideration of personal lifestyle and health goals. Patients who prefer non-invasive procedures may appreciate treatments that produce incremental changes rather than those that yield radical, visible results. On the other hand, individuals with specific aesthetic aspirations might find the surgical method more appealing for the sake of getting the desired look quickly and in the best possible way. Additionally, economic factors influence the choice: non-surgical treatments are more affordable because they entail lower costs and fewer additional expenses related to recovery, rehabilitation, or potential complications. Thus, patient treatment should include careful evaluation by qualified professionals of patients' needs and goals, as well as the potential hazards of each procedure type. Such a collaboration results in an informed decision, allowing individuals to choose the technique best suited to their aesthetic aspirations and lifestyle requirements.

7.3.1. Definition and Examples of Non-Invasive Procedures

In cosmetic dermatology, non-invasive procedures have become increasingly common because they can enhance aesthetic outcomes without surgery. Non-invasive treatments are procedures that do not penetrate the skin surface and are associated with progressive improvement in skin texture, tone, and overall appearance. These treatments are typically associated with lower risks than their invasive counterparts, shorter recovery times, and fewer complications. Examples of non-invasive treatments that are widely used include chemical peels, microdermabrasion, and laser skin resurfacing, which act via various mechanisms to rejuvenate and resurface the skin. Among the numerous non-invasive treatments, injectable procedures such as dermal fillers and botulinum toxin (commonly known as Botox) have transformed the landscape of cosmetic treatments. Dermal fillers introduce biocompatible materials that restore volume and definition to facial contours, reversing the effects of aging. Botox, on the other hand, temporarily paralyzes the muscles involved, basically eliminating wrinkles and fine lines. While these procedures are least invasive, they provide significant cosmetic benefits and are often sought for their rapid action and minimal downtime. Practitioners, nonetheless, should provide these treatments with utmost caution to avoid complications, such as those associated with autologous fat injection, which can have adverse effects if performed incorrectly (Vojdani, A., & Shoenfeld, Y., 2022).

Additionally, the non-invasive therapies, such as electronic brachytherapy, are also altering the treatment pathway of non-melanoma skin cancers, which is a significant evolution in the field of dermatology. This method uses targeted radiation to successfully treat skin lesions with minimal damage to surrounding healthy tissue, thereby maintaining cosmetic outcomes. As mentioned, the Esteya electronic brachytherapy system is one of the most accurate forms of skin cancer treatment that delivers treatments in accordance with patients' beauty expectations and reviving therapeutic efficacy (Pons-Llanas et al., 2015). These advancements not only highlight the evolution of non-surgical treatments but also highlight their increasing significance in maintaining a balance between the aesthetic and medical requirements in cosmetic dermatology (Figure 7.7).

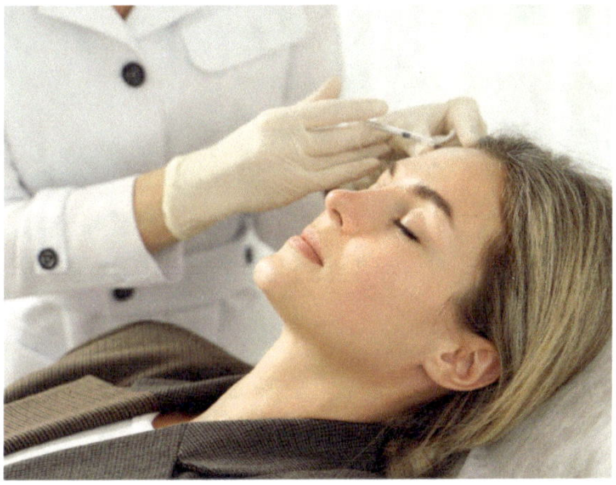

Figure 7.7. Non-invasive procedures have gained substantial popularity due to their ability to enhance aesthetic appearance without requiring surgical intervention.

Source: https://cdn.prod.website-files.com/628ba7e416903d0c51e6fdc4/65c257b0c4cb7f17a473259b_02.webp.

7.3.2. Definition and Examples of Invasive Procedures

In cosmetic dermatology and aesthetic procedures, invasive treatments are techniques that penetrate the skin or underlying tissue, typically via surgery. These treatments are used to alter, transform, or enhance physical appearance and fall under several categories, such as surgical reconstructions, lifts, and more complex dermatological interventions. Interestingly, invasive procedures differ from minimally invasive methods, where the primary concern is achieving a cosmetic outcome with shorter recovery periods and minimal risk. By definition, more risks, such as infection, scarring, and anesthetic complications, are involved in invasive procedures, making patient selection and aftercare critical to achieving the desired outcome (Meghe et al., 2024). With the increasing prevalence of cosmetic dermatology, it is vital that practitioners and individuals undergoing aesthetic procedures are aware of the invasive nature of such treatments. There are numerous examples of invasive treatments available in cosmetic dermatology. Some of these include conventional surgeries in the context of face lifts, tummy tucks, and breast enlargements, all of which involve serious consideration for surgical approach and recuperation time. In addition, procedures such as liposuction and rhinoplasty provide evidence of the effectiveness of body-shaping remodeling and nose reconstruction, respectively, through surgical interventions. Outcomes of such surgical interventions vary with members' experience, particularly in handling complex cases, where multiple surgeries or interdisciplinary approaches may be required (Karel et al., 2022). Identifying these examples helps account for the prevalence of invasive treatments, as they are more likely to produce more dramatic and enduring changes than non-invasive treatments such as fillers or laser treatments, which may provide the patient with a dramatically improved self-image. This shift towards minimally invasive treatment has not diminished the significance of invasive treatment; rather, it has allowed for a revolution in patient care and the advancement of techniques. As the practitioner strives to reach harmony among the desire for beauty and protection, increasing numbers are employing innovative ways to optimize functional, along with cosmetic results. Better technology and surgical methods have established procedural precision, resulting in lowered complication and recovery time rates, which eventually influence patient satisfaction. In this case, the synergy of achieving aesthetic targets with optimal minimization of invasiveness underscores the value of careful procedural selection, patient awareness, and ongoing assessment of outcomes in cosmetic dermatology. Hence, awareness of invasive techniques, as well as their respective innovation, is valuable with a view to avoiding the complexities inherent in aesthetic practice (Meghe et al., 2024) (Figure 7.8).

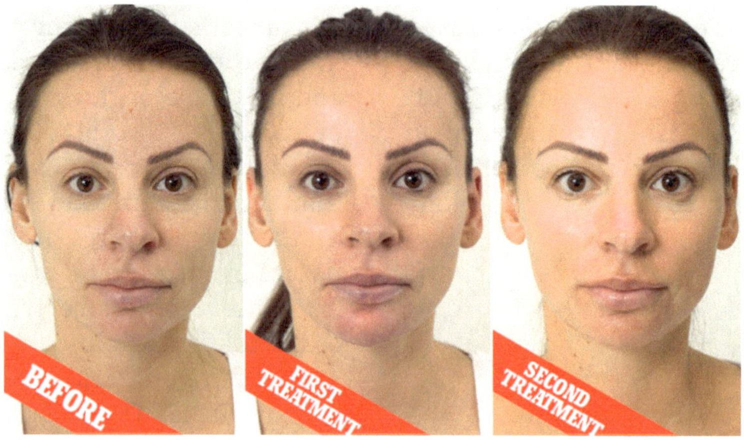

Figure 7.8. A girl's face before and after an invasive procedure.

Source: https://i.dailymail.co.uk/i/pix/2016/11/09/09/3A33092500000578-0-image-a-6_1478684714190.jpg.

7.3.3. Risks and Benefits Associated with Each Type

In the art of cosmetic dermatology and aesthetic therapies, there must be a discreet perception of the advantages and disadvantages of all these modes of therapy. For instance, non-surgical procedures such as chemical peels and microdermabrasion are generally safe, with a low risk of skin allergy or irritation. But the advantages are significant, such as smoothing and improvement of the skin texture and color with minimal downtime. Conversely, more invasive methods, such as surgical operations or laser surgery, are associated with higher risks, including scarring and complications related to anesthesia. Invasive options , such as these, although they provide dramatic results like tightening of the skin or wrinkle removal, require extensive analysis of the patient to ensure that the potential gains outweigh the risk. The use of newer technologies enhances the safety and effectiveness of such interventions and underscores the role of informed consent and patient education in guiding such decisions in cosmetic dermatology (Haykal et al., 2024). Moreover, the integration of artificial intelligence (AI) into cosmetic dermatology has revolutionized the assessment of risks and benefits. AI diagnostic devices provide precise skin analysis, enabling dermatologists to develop treatment plans tailored to individual patients' needs, thereby reducing the risk of unrealistic outcomes. By using algorithms that predict treatment outcomes, AI enhances decision-making, thereby building patient confidence in the predicted outcomes. However, technological dependence also raises critical concerns regarding data privacy and the accuracy of AI predictions. These are risks that need to be monitored strictly and ethically, ensuring that AI is applied as a complement to the clinician's knowledge and not a complete substitution. The balance between embracing new technology and its associated risks is central to advancing the field ethically (Keohane et al., 2020). Finally, the ethics of cosmetic treatment is relevant not only to personal treatment decisions but also to societal challenges at large. With increased availability of cosmetic dermatology by way of various treatments, there is also the greater need to evaluate the stresses of society on beauty standards and their psychological implications for patients. While the benefits of aesthetic enhancements can boost confidence and self-esteem, the desire for idealized beauty can be linked to body dysmorphic disorder risks and unrealistic expectations. Treatment professionals must thus focus on mental well-being as much as cosmetic outcomes, with the patient entering procedures with level-headed expectations and a thorough awareness of the risks (Haykal et al., 2024). As the industry continues to evolve, establishing a culture of inclusivity and body acceptance is essential to mitigate the potential harms of cosmetic dermatology and to recognize its benefits.

Test Your Knowledge

1. What are the key differences between non-invasive and invasive cosmetic dermatology procedures in terms of technique, recovery time, and risk profile?
2. How has the popularity of non-invasive procedures influenced patient preferences and the overall cosmetic industry?

7.4. The Role of Technology in Cosmetic Dermatology

Learning Outcome

1. Focus on advancements in laser technology.
2. Explain the impact of digital imaging and simulation in cosmetic dermatology.
3. Describe emerging trends in aesthetic devices.

Technological adoption in cosmetic dermatology has transformed the aesthetic treatment landscape, influencing advancements toward personalized, data-driven patient care. The core of this revolution is the advent of digital twin technology, which creates an evolving digital replica of an individual's skin by integrating various data points like imaging, genetic markers, and lifestyle characteristics. This new approach entails simulating treatment responses, adapting interventions, and predicting future skin issues. By enhancing the precision of aesthetic treatments, digital twins circumvent the constraints of traditional experimental processes, enabling dermatologists to select optimal treatments tailored to a person's individual skin profile. Future application is promising, as treatment efficacy can be maximized through real-time feedback and individual heterogeneity, leading to improved patient satisfaction and outcomes in cosmetic dermatology (Haykal, 2025).

Once again supporting the role of technology is the application of Artificial Intelligence (AI) in aesthetic treatments, which has changed diagnosis, planning for treatment, and patient interaction. AI technologies can scan large databases and generate insights to inform highly individualized treatment protocols. The technologies enhance the accuracy of skin assessments and predictive analysis, which allows practitioners to identify potential complications at an early stage. Most importantly, AI systems have been shown to outperform human diagnostic performance in certain areas, providing critical support for diagnosing skin conditions and refining treatment regimens in real time. Moreover, the advent of virtual consultations enabled by AI has enabled cosmetic dermatological services to reach wider territories. They have enabled substantial improvements. This not only enhances the patient consultation experience but also enables the rapid delivery of care, facilitating a seamless transition in the delivery of dermatological care (Haykal et al., 2024).

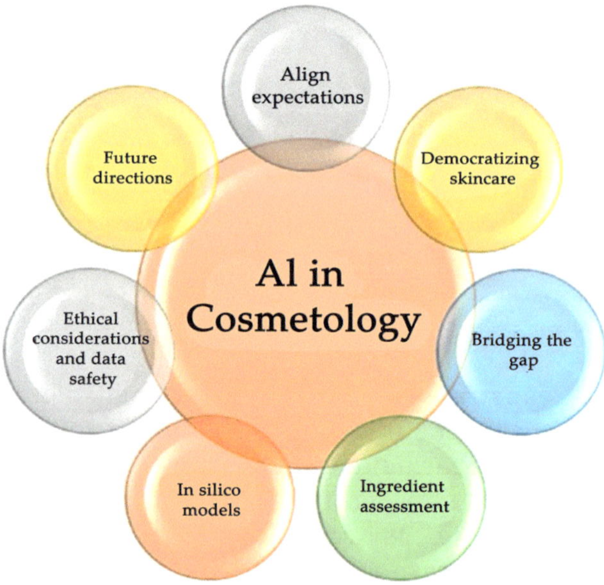

Figure 7.9. AI in cosmetic dermatology.

Source: https://www.mdpi.com/cosmetics/cosmetics-11-00135/article_deploy/html/images/cosmetics-11-00135-g003.png.

Furthermore, technology in cosmetic dermatology plays an important role in enhancing patient outcomes and experiences through enhancing transparency and education. AI-based technology provides patients with realistic representations of potential outcomes across a range of treatments to promote informed decision-making. This not only enhances patient confidence but also fosters an open culture in which patients are more directly engaged in their care procedures. When they interact with more advanced imaging devices, patients become more knowledgeable about their skin conditions and how environmental factors impact them. Accordingly, this technological convergence places power in patients' hands by providing vital information about their rights and responsibilities throughout the treatment process. Overall, technology's role in cosmetic dermatology not only facilitates clinical practices but also transforms patient-provider relationships, instilling an open culture of education and empowerment within the aesthetic practice (Haykal, 2025) (Figure 7.9).

7.4.1. Advancements in Laser Technology

The evolution of laser technology has revolutionized the practice of cosmetic dermatology, bringing new treatments that were not previously possible. Lasers are employed currently for numerous applications, including skin resurfacing, tattoo removal, and depigmentation. The precision of lasers enables dermatologists to target specific tissue with minimal damage to adjacent tissue, thereby reducing recovery time and improving patient satisfaction. More advanced laser technologies, such as fractional lasers, are further developing the science by providing higher penetration and encouraging collagen development with less downtime. This technology enables practitioners to provide individualized treatments tailored to each skin type, reinforcing the concept of personalized medicine in cosmetic dermatology. By understanding the wavelengths and modalities most effective for specific skin conditions, dermatologists can maximize efficacy and minimize side effects, a critical aspect of patient safety (Haykal, 2025). The synergy of contemporary laser technology in aesthetic clinics also mirrors the trend towards non-invasive procedures. Patients increasingly desire solutions that promise excellent outcomes with less downtime, and laser treatments provide this. For instance, the recent introduction of picosecond lasers has significantly improved the efficacy of tattoo and pigmentation treatments, enabling faster procedures with fewer sessions. Additionally, lasers are increasingly combined with other dermatological procedures, such as injectables, to further enhance their combined efficacy. Not only does this synergy provide greater diversity of treatments available to patients, but it also decreases the risks associated with surgical procedures. With further technological advancements, the integration of machine learning and artificial intelligence with laser applications may further enhance treatment planning and outcome prediction accuracy, leading to more dynamic practices in cosmetic dermatology (Haykal et al., 2024). Patient safety and satisfaction remain priorities in the development of laser technology for cosmetic dermatology. Through ongoing research and development, new protocols and technologies are being developed to address safety concerns associated with laser therapy, particularly for patients of diverse ethnic backgrounds with varying skin conditions. Advances in the clinical world have led to improved laser parameters, which enhance safety without hindering optimum treatment outcome. Moreover, practice-based training courses for experts are critical to the judicious use of these technologies, emphasizing the importance of personalized practice models tailored to individual patient needs. With the growing popularity of aesthetic treatments, the safety and efficacy of laser technology will be focal points in shaping the future of cosmetic dermatology. By continually refining approaches and introducing innovative solutions, dermatologists can optimize patient satisfaction with best-quality care that is efficacious and safe (Haykal, 2025) (Figure 7.10).

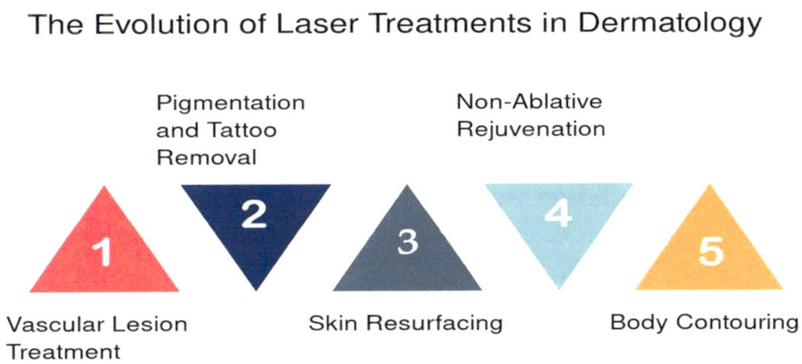

Figure 7.10. The evolution of laser treatments in cosmetic dermatology.

Source: https://fastercapital.co/i/Laser-Skin-Care-Clinic--The-Role-of-Technology-in-Laser-Skin-Care-Clinics--Innovations-and-Trends--The-Evolution-of-Laser-Treatments-in-Dermatology.webp.

7.4.2. The Impact of Digital Imaging and Simulation

The integration of digital imaging and simulation in cosmetic dermatology has revolutionized the way practitioners manage aesthetic treatments. With the help of high-resolution imaging technology, dermatologists are able to create high-resolution visual images of a patients skin and capture high-level detail of texture, pigmentation, and vascularity. The resultant visual data is used to provide the foundation for simulating the potential results of treatment, thereby allowing clinicians and patients to visualize the anticipated result of various interventions. Such pre-treatment simulations can minimize patient anxiety, enhance satisfaction, and facilitate informed decision-making by enabling active engagement in treatment planning. Significantly, these digital solutions also enable dermatologists to standardize practice, reducing variability in results that often derives from subjective estimates of treatment effectiveness. The combination of imaging technology and simulation thus sets a new benchmark in cosmetic dermatology, making aesthetic treatments not only effective but also tailor-made to individual patient needs. Perhaps one of the most significant advancements in digital imaging and simulation is the concept of digital twins, which is being increasingly adopted in dermatological clinics. A digital twin is actually a dynamic, real-time virtual twin of a patient's skin, created by integrating imaging data, genetic data, and lifestyle data. This revolutionary technology enables dermatologists to simulate multiple treatments and predict skin responses, thereby greatly enhancing treatment accuracy. For example, with the use of digital twin technology, dermatologists can simulate how any patient's skin is likely to react to a particular topical agents or energy devices, optimizing treatment plans with customized data. The use of digital twins facilitates the transition to personalized treatment models that significantly improve patient outcomes and eliminate the risks associated with trial-and-error practices in aesthetic treatments (Haykal, 2025). Furthermore, interdisciplinary strategies enabled by digital imaging and simulation within cosmetic dermatology highlight the cooperative strategies of healthcare delivery. By narrowing the gap between dermatology and engineering, as demonstrated by ongoing developments in plastic surgery, clinicians can apply engineering principles to develop sophisticated imaging technologies and simulation strategies. This multidisciplinary collaboration enhances the effectiveness of cosmetic treatments through innovations that integrate technical competence with clinical awareness. Nevertheless, the effective deployment of such integration is constrained by challenges such as the necessity for uniform protocols and trained personnel to navigate these complexities. Solving these issues is crucial for promoting the cosmetic dermatology profession and enabling the full application of digital imaging and simulation technologies to deliver personalized patient care and innovative solutions in aesthetic clinics (Sun et al., 2024).

7.4.3. Trends in Aesthetic Devices in the Future

Recent developments in cosmetic dermatology have ushered in a wave of future trends in aesthetic devices, particularly with the development and use of new dermal fillers. Indeed, these formulations, such as hyaluronic acid fillers, are evolving to incorporate newer technologies like biorthogonal methods and thiomer-based formulations. These breakthroughs not only make treatments more efficient but also improve patient outcomes by achieving longer-lasting results and reducing the number of touch-ups required. Additionally, recent studies indicate that biostimulators, including poly-L-lactic acid and calcium hydroxyapatite, trigger active neo-collagenesis. As more familiar practicing professionals become aware of these products, they design more comprehensive treatment protocols that maximize aesthetic improvement while reducing complications. As more studies are conducted on these products, the cosmetic industry will expand its portfolio to ensure that customers are offered the most cutting-edge and efficient treatments available (Goldust et al., 2024).

The impact of botulinum toxin (BTX) in cosmetic treatment has also been revolutionized by emerging trends that focus on enhancing the safety and efficacy of such treatments. New recombinant toxins and blended preparations promise to enhance BTX potency while minimizing their hazards. Recent advances have opened the door to new methods of delivery and protocols, making practitioners more responsible for therapy outcomes and enabling personalized approaches to meet particular patient needs. Finally, anti-aging treatments now include new drugs targeting cellular aging, such as exosomes and nicotinamide mononucleotide (NMN). Although these treatments are promising, they must be tested and proven in future studies to establish their long-term safety and effectiveness (Goldust et al., 2024). The convergence of these breakthroughs marks a radical transformation in aesthetic therapy, ultimately enhancing the patient experience in cosmetic dermatology. With non-surgical body renewal increasing, clinicians are increasingly using advanced devices and therapies to address a broad array of aesthetic concerns. This is evident in the increased use of dermal fillers, originally developed for facial applications, now used for volumization and skin enhancement in other body regions. Emerging trends highlight the need to use collagen stimulators, such as poly-L-lactic acid (PLLA), which have demonstrated encouraging outcomes in the management of conditions such as skin laxity, cellulite, and striae distensae. Although the effectiveness of the treatments is well established, further studies are necessary to refine injection procedures and maximize patient safety. Additionally, given the high patient satisfaction rate reported, continued interest in body-specific procedures is likely to drive further innovation, ultimately benefiting the field of cosmetic dermatology.

Test Your Knowledge

1. How have advancements in laser technology improved the precision and safety of cosmetic dermatology treatments?
2. What role does digital imaging and simulation software play in patient assessment, treatment planning, and outcome prediction?

7.5. Ethical Considerations

Learning Outcome

1. Focus on patient consent and informed decision-making
2. Explain the role of regulation in cosmetic procedures
3. Focus on psychological implications of aesthetic enhancements

The intersection of ethical questions and cosmetic dermatology is an issue of significant proportion, notably patient safety and the psychological effects of cosmetic procedures. Dermatologists must weigh the benefits and disadvantages of treatments while ensuring complete transparency to patients about the risks associated with certain procedures, including dermal fillers and laser procedures. As defined in contemporary literature, these concerns include the risk of complications such as tissue necrosis and infection when procedures are performed by inadequately trained staff. Moreover, patients must be informed about the quality and type of products used in aesthetic treatments, as non-certified Class 3 Medical devices may pose a health risk. The onus lies with trained doctors to prioritize patient safety, emphasizing the moral responsibility to use only certified products and to remain open to potential outcomes and complications in the cosmetic arena (Keskinbora, K., & Kumbasar, E., 2023). The other equally urgent ethical responsibility is to safeguard the psychological health of patients undergoing cosmetic treatment. There has been a documented link between aesthetic procedures and body dysmorphic disorder (BDD), where an individual gets preoccupied with imperfections in their own looks. Dermatologists must realize that while the cosmetic treatment may meet a patient's desire for improvement, it may subconsciously exacerbate the inherent psychopathological processes. Symptoms of BDD have been reported to deteriorate after the treatment, rendering self-perception challenging and generating emotional distress (Kuhn et al., 2018). Thus, professionals must handle each case with care, conducting careful evaluations through psychological testing. Ethical practice demands that dermatologists not just assess the physical condition of patients but also be sensitive to their mental status, referring those who are at risk of BDD to extensive treatment programs incorporating psychotherapy and treatments (Kuhn et al., 2018). Moreover, social media's influence on cosmetic dermatology warrants consideration in ethical debates. Many patients are increasingly influenced by unattainable beauty standards disseminated through digital media, thereby likely inducing skewed perceptions of self-worth and beauty ideals. As dermatologists work with clients affected by such external factors, it is essential to foster an environment that promotes realistic expectations. Ethical practice calls on professionals to educate patients about the limits of cosmetic procedures, so that they understand that cosmetic treatments can never perfectly rectify individual imperfections or conform to social standards of beauty. A pledge to ethical practice is as much in the enactment of correct cosmetic techniques as in empowering the patient through informed discussion and treatment, enabling them to adopt a more integrated definition of beauty in which mental and emotional health are accorded greater standing than physical appearance (Keskinbora, K., & Kumbasar, E., 2023).

7.5.1. Patient Consent and Informed Decision-Making

In cosmetic dermatology and aesthetic treatments, patient consent is a significant factor that underscores practitioners' ethical responsibility. Patient education must be emphasized because patients undergo procedures not only for cosmetic reasons but also for psychological reasons. Clinicians owe it to themselves and their patients to provide thorough explanations of the benefits, risks, and limitations of available treatments. This discussion presents a scenario in which patients are empowered to make decisions aligned with their expectations and objectives. Furthermore, the innovation of technologies such as generative AI has upended the handling of consent. The software that facilitates realist projections of future outcomes can be used to set realistic expectations, thereby enhancing the informed consent process and minimizing regret after the procedure (Landau et al., 2025). Furthermore, cultural factors must be taken into account to provide informed consent to diverse patient populations. The increasing popularity of aesthetic procedures among Hispanic and Latino populations in the US highlights the importance of ethnic variation in treatment needs and anatomical characteristics. These special needs must be addressed by the clinician with sensitivity and adaptability, and the consent process must reflect this sensitivity to cultural variation. For instance, such patients may prioritize aesthetic qualities differently from their Caucasian counterparts. Fulfilling this diversity not only dignifies the patient-clinician interaction but also increases patient satisfaction and confidence. Through culturally sensitive communication strategies, aesthetic dermatology practitioners are better positioned to manage the informed consent process effectively, thereby ensuring that their patients are well informed and aligned with their aesthetic choices (Sabrina et al., 2022). Informed decision-making extends beyond consent; it continues throughout the patient's aesthetic journey. Providing patients with ongoing education about their procedure, including potential long-term outcomes and follow-up care, is essential for fostering a sense of agency. Moreover, technology-based instruments can help keep patients continuously informed about their treatment plans, outcomes, and planned changes, thereby enhancing informed decision-making. Such continuous communication not only generates trust but also cultivates an open culture between the practitioners and patients.

With increased use of cosmetic treatments, patient consent and informed choice should remain a top priority to maintain patient welfare and ensure ethical practice in cosmetic dermatology (Landau et al., 2025) (Figure 7.11).

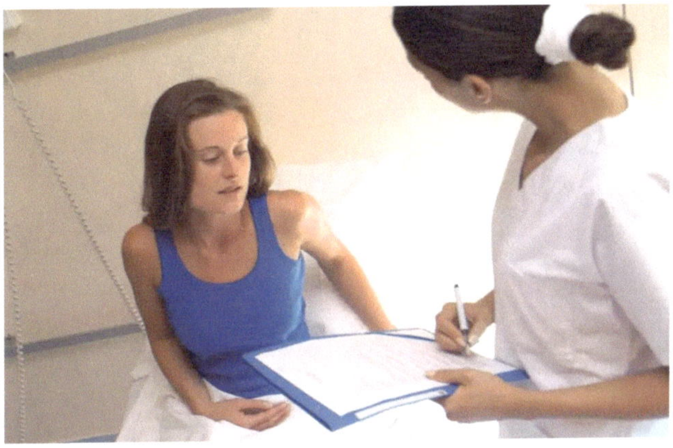

Figure 7.11. Patient consent is a critical component that underscores the ethical responsibility of practitioners.

Source: https://pharmaceutical-journal.com/wp-content/uploads/2021/01/patient-woman-hospital-consent-form-15-927x617.jpg.

7.5.2. The Role of Regulation in Cosmetic Procedures

Regulation of cosmetic procedures is of paramount significance in ensuring patient safety and effectiveness in the practice of cosmetic dermatology. Due to the growing demand for these procedures, control measures need to be set by regulatory bodies and enforced in order to protect consumers against potential risks that may be caused by uncontrolled practice. This legislation typically addresses a series of issues, from ensuring qualifications for practitioners to the safety profiles of cosmetic products and the procedures necessary to carry out specific procedures. The enforcement of stringent regulatory standards helps prevent malpractice and ensures that cosmetic treatments are performed by certified personnel. In the absence of regulation, patients may be exposed to cosmetic treatments that not only fail to meet their expectations but also cause severe side effects, underscoring the need for regulation to ensure safety and quality (Haykal et al., 2024). Apart from patient protection, regulation assures a higher level of professionalism in the profession of cosmetic dermatology. By ensuring that practitioners receive specific training and certification, regulatory norms foster a culture of accountability and professionalism. The use of advanced technologies, such as Artificial Intelligence, in beauty treatments entails that existing regulatory norms have to be re-examined. As practitioners increasingly use AI for accurate skin evaluation and personalized treatment protocols, regulatory authorities must adapt to ensure that these technologies are used ethically and effectively.

By issuing clear directions regarding the application of new technologies, regulations can encourage innovation without risking patients to potential misuse or excessive reliance on untested methods. Thus, effective regulation not only encourages the growth of cosmetic treatments but also instills confidence in patients in the expertise of the treatments they receive (Richard et al., 2022). In addition, heightened awareness of the prevalence of skin disorders necessitates regulation to address public health challenges in cosmetic dermatology.

Existing research has revealed that a significant rate of the population is afflicted with skin disorders, and the majority of them desire to seek cosmetics to mend discomfort and enhance appearance (Richard et al., 2022). By regulating the cosmetics industry, policymakers can ensure greater access to effective and safe treatments for such ailments, thereby meeting health needs alongside beauty requirements. Second, regulatory systems can ensure that market competition does not compromise patient safety, enabling the delivery of diverse choices while maintaining high-quality care.

This type of regulation not only protects individual patients but also a healthier population by encouraging that easily accessible evidence-based cosmetic dermatologic treatments be made available to meet evolving public needs (Haykal et al., 2024) (Figure 7.12).

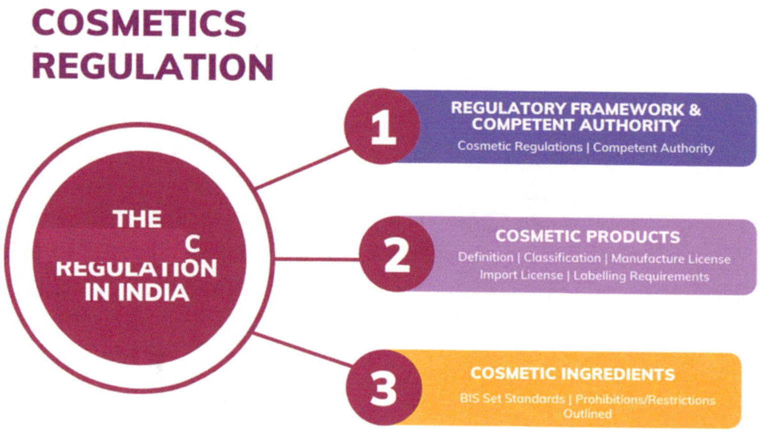

Figure 7.12. Cosmetic regulation.

Source: https://cliniexperts.com/wp-content/uploads/2022/04/image1.png.

7.5.3. Psychological Implications of Aesthetic Enhancements

The psychological impact of aesthetic enhancements is multifaceted, particularly as patient volumes for cosmetic procedures increase. Patients seek these enhancements, hoping that a new appearance will increase their self-esteem and social acceptance. This, however, may mask underlying psychological issues. The growth of body dysmorphic disorder (BDD) patients has become evident in cosmetic dermatology practices, resulting in ethical concerns regarding the appropriateness of the treatment for such patients. Proper identification of BDD patients is necessary to avoid increasing their psychological agony through aesthetic treatments and ensure professionals take into account mental health alongside physical alterations (Susan et al., 2017). It is imperative that practitioners provide holistic and ethical care by understanding the psychological drivers of aesthetic enhancements. The phenomenon of beauty apps only complicates the psychological context of aesthetic enhancement further by heightening societal pressure related to appearance. Apps reinstate a digital regime of self-scanning in which clients tend to constantly monitor and modulate their appearance to sustain prevailing standards of beauty, thereby becoming a primary agent in compounding self-scrutiny. This has the potential to generate an internalized understanding of the regulative gaze that especially affects women's perceptions of their bodies. From a feminist-Foucauldian perspective, beauty apps generate a new form of subjectivity, reassembling users into entrepreneurial selves that are perpetually judged against societal beauty norms (Elias, A. S., & Gill, R., 2017). As technology becomes more aesthetically engaged, there is a need for critical thinking about the psychological impact of such devices on self-esteem and self-concept. Furthermore, cross-talk between aesthetic interventions and psychological well-being necessitates greater caution among practitioners regarding the potential impact of treatments. While some patients become more self-assured and satisfied with procedures, others become increasingly worried and develop unreasonably high expectations regarding their appearance. Such a disparity indicates the importance of requiring cosmetic dermatologists to have thorough psychological testing before referring patients for treatment. In being educated on the psychological risks of cosmetic enhancements, providers are better equipped to address the ethical dilemmas posed by their field. Engaging patients in discussions of realistic treatment outcomes can minimize adverse psychological effects and foster a healthier relationship with their bodies, ultimately improving treatment experiences (Susan et al., 2017).

Test Your Knowledge

1. Why is informed consent especially important in cosmetic dermatology?
2. How do national and international regulations govern the practice of cosmetic dermatology?

7.6. The Future of Cosmetic Dermatology

Learning Outcome

1. Understand the predictions for new treatments and technologies.
2. Discuss the growing demand for personalized aesthetic care.
3. Focus on potential challenges facing the industry.

The global cosmetic dermatology market stands on the precipice of a revolutionary era, with technology and changing attitudes to beauty at its center. As aesthetic treatments gain popularity, a sophisticated model of cosmetic consultation is developing. Face-to-face consultations, previously the staple of patient-physician encounters, are more and more being complemented by teleconsultations and metaconsultations, which leverage virtual technology to enhance patient convenience and access. This shift also reflects a change in society and addresses logistical issues, such as during the pandemic. Teledermatology, in particular, enables practitioners to reach a larger audience without compromising the provision of individualized care. Patients can now engage with healthcare professionals across various platforms, improving understanding of procedures while fostering a sense of familiarity necessary for informed choice (Haykal et al., 2023).

The aesthetic world is also transforming with the integration of medical and aesthetic practices. Recent advances reflect a multidimensional appreciation of the common value of laser and energy-based treatments, both aesthetic and medical. Crossover underscores the fundamental focus on the health and integrity of the skin, combined with cosmetic enhancement, opening a window for patient treatment that is novel and exciting. Increasingly, cosmetic dermatologists are embracing the duality, encouraging treatments that aim for both aesthetic outcomes and skin health. These integrative strategies prioritize the delivery of ongoing education to practitioners to keep up with best practice, particularly when patient education is paramount. The commitment to better treatment methods reflects a greater recognition of patient-centered care, hence establishing trust and adherence to the treatment protocol (Rossi, 2023). Furthermore, the future of cosmetic dermatology will be characterized by new technologies that have the potential to significantly improve patient outcomes. The advent of artificial intelligence and virtual reality-based solutions in dermatology practice will lead to the replacement of conventional methods by more sophisticated diagnostic tools and treatment-planning options. For instance, recent studies have shown that medical procedures enhanced by artificial intelligence achieve significantly higher success rates than conventional procedures. These advancements, along with increased efficiency, enable patients to observe outcomes, thereby enhancing informed decision-making regarding cosmetic treatments. As this field continues to advance technologically, the collaborative aspect of physician-patient interactions will be crucial to establishing a paradigm grounded in ethical practice, patient safety, and patient satisfaction in the ever-changing landscape of cosmetic dermatology (Haykal et al., 2023).

7.6.1. Predictions of New Treatments and Technologies

The future of cosmetic dermatology will witness significant advancements in treatments and technologies, driven primarily by ongoing innovation in medical devices. Advances in laser technology are expected to make aesthetic treatments more effective and safer, enabling practitioners to treat a wider range of skin conditions with greater precision. Current research highlights the need to close regulatory loopholes in the laser industry, as uncontrolled cosmetic laser treatments can expose patients and experts alike to potential harm. A close examination of existing practices is necessary to avoid compromising safety while enhancing treatment outcomes through these technologies. By promoting rigorous regulatory frameworks, players can foster an innovation-friendly environment that maintains patient safety, leading to a new era of cosmetic treatments driven by scientific integrity and best practices (Youngerwood, 2012).

Technological advancements are also enabling the use of artificial intelligence (AI) in cosmetic dermatology, which holds significant promise for personalizing patient care. AI application examples can enable practitioners to provide tailored treatment recommendations based on one's specific skin type, background, and individual interests. Individualized care through this shift enhances patient satisfaction and treatment efficacy by allowing solutions to be tailored to individuals' unique needs. Furthermore, machine learning models can analyze large volumes of clinical outcome data to improve existing treatments and identify emerging technologies. As the business of this line increases, there is a necessity for professionals to keep abreast with emerging AI-based techniques, thereby being capable of capitalizing on technological innovation to enhance the quality of care provided (Ambrosio, 2018). Moreover, the trend towards non-surgical treatments in aesthetics is likely to continue as advances in materials and methods accelerate. The use of biocompatible fillers and implant materials will likely result in longer-lasting, safer effects with less recovery time for the patient. This demand for non-surgical interventions is a byproduct of changes in attitudes toward beauty and the ideal of achieving natural results, making ongoing education for professionals paramount. For instance, the creation of higher-level aesthetic somatology recognizes an area in which beauty therapists can specialize their knowledge and skills and bridge the gap between cosmetology and medical care. A nationwide curriculum grounded in the latest techniques will not only enhance practitioners' professionalism but also ensure that consumers receive the highest-quality care that reflects the latest developments in the industry (Ambrosio, 2018).

7.6.2. The Growing Demand for Personalized Aesthetic Care

The increased emphasis on individualized notions of beauty is a major driver of the emerging trend toward individualized aesthetic treatments in cosmetic dermatology. Today's consumers are more interested in treatments that are tailored to their personal profiles, lifestyles, and interests. This is a function of the pervasive influence of social media, in which the idealized image of beauty fuels the call for customized treatments responsive to personal identity. Patients are more educated and more assertive in seeking procedures that meet their individual aesthetic needs, ultimately insisting that practitioners provide a tailored solution. This trend necessitates that dermatologists not only improve technical proficiency but also hone the communication skills necessary to interact effectively with patients. Consequently, the expansion of customized aesthetic treatments guides a collective endeavor toward higher self-concept and self-esteem, compelling practitioners to adapt their services to evolving consumer needs, thereby redefining the landscape of cosmetic dermatology. Additionally, the advent of digital technology has played an important role in making the trend towards custom-made aesthetic care more viable. With the advent of newer diagnostic tools and tailor-made skincare products, dermatologists can now make personalized suggestions based on individual skin type and concerns. Artificial intelligence and machine learning are being used in marketing strategies as well as in treatment protocols so that the consumer's behavior and choice can be monitored with more precision. As noted in today's market analyses, the availability of over-the-counter drugs and advanced aesthetic procedures indicates a profound shift in consumer behavior toward customized self-care routines (Dingre et al., 2025). This technology revolution intensifies the patients' experience, making services not only customized but also convenient. These advances bridge the gap between consumer demand and medical specialism, ultimately reconfiguring the scope and assumptions of aesthetic care in dermatology. But the greater focus on customized aesthetic care raises ethical concerns that should be handled with care by clinicians. Commodification of care, however, can lead to a scenario where corporate interests compromise patient health, for example, over-treatment due to aggressive marketing strategies (Rostamzadeh, M., & Rahimi, F., 2025). Ethical business behavior should obtain informed consent from patients and prioritize patients' autonomy over profit. Whereas the market is flooded with options, practitioners are faced with the burden of educating patients about the potential benefits and risks of treatments and creating an open patient-practitioner relationship. Regulatory bodies may be compelled to implement stringent ethical standards and regulations that discourage deceptive marketing tactics that promote unattainable beauty standards. This mandate stresses the need to balance the commercialization of aesthetic treatments with a patient-centered mission. Ultimately, addressing these ethical issues is critical to building trust and ensuring that the expansion of individualized aesthetic care continues to benefit consumers and healthcare professionals (Figure 7.13).

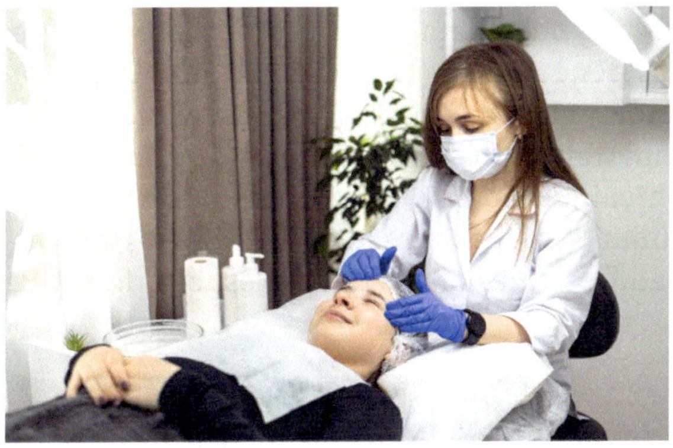

Figure 7.13. Personalized aesthetic care within cosmetic dermatology.

Source: https://ranimd.com/images/blog/6fca2d7c5b413512016aa5eb2e3dd2db6971a3af.jpg.

7.6.3. Potential Challenges Facing the Industry

The cosmetic dermatology and aesthetic procedures industry is under constant threat from the burgeoning medical tourism, particularly non-surgical aesthetic treatments. Though Thailand is becoming a prime destination for these services, most risks associated with medical tourism may discourage consumer confidence. Research indicates that there are six established categories of risk, including functional, financial, psychological, and social risk, which may serve as entry barriers to incoming patients who wish to receive aesthetic treatments abroad (Simpattanawong., 2016). These risk perceptions complicate individuals' decisions about whether to forgo the savings in favor of greater safety and health. Hence, it becomes essential for clinics and physicians to go through these problems, making sure that they deliver high standards of care and also make it transparent to potential patients. Another important issue for the cosmetic dermatology industry concerns the formulation and use of active ingredients such as hyaluronic acid (HA). While HA has been a cornerstone of many skincare treatments due to its purported water-holding and anti-wrinkle effects, its clinical use has long been hampered by instability and poor skin penetration (Kapadiya et al., 2025). Such factors can compromise treatment efficacy, ultimately influencing patient satisfaction and clinical outcomes. As demand for HA-based products surges, practitioners must not forget to address these formulation issues innovatively, through the use of newer technologies such as HA derivatives and nanotechnology to enhance delivery systems. Such breakthroughs are required not only to meet consumers' demands but also to sustain competitive advantages in a rapidly evolving market. Lastly, the rapid growth in aesthetic treatments poses regulatory challenges that vary widely across regions, making industry-wide standardization challenging. Regulatory bodies are increasingly under pressure to police aesthetic treatments, particularly on grounds of safety and efficacy. The absence of regulation harmonization threatens to create uneven practice and an uneven playing field that chills consumers and dissolves faith in professional services. As new technologies and methods emerge regularly, regulators cannot always keep pace, creating a twilight zone in which practitioners labor without clear guidelines. This vagueness poses risks not only to patients but also to clinicians, who may be concerned about liability as the regulatory landscape evolves. Overcoming these regulatory challenges is essential for the industry because it shapes public perceptions of safety and the long-term viability of aesthetic dermatology.

Test Your Knowledge

1. What new treatments and technologies are expected to shape the next decade of cosmetic dermatology?
2. How is the demand for personalized aesthetic care influencing product development and treatment planning in cosmetic dermatology?

SUMMARY

The landscape of aesthetic treatments and cosmetic dermatology continues to evolve in line with an evolving society and advancing technology. As interest in such treatments grows, particularly among a heterogeneous population, it is essential to critically assess both their benefits and pitfalls. Though non-invasive therapies , such as injectables and laser treatments have become very popular due to their minimal downtime and fast results, the rising prevalence of side effects underscores the need for greater caution on the part of consumers as well as practitioners. Educational campaigns, as suggested, should emphasize patient safety and informed choice in cosmetic transformation (Mihova et al., 2025). Furthermore, the implications of hormonal impact upon pain sensing during cosmetic procedures reveal an avenue of enormous under-tapped potential. Recent studies have demonstrated that understanding the interaction between pain during treatment and the menstrual cycle can enable practitioners to individualize interventions according to specific patient requirements. Growing awareness of the effects of demographic factors, including age and sex, on treatment results opens room for patient-specific care in cosmetic dermatology. Addressing these nuances will not only improve patient satisfaction but also enhance the success of aesthetic treatments overall (Nouf et al., 2025). Finally, a culture of transparency and ongoing education in cosmetic dermatology should be encouraged. As technology continues to develop and new procedures are created, there needs to be constant training for the professionals. This emphasis on professional training will make sure that the experts are up to date with the safety profiles and efficacy of the various cosmetic interventions. Furthermore, promoting a better understanding of the dangers involved with cosmetic procedures can create stronger safety measures and regulations. All these can ultimately promote the integrity of the profession, building confidence between providers and clients while protecting public health (Mihova et al., 2025; Nouf et al., 2025).

Aesthetic medicine and cosmetic dermatology is a diversified field of treatments for enhancing physical appearance and addressing some issues related to the skin. The recent research findings indicate that minimally invasive aesthetic procedures, such as injectables and laser depilation, are prevalent in clinics and beauty clinics, hence the need for proper control and compliance with regulatory standards. Most malpractice claims for such dermatological treatments arise from deficiencies in procedural monitoring and informed consent, and the majority have been overturned due to deficiencies in expert evaluation. This suggests that clients should be well informed about potential risks and benefits, with an emphasis on practitioners' right to full disclosure throughout the treatment process (Dereli et al., 2025). The evidence again indicates that patient interests need not take a back seat as the development of cosmetic dermatology continues. Recent advances have ushered in a revolutionary era in aesthetic treatments, particularly exosome-based treatments. Exosomes derived from human stem cells have emerged as agents for managing skin aging, scars, and other dermatological diseases. Evidence points to promising results in the use of inflammatory skin conditions and as biomarkers for major diseases such as melanoma and psoriasis. Still, the transition of exosome treatments from study to therapy will require overcoming significant challenges, including regulatory issues and harmonization of production protocols (William et al., 2025). As demand for exosome-based products increases, particularly in the United States, it is imperative that practitioners and scientists collaborate to develop robust guidelines that ensure the safety and efficacy of these novel treatments. The synergy between the rapid progress of cosmetic dermatology and the increasing sophistication of aesthetic treatments necessitates a reevaluation of practitioner training and certification. When techniques grow more sophisticated, so must the laws that regulate their provision. An overview of current practices indicates that aesthetic therapies are not merely technical but also involve ethical considerations in patient care and informed consent (Dereli et al., 2025). Based on this, educational programs must adapt to include comprehensive training in new technologies, legal implications, and patient interactions. This critical shift is necessary to establish a culture of responsibility and safety, ultimately resulting in greater patient trust and satisfaction as the practice of cosmetic dermatology expands.

KEY TERMS FROM THIS CHAPTER

Advanced aesthetic treatments
Aesthetic procedures
Aesthetic treatments
Beauty norms
Body dysmorphic disorder (BDD)
Cosmetic procedures
Cosmetic treatments
Customized treatment
Dermatological treatment
Aesthetic dermatology
Aesthetic somatology
Artificial Intelligence (AI)
Beauty standards
Cosmetic dermatology
Cosmetic Readiness Questionnaire (CRQ)
Cosmetics industry
Dermabrasion
Dysmorphic disorder

CRITICAL THINKING QUESTIONS

1. **Which of the following is a common non-invasive cosmetic dermatology procedure?**
   a. Facelift surgery
   b. Dermal filler injection
   c. Liposuction
   d. Hair transplant
2. **Which of the following best distinguishes non-invasive from invasive aesthetic procedures?**
   a. Non-invasive procedures require general anesthesia
   b. Invasive procedures use topical creams only
   c. Non-invasive procedures do not require incisions or downtime
   d. Invasive procedures are only performed by plastic surgeons
3. **Which procedure is considered invasive in cosmetic dermatology?**
   a. Chemical peel
   b. Botox injection
   c. Laser resurfacing
   d. Rhytidectomy (facelift)
4. **Which technological advancement has significantly improved precision in non-invasive cosmetic treatments?**
   a. Fractional laser technology
   b. Ultrasound imaging
   c. Artificial intelligence
   d. X-ray radiation
5. **What is a key trend shaping the future of cosmetic dermatology?**
   a. Increase in surgical interventions
   b. Decline of injectable treatments
   c. Rise of personalized treatments using AI and genetic profiling
   d. Discontinuation of laser-based treatments

Short Answer Questions

1. How has the field of cosmetic dermatology evolved from ancient beauty practices to a modern medical specialty?
2. What are the most common cosmetic dermatology procedures today, and how do they address different aesthetic concerns?
3. What are the key differences between non-invasive and invasive cosmetic procedures in terms of risk, recovery, and patient outcomes?
4. How has technology revolutionized cosmetic dermatology, particularly in areas like laser treatments, digital imaging, and skin diagnostics?
5. In what ways have digital simulation and artificial intelligence enhanced patient experience and clinical decision-making in cosmetic dermatology?
6. What ethical issues must practitioners consider when performing aesthetic procedures, especially regarding informed consent and patient mental health?

Answer to Critical Thinking Questions

1. (b); 2. (c); 3. (d); 4. (a); 5. (c)

REFERENCES

1. Alsatti, H., Samarkandy, S. J., Albogami, D. B., Alrajhi, R. K., Alahmadi, R. A., Alturkistani, R., & Alzahrani, S. (2023). The impact of social media on seeking dermatological care. *Cureus, 15*(12), e49941. https://doi.org/10.7759/cureus.49941Ambrosio, D. V. (2018). Incidence and need of advanced aesthetic somatology in South Africa. https://core.ac.uk/download/222968033.pdf (accessed on 21st July 2025).
2. Arian, H., Alroudan, D., Alkandari, Q., & Shuaib, A. (2023). Cosmetic surgery and the diversity of cultural and ethnic perceptions of facial, breast, and gluteal aesthetics in women: A comprehensive review. *Clinical Cosmetic and Investigational Dermatology, 16*, 1443–1456. https://doi.org/10.2147/ccid.s410621 (accessed on 21st July 2025).
3. Bin Rubaian, N. F., Alghamdi, N. J., AlHemli, H. A., Alhuraish, D. S., Bukhari, A. E., & Amir, B. (2025). Assessment of pain perception of aesthetic procedures during menstrual period in comparison to non-menstrual period days. *International Journal of Women's Health, 17*, 235–243. https://www.semanticscholar.org/paper/0e8317c00b5736cc5b3ed95ccb67b058b96f2d73 (accessed on 21st July 2025).
4. Burger, P., Landreau, A., Azoulay, S., Michel, T., & Fernàndez, X. (2016). Skin whitening cosmetics: Feedback and challenges in the development of natural skin lighteners. *Cosmetics, 3*, 36–36. https://doi.org/10.3390/cosmetics3040036 (accessed on 21st July 2025).
5. Calik, J., Sauer, N., Woźniak, B., Wojnar, A., Pietkiewicz, P., & Dzięgiel, P. (2024). Pilot study on high-intensity focused ultrasound (HIFU) for basal cell carcinoma: Effectiveness and safety. *Journal of Clinical Medicine, 13*, 3277–3277. https://doi.org/10.3390/jcm13113277 (accessed on 21st July 2025).
6. Christen, M. O. (2022). Collagen stimulators in body applications: A review focused on poly-L-lactic acid (PLLA). *Clinical Cosmetic and Investigational Dermatology, 15*, 997–1019. https://doi.org/10.2147/ccid.s359813 (accessed on 21st July 2025).
7. Corbu, V. M., Gheorghe-Barbu, I., Dumbravă, A. Ş., Vrâncianu, C. O., & Şesan, T. E. (2023). Current insights in fungal importance—A comprehensive review. *Microorganisms, 11*, 1384–1384. https://doi.org/10.3390/microorganisms11061384 (accessed on 21st July 2025).
8. Crişan, D., Tarnowietzki, E., Bernhard, L., Møller, M. L., Scharffetter-Kochanek, K., Crişan, M., & Schneider, L. (2024). Rationale for using high-frequency ultrasound as a routine examination in skin cancer surgery: A practical approach. *Journal of Clinical Medicine, 13*, 2152–2152. https://doi.org/10.3390/jcm13072152 (accessed on 21st July 2025).
9. Dereli, A. K., İzci, A., Cenk, H., Şanlı, B., & Acar, K. (2025). Evaluation of medical malpractice claims arising from minimally invasive cosmetic procedures in the context of supreme court decisions. *TURKDERM*. https://www.semanticscholar.org/paper/d629cc666684f191a8b8642785afab0e16ca317e (accessed on 21st July 2025).
10. Dingre, S., Girbane, V., Tekavade, G., Todakari, P., Borawake, D., & Deshmukh, M. (2025). Strategic sales and marketing approaches in the dermatology product segment. *World Journal of Biology Pharmacy and Health Sciences*. https://www.semanticscholar.org/paper/18956009b1b74acf7c2b68586b945f9a42e529f6 (accessed on 21st July 2025).
11. Elias, A. S., & Gill, R. (2017). Beauty surveillance: The digital self-monitoring cultures of neoliberalism. *European Journal of Cultural Studies, 21*, 59–77. https://doi.org/10.1177/1367549417705604 (accessed on 21st July 2025).

12. Fabi, S. G., Hernandez, C. A., Montes, J. R., Cotofana, S., & Dayan, S. (2022). Aesthetic considerations when treating the Latin American patient: Thriving in diversity international roundtable series. *Journal of Cosmetic Dermatology, 22*, 593–602. https://doi.org/10.1111/jocd.15516 (accessed on 21st July 2025).

13. Fabi, S., Boen, M., Weinstein Velez, M., Woodward, J. A., Hui Austin, A., & Dayan, S. (2024). Expert roundtable on skin care integration after aesthetic procedures: Consensus recommendations. *Journal of Drugs in Dermatology: JDD, 24*(1), 47–53. https://www.semanticscholar.org/paper/ac2c330163fd8948432db9fe23a198403b551230 (accessed on 21st July 2025).

14. Fonfría, E., Maignel, J., Lezmi, S., Martin, V., Splevins, A., Shubber, S., Kalinichev, M., et al. (2018). The expanding therapeutic utility of botulinum neurotoxins. *Toxins, 10*, 208–208. https://doi.org/10.3390/toxins10050208 (accessed on 21st July 2025).

15. Goldust, M., Baumann, L., Gold, M. H., & Landau, M. (2024). Advancements in cosmetics and aesthetics: A comprehensive review. *Dermatological Reviews, 5*. https://doi.org/10.1002/der2.245 (accessed on 21st July 2025).

16. Haykal, D. (2025). Digital twins in dermatology: A new era of personalized skin care. *Frontiers in Digital Health, 7*. https://doi.org/10.3389/fdgth.2025.1534859 (accessed on 21st July 2025).

17. Haykal, D., Cartier, H., Rossi, A., Margara, A., & du Crest, D. (2023). The art of a successful cosmetic consultation in 2023. *Journal of the European Academy of Dermatology and Venereology, 37*. https://www.semanticscholar.org/paper/8198541f124c4fda1b47b839612867b10073daa6 (accessed on 21st July 2025).

18. Haykal, D., Garibyan, L., Flament, F., & Cartier, H. (2024). Hybrid cosmetic dermatology: AI generated horizon. *Skin Research and Technology, 30*. https://doi.org/10.1111/srt.13721 (accessed on 21st July 2025).

19. Heilman, E., Isseroff, R. R., Jagdeo, J. R., Jakus, J., et al. (2019). A dose-ranging, parallel group, split-face, single-blind phase II study of light emitting diode-red light (LED-RL) for skin scarring prevention: Study protocol for a randomized controlled trial. https://core.ac.uk/download/323070347.pdf (accessed on 21st July 2025).

20. Higgins, S. A., & Wysong, A. (2017). Cosmetic surgery and body dysmorphic disorder–An update. *International Journal of Women's Dermatology, 4*, 43–48. https://doi.org/10.1016/j.ijwd.2017.09.007 (accessed on 21st July 2025).

21. Hogan, S., Zachary, C., & Arndt, K. (2021). Prejuvenation: Definition of the term and evolution of the concept. *Dermatologic Surgery*. https://www.semanticscholar.org/paper/629eea70100e7454344439012a8ec241c7e979a7 (accessed on 21st July 2025).

22. Joshi, M., Korrapati, N. H., Reji, F., Hasan, A., & Kurudamannil, R. A. (2022). The impact of social media on skin care: A narrative review. *Lviv Clinical Bulletin, 1, 2*, 85–96. https://doi.org/10.25040/lkv2022.01-02.085 (accessed on 21st July 2025).

23. Kapadiya, D., Mitul, M., & Prajapati, B. (2025). From science to skincare: The efficacy of hyaluronic acid in cosmeceuticals. https://core.ac.uk/download/658783629.pdf (accessed on 21st July 2025).

24. Keohane, S., Botting, J., Budny, P. G., Dolan, O. M., Fife, K., Harwood, C. A., Mallipeddi, R., et al. (2020). British Association of Dermatologists guidelines for the management of people with cutaneous squamous cell carcinoma 2020*. *British Journal of Dermatology, 184*, 401–414. https://doi.org/10.1111/bjd.19621 (accessed on 21st July 2025).

25. Keskinbora, K., & Kumbasar, E. (2023). Ethical concerns in dermatology and cosmetic applications. *Medical Research Archives*. https://www.semanticscholar.org/paper/888f1ad9b5a0c236c51f83cb5213b5e1b2859908 (accessed on 21st July 2025).

26. Kuhn, H., Cunha, P. R., Matthews, N. H., & Kroumpouzos, G. (2018). Body dysmorphic disorder in the cosmetic practice. *Giornale Italiano di Dermatologia e Venereologia, 153*(4), 506–515. https://www.semanticscholar.org/paper/cc09091cc75a43ab3ed1395517f3ccf39ea53b33 (accessed on 21st July 2025).

27. Kurtoğlu Necef, Ö., Öndoğan, Z., Tama, D., Boz, S., Şen Kılıç, A., Boyacı, B., & Ertam, İ. (2024). Evaluating the efficacy of cosmetic textiles in skin hydration and cellulite management through wear trials. *Applied Sciences, 14*, 11874–11874. https://doi.org/10.3390/app142411874 (accessed on 21st July 2025).

28. Landau, M., Kassir, M., & Goldust, M. (2025). Transforming aesthetic medicine with generative artificial intelligence. *Journal of Cosmetic Dermatology, 24*. https://doi.org/10.1111/jocd.70015 (accessed on 21st July 2025).

29. Lipozenčić, J., & Bukvić-Mokos, Z. (2010). Korektivna dermatologija danas. https://core.ac.uk/download/14451790.pdf (accessed on 21st July 2025).

30. Löhr, F., Papakonstantinou, E., & Raap, U. (2017). Photodynamic therapy and skin cancer. https://core.ac.uk/download/322432943.pdf (accessed on 21st July 2025).

31. Meghe, S., Ramapure, R., Jaiswal, S., Jawade, S. A., & Singh, S. (2024). A comprehensive review of minimally invasive dermatosurgical procedures. *Cureus, 16*. https://www.semanticscholar.org/paper/149d288c697c63903a0997fd7b09d082e7b377a3 (accessed on 21st July 2025).

32. Mihova, T., Georgieva, E., & Trifonova-Laskova, S. (2025). Study of eye health risks associated with decorative cosmetics and aesthetic procedures. *Trakia Journal of Sciences*. https://www.semanticscholar.org/paper/663bf23ec0d503e06c0a42f0fb7616378190bb6b (accessed on 21st July 2025).

33. Nahm, W. J., Nikas, C., Goldust, M., Horneck, N., Cervantes, J. A., Burshtein, J., & Tsoukas, M. (2025). Exosomes in dermatology: A comprehensive review of current applications, clinical evidence, and future directions. *International Journal of Dermatology*. https://www.semanticscholar.org/paper/c8e306dd7e9cededa906bf6dab9d46ae0954b1d0 (accessed on 21st July 2025).

34. Papadopoulos, K., Piperi, C., & Korkolopoulou, P. (2024). Clinical applications of adipose-derived stem cell (ADSC) exosomes in tissue regeneration. *International Journal of Molecular Sciences, 25*, 5916–5916. https://doi.org/10.3390/ijms25115916 (accessed on 21st July 2025).

35. Pearlman, R., Wilkerson, A. H., Cobb, E. K., Morrissette, S., Lawson, F. G., Mockbee, C. S., Humphries, L. S., et al. (2022). Factors associated with likelihood to undergo cosmetic surgical procedures among young adults in the United States: A narrative review. *Clinical Cosmetic and Investigational Dermatology, 15*, 859–877. https://doi.org/10.2147/ccid.s358573 (accessed on 21st July 2025).

36. Pikoos, T. D., Buchanan, B., Hegarty, D., & Rossell, S. L. (2024). The Cosmetic Readiness Questionnaire (CRQ): Validation of a pre-operative psychological screening tool for aesthetic procedures. *Aesthetic Surgery Journal*. https://www.semanticscholar.org/paper/a6d347e5df27d403a407019138c2dfe560e1f698 (accessed on 21st July 2025).

37. Pons-Llanas, O., Ballester-Sánchez, R., Celada-Álvarez, F., Candela-Juan, C., García-Martínez, T., Llavador-Ros, M., Botella-Estrada, R., et al. (2015). In reply to the Letter to the Editor titled: "Comments on: Clinical implementation of a new electronic brachytherapy system for skin brachytherapy." *Journal of Contemporary Brachytherapy, 7*, 319–320. https://www.semanticscholar.org/paper/3483bf0b86ce2e943484134b13a5c08707f3820f (accessed on 21st July 2025).

38. Richard, M. A., Paul, C., Nijsten, T., Gisondi, P., Sălăvăstru, C., Taïeb, C., Trakatelli, M., et al. (2022). Prevalence of most common skin diseases in Europe: A population-based study. *Journal of the European Academy of Dermatology and Venereology, 36*, 1088–1096. https://doi.org/10.1111/jdv.18050 (accessed on 21st July 2025).

39. Rossi, A. (2023). Introduction to special dermatology plastic surgery issue. *Lasers in Surgery and Medicine, 55*. https://www.semanticscholar.org/paper/26f3564fdcdccef6c0a0796aa27457b9dc2b077f (accessed on 21st July 2025).

40. Rostamzadeh, M., & Rahimi, F. (2025). Aesthetic dentistry and ethics: A systematic review of marketing practices and overtreatment in cosmetic dental procedures. *BMC Medical Ethics, 26*. https://www.semanticscholar.org/paper/b9651d439d9cdc44e7c5e7fc749d454ac90669cd (accessed on 21st July 2025).

41. Samizadeh, S., & De Boulle, K. (2018). Botulinum neurotoxin formulations: Overcoming the confusion. *Clinical Cosmetic and Investigational Dermatology, 11*, 273–287. https://doi.org/10.2147/ccid.s156851 (accessed on 21st July 2025).

42. Schlesinger, T. (2023). GE introduction: Injectables—Dermal fillers part A. *Dermatological Reviews, 4*. https://www.semanticscholar.org/paper/cb415127715cb2e4eab4feeed98063a795185217 (accessed on 21st July 2025).

43. Simpattanawong, D. (2016). Non-invasive aesthetic medical tourism in Bangkok: A qualitative analysis of stakeholder risk. https://core.ac.uk/download/341769488.pdf (accessed on 21st July 2025).

44. Sun, Y., Mao, J., Su, Y., Xia, W., Li, Q., & Zan, T. (2024). Application and exploration of interprofessional education in the teaching of plastic and reconstructive surgery: A narrative review. *BMC Medical Education, 24*. https://doi.org/10.1186/s12909-024-06423-w (accessed on 21st July 2025).

45. Van Praet, K. M., Kofler, M., Akansel, S., Montagner, M., Meyer, A., Sündermann, S., Falk, V., et al. (2022). Periareolar endoscopic minimally invasive cardiac surgery: Postoperative scar assessment analysis. *Interactive Cardiovascular and Thoracic Surgery, 35*. https://www.semanticscholar.org/paper/be717e587077a26b87872d1311f0f2effa9fbc9f (accessed on 21st July 2025).

46. Vojdani, A., & Shoenfeld, Y. (2022). Catastrophic embolism following cosmetic injection of autologous fat: Are silicone-treated syringes the only suspects on the crime scene? *Frontiers in Surgery, 9*. https://www.semanticscholar.org/paper/0de75ff56b330c3e3337b823eb6044ca66f17e73 (accessed on 21st July 2025).

47. Youngerwood, A. (2012). From creams to lasers: Regulating the beauty industry in the new millennium. https://core.ac.uk/download/28938988.pdf (accessed on 21st July 2025).

LASERS AND LIGHT-BASED THERAPIES IN DERMATOLOGY

8

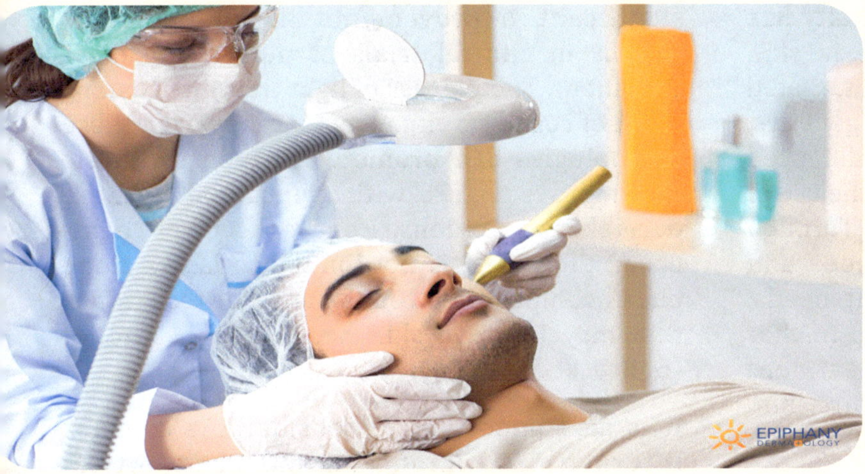

LEARNING OBJECTIVES

After studying this chapter, you will be able to:

1. Understand the mechanism of action underlying lasers and light-based therapies
2. Define types of laser therapies
3. Describe light-based therapies
4. Discuss the applications of lasers and light-based therapies in dermatology
5. Explain the benefits of laser and light therapies
6. Focus on risks and side effects associated with lasers and light-based therapies

Introduction

Laser and light therapy have changed the science of dermatology by introducing new means of managing multiple skin ailments. These therapies leverage the unique properties of light to target specific tissues with minimal harm to surrounding healthy tissue. These developments allow dermatologists not only to treat cosmetic conditions such as hair removal and skin rejuvenation but also to treat severe dermatological disorders such as psoriasis and acne scarring. Laser therapy has increased significantly and has now become a fundamental part of dermatological practice, as it continues to evolve to meet the growing demands of patients seeking aesthetic and therapeutic outcomes. One of the key advantages of laser treatments is their ability to achieve significant effects with minimal invasiveness, which in some cases can lead to faster recovery than with conventional surgical procedures. For instance, photodynamic therapy (PDT) has emerged as a useful treatment modality for conditions oral lichen planus (OLP), which is defined by chronic inflammation and mucosal lesions. Quoted in recent literature,

PDT is characterized by low side effects and promising results, reflecting its growing utility in a variety of dermatologic conditions. This improvement not only demonstrates advances in dermatologic therapeutic modalities but also underscores the need for ongoing research to further establish laser and light therapies as mainstream treatments. Moreover, the use of lasers in dermatology reflects broader technological and scientific advances in medicine, which capture the interest of both patients and dermatologists. The specialty has also experienced enormous advances in skin physiology, enabling more effective and targeted therapies. As suggested, advances in genetics, immunology, and pharmacology have influenced the treatment of skin disease, enabling the use of novel procedures such as laser therapy. Through continuous refinement of these methods and their extension to specialized patient needs, dermatology stands poised to undergo further developments that can reshape treatment models, offer patients a brighter future, and leave behind otherwise incapacitating skin disease.

Definition of Lasers and Light-Based Therapies

The term laser stands for Light Amplification by Stimulated Emission of Radiation and refers to a light source that emits light at specific wavelengths. In dermatology, lasers are now valuable assets to a range of therapeutic interventions, from ablative skin resurfacing to hair removal and the removal of vascular lesions. The precision in wavelength and deposited energy enables therapists to selectively target skin layers and conditions. For instance, lasers can selectively target the heating of cells that transport pigments or vascular structures, thereby reducing tissue damage during procedures. With the growing demand for non-invasive cosmetic procedures, awareness of the principles of how lasers work has become a requisite for patients and their dermatologists as they sort through the myriad of options in light-based treatments. Light therapies, including lasers, use a range of wavelengths to produce therapeutic effects in the skin. One of the foremost applications is photodynamic therapy (PDT), which uses light-activated photosensitizing agents to treat conditions such as acne vulgaris. Research has suggested that the application of PDT with agents 5-aminolevulinic acid (ALA) can significantly reduce the severity of acne, based on statistically significant improvements in inflammatory lesions in clinical trials of pulsed dye laser treatment. The physics of light treatments stops short of cosmetic enhancement; however, these technologies can promote collagen synthesis and improve texture, with applications for more dermal interventions. Hence, the term "light-based therapies" is not limited to lasers alone but encompasses a broad range of techniques that may improve skin health and aesthetics (Bailey et al., 2010).

It is also important to consider the complex interactions among numerous optical characteristics of the skin when evaluating light-based therapies. The interaction between light and the skin is fundamental to making treatment as effective as possible. Heterogeneity in skin content may lead to substantial differences in light absorption and scattering, posing a challenge for precisely forecasting treatment outcomes. A recent publication emphasized that the optical characteristics of human skin compartments can vary by orders of magnitude, and measurements have revealed discrepancies up to 100-fold in published values. These findings underscore the value of using robust datasets to better replicate *in vivo* conditions when simulating light interactions with skin. Use of a well-defined dataset can enhance treatment precision and predictability of outcomes across various therapeutic applications, thereby further advancing the field of dermatology through new light-related technologies (Altshuler et al., 2017) (Figure 8.1).

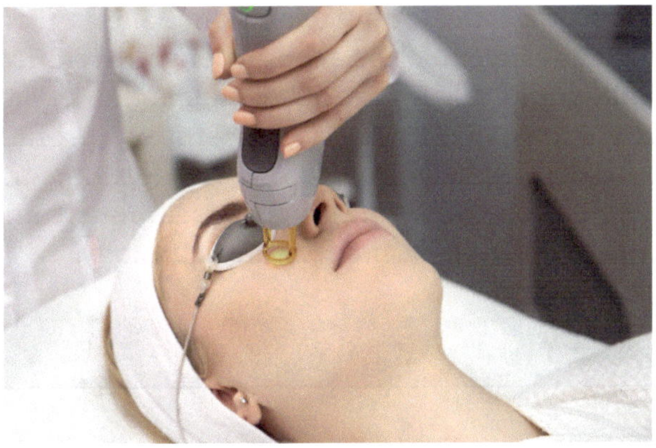

Figure 8.1. Skin laser treatment.

Source: https://cdn.prod.website-files.com/601780d2b928498177696784/64ae816f30fc94b79a9c81d3_BBL%20Laser.jpeg.

Historical Context of Their Use in Dermatology

The development of lasers and light therapies in dermatology over time clearly demonstrates substantial progress in medical technology and in the knowledge base on skin disorders. Traditional dermatologic management previously relied on topical and systemic medications, along with numerous forms of physical therapy. The introduction of lasers in the 1960s opened new avenues that revolutionized dermatology. The use of the first continuous-wave laser, the ruby laser, enabled accurate treatment of vascular and pigmentary lesions, providing clinicians with unprecedented precision. The use of these modalities spread, leading to the development of laser-assisted treatments for conditions like hemangiomas, melasma, and acne scars, ultimately establishing the modern basis of aesthetic dermatology. Over the decades since the invention of laser technology, advances have enabled the diversification of light therapies for various skin conditions and types. In the 1980s and 1990s, pulsed dye lasers emerged and proved particularly effective for treating vascular lesions due to their ability to selectively target hemoglobin. This was when dermatology reached a turning point, as professionals recognized the advantages of non-surgical methods that minimized scarring and facilitated healing. Additionally, the introduction of fractional laser technology was a paradigm shift towards enhancing tissue remodeling processes with fewer side effects. By integrating technology with dermatologic expertise, dermatologists can provide patients with more efficient and safer treatments and establish a new standard for dermatologic care. As the field evolved, studies and clinical trials continued to expand our understanding of the mechanisms of laser and light treatments. Improvements, such as the advent of intense pulsed light (IPL) machines, further expanded treatment capability by addressing several skin conditions with one visit and providing flexible uses like hair removal and photo-rejuvenation. Researchers have observed the interaction between light and biological tissues and have contributed to the body of knowledge that informs contemporary clinical practice. The history of dermatological light-based therapies chronicles the advancement of technologies and their meaningful integration into patient care, indicating that further research will soon yield even more sophisticated treatments. Knowledge of these trends gives a better understanding of how dermatology has continued to develop in reaction to both patients' needs and available technologies as it strives to meet the objectives of improving therapeutic results for various skin disorders.

Significance of the Subject in Contemporary Dermatology Practices

The role of lasers and light treatments in modern dermatology cannot be overstated. The newer modalities offer new approaches for treating a vast array of skin diseases, ranging from cosmetic conditions photoaging and hyperpigmentation to more problematic lesions, including acne and vascular lesions. The precision of laser technology enables practitioners to deliver energy to specific skin layers accurately without damaging adjacent tissues, a substantial advantage over conventional therapy. This characteristic not only ensures maximal therapeutic efficacy but also reduces recovery time and the risk of complications. As dermatology continues to evolve, the use of lasers and light therapies reflects a commitment to improved outcomes and patient satisfaction and underscores their central role in contemporary practice. Moreover, the evolution of nanotechnology through laser treatment offers a unique opportunity to further enhance treatment efficacy. Nanocarrier systems can be engineered to deliver medications to specific sites, thereby significantly increasing therapeutic efficacy by overcoming the limitations of traditional methods. One can design these systems to release medications directly at the site of a dermatological disorder to minimize systemic side effects associated with conventional treatments. By combining targeted nanocarriers with laser therapy, healthcare practitioners can treat skin ailments more effectively, meeting the demand for high-efficacy, low-toxicity treatments that are favorable to patients' overall health (Qu et al., 2022). Not only does this combination revolutionize patient care, but it also maintains dermatology at the pinnacle of technological advancement in medicine. Laser and light-based therapies have a broader impact beyond conventional treatments on the psychological and social dimensions of patient care. Skin diseases usually have a heavy psychological impact on the patients, affecting their self-esteem and quality of life. By using effective modalities such as laser therapy, dermatologists can mitigate adverse effects to some extent, thereby healing the patient not only physically but also emotionally. The procedure for refining the look of the skin promptly enhances patients' self-confidence, thereby improving their overall psychological well-being. As such treatments become widespread, the dermatological industry is compelled to focus on patient education and accessibility to ensure that the population can benefit from these advancements. Secondly, ongoing clinical studies and investigations will be the key to substantiating the safety and efficacy profiles of new laser technology, thereby forming the grounds for their continued development and implementation in modern dermatology.

8.1. Mechanism of Action

Learning Outcome

1. Explain the principles of laser technology
2. Understand the interaction of light with skin tissues
3. Explain the types of light used in dermatological treatments

The mechanism of action of lasers and light therapy in dermatology is based on the interaction between light and biological tissue. When laser light is absorbed by chromophores in the skin, such as melanin, hemoglobin, or water, it creates a range of effects based on wavelength and time exposure. For instance, shorter wavelengths tend to be absorbed by superficial structures , such as the epidermis, while longer wavelengths penetrate deeper layers and reach structures , such as blood vessels and collagen fibers. Such selectivity allows dermatologists to tailor treatments to treat particular skin conditions, such as pigmentation disorders, vascular lesions, or signs of aging. This specificity not only makes it highly effective but also minimizes harm to surrounding tissues, thereby ensuring greater patient comfort and safety (Lucas et al., 2022). Another important aspect of the treatments is the photobiomodulation concept, which involves the application of non-thermal light to modulate cellular activity. Photobiomodulation facilitates multiple biological processes, such as increased ATP production and enhanced cellular metabolism, ultimately promoting wound healing and tissue regeneration. Directly applicable to post-viral complications, like those seen in COVID-19 survivors, these light therapies are promising forms of rehabilitation. By understanding the mechanisms of light-induced cellular responses, therapy professionals are better able to plan therapeutic regimens to prevent dermatological outcomes, particularly those arising from long-term health effects (Lucas et al., 2022). This use of photobiomodulation indicates the capability of lasers not only to address cosmetic concerns but also to enhance recovery from more complex dermatological conditions. Furthermore, the efficacy of laser treatments is highly contingent on an intimate understanding of skin anatomy and light physics. Parameters laser fluence, pulse duration, and wavelength play a pivotal role in determining outcome and safety profiles. A clinician must appreciate how these parameters affect laser-tissue interaction across skin types to determine optimal treatment protocols. It is necessary for optimal therapeutic results with fewer side effects, such as burns or post-inflammatory hyperpigmentation. One cannot advance with existing or develop novel therapeutic methods without adequate knowledge of the fundamentals of laser technology and skin interactions. Working with the complex interaction between the physics of lasers and dermatological applications ultimately reinforces the field's capacity to deliver effective, evidence-based treatments (Alhallak, 2021).

8.1.1. Principles of Laser Technology

Laser technology relies on the principles of light and its interaction with tissue. At the center of laser action is the phenomenon of stimulated emission, in which photons cause electrons in a medium to emit more photons of the same energy. This results in a monochromatic beam of highly concentrated and coherent light. The unique properties of laser light render it particularly appropriate for a broad array of dermatologic applications, such as the elimination of tattoos, skin resurfacing, and therapy for vascular lesions. By targeting distinct chromophores within the skin with precise accuracy, lasers selectively heat and destroy the undesired tissue with minimal injury to nearby normal cells. Wavelength selection is critical to determining the lasers' effectiveness and safety profile because, depending on wavelength, different wavelengths penetrate skin tissues to varying depths and thus affect treatment outcomes. Secondly, the development of diverse laser types has enabled significant advances in dermatologic light treatments. The most prevalent types are ablative and non-ablative lasers, which have diverse therapeutic applications. Ablative lasers, for example, carbon dioxide (CO_2) and erbium YAG, function by ablating layers of skin, hence promoting the generation of new tissue and enhancing skin texture. Non-ablative lasers, for example, pulsed dye and Nd:YAG, function primarily in the deeper skin structures without damaging the epidermis and are therefore best suited for conditions such as pigmentation, vascular lesions, and overall skin rejuvenation. Recognizing these variations is essential to clinicians because it allows for the best laser modality to be chosen based on the patients' own skin issues, desired results, and rehabilitation time. With the prospect of utilizing the advantages of both types of lasers, practitioners can optimize treatment protocols to meet individual patient needs. In addition to the evolution of laser technology, ongoing research on the integration of nanotechnology is the most promising avenue for enhancing the effectiveness of laser treatment. Nanoparticles can be engineered to act as targeted delivery systems for drugs or imaging agents, permitting more focused treatment strategies in dermatology. The integration of nanotechnology and laser therapy has the potential to enhance the specificity of cancer-cell targeting and reduce collateral damage to healthy tissues. Studies have shown that such combinations are likely to yield improved therapeutic outcomes and patient experience. However, despite optimism about such breakthroughs, translating laboratory findings to the clinic has proven difficult. It should be noted that ongoing research is addressing these translational hurdles, enabling the benefits of this technology to reach patients and illustrating the potential of lasers and nanotechnology to revolutionize dermatological treatment (Chehelgerdi et al., 2023; Teede et al., 2023) (Figure 8.2).

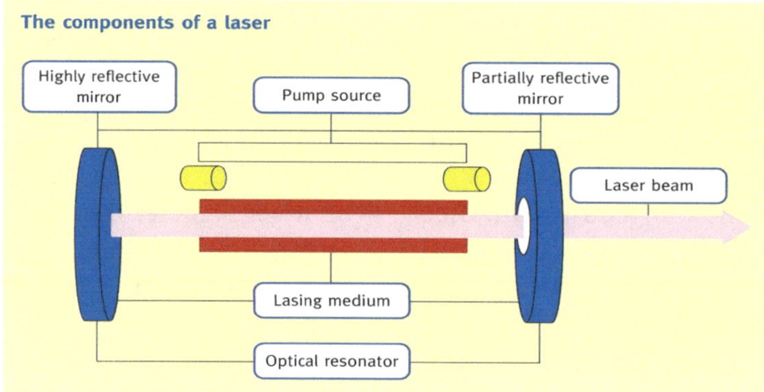

Figure 8.2. The principles of laser technology.

Source: https://ars.els-cdn.com/content/image/1-s2.0-S1472029914002410-gr1.jpg.

8.1.2. Interaction of Light with Skin Tissues

The behavior of light on skin tissues is a complex phenomenon that is important to the efficacy of laser and light treatments in dermatology. During phototherapy, the transmission, scattering, and absorption of light by the skin depend to a great extent upon the applied wavelength and the provided components of the skin. Several chromophores, such as melanin and hemoglobin, absorb at certain wavelengths with different patterns and cause various therapeutic effects. For instance, melanocytes in skin tissue absorb UV light, which is a factor in pigmentation disorders, whereas hemoglobin absorbs visible light, which is necessary for selective vascular lesion targeting. The selective targeting ability of these chromophores enables more precise and effective therapy without harming surrounding tissues, resulting in better patient outcomes. These features emphasize the necessity to investigate these interactions in order to make best therapeutic use of them in dermatology. Over the past several years, developments in photodynamic therapy (PDT) have revealed the therapeutic utility of using specific wavelengths of light in combination with photosensitizing agents. For example, therapy of common warts using PDT as 5-aminolevulinic acid (5-ALA) indicates the manner in which light will induce photosensitizers that damage cells within virus-infected skin sites. Research has shown that, when coupled with water-filtered infrared A (wIRA), the efficacy of PDT is significantly enhanced due to increased tissue penetration, leading to improved clinical outcomes in the management of conditions such as HPV-related skin lesions. Significantly, the incorporation of wIRA not only enhances the efficacy of PDT by targeting deeper skin layers but also provides a non-invasive approach, thereby improving patient comfort. The findings of such interactions underscore the increasing volume of knowledge around light's role in dermatological treatments, as well as the importance of maximizing treatment modalities. Furthermore, the role of photobiomodulation (PBM) is increasingly recognized for its multifaceted applications in healing enhancement, skin rejuvenation, and hair growth. Research has revealed that a variety of optical parameters play a significant role in the overall effectiveness of PBM in clinical settings. Above all, differences in the selection of these parameters can yield varying results and indicate the need for standardized protocols in clinical practice. The role of photoreceptors, for instance, cytochrome c oxidase, and the mechanisms associated with them make it even more complex to analyze light's interaction with skin tissue. A more systematic methodology that can correlate optical parameters with biological constructs can result in targeted therapies and improved clinical outcomes. Future studies in this area are to further clarify the interaction between light and tissue and improve the efficacy of light treatments in dermatology (Bankova et al., 2005; Anders et al., 2016) (Figure 8.3).

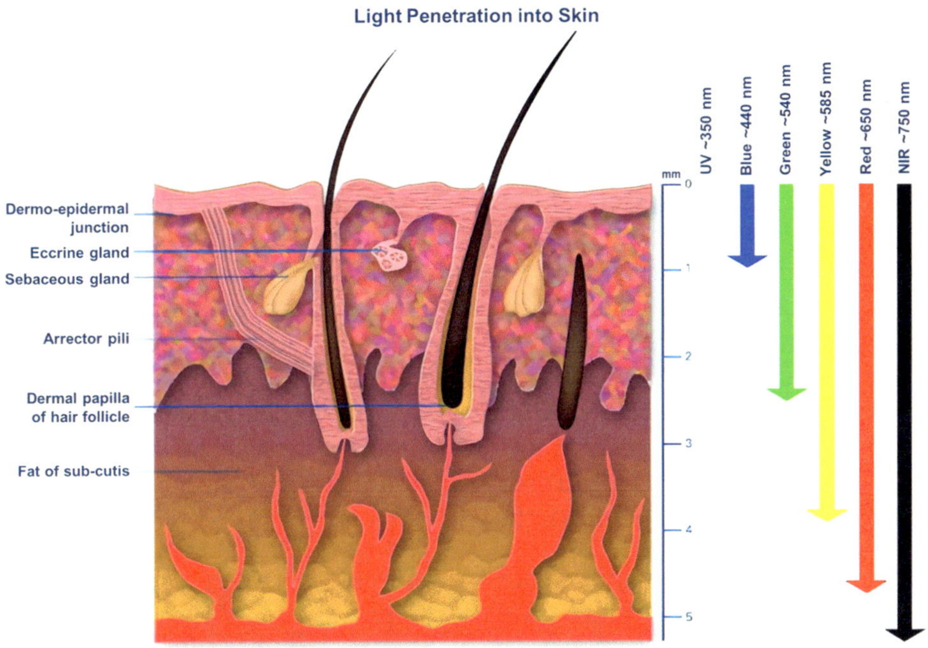

Figure 8.3. Light-tissue interaction. Depth of light penetration into human skin; as the wavelength of light increases, the penetration depth becomes deeper.

Source: https://www.researchgate.net/profile/Angela-Kwan/publication/349703073/figure/fig1/AS:1019520575602688@1620084055147/Light-tissue-interaction-Depth-of-light-penetration-into-human-skin-as-the-wavelength.jpg.

8.1.3. Types of Light Used in Dermatological Treatments

In dermatology, the evolution of various light therapies has made them essential tools for treating a range of skin diseases. Amongst them, lasers have also gained prominence for precision and effectiveness. The various wavelengths of lasers are employed to treat individual chromophores in the skin, enabling tailored treatments for conditions such as acne scars, pigmentation disorders, and vascular lesions. For instance, the 1064 nm Nd:YAG laser is suitable for the management of deeper vascular lesions, while the 532 nm laser is commonly used for superficial cutaneous disease, including lentigines and cherry angiomas. Fractional laser technology has further revolutionized dermatologic therapy by enabling selective ablation of skin tissue with minimal harm to surrounding tissues. By fractionating therapy to columns, the technique minimizes downtime and accelerates healing, a fundamental shift from patient treatment in dermatology. Another important advance in light treatments is the use of non-ablative lasers, which deliver energy that induces collagen synthesis rather than removing the skin's outer layer. Such lasers are particularly beneficial for addressing skin laxity, lines, and overall textural anomalies. The erbium laser at 1540 nm is an excellent example of this approach by inducing remodeling of collagen without injuring the epidermis. Furthermore, light-emitting diodes (LEDs) have gained widespread acceptance for their use in photomodulation and are now commonly used in conjunction with other dermatologic treatments. Blue light, in this context, targets bacteria that cause acne and therefore represents a beneficial adjunctive treatment for patients with acne vulgaris, particularly those with skin of color, according to recent studies (Pathmarajah et al., 2022). This advancement represents a promising development in the specialty that expands access to and efficacy of therapy. Photodynamic therapy (PDT) is another significant light-based treatment in which light is combined with a photosensitizing agent to treat a range of skin conditions, including non-melanoma skin cancers and acne. This treatment uses specific wavelengths to activate photosensitizers, thereby inducing cytotoxic effects in pathologic cells. The benefits of laser-induced photodynamic therapy, as discussed in recent technological advances, have been particularly advantageous for treating diseases characterized by actinic keratoses and other precancerous lesions (Paasch, U., & Grunewald, S., 2020). PDT is important for treating large skin surfaces without causing damage to adjacent tissues. Moreover, the advancements of new technologies, such as daylight-activated systems, enhance the adaptability of PDT for customizing treatment protocols for better patient comfort. Taken together, these phototherapies indicate ongoing innovation in dermatology, reflecting an unwavering commitment to improving patient outcomes through advanced treatment modalities.

Test Your Knowledge

1. What are the fundamental principles of laser technology, and how do they apply to dermatological treatments?
2. What are the main types of lasers used in dermatology, and what conditions are they best suited to treat?

8.2. Types of Laser Therapies

Learning Outcome

1. Differentiate between ablative and non-ablative lasers.
2. Describe commonly used laser types.
3. Address indications for various laser therapies.

A variety of laser therapies are now important tools in dermatology practice, employed for the treatment of various dermatoses with varying degrees of effectiveness. Most well-known is low-level laser therapy (LLLT), which found more and more applications for the treatment of diseases like androgenetic alopecia. Evidence indicates that LLLT stimulates hair follicles, promoting hair growth and increased hair density, offering a non-surgical alternative to traditional treatments for baldness. Clinically apparent baldness patients are likely to experience psychological disturbance, and the onset of such therapies is thus opportune. Studies demonstrate the efficacy of fractional lasers, another type of laser therapy, not only in alopecia but also in scar treatment and skin rejuvenation, thereby making them increasingly significant in dermatological procedures (Christina et al., 2024). In addition to LLLT, the pulsed dye laser has also been proven effective in the treatment of an array of vascular lesions, such as rosacea and port wine stains. These lasers operate on the principle of selective photothermolysis, which targets a specific chromophore in the skin. By targeting intravascular oxyhemoglobin, pulsed dye lasers can be used to remove vascular lesions, thereby significantly improving cosmetic appearance with minimal collateral damage to surrounding tissues. Moreover, calming and efficient, these lasers are currently regarded as the gold standard for treating disorders related to abnormal blood vessels. They therefore emphasize the potential of laser therapy in enhancing patient satisfaction and quality of life by offering relief from physical as well as psychological effects of dermatological conditions (Janocha et al., 2024). The uses of laser treatments also extend to their application in scar management, either in the form of hypertrophic scars, keloids, or acne scarring. Fractional ablative lasers enable precise remodeling of the skin surface by delivering focused energy to induce microinjuries, thereby markedly stimulating collagen remodeling and skin regeneration. Not only is scar size and visibility minimized, but the overall skin texture is also enhanced, resulting in a dramatic aesthetic difference for patients. Laser-treated scars demonstrate the latest technological advancements in dermatology and how laser procedures can make a significant difference in patients' lives. Ongoing investigation of these laser devices has the potential to yield further advances in efficacy, safety, and patient satisfaction, further entrenching the position of laser treatments as a mainstay of contemporary dermatologic practice (Janocha et al., 2024).

8.2.1. Ablative Versus Non-Ablative Lasers

Laser treatments have become integral to dermatological practice, particularly in distinguishing ablative from non-ablative lasers. Ablative lasers, such as carbon dioxide (CO_2) and erbium YAG lasers, do this by causing ablation of the outer skin layers of damaged skin, thus triggering new skin development during the healing process. This is what makes it possible to observe dramatic improvements in skin texture, coloration, and wrinkles, particularly in more complex cases such as deep scars and photoaging. The recovery period after ablative laser treatment is longer and can take a few weeks, which may be a significant limiting factor for most patients. However, success in providing extensive skin damage renders it an important reason for those wanting considerable aesthetic improvements (Morton et al., 2019). Non-ablative lasers, on the other hand, don't remove layers of skin but go through the dermis to stimulate collagenesis, with resulting enhancement of the appearance of the skin in the long term. Treatments , such as pulsed dye lasers and Nd:YAG lasers are a more typical example of this category since they tend to hurt less and aren't so time-consuming. Non-ablative lasers are ideal for conditions such as melasma, rosacea, and light-to-moderate photoaging, offering a balance between effectiveness and time off (Passeron et al., 2019). While the results are not as dramatic as with ablative lasers, non-ablative treatment is generally more appealing to those seeking a more conservative procedure, allowing them to maintain skin integrity while achieving cosmetic improvement. The choice between ablative and non-ablative lasers is largely based on patient-specific factors, including skin type, desired outcome, and tolerance for downtime. For instance, ablative lasers may be selected for younger patients requiring maximal skin rejuvenation, whereas non-ablative treatments may be selected for patients with thinner skin to reduce the risk of complications. Furthermore, advances in laser technology and improved protocols enhance the safety and efficacy of both modalities, enabling more tailored therapies that target skin concerns effectively. With continued advances in dermatology, it is important to deepen understanding of the distinctions among these lasers for patients and clinicians alike to achieve optimal therapeutic outcomes (Morton et al., 2019; Passeron et al., 2019) (Figure 8.4).

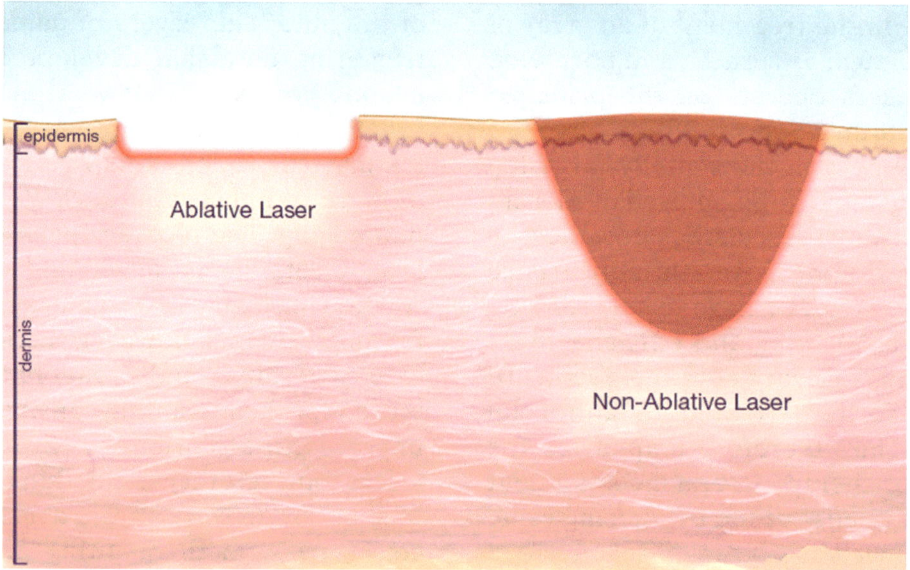

Figure 8.4. Ablative versus non-ablative lasers.

Source: https://estheticformula.com/wp-content/uploads/2022/10/AblativeVSNonAblativeIllustration.png.

8.2.2. Commonly Used Laser Types (e.g., CO_2, Er:YAG, Nd:YAG)

Applications of lasers in dermatology include various types for different treatment purposes, with the CO2 laser being among the most widely recognized. The CO_2 laser emits a steady beam at 10,600 nm and is ideal for ablative procedures. This laser vaporizes tissue, thereby making the damaged layers of the skin readily removable while initiating collagen remodeling in the underlying layers. Its characteristics make CO2 lasers highly valuable for the treatment of skin diseases such as wrinkles, scars, and keloids. In more recent studies, a combined protocol using CO2 lasers supplemented by other modalities, such as dye lasers, has been highly effective in reducing keloid recurrence rates, demonstrating the efficacy of multimodal laser therapy in achieving more satisfactory outcomes (Domenico et al., 2023). The Erbium:YAG (Er:YAG) laser, meanwhile, operates at 2940 nm wavelength, making it possible to target more specifically with minimal thermal damage to the surrounding tissues. Such precision makes the Er:YAG laser a viable choice for skin resurfacing and rejuvenation procedures, particularly ideal for patients with sensitive or fragile skin. Selective water absorption within the skin enables effective management of superficial skin flaws , such as wrinkles, pigmentation, and textural blemishes. Its effectiveness is further enhanced by fewer side effects and shorter recovery times than CO_2 lasers. Ongoing development of this technology further underscores its relevance in modern dermatology, particularly as demand grows for minimally invasive treatments that yield dramatic cosmetic outcomes. The 1064 nm Nd:YAG laser has another application, that being the targeting of deeper vascular lesions and pigmentary concerns. It is ideally suited to treating conditions such as rosacea, in which vascular abnormalities cause significant pain and aesthetic disruption. Its ability to penetrate deeper layers of skin with minimal destruction of the epidermis renders it particularly valuable for the management of a variety of dermal and vascular lesions. Nd:YAG lasers are also popularly employed in hair removal, utilizing the phenomenon of selective photothermolysis, whereby hair follicles are destroyed with minimal injury to the surrounding tissues. With advances in dermatological research, the medical applications of Nd:YAG lasers continue to be developed to maximize treatment efficacy and patient comfort (Chen et al., 2023). The variety of lasers suggests that they play an important role in the continuously evolving field of dermatological therapy (Figure 8.5).

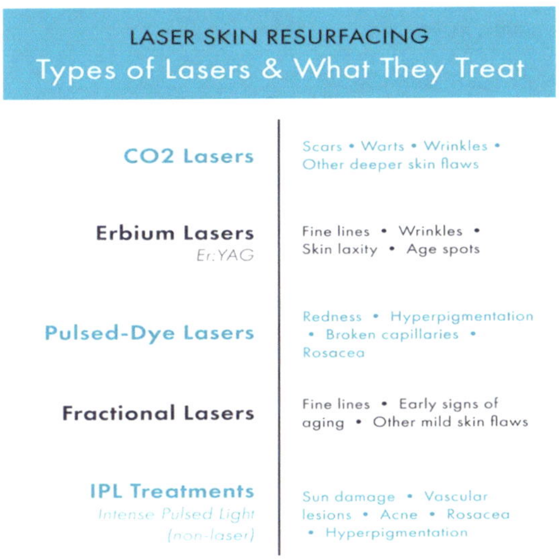

Figure 8.5. Types of lasers.

Source: https://www.americanboardcosmeticsurgery.org/wp-content/uploads/2024/05/4261-acd03db155-819x1024.png.webp.

8.2.3. Indications for Different Laser Therapies

The use of laser treatments in dermatology has expanded significantly, enabling precise treatment of many skin disorders. Various types of lasers have been developed, and each one has unique indications owing to its varied mechanisms of action. Some examples include ablative lasers, such as carbon dioxide (CO_2) and erbium:yttrium-aluminum-garnet (Er:YAG), which are ideal for scars and resurfacing of the skin. These lasers remove the epidermal and superficial dermal layers of the skin and stimulate collagen remodeling in the deeper tissues. These laser devices are used for hypertrophic scars, keloids, and photoaging, with the objective of thinning the scars, enhancing skin texture, and improving overall cosmetic appearance. However, side effects, for instance, post-inflammatory hyperpigmentation, should be considered when selecting appropriate cases for ablative laser treatment (Juh Mász et al., 2021). Non-ablative lasers, including pulsed dye and Nd:YAG lasers, offer treatment options for specific conditions with less downtime than their ablative counterparts. These lasers are applied primarily on vascular lesions, such as hemangiomas and rosacea, because they selectively coagulate the blood vessels without damaging the rest of the skin. The pulsed dye laser is effective in that it creates wavelengths of light that specifically target vascular lesions only, which leads to a drastic cutting off of the blood flow and improved look of the skin. Similarly, Nd:YAG laser is employed in deeper skin issues, such as leg veins and certain types of scars, with the capacity to work on various types of skin and states. With appropriate patient selection and adherence to strict recommended laser settings, these non-ablative devices can yield good results in minimizing adverse effects (Nast et al., 2020). Another important use of laser treatment is the use of fractional laser technology, which has found broad acceptance for its therapeutic benefits in treating a variety of conditions, from acne scars to melasma. Fractional lasers deliver energy in a pattern that creates microthermal zones, initiating healing while leaving the surrounding healthy skin intact. This new method provides significant skin texture and color enhancement without prolonged recovery time and is a useful option for patients requiring cosmetic therapy. It has indications that are broad-based, particularly in patients with damaged skin types who will be more susceptible to hyperpigmentation with traditional laser therapies. With ongoing research development, the understanding of nuances in various laser treatments will help clinicians individualize treatment plans to suit patient needs appropriately, maximizing both safety and effectiveness (Juh Mász et al., 2021) (Table 8.1).

Table 8.1. Indications Amenable to Treatment By Nonablative Lasers

Skin Tightening	Neck laxity, periorbital rhytides, jowls, nasolabial lines- Using RF devices
Photodamaged skin	Uneven pigmentation, freckles, lentigines, rhytides, textural changes- Using IPL devices for pigmentation and RF for rhytides
Body sculpting	Focused inch loss, fat reduction/ remodeling, treatment of cellulite- Using RF devices
Scar remodeling	Post acne scars, traumatic scars, post surgical scars- Using long pulsed Nd:YAG, pulsed dye laser and NAFL

Source: https://www.researchgate.net/publication/51066057/figure/tbl1/AS:996704501395456@1614644279257/Indications-amenable-to-treatment-by-nonablative-lasers.png.

Test Your Knowledge

1. What are the key differences between ablative and non-ablative laser therapies in terms of mechanism, recovery time, and typical applications?
2. What are the characteristics and clinical uses of the CO_2 and Er:YAG lasers in dermatological treatments?

8.3. Light-Based Therapies

Learning Outcome

1. Define photodynamic therapy (PDT).
2. Understand intense pulsed light (IPL) therapy.
3. Discuss blue light therapy for acne treatment.

The development of light-based treatments, particularly lasers, has significantly transformed dermatology clinics, offering new therapeutic options for a wide range of skin diseases. These treatments employ specific wavelengths of light to treat and modify various structures in the skin and to cure conditions such as pigmentation, vascular lesions, and scars. One of the most advanced technologies used is the Q-switched laser, which has been demonstrated to be effective for the treatment of dermal pigmentation disorders, particularly in individuals of color. Studies have found that sequential treatments with Q-switched lasers have produced substantial reductions in pigmentation across various conditions, not only validating efficacy and safety but also maximizing quality of life for patients. This paradigm shift reflects the increasing reliance on laser technology for augmenting treatment outcomes in dermatology and the necessity for continued innovation in the field (Garg et al., 2024). Dermatology-specific light treatments provide tailored solutions for hyperpigmentation and keloid formation issues. Fractional ablative lasers have enabled clinicians to deliver targeted therapy with minimal damage to adjacent tissues. This method preserves healthy tissue while effectively degrading pathological tissue, as demonstrated in landmark studies on hypertrophic scar and keloid therapy. Emerging guidelines emphasize the need for individualized treatment protocols based on patient-specific characteristics and scar responses, underscoring the merit of individualized laser therapies. Furthermore, light treatment in the guise of Intense Pulsed Light (IPL) has revolutionized the management of photoaging and vascular lesions, with repeatable outcomes in varied skin types and safety profiles that ensure extensive clinical application (Nast et al., 2020).

As laser technology continues to advance, the future of light therapy in dermatology is promising. Picosecond lasers are a breakthrough, offering greater precision and shorter recovery times for patients. Pulse lasers employ extremely short bursts of energy, resulting in the effective elimination of pigmented lesions and acne scars and a reduction in the risk of post-inflammatory hyperpigmentation, which is a prevalent complication in darker skin types. The persistent effort to improve these techniques by ongoing research and clinical trials will hopefully yield better methodologies and treatment regimens, with enhanced patient satisfaction and safety. Systematic reviews also attest that combination therapy using laser treatments along with medications , such as 5-fluorouracil and triamcinolone largely contributes to better outcomes for keloid and hypertrophy scar management. Overall, light-based treatments are poised to be at the forefront of dermatological advancement, driving future technologies and applications to benefit diverse patient populations.

8.3.1. Photodynamic Therapy (PDT)

Photodynamic therapy (PDT) has been a significant advance in dermatologic surgery, playing a central role in the class of light-based therapies. PDT therapy relies on the integration of photosensitizing agents and specific wavelengths of light, which induce selective cytotoxicity in cells. Notably, PDT can treat a range of neoplastic and inflammatory cutaneous disorders, including actinic keratosis and non-melanoma cutaneous malignancies. Its application represents a significant advance in dermatology, offering an alternative to traditional surgery, which is typically invasive and associated with prolonged recovery times. The shift from more aggressive, riskier procedures to less aggressive, safer ones is a paradigm of PDTs in dermatology, where their ability to target affected tissues with precision without damaging surrounding healthy tissues is their hallmark (Jeffrey et al., 2025). The capacity of PDT is also optimized by emerging technologies that have transformed its use in dermatology. Laser-assisted photodynamic therapy (LAPDT) is a novel approach that combines the use of lasers with conventional PDT techniques. The new concept enables controlled light distribution, thereby maximizing the efficacy of treatments for diseases such as non-melanoma skin cancer and field cancerization. With the aid of artificial and natural light sources, LAPDT has been proven to facilitate better patient outcomes as it facilitates penetration of the photosensitizing agents into the infected tissues. This subtle application underscores the dermatologic community's commitment to enhancing therapeutic options and adapting new technologies to improve clinical practice (Paasch, U., & Grunewald, S., 2020). Although it has numerous advantages, the efficacy of PDT in dermatology depends on careful evaluation of several parameters. Treatment efficacy depends on the judicious selection of photosensitizing agents, light sources, and treatment modalities, tailored to the patient's individual requirements.

Furthermore, the possibility of side effects, ranging from erythema to severe forms of dermatitis, necessitates appropriate patient management and counseling. While continued studies endeavor to realize the possibility of enhancing PDT's efficacy and minimizing its risks, the demand for individualized treatment plans grows. These achievements not only establish PDT's position as a cornerstone of light therapy but also demonstrate the ongoing evolution of dermatological treatments, thereby expanding the arsenal available to dermatologists (Jeffrey et al., 2025) (Figure 8.6).

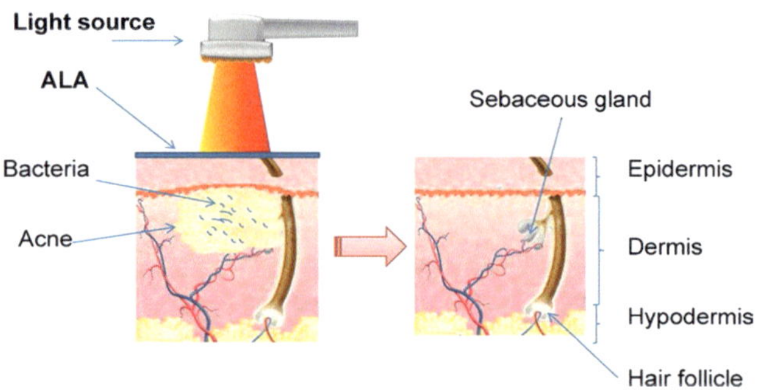

Figure 8.6. Schematic depiction of ALA-PDT for acne. The inflammation and the bacteria in the sebaceous gland are destroyed.

Source: https://www.researchgate.net/profile/Tianhong-Dai/publication/40025810/figure/fig8/AS:341340769538060@1458393389903/Schematic-depiction-of-ALA-PDT-for-acne-The-inflammation-and-the-bacteria-in-the.png.

8.3.2. Intense Pulsed Light (IPL) Therapy

In dermatology, Intense Pulsed Light (IPL) therapy has gained recognition for its versatility and efficacy in treating a range of skin conditions. IPL utilizes a broad spectrum of light wavelengths, which distinguishes it from laser therapies that typically focus on individual wavelengths. This attribute enables IPL to target a range of skin concerns, including photodamage, acne, and vascular lesions, demonstrating its utility as a comprehensive treatment option. The technology operates by emitting light pulses that penetrate the skin and subsequently target hemoglobin and melanin.

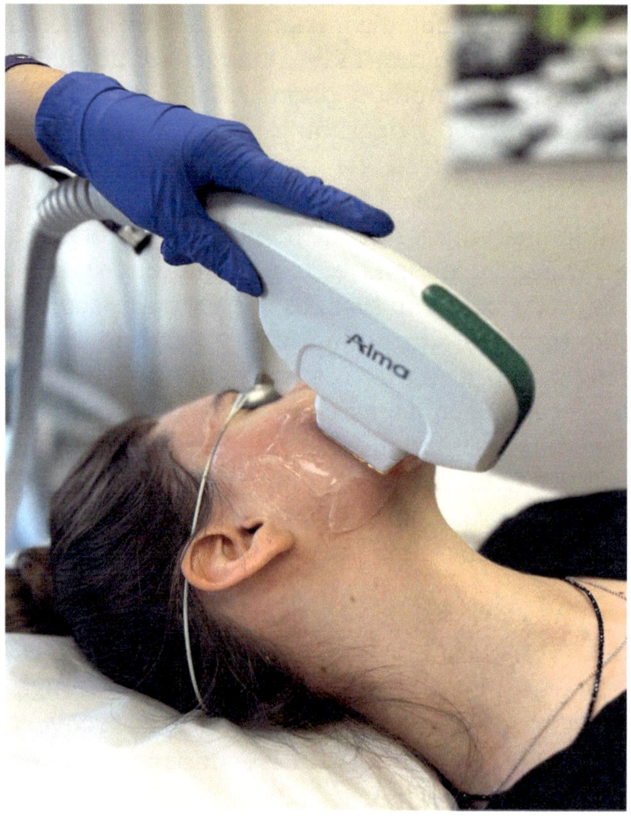

Figure 8.7. Intense pulsed light (IPL) therapy has gained recognition for its versatility and efficacy in treating a variety of skin conditions.

Source: https://www.edgebrookdermatology.com/wp-content/uploads/2023/06/50CD2B9F-6014-4B61-A9B9-5A9949E1A434-scaled.jpg.

This mechanism makes it particularly effective for addressing conditions rosacea and sunspots, thereby improving the skin's texture and tone, reflecting the increasing interest among both practitioners and patients in achieving aesthetic enhancement through non-invasive means. Despite its many benefits, IPL therapy also presents considerations regarding treatment protocols and patient experience. The treatment generally requires multiple sessions to achieve optimal results, with some patients experiencing temporary erythema and swelling post-procedure. It is essential for practitioners to conduct comprehensive consultations to assess skin type, severity of skin condition, and treatment goals. Understanding individual variability in response is essential, as factors such as skin thickness and pigmentation may influence outcomes. To enhance patient comfort, pre-treatment assessments may include the application of topical anesthetics or cooling devices to minimize discomfort during treatment. Thus, patient education surrounding potential side effects and recovery times is crucial for fostering informed decision-making and ensuring a high level of satisfaction with the therapy's outcomes (Figure 8.7).

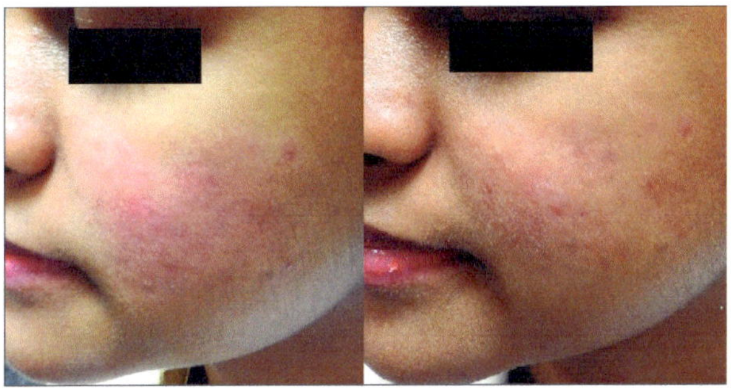

Figure 8.8. A 23-year-old female is showing good improvement following three sessions of IPL.

Source: https://www.researchgate.net/publication/325521181/figure/fig1/AS:11431281152863542@1682181987137/A-23-year-old-female-showing-good-improvement-following-three-sessions-of-IPL.png.

The efficacy of IPL therapy is also supported by its use in aesthetic and therapeutic dermatology, particularly for conditions related to abnormal vascularity and skin pigmentation. Evidence supports its use in rejuvenating aged skin by reducing the effects of sun damage, such as fine lines and open pores, thereby improving overall skin quality. Further, recent studies suggest that the combined use of IPL with other modalities, such as topical therapies, may maximize therapeutic outcomes. The combined approach reflects a growing trend in dermatologic treatment toward customized protocols that employ multimodal strategies to address complex skin conditions with high efficacy. As guidelines evolve, an understanding of the full scope of IPLs capabilities will become essential to clinicians striving to provide evidence-based care sensitive to their patients' diverse needs, particularly in the context of ongoing advancements in laser and light-based therapies, as highlighted by recent developments within the field (Morton et al., 2019; Teede et al., 2023) (Figure 8.8).

8.3.3. Blue Light Therapy for Acne Treatment

The addition of blue light therapy as an acne treatment has attracted considerable interest in dermatology, particularly given its promise of efficacy and non-invasiveness. Blue light therapy is based primarily on the observation that blue light wavelengths will destroy *Propionibacterium acnes*-synthesized porphyrins, a primary causative factor of acne vulgaris. Photodynamic activation of these porphyrins generates reactive oxygen species that kill bacteria while simultaneously inhibiting inflammation. In clinical trials, patients receiving blue light therapy were found to have a notable reduction in inflammatory lesions and, consequently, an overall improvement in skin condition. This is consistent with current trends in laser and light treatments, as dermatologists increasingly turn to alternative therapies that have the potential to reduce antibiotic use and associated resistance issues. However, while blue light therapy has clinical promise, its use is not absolute. Treatment is often multiple sessions in order to maximize effects, with patients potentially requiring further treatments to full manage. Evidence indicates that while blue light therapy has a significant decrease in acne lesions, the duration of its effectiveness is inconsistent for various patients. Additionally, darker-skinned patients may experience post-inflammatory hyperpigmentation after treatment, and dermatologists should exercise caution and adopt individualized approaches. In addition, understanding the pathophysiology of acne vulgaris—microcomedones, seborrhea, and bacterial growth—is critically important when blue light therapy is considered for treatment (Ashton, R., & Weinstein, M., 2019). Finally, blue light therapy is an important addition to the dermatologic armamentarium in the management of acne. Its targeted approach and low side-effect profile make it attractive to both patients and practitioners, reflecting a commitment to safer, more efficient therapeutic options. As the field continues to evolve, ongoing studies are needed to simplify treatment regimens, assess long-term efficacy, and investigate combination therapies that may enhance outcomes. The increasing incidence of antibiotic resistance in acne treatment underscores the importance of alternative treatments, such as blue light, which may enable its future use as a leading dermatologic therapy (Attia et al., 2019) (Figure 8.29).

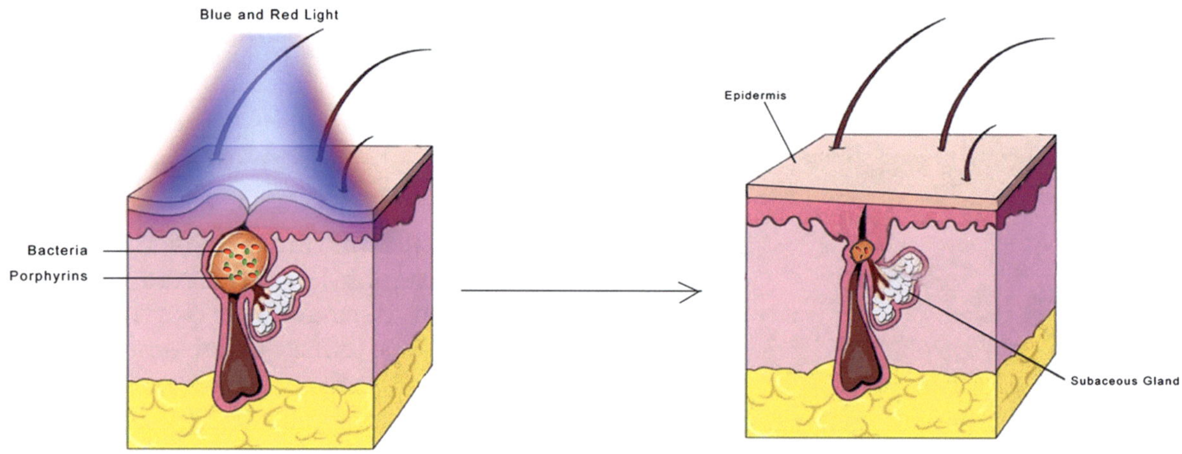

Figure 8.9. Illustration of acne treatment with red and blue light.

Source: https://www.researchgate.net/profile/Michael-Hamblin/publication/256835631/figure/fig4/AS:297904859303948@1448037461251/llustration-of-acne-treatment-with-red-and-blue-lightWhen-used-in-combination-red-light.png.

Test Your Knowledge

1. ow does Photodynamic Therapy (PDT) work, and what skin conditions is it most commonly used to treat?
2. What distinguishes Intense Pulsed Light (IPL) therapy from laser treatments in terms of light emission and clinical applications?
3. What is the mechanism by which blue light therapy helps in the treatment of acne?

8.4. Applications in Dermatology

Learning Outcome

1. Treat skin lesions and scars.
2. Use to hair removal and skin rejuvenation.
3. Manage vascular lesions and pigmentation disorders.

Laser and light therapy have revolutionized dermatology, with numerous applications for a variety of skin conditions. Perhaps their most obvious use is treating dermal pigmentation disorders, particularly among patients of color. Such patients tend to have difficulty with hyperpigmentation, which can significantly impact the quality of their lives since traditional treatment has limitations. Notably, advances in laser technologies, such as Q-switched and picosecond lasers, have revolutionized modalities for the treatment of conditions such as melasma and post-inflammatory hyperpigmentation. There is substantial evidence that these treatments are effective and can cause significant improvement in patients when used appropriately. Additionally, the versatility of laser treatments allows clinicians to tailor protocols to each patient's individual needs, optimizing outcomes and reducing risks, particularly for darker Fitzpatrick skin types, as recent evidence indicates (Garg et al., 2024). In addition to correcting pigmentation disorders, light-based therapies also treat conditions such as acne, rosacea, and vascular lesions. Laser therapies, such as pulsed dye lasers and fractional ablative lasers, offer effective solutions to multifaceted skin conditions. For instance, fractional lasers address issues by delivering energy to targeted skin layers, thereby promoting collagen production and facilitating acne scar repair. Similarly, pulsed dye lasers are specifically designed to treat vascular lesions by inducing selective photothermolytic damage, thereby significantly improving appearance and symptoms. The physics behind the aforementioned technologies is crucial to comprehend because practitioners must masterfully manage the complexity of skin-laser interactions to maximize the success of treatments as well as avoid causing injury to patients (Alhallak, 2021). As research advances, so too will the applications of these cutting-edge treatments for a broad range of dermatologic conditions. In addition to their therapeutic uses, light treatments and lasers also have significant application in cosmetic surgery procedures aimed at enhancing the attractiveness of the skin. Treatments laser hair removal and non-ablative resurfacing have become very popular among patients seeking ways to improve their appearance with little downtime. Laser hair removal targets multiple wavelengths to selectively eliminate the hair follicle with long-term effective hair reduction. Non-ablative lasers also stimulate skin rejuvenation by inducing collagen synthesis in the deeper layers of the skin with minimal disruption to the surface layer. These advancements not only cater to the growing demand for cosmetic treatments but also demonstrate the demand for an ideal comprehension of laser parameters and safety profiles to produce maximum outcomes. Furthermore, as ongoing research provides practitioners with greater knowledge, they can refine existing protocols and develop new methods that progressively improve patient satisfaction and outcomes (Alhallak, 2021).

8.4.1. Treatment of Skin Lesions and Scars

The treatment of skin lesions and scars has been revolutionized by lasers and light-based modalities, which offer effective alternatives to traditional methods. Among the various treatments available, ablative lasers CO2 and Er:YAG have been shown to be important in scar treatment. These lasers function by causing micro-injuries to the skin, which trigger natural wound healing and collagen remodeling, resulting in improved scar texture and appearance. Ablative lasers not only thin the scars but can also alleviate secondary symptoms , such as erythema and pruritus. But post-inflammatory hyperpigmentation, particularly in darker skin types, is a risk that must be addressed with proper patient selection and cautionary treatment planning. With overwhelming evidence of their effectiveness, ablative lasers have gained a foothold in dermatologic practice for the management of keloids and hypertrophic scars, enhancing not only cosmetic outcomes but also patients' quality of life (Nast et al., 2020). Non-ablative laser resurfacing has become an increasingly favored option for less invasive treatment of scarring and skin lesions, particularly for patients seeking low downtime. Pulsed dye laser (PDL) and Nd:YAG lasers are well-illustrated examples of this technique, employing vascular targeting to reduce redness and improve scar appearance. By delivering energy at specific wavelengths, these lasers induce thermocoagulation of target tissue, reducing blood supply to the scar, and evidence further suggests reduced fibroblast proliferation and collagen production. Non-ablative treatments are typically performed in multiple sessions to achieve the desired outcomes and are thus an ideal choice for those patients who have a fear of post-procedure pain and downtime of ablative treatments. Advances in technology and understanding scar physiology have made the procedures more acceptable, and the treatment options would be tailored to each patient's needs (Attia et al., 2019). In addition to laser treatments, combination therapy has also been an effective means in dealing with complex scarring and skin lesions. For instance, combining microneedling with laser therapy leverages the benefits of enhanced collagen stimulation and deeper penetration of topical medications, thereby maximizing therapeutic response. In combination with laser therapy, adjunct treatments , such as intralesional corticosteroids or 5-fluorouracil have also been employed to decrease excess scar tissue, particularly keloids and hypertrophic scars. This multidisciplinary approach promotes a more comprehensive treatment paradigm, fostering an understanding of the multifactorial etiology of scarring, influenced by genetic background, skin type, and prior treatments. As the field evolves, ongoing research into the safety and efficacy of combined modalities promises to refine and expand the potential for the treatment of skin lesions and scars toward an ultimate goal of increased patient satisfaction and aesthetic outcome (Nast et al., 2020) (Figure 8.10).

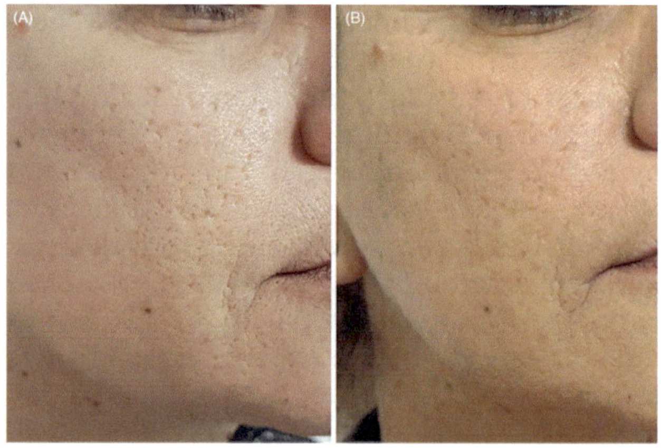

Figure 8.10. Treatment of acne scars with a fractional laser (two sessions). (A) Before treatment, (B) after treatment.

Source: https://www.researchgate.net/publication/347897097/figure/fig5/AS:11431281173864283@1689056664886/Treatment-of-acne-scars-with-fractional-laser-two-sessions-A-Before-treatment-B.png.

8.4.2. Hair Removal and Skin Rejuvenation

The demand for rapid and efficient hair removal has made the use of many laser and light treatments increasingly common in dermatology. Shaving, waxing, and tweezing, traditional methods, have too many drawbacks, being painful, skin-irritating, and temporary in action. Laser hair removal, by contrast, is a long-term solution that targets the hair follicles specifically without damaging the surrounding tissue. This method employs selective photothermolysis, in which light of specific wavelengths is absorbed by pigments in hair follicles, thereby destroying them. With enhanced understanding of skin physiology, the efficacy of these treatments continues to improve, leading to higher patient satisfaction among those who undertake these procedures in pursuit of not only aesthetic value but also functional improvement. Technological improvement in lasers has enabled body hair removal in a safer and more effective manner, which has become common among diverse populations. Skin rejuvenation is another field in which lasers and light therapy have been transformative. Procedures such as fractional laser resurfacing and intense pulsed light therapy (IPL) are commonly used to enhance the skin's texture, tone, and elasticity, correcting concerns such as fine lines, sun spots, and hyperpigmentation. By stimulating collagen production and skin cell turnover, these treatments produce a more youthful appearance with minimal downtime. Moreover, the adaptability of these technologies enables practitioners to tailor treatments to address unique patient needs, thereby enhancing their effectiveness. The body of evidence supporting the benefits of light-based treatments also reiterates their role in cosmetic dermatology. As noted, IPL devices not only facilitate hair removal but also enable efficient treatment of various dermatological conditions, making them important for both therapeutic and cosmetic use (Hüseyin et al., 2019). Furthermore, advancing technology continues to improve the efficacy and safety of laser and light treatments in dermatology. Advances such as sophisticated cooling devices and variable treatment parameters enable accurate and acceptable procedures with a reduced risk of adverse effects. With technological progress, the safety profiles of these technologies require thorough evaluation. For instance, recent studies emphasize the importance of understanding the responses of energy-based devices to skin types, which can facilitate appropriate treatment decisions and ensure patient safety (Heather et al., 2019). Moreover, as practitioners become more knowledgeable about skin anatomy and physiology, they can apply these advances to deliver more accurate therapies, ultimately improving patient outcomes for hair removal and skin rejuvenation. The future of dermatology will see further advances as research and clinical practice continue to evolve in this ever-changing landscape (Figure 8.11).

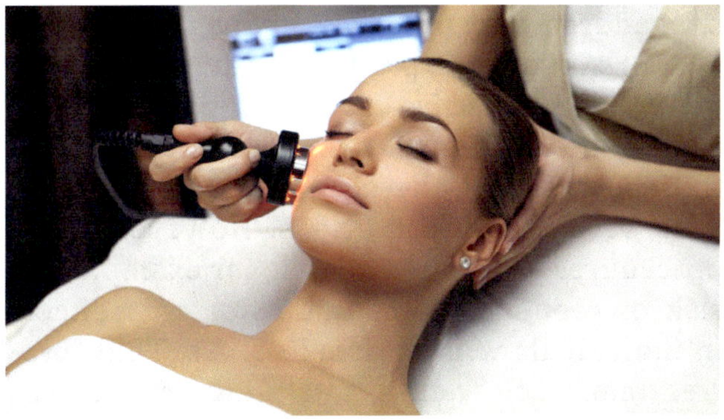

Figure 8.11. Laser Skin Rejuvenation.

Source: https://dermsurgery.net/wp-content/uploads/2024/09/Untitled-design-2024-09-12T105216.382.png.

8.4.3. Management of Vascular Lesions and Pigmentation Disorders

The management of vascular lesions and pigmentation disorders in dermatology has been revolutionized by the advent of laser and light therapy. These newer modalities offer selective, minimally invasive treatments that address the causative pathophysiology of these diseases. For vascular lesions, such as therapies with pulsed dye lasers (PDL) and Nd:YAG lasers, have become standards of care since these can selectively ablate vascular structures with minimal disruption to the overlying tissues. The principle of selective photothermolysis enables practitioners to achieve effective outcomes with reduced discomfort and scarring. Such advancements have enhanced patient satisfaction and quality of life, as they can, in most cases, provide high-quality results with shorter treatment durations than traditional therapeutic interventions, which tend to have longer treatment durations and more frequent side effects (Qu et al., 2022). Pigmentation disorders, such as melasma and post-inflammatory hyperpigmentation, also benefit immensely through the application of laser technology. Fractional ablative laser treatments enable dermatologists to correct hyperpigmented areas and stimulate collagen remodeling. This not only addresses pigmentation but also improves overall skin texture, providing a dual benefit for patients. The selective use of light-based therapy can significantly improve skin color uniformity, thereby reducing the shame often associated with severe skin conditions. However, these procedures carry risks as well, for example, the risk of rebound pigmentation or side effects in individuals with dark skin types. Thus, pre-treatment counseling and judicious patient selection are critical for optimizing outcomes (Nast et al., 2020). A multimodal approach is typically necessary to optimize outcomes in the treatment of vascular lesions and pigmentation. Its use in combination with adjuvant therapy, such as the application of topical agents or systemic medication, is beneficial in enhancing efficacy and minimizing recurrence. For instance, the use of 5-fluorouracil in combination with laser treatment of hypertrophic scars has been shown to be beneficial, illustrating the potential of combination therapy to maximize therapeutic outcomes. Additionally, further studies on the environmental and genetic factors that influence the pathogenesis of these conditions are essential, as they provide opportunities for more targeted treatments. By being foresighted in addressing treatment challenges and acquiring patient-specific information, practitioners can enhance effectiveness and satisfaction by making interventions more specifically tailored, thus innovating the dermatology domain (Qu et al., 2022) (Figure 8.12).

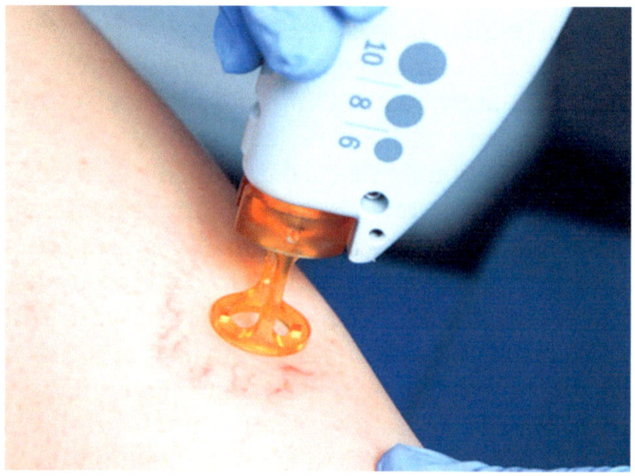

Figure 8.12. Managing vascular lesions by laser.

Source: https://drypskin.com/assets/frontend/img/vascular2.jpg.

Test Your Knowledge

1. How are lasers and light-based therapies utilized in the treatment and remodeling of skin lesions and scars?
2. What types of lasers and light-based devices are most effective for permanent hair removal?

8.5. Benefits of Laser and Light Therapies

Learning Outcome

1. Embrace minimally invasive treatments.
2. Reduce recovery time compared to traditional methods.
3. Treat various skin conditions flexibly.

The addition of laser and light therapy to dermatology has revolutionized treatment, primarily because they can treat a variety of skin diseases with specificity and efficiency. The benefit of such therapies is that they can act specifically, that is, they can treat a specific location without affecting surrounding tissues. Methods such as photobiomodulation (PBM) use light of specific wavelengths to induce cellular responses that promote cell healing and regeneration. The procedure is widely established in various applications, with successful outcomes in wound healing, inflammation reduction, and overall tissue rehabilitation, and thus forms the foundation of contemporary dermatological treatments (Ratnani, G. R., & Vardhan, V., 2022). Additionally, laser and light therapies are not only beneficial for physical dermatological conditions but also integral to enhancing cosmetic outcomes by firming the skin, improving tone, and sharpening the appearance. Modalities such as fractionated laser therapy and intense pulsed light (IPL) have gained popularity due to their effectiveness in reducing pigmentation, vascular irregularities, and signs of aging. By targeting melanin or hemoglobin in the skin, these modalities can significantly diminish unwanted coloration and vascular lesions and restore a more uniform complexion. Furthermore, these non-invasive treatments typically require only brief episodes of downtime, an important consideration for those seeking successful treatments with recovery time concerns (Loyal et al., 2021). The versatility of laser and light treatments is also underscored by their development for a range of dermatological diseases. These include the effective treatment of conditions such as acne, rosacea, and psoriasis, as well as applications in cosmetic interventions. Evidence of this is the mounting evidence regarding the safety and efficacy of these therapies, which underpins their credibility in the practitioner's and patient's eyes. By applying a biphasic dose-response model, treatments can be personalized based on pathology and patient characteristics to maximize therapeutic benefit. With the constant evolution of technology, there is immense scope for new dermatological applications of laser and light therapies, with the potential for continuous improvement in patient care (Ratnani, G. R., & Vardhan, V., 2022).

8.5.1. Minimally Invasive Nature of Treatments

The art of dermatology has come to more fully incorporate minimally invasive procedures that offer significant outcomes with less patient discomfort and downtime. Among the most notable of these are lasers and light therapy, which have become powerful tools for rejuvenating skin and treating other dermatological problems. These methods use advanced technology to target specific skin layers without causing significant trauma to surrounding tissues. For instance, the use of plasma radiofrequency (PRF) ablation, along with topical treatments like resorcinol, is proof of how accuracy leads to enhanced patient satisfaction. In a study, 92% of participants demonstrated significant wrinkle reduction after a single PRF session, supporting the therapeutic efficacy of minimally invasive treatments in addressing skin aging (Giorgio et al., 2025). In addition, the ability of laser treatments to treat many dermatologic disorders attests to the modality's minimally invasive nature. Treatments are usually customized to an individual basis, allowing practitioners to choose specific wavelengths and modulations to suit each patient's unique dermatologic features.

Laser methods, such as the Alexandrite and neodymium-doped yttrium aluminum garnet (Nd: YAG) lasers, have been preferred not just for the extraction of hair, but also because of how well lasers treat hyperpigmentation and vascular lesions. This underscores how laser technology emphasizes the substantial benefits of lasers in delivering results while being conservative toward healthy tissue. Such an approach can lead to shorter recovery times, a lower likelihood of complications, and improved overall patient satisfaction, consistent with growing patient interest in less invasive medical therapies (Gomez et al., 2024). Dermatologic practice is being transformed by the integration of light-based treatments with traditional approaches, thereby enhancing treatment modalities for a variety of disorders. For instance, the use of combination therapies—such as photodynamic therapy (PDT) or cryoinsufflation — for hidradenitis suppurativa (HS) demonstrates the efficacy of minimal invasiveness. These therapies provide relief to patients who otherwise would be afraid of more invasive procedures. By using in-office treatments compatible with local anesthesia and minimal disruption to daily activities, practitioners can better tailor treatments to specific needs. With the rising demand for high-quality, minimally invasive treatments, the continued advancement of laser and light therapy will be a core component of the future of dermatology, thereby maximizing therapeutic outcomes and patient quality of life (Gomez et al., 2024).

8.5.2. Reduced Recovery Time Compared to Traditional Methods

The availability of lasers and light therapies has revolutionized procedures in dermatology, particularly with respect to healing times. Traditional treatments are known to take longer periods of time for healing due to the invasive nature of the surgical procedure. This is as opposed to non-surgical procedures Intense Pulsed Light (IPL) and Ablative Fractional CO2 Lasers (AFCL), which drastically reduce recovery time with good results. For instance, one of the studies on the efficacy of combination IPL-AFCL treatments on burn hypertrophic scars provided evidence of significant reductions in Modified Vancouver Scar Scale (MVSS) scores, which are measures of the effectiveness of scar treatment, along with shorter recovery times compared with conventional procedures. Not only does this technology provide patients with cosmetic improvements, but it also enhances their quality of life, as shorter recovery times allow them to promptly resume their activities (Elkady et al., 2024). Moreover, the quick recovery that accompanies laser treatments reduces significant psychological and physical burdens that patients face following dermatological interventions. Traditional excisional methods involve much pain and lengthy healing time, which leads to patient dissatisfaction and increased healthcare costs due to follow-up appointments and longer care. The reduced recovery time offered by laser treatment is associated with decreased postoperative pain, fewer complications, and a more rapid return to normal daily activities. Comparative studies of surgical techniques, including one examining vulvar cancer, have shown that newer techniques, such as FSDE, can reduce positive margin rates and shorten recovery time. This integrative practice thus enhances healing outcomes and overall patient satisfaction in dermatological treatment (Mujumdar et al., 2024). With the continuous advancement in health, the integration of lasers and light-based technologies into dermatology is likely to unlock further progress in patient care, with emphasis on minimizing recovery times. The promising results achieved in trials made for hypertrophic scars and cancerous lesions indicate a powerful move from traditional surgical procedures towards new treatments with emphasis on patients' healing. As practitioners become more inclined to use these new modalities, they not only facilitate accelerated patient recovery but also improve long-term control of skin disease.

Finally, this new era constitutes a dramatic advance in dermatologic practice; therefore, it is crucial that professionals keep up with training and education on such innovative treatments to offer their patients the best possible care (Elkady et al., 2024; Mujumdar et al., 2024).

8.5.3. Flexibility in the Treatment of a Range of Skin Disorders

Lasers and light treatments are versatile modalities in dermatology, capable of treating a wide range of skin conditions. The reason for their versatility is that they can address various chromophores of the skin, including melanin and hemoglobin, to deliver precise treatment for pigmentation disorders, vascular lesions, and acne. By adjusting parameters such as wavelength, pulse duration, and energy density, treatments can be tailored to the unique needs of each patient and the specific skin condition at hand. The efficacy of lasers, particularly in conditions such as acne and rosacea, not only enhances patient satisfaction but also reduces downtime compared with traditional methods, thereby highlighting their growing role in contemporary dermatology practice. In addition to superficial disorders, light treatments and lasers play a role in the treatment of more serious skin conditions, including photoaging and scarring.

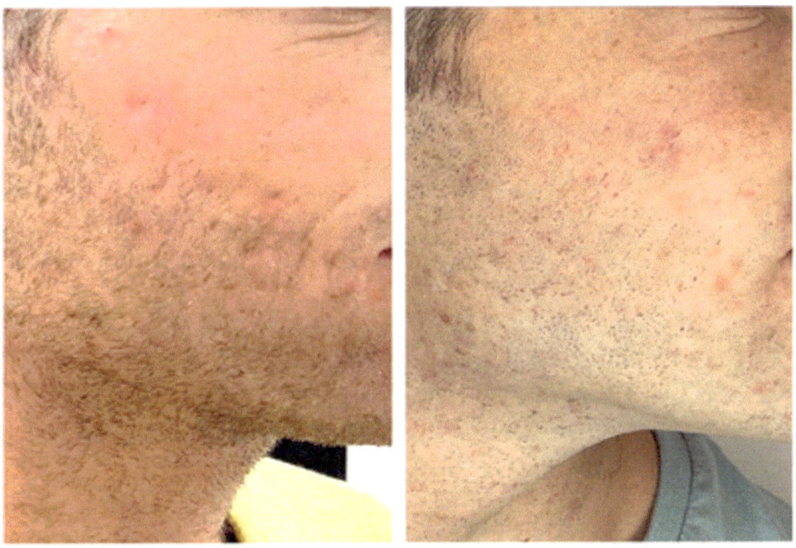

Figure 8.13. Treatment with the 675 nm laser was performed on a male patient in the cheek area. The baseline and the follow-up 3 months after the last treatment are shown.

Source: https://www.researchgate.net/publication/375048152/figure/fig3/AS:114312812456859 37@1716206089252/Treatment-with-the-675nm-laser-performed-on-a-male-patient-cheek-area-The-baseline-and.png.

Fractional laser therapy, for example, has significantly advanced the treatment of atrophic scars by promoting collagen remodeling and skin rejuvenation. Furthermore, light-sensitive biomaterials have expanded the range of dermatologic treatments, enabling new applications such as photodynamic therapy for precancerous lesions and skin cancer. The integration of light-powered materials has been instrumental in the development of non-invasive, patient-friendly treatment protocols that enhance the therapeutic experience, reduce complications, and shorten recovery time. Such flexibility enhances applicability, enabling the design of patient- and skin-type-specific intervention strategies. Continued advances in laser technology and the discovery of new light-sensitive materials foreshadow a promising future for dermatological applications. Nanotechnology discoveries further complicate this field by enabling researchers to explore novel material properties and behaviors that can be used in skin treatments. The case of zinc oxide nanoparticles (ZnO NPs) illustrates how emerging compounds can be used for their novel therapeutic properties, thereby promoting the treatment of many skin ailments. Light-responsive biomaterials also enable the design of noninvasive instruments that modulate drug delivery with specificity and control cell behavior. As these advancements continue, the future of dermatology is poised to undergo revolutionary transformations, encompassing not only efficacy but also the personalization and safety required in patient care (Lee, H. P., & Gaharwar, A. K., 2020; Raha, S., & Ahmaruzzaman, M., 2022) (Figure 8.13).

Test Your Knowledge

1. How does the minimally invasive nature of laser and light therapies benefit patients compared to traditional surgical dermatology treatments?
2. In what ways do laser and light-based treatments offer shorter recovery times and downtime for patients?

8.6. Risks and Side Effects

Learning Outcome

1. Understand common side effects of lasers and light-based therapies.
2. Describe potential complications (e.g., scarring, hyperpigmentation).
3. Explain the importance of patient selection and pre-treatment assessment.

The use of lasers and light-based therapies in dermatology has revolutionized the treatment of numerous skin disorders; however, these modalities are associated with side effects and risks. The patient may develop any one of a range of side effects including erythema, edema, and hyperpigmentation as a result of techniques like laser resurfacing or intense pulsed light therapy. These reactions typically manifest as skin responses to energy delivered during treatment; although they are usually transient, they can affect long-term facial appearance. It is essential for dermatologists to clearly inform patients of these risks and set realistic expectations regarding recovery and outcomes. More specifically, information regarding an individual's response to treatment, as well as past skin problems, can rule out extreme reactions to therapy. In addition, one of the greatest concerns with many laser therapies is the formation of scarring, potentially brought about by improper protocols. Scarring can result from unskilled technique, excessive energy input, or negligence in post-treatment care, underscoring the importance of skilled practitioners in their administration. In addition, certain patients, particularly those who possess darker skin tones, are at risk of developing post-inflammatory hyperpigmentation complications. To address such issues, professionals also recommend pre-treatment assessment to determine skin types and tailor interventions to the respective conditions. Therefore, encouraging individualized treatment can significantly reduce the incidence of side effects and optimize therapeutic outcomes in laser and light therapy in dermatology. Furthermore, the unique side effects of separate treatments, such as PUVA treatment, place additional emphasis on intensive patient education prior to treatment onset. PUVA, combining the use of psoralen medication with exposure to UVA radiation, is a potent therapy for psoriasis but carries risks in the way of photoaging and increased susceptibility to skin cancers with prolonged use. This necessitates ongoing diligence in post-treatment patient monitoring to mitigate risks. Current initiatives, such as the creation of teaching videos and step-by-step guides, are intended to further inform patients regarding PUVA therapy, discussing both the advantages and risks of receiving it. By informing patients, they can actively participate in their care, thereby increasing adherence and satisfaction with outcomes, which are crucial elements in managing long-term dermatologic conditions such as psoriasis, which require continuous therapy (Abrouk et al., 2016).

8.6.1. General Side Effects (e.g., Redness, Swelling)

In dermatology, light-based and laser treatments are increasingly used to treat a range of skin diseases. As with every type of therapeutic therapy, however, the treatments do have side effects, which in most cases are swelling and redness. These tend to be indicators of the skin's inflammatory response to the energy delivered in the process.

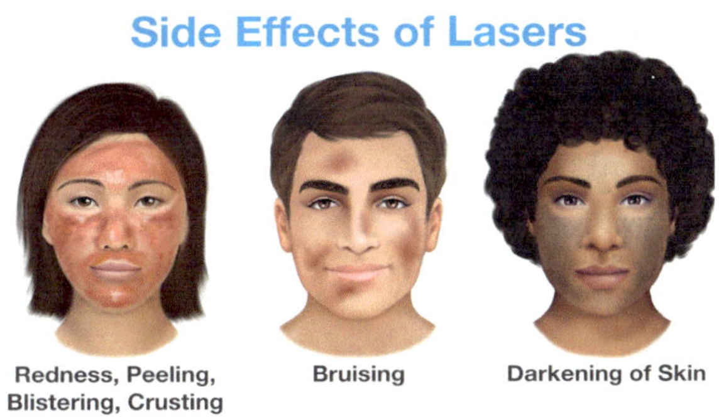

Figure 8.14. Side effects of lasers.

Source: https://www.acne.org/wp-content/uploads/2022/08/Article-124-Image-4.1.jpg.

Redness (erythema) can result from selective heating of the dermal layers, which stimulates blood flow to the affected area as part of the healing process. While these reactions could be alarming for the patients, these tend to subside within a few days, depending on the patient's skin type and the level of treatment administered. Understanding these common reactions is valuable for both practitioners and patients, enabling the negotiation of expectations and a smoother post-procedural experience. Edema, or swelling, is also a common side effect following laser and light treatments. It results from localized inflammation, most often an essential response to start the healing process. The extent of swelling may also vary with the type of treatment used and the patient's specific skin type. A more intense treatment that penetrates deeper into the skin, for instance, can cause greater skin swelling than a less intensive treatment focused on surface-level spots. Knowledge of such potential side effects enables practitioners to provide appropriate pre- and post-procedural care, thereby improving outcomes. Exercising caution, such as the application of cold compresses, can also greatly reduce pain and the persistence of these effects following treatment (Dhawn et al., 2022). Complicating the issues with laser and light treatments are additional potential side effects, including scarring and changes in pigmentation. Though the vast majority of patients develop only transient redness and swelling, patients with darker complexions are potentially at higher risk of developing post-inflammatory hyperpigmentation. That is when the skin releases excess melanin due to inflammation, which can raise aesthetic concerns. Thus, both patients and dermatologists must weigh the benefits of each treatment against the risks. Research has established that the use of specific light-emitting technologies pre-, intra-, and post-treatment may counteract harmful effects, including fibrosis and extensive scarring, thereby optimizing patient outcomes and overall treatment satisfaction (Heilman et al., 2019). Intentional side effect planning and corresponding mitigation remain relevant to the evolution of aesthetic dermatology (Figure 8.14).

8.6.2. Potential Complications (e.g., Scarring, Hyperpigmentation)

In dermatological laser treatments, scarring and hyperpigmentation remain potential complications to be treated by practitioners. Scarring, particularly hypertrophic scarring and keloiding, can occur after laser treatment because of an overwound healing response. Not only do these complications influence the cosmetic outcome of the treatments, but the patient's psyche is also involved. Risk of scarring can also be defined by multiple factors like the skin type, the kind of laser employed, and the condition being treated. Practitioners then need to employ rigorous techniques and modulate their practice based on patient-by-patient evaluation to minimize these risks. Investigation of the mechanisms of scar formation is required to integrate effective laser therapy and ensure both safety and optimal clinical outcomes (Garg et al., 2024). This delicate balance between efficacy and managing complications improves the quality of overall care in dermatology. Scarring is not the only complication that is a frequent result of laser procedures, as hyperpigmentation is also a common effect, especially in darker-skinned patients. Hyperpigmentation can take the form of post-inflammatory discoloration, which poses a challenge in the treatment of skin diseases such as melasma or post-inflammatory hyperpigmentation. The risk is higher in situations in which lasers penetrate the dermal layers and activate melanocytes to produce excess melanin. Existing evidence shows that some laser modalities, such as Q-switched and picosecond lasers, are effective in treating dermal pigmentary disorders but have the potential to cause post-treatment hyperpigmentation, especially on Fitzpatrick skin types IV-VI (Garg et al., 2024).

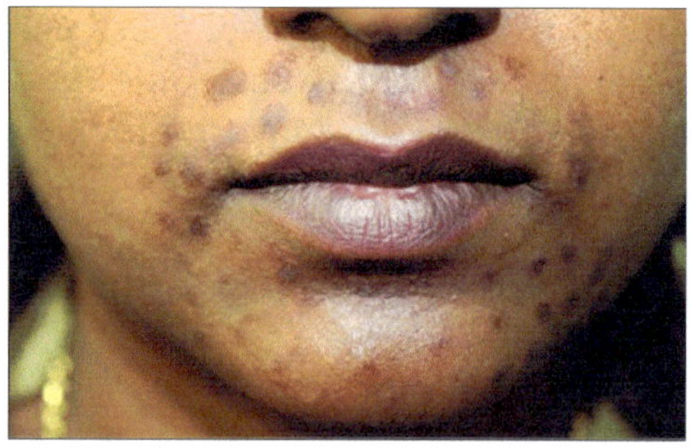

Figure 8.15. Postinflammatory hyperpigmentation after diode laser for hair removal.

Source: https://www.researchgate.net/publication/329727847/figure/fig2/AS:1023654955597825@1621069768365/Postinflammatory-hyperpigmentation-after-diode-laser-for-hair-removal.png.

Hence, professionals must possess a sound understanding of appropriate laser technologies and protocols to minimize the risk of hyperpigmentation and maximize therapeutic outcomes. The risk of complications, such as scarring and hyperpigmentation, causes laser methods and protocols to change dynamically in dermatology. For instance, as outlined in recent publications, enhancing efficacy while minimizing side effects is a focus of progress in laser technologies. Research on sequential laser therapy highlights its capacity to decrease dermal pigmentation at a safer treatment pathway, particularly in hyperpigmentation-susceptible skin types (Janocha et al., 2024). Practitioners are also encouraged to apply pre-treatment screening that rigorously assesses patient history and skin type, enabling tailored treatment options in accordance with individual risk factors. As studies continue and clinical trials focus on refining laser protocols, the dermal community is well positioned to further refine techniques that effectively reduce the incidence of complications, producing a more positive patient experience for those seeking resolution of skin issues (Figure 8.15).

8.6.3. Importance of Patient Selection and Pre-Treatment Assessment

Patient selection and preoperative assessment are most important to successful outcomes in dermatologic therapy using lasers and light. Efficacy and safety with these modalities largely rely upon patient-specific characteristics, including skin type, medical illness, and specific dermatologic illnesses. For instance, certain laser treatments may function less well or have greater dangers for patients with more melanized skin due to increased absorption of the laser wavelength by the pigmentation, highlighting the necessity for individualized evaluation to prevent complications. In addition, a thorough evaluation can identify contraindications , such as photosensitivity or skin condition, allowing treatment programs to be individualized for optimal results with minimal side effects in patients who are suitable candidates for such treatments. Not only does pre-treatment evaluation assess patient suitability, but it also provides a valuable basis for education and informed consent. Patients must be informed about the benefits, risks, and anticipated outcomes of their desired therapy. In this regard, the doctor is responsible for establishing realistic expectations and conditioning the patient to the procedure process. For example, prospective patients must be counseled on potential side effects and the recovery period, thereby enabling better informed decisions. This interaction enhances patient adherence to treatment and follow-up care, ultimately resulting in improved therapeutic outcomes and safer patient care. Combined, effective communication at this stage is critical for establishing confidence and ensuring a smooth transition to the treatment process. Furthermore, the significance of an efficient patient selection process is promoted by advancements in recent laser technology that permit an increased scope of applications for various dermatological disorders. But as treatments become more diverse and complex, so also does the opportunity for abuse or over-treatment, necessitating more rigorous selection parameters. The use of novel nanotechnology-based carriers for laser treatment of skin cancer, for instance, is an example of particular patient criteria in optimizing therapeutic potential while minimizing risk from highly aggressive treatment protocols (Chehelgerdi et al., 2023). As the field advances, standardized parameters for patient choice and pre-treatment assessment will become important for effectively addressing the complexities of laser and light-based therapy, ensuring that patients receive personalized care based on the latest scientific evidence (Northrup et al., 2021).

Test Your Knowledge

1. What are the most common side effects experienced after cosmetic dermatology procedures?
2. What steps can practitioners take to minimize the risks of adverse effects during and after dermatological treatments?

SUMMARY

In concluding the analysis of lasers and light-based treatments in dermatology, it is evident that these technologies represent a significant breakthrough in the treatment of a wide range of skin conditions. The effectiveness of laser treatment, particularly in treating pigmentation disorders, supports the pivotal role of such technologies in clinical practice. A thorough review identifies that picosecond and Q-switched lasers have been invaluable technologies, particularly for the treatment of hyperpigmentation prevalent in skin-of-color patient populations. This is something that has been reinforced by studies that recommend personalized protocols for individual skin types and diagnoses, commenting on how critical it is to understand the mechanisms behind these therapies as well as the intricacies of skin reaction to light therapy (Garg et al., 2024). Its ongoing development promises more safety and effectiveness, thereby expanding the way for more efficient treatment modalities that are custom-fit to address the different needs of patients. Not limited to pigmentation problems, light therapies also encompass inflammatory dermatoses such as acne vulgaris. This systematic review of the prevalent disorder across skin types demonstrates that, despite the suggestion that laser and light treatments are potent interventions, there remains a significant lacuna in the literature, particularly regarding their efficacy in patients with skin of color. This underscores the need for ongoing research that accounts for the unique physiological characteristics of darker skin tones, as most existing recommendations rely to a considerable extent on studies that predominantly involve Caucasian participants (Pathmarajah et al., 2022). In their bid to optimize treatment results, this deficit further underscores the need for evidence-based practice to accommodate different ethnicities and enhance the quality of care across all patients. In summary, the inclusion of laser and light treatments in dermatology is a milestone in the management of skin disorders. They have both been shown to be effective across a range of indications, from hyperpigmentation to acne vulgaris, but further research is required to develop evidence-based treatment plans that account for the heterogeneity of skin types among patients. As barriers to effective treatment continue to emerge, the dermatology clinic stands at a juncture at which the development of patient-tailored protocols can significantly improve quality of life. A commitment to advancing knowledge and practice in this area will equip dermatologists with the tools to provide high-quality care to all patients in accordance with their skin type, thereby creating a more levelled healthcare ecosystem (Pathmarajah et al., 2022; Garg et al., 2024).

In dermatology, laser and light therapies are a significant advancement in treatment modalities that have proven to have a host of applications for hair removal, tattoo removal, and the management of other skin conditions , such as acne and rosacea. These therapies harness the unique properties of light to treat superficial and deeper skin structures with precision and efficacy. The therapy of these treatments typically discusses both the science behind their mechanisms, such as selective photothermolysis, and the clinical outcomes derived from various studies. Therefore, understanding the efficacy and safety profiles of various laser systems has become essential for practitioners seeking to maximize patient satisfaction while minimizing side effects. Along with this, progress in laser technology, and specifically in the development of fractional laser systems, has revolutionized the method of treating dermatological diseases. Fractional lasers enable the selective delivery of laser energy to discrete areas of the skin, thereby promoting faster healing and reducing recovery times compared with conventional ablative techniques. This improved strategy has increased demand for patient laser treatments, thereby strengthening the incentive for clinicians to maintain familiarity with emerging technologies and their implications. Increasing evidence in the literature indicates the importance of tailored treatment protocols that incorporate individual patient variables to optimize outcomes and successfully treat diverse dermatological diseases. The integration of new research and clinical practice is essential to the continued evolution of lasers and light-based treatments in dermatology. Ongoing research aims to establish stronger evidence-based guidelines for treatment protocols, emphasizing recommendations to enhance clinical decision-making. Additional discussion highlights the integration of nanotechnology into dermatological laser therapy, specifically the use of nanoparticles for targeted drug delivery to patients, thereby enhancing the efficacy of phototherapy. Collectively, these observations reinforce the merits of multidisciplinary practice and a commitment to implementing the best available evidence to inform practice in dermatology and to maximize patient care outcomes (Raha, S., & Ahmaruzzaman, M., 2022; Teede et al., 2023).

KEY TERMS FROM THIS CHAPTER

- 5-aminolevulinic acid (5-ALA)
- Adjuvant therapy
- Cellular metabolism
- CO2 laser
- Cosmetic enhancement
- Cytotoxic effects
- Dermatological conditions
- Dermatological industry
- Evidence-based care
- Actinic keratoses
- ATP production
- Chronic inflammation
- Combination therapy
- Cosmetic treatments
- Dermatologic armamentarium
- Dermatological diseases
- Dermatology domain
- Fractional ablative lasers

CRITICAL THINKING QUESTIONS

1. **What is the primary mechanism of action for lasers used in dermatology?**
   a. Chemical alteration of skin cells
   b. Selective photothermolysis targeting specific chromophores
   c. Increasing skin temperature uniformly
   d. Mechanical removal of skin layers
2. **Which of the following is a commonly used laser type for hair removal in dermatology?**
   a. CO_2 laser
   b. Excimer laser
   c. Nd:YAG laser
   d. Pulsed dye laser
3. **Intense Pulsed Light (IPL) therapy is best described as:**
   a. A laser emitting a single wavelength of light
   b. A type of cryotherapy
   c. Ultrasound-based skin therapy
   d. A broad-spectrum light source with multiple wavelengths
4. **Which dermatological condition is most effectively treated using pulsed dye laser therapy?**
   a. Acne vulgaris
   b. Port-wine stains (vascular lesions)
   c. Melasma
   d. Onychomycosis
5. **One of the key benefits of laser and light-based therapies in dermatology is:**
   a. Complete elimination of all skin disorders without side effects
   b. Instantaneous skin regeneration
   c. Targeted treatment with minimal damage to surrounding tissues
   d. Ability to treat only deep tissue disorders

Short Answer Questions

1. What is the basic mechanism of action by which lasers and light-based therapies target skin tissues in dermatological treatments?
2. What are the main types of lasers used in dermatology, and how do their wavelengths and target chromophores differ?
3. How do non-laser light-based therapies, such as intense pulsed light (IPL) and photodynamic therapy (PDT), differ from traditional laser treatments?
4. What are the primary dermatological conditions and applications for which laser therapies are commonly used?
5. How do light-based therapies benefit patients compared to traditional dermatological treatments?
6. What are the common short-term and long-term risks or side effects associated with laser and light-based dermatological treatments?

Answer to Critical Thinking Questions

1. (b); 2. (c); 3. (d); 4. (b); 5. (c)

REFERENCES

1. Farahnik, B., Nakamura, M., Singh, R. K., Abrouk, M., Zhu, T. H., Lee, K. M., Jose, M. V., DaLovisio, R., Koo, J., Bhutani, T., & Liao, W. (2016). The Patient's Guide to Psoriasis Treatment. Part 2: PUVA phototherapy. *Dermatology and Therapy, 6*(3), 315–324. https://doi.org/10.1007/s13555-016-0130-9Alhallak, K. (2021). Skin, light and their interactions: An in-depth review for modern light-based skin therapies. *Clinical Dermatology and Therapy, 7*, 1–15. https://doi.org/10.24966/cdt-8771/100081 (accessed on 21st July 2025).
2. Altshuler, G. B., Anderson, R. R., Bashkatov, A. N., Booth, S., Buscone, S., Chung, J. H., et al. (2017). Shedding light on the variability of optical skin properties: Finding a path towards more accurate prediction of light propagation in human cutaneous compartments. https://core.ac.uk/download/153515826.pdf (accessed on 21st July 2025).
3. Anders, J. J., Arany, P. R., Azevedo, L. H., Babilas, P., Barolet, D., Basso, F. G., Bellono, N. W., et al. (2016). Photobiomodulation devices for hair regrowth and wound healing: A therapy full of promise but a literature full of confusion. https://core.ac.uk/download/76945843.pdf (accessed on 21st July 2025).
4. Anzalone, A., Carlesimo, M., Caro, G., Fortuna, M. C., et al. (2016). Multi-therapies in androgenetic alopecia: Review and clinical experiences. https://core.ac.uk/download/54535222.pdf (accessed on 21st July 2025).
5. Ashton, R., & Weinstein, M. (2019). Acne vulgaris in the pediatric patient. *Pediatrics in Review, 40*, 577–589. https://doi.org/10.1542/pir.2018-0137 (accessed on 21st July 2025).
6. Attia, A. B. E., Balasundaram, G., Moothanchery, M., Dinish, U. S., Bi, R., Ntziachristos, V., & Olivo, M. (2019). A review of clinical photoacoustic imaging: Current and future trends. *Photoacoustics, 16*, 100144–100144. https://doi.org/10.1016/j.pacs.2019.100144 (accessed on 21st July 2025).
7. Bailey, E. C., Hamilton, T. A., Kang, S., Orringer, J. S., et al. (2010). Photodynamic therapy for acne vulgaris: A randomized, controlled, split-face clinical trial of topical aminolevulinic acid and pulsed dye laser therapy. https://deepblue.lib.umich.edu/bitstream/2027.42/79403/1/j.1473-2165.2010.00483.x.pdf (accessed on 21st July 2025).
8. Bankova, L., Elsner, P., Fluhr, J. W., Fuchs, A., et al. (2005). Photodynamische Therapie (PDT) und wassergefiltertes Infrarot A (wIRA) bei Patienten mit therapierefraktären vulgären Hand- und Fußwarzen. https://core.ac.uk/download/14504309.pdf (accessed on 21st July 2025).
9. Benson, H. A. E., Grice, J. E., Mohammed, Y., Namjoshi, S., & Roberts, M. S. (2019). Topical and transdermal drug delivery: From simple potions to smart technologies. *Current Drug Delivery, 16*, 444–460. https://doi.org/10.2174/1567201816666190201143457 (accessed on 21st July 2025).
10. Boffa, M. J. (2004). *Dermatology*. https://core.ac.uk/download/46601884.pdf (accessed on 21st July 2025).
11. Chehelgerdi, M., Chehelgerdi, M., Allela, O. Q. B., Cosme Pecho, R. D., Narayanan, J., Rao, D. P., Thamaraikani, T., et al. (2023). Progressing nanotechnology to improve targeted cancer treatment: Overcoming hurdles in its clinical implementation. *Molecular Cancer, 22*. https://doi.org/10.1186/s12943-023-01865-0 (accessed on 21st July 2025).

12. Chen, C., Wang, P., Zhang, L., Liu, X., Zhang, H., Cao, Y., Wang, X., et al. (2023). Exploring the pathogenesis and mechanism-targeted treatments of rosacea: Previous understanding and updates. *Biomedicines, 11*, 2153–2153. https://doi.org/10.3390/biomedicines11082153 (accessed on 21st July 2025).
13. Cramer, S. W., & Chen, C. C. (2020). Photodynamic therapy for the treatment of glioblastoma. *Frontiers in Surgery, 6*. https://doi.org/10.3389/fsurg.2019.00081 (accessed on 21st July 2025).
14. Dhawan, S., Kandhari, R., Madnani, N., Nischal, K., et al. (2022). Expert opinion on pre and post procedure care in aesthetic dermatology. https://core.ac.uk/download/539912253.pdf (accessed on 21st July 2025).
15. Dias, L. D., Blanco, K. C., de Faria, C. M. G., Dozza, C., Zanchin, E. M., Paolillo, F. R., Zampiéri, K. R., et al. (2022). Perspectives on photobiomodulation and combined light-based therapies for rehabilitation of patients after COVID-19 recovery. *Laser Physics Letters, 19*, 045604–045604. https://doi.org/10.1088/1612-202x/ac52f5 (accessed on 21st July 2025).
16. Dover, J. S., Liu, C., Watchmaker, J., Wang, J. V., Geronemus, R. G., Arndt, K. A., & Anderson, R. R. (2025). The history and advancement of light, lasers, and energy-based devices in dermatologic surgery. *Dermatologic Surgery, 51*, 113–122. https://www.semanticscholar.org/paper/c0ab7c098beaec3b99d2b1a428ff39850fc8859e (accessed on 21st July 2025).
17. Durmuş, H. O., Çetin, E., Karaböce, B., & Seyidov, M. H. Y. (2019). Investigation of the temperature effect of the IPL therapy device on tissue-mimicking material. *AIP Conference Proceedings*. https://doi.org/10.1063/1.5135399 (accessed on 21st July 2025).
18. Elkady, D., Larson, B. M., Sharma, S., Lou, R., & Khandelwal, A. (2024). 81 Effectiveness of simultaneous intense pulsed light and fractional CO_2 laser therapy in hypertrophic burn scars. *Journal of Burn Care & Research: Official Publication of the American Burn Association, 45*, 64–64. https://www.semanticscholar.org/paper/6d552524786f2e87db57179cd27a6d2f60b63da1 (accessed on 21st July 2025).
19. Garg, S., Vashisht, K. R., Garg, D., Oberoi, B., & Sharma, G. (2024). Advancements in laser therapies for dermal hyperpigmentation in skin of color: A comprehensive literature review and experience of sequential laser treatments in a cohort of 122 Indian patients. *Journal of Clinical Medicine, 13*, 2116–2116. https://doi.org/10.3390/jcm13072116 (accessed on 21st July 2025).
20. Georgescu, S. R., Mitran, C. I., Mitran, M. I., Popa, D., et al. (2019). Photodynamic therapy as a new therapeutic approach of oral lichen planus. https://core.ac.uk/download/216811053.pdf (accessed on 21st July 2025).
21. Giorgio, C. M., Licata, G., Di Brizzi, E. D., Babino, G., Fulgione, E., Moscarella, E., Lodi, G., et al. (2025). Facial skin rejuvenation through plasma radiofrequency ablation combined with 5% resorcinol cream: Clinical and LC-OCT evaluation. *Dermatology Reports*. https://www.semanticscholar.org/paper/310bfc483c3f270374490acd9da33fdc3e5221cf (accessed on 21st July 2025).
22. Gomez, J., Fonjungo, F. E., Chen, S. X., Aleshin, M. A., Naik, H., Wadhera, A., Sayed, C. J., et al. (2024). In-office procedures for dermatologists managing hidradenitis suppurativa. *Current Dermatology Reports*. https://www.semanticscholar.org/paper/a24d057d408a35b25e3c14341b49a80b2755e90f (accessed on 21st July 2025).

23. Heilman, E., Isseroff, R. R., Jagdeo, J. R., Jakus, J., et al. (2019). A dose-ranging, parallel group, split-face, single-blind phase II study of light emitting diode-red light (LED-RL) for skin scarring prevention: Study protocol for a randomized controlled trial. https://core.ac.uk/download/323070347.pdf (accessed on 21st July 2025).

24. Janocha, A., Ziemba, P., Jerzak, A., & Jakubowska, K. (2024). Clinical use of lasers and energy-based devices in selected skin diseases. *Journal of Education, Health and Sport.* https://www.semanticscholar.org/paper/1c24dc05e4cc811f7fb4565fe765682b6dc58923 (accessed on 21st July 2025).

25. Juhász, M., Zachary, C. B., & Cohen, J. L. (2021). Ocular complications after laser or light-based therapy—Danger's dermatologists should know. *Dermatologic Surgery, 47*, 624–629. https://doi.org/10.1097/dss.0000000000002974 (accessed on 21st July 2025).

26. Lee, H. P., & Gaharwar, A. K. (2020). Light-responsive inorganic biomaterials for biomedical applications. *Advanced Science, 7.* https://doi.org/10.1002/advs.202000863 (accessed on 21st July 2025).

27. Loyal, J., Carr, E., Almukhtar, R., & Goldman, M. (2021). Updates and best practices in the management of facial erythema. *Clinical, Cosmetic and Investigational Dermatology, 14*, 601–614. https://www.semanticscholar.org/paper/31b4dcfd57b69cd3b578f85a36b91e0980fdeba4 (accessed on 21st July 2025).

28. Morton, C. A., Szeimies, R. M., Basset-Séguin, N., Calzavara-Pinton, P., Gilaberte, Y., Hædersdal, M., Hofbauer, G. F. L., et al. (2019). European Dermatology Forum guidelines on topical photodynamic therapy 2019 Part 1: Treatment delivery and established indications–Actinic keratoses, Bowen's disease and basal cell carcinomas. *Journal of the European Academy of Dermatology and Venereology, 33*, 2225–2238. https://doi.org/10.1111/jdv.16017 (accessed on 21st July 2025).

29. Mujumdar, V., Brown, J., Crane, E. K., Lees, B., Puechl, A., Casablanca, Y., & Naumann, R. W. (2024). A prospective, randomized, single-blinded study evaluating the effect of frozen-section directed excision on positive surgical margins in high-grade vulvar dysplasia. *Journal of Clinical Oncology*. https://www.semanticscholar.org/paper/792f30244a9f4e090bbbd2a47693653d90e2a96a (accessed on 21st July 2025).

30. Nast, A., Gauglitz, G. G., Lorenz, K., Metelmann, H. R., Paasch, U., Strnad, V., Weidmann, M., et al. (2020). S2k guidelines for the therapy of pathological scars (hypertrophic scars and keloids) – Update 2020. *JDDG Journal der Deutschen Dermatologischen Gesellschaft, 19*, 312–327. https://doi.org/10.1111/ddg.14279 (accessed on 21st July 2025).

31. Northrup, H., Aronow, M. E., Bebin, E. M., Bissler, J. J., Darling, T. N., de Vries, P. J., Frost, M., et al. (2021). Updated international tuberous sclerosis complex diagnostic criteria and surveillance and management recommendations. *Pediatric Neurology, 123*, 50–66. https://doi.org/10.1016/j.pediatrneurol.2021.07.011 (accessed on 21st July 2025).

32. Oh, C. S., Karim, M., Klein, E. J., Yin, L., Gutierrez, D., Shapiro, J., & Sicco, K. (2024). Light-based therapies in the treatment of alopecia. *Dermatology Online Journal, 30*(5). https://www.semanticscholar.org/paper/a7469993b42218cbb6a7b03d3b06abf91cc8ecb7 (accessed on 21st July 2025).

33. Paasch, U., & Grunewald, S. (2020). Update on dermatologic laser therapy II–Advances in photodynamic therapy using laser-assisted drug delivery. *JDDG: Journal der*

Deutschen Dermatologischen Gesellschaft, 18. https://www.semanticscholar.org/paper/add43ee0b6ebd1aa63e351af4896424ba86a8e03 (accessed on 21st July 2025).

34. Paasch, U., & Grunewald, S. (2020). Update on dermatologic laser therapy II–Advances in photodynamic therapy using laser-assisted drug delivery. *JDDG Journal der Deutschen Dermatologischen Gesellschaft, 18*, 1370–1377. https://doi.org/10.1111/ddg.14339 (accessed on 21st July 2025).
35. Passeron, T., Genedy, R. M., Salah, L. A., Fusade, T., Kositratna, G., Laubach, H. J., Marini, L., et al. (2019). Laser treatment of hyperpigmented lesions: Position statement of the European Society of Laser in Dermatology. *Journal of the European Academy of Dermatology and Venereology, 33*, 987–1005. https://doi.org/10.1111/jdv.15497 (accessed on 21st July 2025).
36. Pathmarajah, P., Peterknecht, E., Cheung, K., Elyoussfi, S., Muralidharan, V., & Bewley, A. (2022). Acne vulgaris in skin of color: A systematic review of the effectiveness and tolerability of current treatments. *PubMed, 15*, 43–68.
37. Piccolo, D., Crisman, G., Bollero, D., Bovani, B., Gennai, A., Melfa, F., Matteo, T., et al. (2023). Ear keloids: An innovative 3-steps combined treatment. *Skin Research and Technology, 29*. https://doi.org/10.1111/srt.13506 (accessed on 21st July 2025).
38. Qu, F., Geng, R., Liu, Y., & Zhu, J. (2022). Advanced nanocarrier- and microneedle-based transdermal drug delivery strategies for skin diseases treatment. *Theranostics, 12*, 3372–3406. https://doi.org/10.7150/thno.69999 (accessed on 21st July 2025).
39. Raha, S., & Ahmaruzzaman, M. (2022). ZnO nanostructured materials and their potential applications: Progress, challenges and perspectives. *Nanoscale Advances, 4*, 1868–1925. https://doi.org/10.1039/d1na00880c (accessed on 21st July 2025).
40. Ratnani, G. R., & Vardhan, V. (2022). A mini review on photo-biomodulation: Novel approach. *Journal of Pharmaceutical Negative Results*. https://www.semanticscholar.org/paper/b1366f34285e53de4d5bbac7702a928a7d747b73 (accessed on 21st July 2025).
41. Taşaltın, N., Nnamchi, P. S., & Saud, S. (2020). *Advanced Functional Materials*. IntechOpen eBooks. https://doi.org/10.5772/intechopen.87879 (accessed on 21st July 2025).
42. Teede, H., Tay, C. T., Laven, J. J. E., Dokras, A., Moran, L., Piltonen, T., Costello, M., et al. (2023). Recommendations from the 2023 International evidence-based guideline for the assessment and management of polycystic ovary syndrome. *The Journal of Clinical Endocrinology & Metabolism, 108*, 2447–2469. https://doi.org/10.1210/clinem/dgad463 (accessed on 21st July 2025).

CRYOTHERAPY, ELECTROSURGERY, AND CHEMICAL PEELS

9

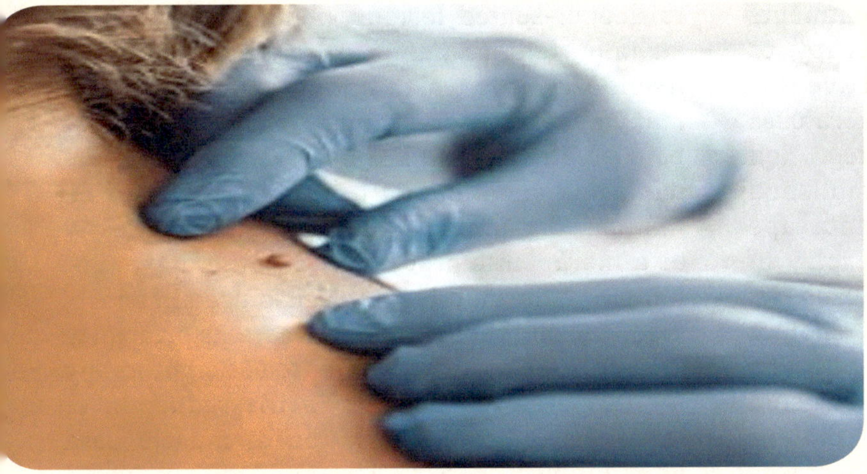

Introduction

Management of skin diseases has evolved to a large degree, with multiple techniques to address various dermatological issues in an effective manner. Among such procedures, cryotherapy, electrosurgery, and chemical peeling are widely practiced for their efficacy in removing abnormal skin growths, enhancing cosmetic appearance, and treating a range of skin disorders. Cryotherapy entails the application of extreme cold to freeze and destroy abnormal cells, and is particularly effective for removing lesions such as warts and precancerous lesions. Electrosurgery applies high-voltage electrical currents to ablate and kill tissue, and is beneficial for precise excisions and targeted treatment of skin cancers. Chemical peeling involves the application of a chemical solution to the scraping of the skin, resulting in the skin being smoother and having improved tone. All these modalities share the same ultimate goal: improving skin health, and they employ distinct mechanisms to address various dermatologic conditions. In recent years, clinicians have sought new avenues alongside traditional treatment methods

LEARNING OBJECTIVES

After studying this chapter, you will be able to:

1. Understand historical background of cryotherapy, electrosurgery, and chemical peels
2. Discuss about mechanisms of action underlying cryotherapy, electrosurgery, and chemical peels
3. Describe the application of cryotherapy, electrosurgery, and chemical peels in medicine
4. Explain benefits of cryotherapy, electrosurgery, and chemical peels in dermatological treatments
5. Deal with risks and side effects associated with cryotherapy, electrosurgery, and chemical peels
6. Focus on comparative effectiveness of cryotherapy, electrosurgery, and chemical peels

due to the growing need for safe, effective, and non-invasive therapies. For instance, hyperspectral imaging systems are becoming powerful adjuvants in the early diagnosis and evaluation of skin cancers, demonstrating the utility of accurate pre-surgical assessments. These technologies enhance treatment precision, enabling better control of skin conditions with fewer unnecessary procedures. Moreover, advancements in photosensitizer formulation in photodynamic therapy have provided new avenues to enhance the efficiency of treatments , such as daylight photodynamic therapy, to make them feasible and cost-effective for managing conditions , such as actinic keratoses (Fang et al., 2022). Therefore, the integration of innovative technologies with established techniques continues to reshape the landscape of dermatological treatment. The interplay of cryotherapy, electrosurgery, and chemical peels reveals not only the magnitude of the choices that are available to dermatologists, but also the sheer imperative of carefully constructed regimes tailored to meet individual patient needs. While the incidence of skin cancer rises globally, effective early diagnosis and treatment regimens are essential in the ongoing fight against skin malignancies. It could become a standard factor for improved patient outcomes and to reduce the burden on healthcare systems (Fang et al., 2022). By understanding the unique properties and applications of each technique, practitioners can more effectively address challenging skin conditions, thereby enabling more successful therapy protocols. The remainder of this chapter will elaborate on the mechanisms, indications, and developments of cryotherapy, electrosurgery, and chemical peels, presenting a synoptic overview of their roles in contemporary dermatological practice.

Definition of Cryotherapy

Cryotherapy, in its definition, is the process of using extremely low temperatures to kill specifically abnormal or diseased tissue. Cryotherapy has been used extensively in the medical specialties, but particularly in dermatology, wherein it is employed as a therapeutic modality for a range of skin lesions. The mechanism of action of cryotherapy is controlled freezing, followed by cell destruction. During this process, the formation of intracellular ice leads to osmotic lysis and secondary necrosis. With localized targeting, clinicians can efficiently address such conditions ranging from individual warts and skin tags to deeper-seated lesions, making cryotherapy an important resource in dermatology. Given its efficacy, it is worth noting that, despite the many benefits of cryotherapy, the process must be correctly applied if the risk of inadvertently damaging surrounding healthy tissue is to be minimized, pointedly underlining its complexity as a therapeutic procedure. Cryotherapy is not limited to dermatology; it is also used in sports medicine and rehabilitation, where its principles are applied. Sportsmen prefer to use cryotherapy for its perceived benefits in the reduction of inflammation and alleviation of muscle pain after intense exercise. Its application is based on the physiological effects of cold, which can lead to vasoconstriction and, subsequently, reduced metabolic activity and inflammation in the affected tissues. Cryotherapy is applied in postoperative management to assist recovery through pain relief and edema reduction. However, clinical application of cryotherapy introduces a number of concerns, that is, timing, duration, and temperature used, that critically influence outcome. These variables present challenges to therapists to maintain an optimal balance between optimizing therapeutic effect and preventing potential side effects.

Despite its various applications, cryotherapy remains a topic of debate and investigation among medical practitioners regarding its safety and effectiveness. A detailed understanding of the mechanisms behind is crucial to describe its use in various clinical situations. For instance, although cryotherapy has been associated with rapid recovery in certain ailments, concerns regarding tissue injury and the potential for adverse responses remain valid. Secondly, as proposed in the literature, practitioners must be well informed about the indications and contraindications of cryotherapy to prevent patient injury and ensure desired outcomes. Complete overviews of cryotherapy's benefits and drawbacks are capable of building clinical policies and informing patients about the dangers of this kind of therapy. Thus, a balanced discussion of cryotherapy's definition and implementation is necessary to establish its use in medical treatment, both therapeutic and cosmetic (Figure 9.1).

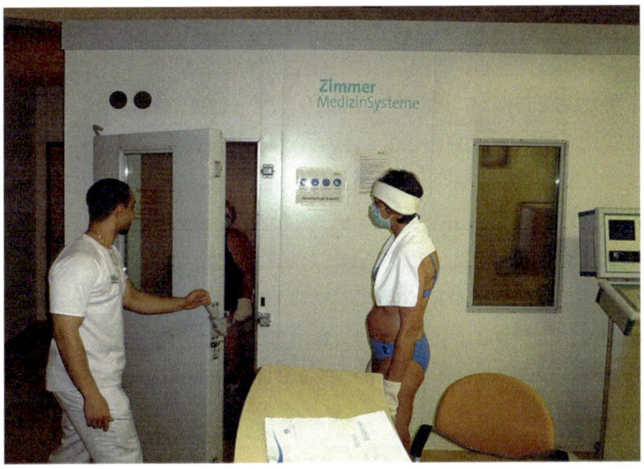

Figure 9.1. Cryotherapy patients during preparation of treatment.

Source: https://upload.wikimedia.org/wikipedia/commons/thumb/a/a8/Cryo-Therapy_Chamber_Entry.JPG/800px-Cryo-Therapy_Chamber_Entry.JPG.

Overview of Electrosurgery

Electrosurgery is now a mainstay technique in contemporary medical practice, employing electrical energy to induce tissue coagulation and hemostasis. Electrosurgical devices operate under the delivery of high-frequency electrical currents that may either cut or coagulate soft tissues, depending on the waveform and mode used. This modality is particularly useful for minimizing blood loss, a significant problem in most surgical interventions. By efficiently cauterizing vessels at the cut site, surgeons can enhance visibility and reduce operative time, making electrosurgery imperative in both minor cuts and major incisions. In response, technological advancements in monopolar and bipolar system integration have broadened its utility, from dermatological procedures to complex internal organ operations, thereby emphasizing its adaptability in the surgeon's toolkit. In dermatological practice, electrosurgery is used to treat a variety of skin diseases in the most effective way for the removal of neoplasms and cosmetic surgery. The method is not only efficient in removing benign and malignant lesions but also reduces the severity of surrounding tissue damage, thereby facilitating faster recovery. Using instruments like the radiofrequency electrosurgical unit, doctors are able to target and destroy unwanted lesions in a most accurate manner without requiring deep incisions. This is particularly useful in patients with actinic keratosis or seborrheic keratosis, in whom standard surgical treatments have a high complication rate or result in more visible scarring. Electrosurgery also synergizes with other forms of treatment, such as cryotherapy and chemical peeling, to provide total therapies in the management of numerous skin conditions. The synergy among these techniques enables customized patient therapy with maximal clinical benefit and cosmetic preservation. With the evolving skin cancer treatment landscape, electrosurgery has emerged at the forefront for its potential to preventively treat precancerous conditions using advanced imaging techniques. Sophisticated imaging devices , such as hyperspectral imaging systems (HIS) allow accurate and minimally invasive diagnosis of skin lesions based on enhanced visual discrimination of tissue characteristics, as mentioned in recent reports. This provides the opportunity for electrosurgery not only to heal clinically apparent lesions but also to restore skin cancer in earlier stages of development, in line with research emphasizing the need for timely and effective measures for growing cases of skin cancer (Neittaanmäki-Perttu, 2015). Furthermore, the integration of electrosurgery with modalities such as HIS represents a new trend toward the convergence of diagnostic and therapeutic procedures, significantly enhancing the precision and reliability of pre-surgical assessments. These advances portend an era of teamwork for electrosurgery, positioning it as a foundation in dermatological practice and oncologic procedures (Figure 9.2).

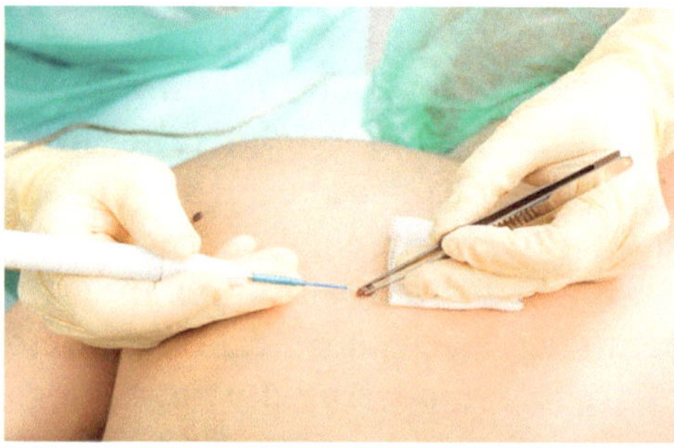

Figure 9.2. Electrosurgery for warts.

Source: https://i0.wp.com/azaleahealthandskin.com/wp-content/uploads/2022/02/ashland-kentucky-electrosurgery-doctor.jpg?fit=600%2C397&ssl=1.

Explanation of Chemical Peels

Chemical peels are a complete dermatologic treatment to enhance the appearance and texture of the skin using various chemical solutions. These chemicals induce the controlled removal of the epidermis and, occasionally, the dermis, thereby stimulating skin regeneration and collagen production. The depth of the chemical peel—superficial, medium, or deep—is determined by the type of agents used and the desired result. Superficial peels usually use alpha hydroxy acids (AHAs), such as glycolic acid, to treat superficial skin issues, while deeper peels may use trichloroacetic acid or phenol for more severe skin imperfections. The adaptability of chemical peels in treating a wide range of conditions makes them desirable for correcting acne, hyperpigmentation, and photoaging, underscoring their place in current skin rejuvenation procedures. The efficacy of chemical peels is demonstrated in the treatment of several skin disorders, and they are increasingly employed in dermatological procedures. For instance, in the management of hyperpigmented lesions, chemical peels can serve as an adjunct to or alternative to laser treatment, particularly when the use of high-energy equipment poses a risk of exacerbating the skin disorder. While chemical peels significantly improve tone and texture of the skin, clinicians must carefully evaluate the patient's skin type and history to avoid undesirable side effects, such as hypopigmentation or inflammation. It is the significance of this evaluation that is highlighted in guidelines for laser treatment, whereby subtle information regarding the individual's skin condition directly determines treatment selection (Passeron et al., 2019). Therefore, understanding the mechanisms and potential implications of chemical peels is important to practitioners wishing to optimize patient satisfaction and safety. Chemical peels can also be integrated into comprehensive skincare regimens, which, in many situations, would make topical products such as retinoids more effective. The combination of chemical peels with these therapies has been demonstrated in various studies on conditions such as actinic keratosis, in which retinoids are used to prevent skin cancer (Ianhez et al., 2013). This combination exemplifies the holistic approach to dermatology, combining procedural and topical therapies. As science evolves, ongoing research and clinical trials will continue to determine optimal regimens for combining chemical peels with other treatments, thereby enriching the practice of dermatologic skin care. With advances in knowledge, practitioners can provide customized therapy plans that meet dermatological standards to produce successful, safe, and rewarding outcomes for patients seeking skin rejuvenation (Figure 9.3).

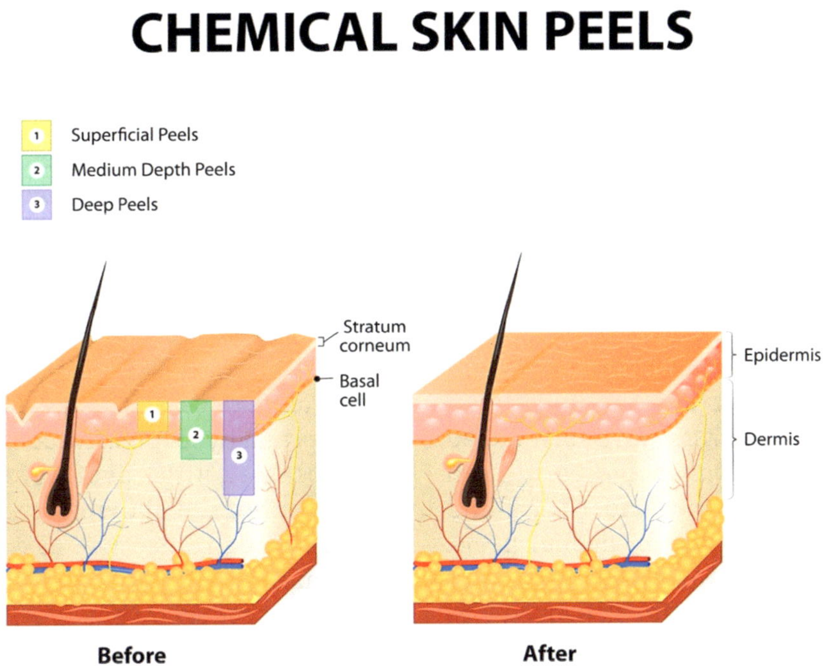

Figure 9.3. Chemical peel skin.

Source: https://dermalife.co.in/blog/wp-content/uploads/2020/06/chemical-peel-skin-1.jpg.

9.1. Historical Background

Learning Outcome

1. Understand the origins of cryotherapy.
2. Focus on the development of electrosurgery techniques.
3. Deal with the evolution of chemical peel methods.

Cryotherapy has its roots in ancient history, with cold treatments being administered as primitive curative measures. The Greeks and Romans were particularly famous for experimenting with cold therapy for disease, applying ice and snow to alleviate pain and inflammation. The first method established a foundational model that endured for centuries to guide the medical use of cryotherapy. By the first two decades of the 20th century, improvements in refrigeration technology enabled more controlled and potent uses of cold, such that it was more widely incorporated in medical practices. The understanding of the efficacy of cryotherapy in the management of localized tumors and skin lesions at the time created a paradigm shift, moving it from an anecdotal treatment to a scientifically validated modality in contemporary medicine. Electrosurgery, which employs high-frequency electrical currents to incise tissue and control bleeding, shares similarly deep historical roots. The science traces back to the findings of Nikola Tesla and the early electrical scientists of the late 19th century. These pioneers demonstrated that electricity could generate sufficient heat to sever soft tissue, thereby improving surgical engineering. The practical clinical use of electrosurgery finally began to take hold in the mid-20th century, as methods and equipment improved, becoming more precise and less traumatic for patients. Surgeons became more supportive of electrosurgical units because they could combine cutting and coagulation into a single instrument, thereby revolutionizing surgical procedures across a variety of specialties. Of particular note is that the technique has undergone continuous improvement, and one of the resulting technologies is radiofrequency ablation (Richard et al., 2011-09-21). Chemical peeling, which aims to impart a youthful appearance through controlled exfoliation, also has a rich history. The use of natural acids in cosmetics dates back to ancient Egypt, when women applied milk and honey to achieve smoother skin, demonstrating a primitive appreciation for the beneficial effects of chemical exfoliants. More formalized processes became prevalent in the early 20th century, with trichloroacetic acid (TCA) and phenol used by dermatologists for deeper peels. With increased research, information on skin types and peel depths has enhanced procedures in cosmetic dermatology. Today, chemical peels are classified as superficial, medium, or deep to allow practitioners to tailor procedures to individual patient needs. This development underscores the growing scientific support and aesthetic applications of chemical peels in dermatological practice (Richard et al., 2011).

9.1.1. Cryotherapy Origins

The origins of cryotherapy date back thousands of years, and there is evidence from various ancient cultures that enjoyed the therapeutic effects of cold. Egyptians, for example, used ice and snow to relieve pain and treat injuries, and Hippocrates, the father of medicine, wrote in support of cold baths as a therapeutic agent. This initial application of cold therapy laid the groundwork for the modern concept of cryotherapy, which has since evolved significantly in medical science. Cryotherapy is now characterized by more precise, technologically advanced methods, a shift from anecdotal use to evidence-based application. As scientists continue to explore the physiological effects of cold stress on the human body, the historical roots of cryotherapy suggest its long-standing acceptance as a viable medical modality. Over the course of the 20th century, developments in medical science propelled cryotherapy into new avenues, taking it from ancient practices to a formalized therapeutic application. The advent of liquid nitrogen in the mid-1900s marked a turning point, enabling more efficient and controlled procedures in dermatology and surgery. This enabled practitioners to precisely target specific tissues while causing minimal damage to the surrounding areas. The establishment of cryosurgical methods gave a significant boost to treating skin lesions, tumors, and certain hyperpigmented disorders, absolutely complementing available dermatological interventions. Following the establishment of the European Society of Laser Dermatology and the emphasis on evidence-based practice, clinical use of cryotherapy has grown significantly. It is nowadays integrated into a wider variety of dermatologic procedures, adding to treatment with methods like electrosurgery and chemical peels (Passeron et al., 2019).

In contemporary clinical practice, cryotherapy is not only a popular analgesic but also a preservative and a tissue-regenerative agent. The two benefits of cryotherapy—its immediate symptomatic relief from inflammation and its long-term healing—are most evident in both cosmetic and therapeutic applications. In dermatology, the therapy is effective in treating a broad range of conditions, from benign skin lesions to precursor lesions, and it augments the efficacy of lasers and chemical peeling. As more insight into cryotherapy is disseminated, practitioners are increasingly seeking its synergistic use with other therapeutic modalities, highlighting its complexity and versatility. Through ongoing clinical research and investigation, the origins of cryotherapy continue to evolve, revealing more about how cold exposure can be used to promote healing and enhance aesthetic outcomes in medicine (Amornyotin et al., 2022) (Figure 9.4).

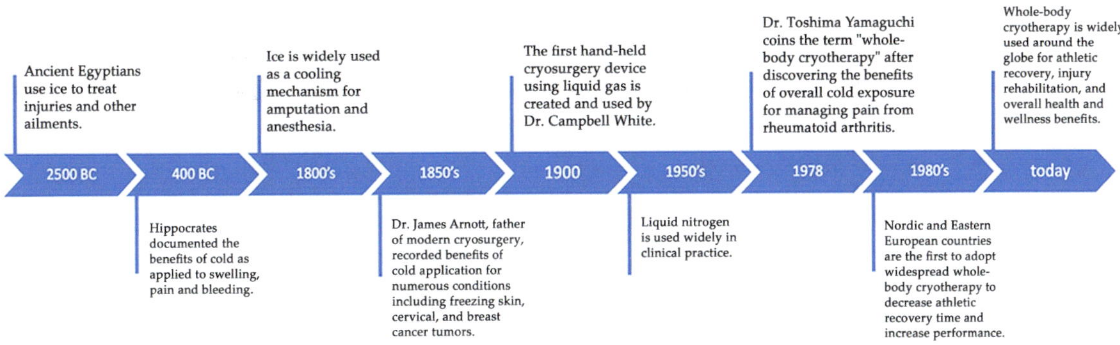

Figure 9.4. The history of cryotherapy.

Source: https://bodyforlife.com.au/wp-content/uploads/timeline.webp.

9.1.2. Development of Electrosurgery Techniques

Advancements in electrosurgery techniques have significantly affected the practice of dermatologic surgery, particularly the management of skin neoplasms. Electrosurgery has changed the course of surgical procedures by providing an alternative to conventional cutting instruments, in which electrical currents are used to incise tissue while coagulating blood vessels simultaneously. Not only does it reduce bleeding, but it also minimizes the time required for surgery, making the procedures more efficient and safer for the patient. As physicians and scientists began to explore the potential of electrosurgery, technological advancements in equipment and methods followed, enabling more precise treatments. These technological advancements have taken on particular significance in managing conditions such as actinic keratosis, which electrosurgery has been able to treat with high clinical study success rates. These improvements portray how electrosurgical methods are modified to manage patients' needs and are a valuable addition to the dermatologist's toolkit. In recent years, the use of specialized electrosurgical devices, such as high-frequency generators, has widened the scope of application of procedures in many dermatological diseases. For instance, electrosurgery is particularly valuable in the elimination of benign neoplasia's , such as syringomas, where patients are most often confronted with cosmetic problems. Studies have found that even though traditional excision remains the most dominant procedure, electrosurgical procedures offer minimally invasive methods with improved outcomes and shorter recovery time. The use of equipment that enables precise energy delivery has also played an important role in minimizing thermal damage to surrounding tissues. The popularity of electrosurgery in cosmetic dermatology, therefore, continues to increase, showing the direction towards effectiveness as well as aesthetics. The trend indicates the need to continue research to establish and simplify electrosurgical applications specific to certain dermatological disorders. With the increasing use of electrosurgery, it is crucial to compare its application with other current therapies, such as cryotherapy and chemical peels. Proof shows that electrosurgical treatments tend to outdo traditional methods in some instances actinic keratosis treatment, in which cryotherapy was found to have an effect rate of 72.8% compared to just 40.9% by trichloroacetic acid peels (Ridha, I. M., & Sabir, H. J., 2019). Furthermore, persistent reports in the medical literature support the comparative efficacy of various electrosurgical applications for tumors and delineate promising knowledge gaps for therapeutic decision-making (Haddad et al., 2022). These results encourage critical evaluation of treatment choices and emphasize evidence-based practice in dermatologic decision-making. The integration of these modalities underscores a trend toward individualized medicine, in which patient outcomes drive the ongoing evolution of electrosurgical techniques and their integration into overall treatment regimens (Figure 9.5).

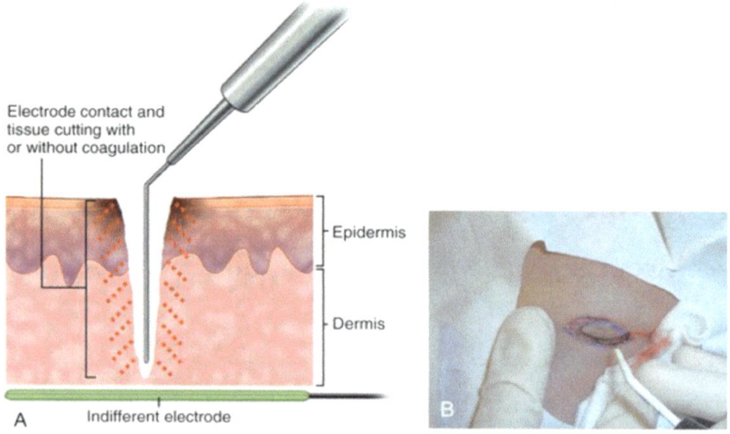

Figure 9.5. (A) In electrosection, the unit is set so that the electrode cuts the tissue. This mode requires an indifferent electrode. (B) Electrosection is being performed with a very thin tip electrode attached to a Surgitron. An indifferent electrode is placed under the patient near the surgical site.

Source: https://plasticsurgerykey.com/wp-content/uploads/2016/03/B9781437705805000145_f014-004ab-9781437705805.jpg.

9.1.3. Evolution of Chemical Peel Methods

Advances in chemical peel techniques reflect ongoing improvements in cosmetic dermatology, enhancing skin appearance and addressing various cutaneous disorders. Mild peels with alpha-hydroxy acids (AHAs) were initially popularized for their lower invasiveness and reduced risk. These peels were used to address surface defects such as fine lines and superficial pigmentation and were made available to the general patient population. As treatment demand rose, practitioners began to formulate deeper peels using trichloroacetic acid (TCA) and phenol to treat more severe skin conditions, such as deep wrinkles and moderate scarring. The introduction of these new formulations marked a watershed moment in the approach to skin rejuvenation, enabling tailored treatment to meet individual patient requirements. Knowledge of the skin's biochemical response to these procedures has played an important role in advancing chemical peel techniques. Research into why particular agents penetrate to varying depths within the skin has led to greater safety and effectiveness. As skin reactions were learned by dermatologists, they began introducing combination treatments, pairing chemical peels with other technologies, such as laser therapies, in order to further enhance aesthetic outcomes. Laser, as it was discussed by experts, has been found effective for problems that chemical peeling is unable to correct on its own, such as certain pigmentary disorders (Passeron et al., 2019). This suggests a multimodal approach in which chemical peels must be combined with other methods to maximize patient satisfaction and achieve optimal results. The practice of chemical peels today is characterized by more individualized treatment planning. Today's dermatologists weigh the patient's skin type, personal skin concerns, and cosmetic goals before prescribing a specific chemical peel. This alteration has enabled careful tailoring of agents and peel strengths to address each patient's needs. Furthermore, as understanding of potential side effects has increased, so has emphasis on proper patient selection and pre-treatment education. The indications for chemical peels now extend beyond beautification to encompass broader dermatological concerns, including malignancy prevention in certain skin types (Fathi et al., 2019). This expansion reflects a deeper understanding of chemical peel application in general skin care, further solidifying their place within the broader practice of dermatology (Figure 9.6).

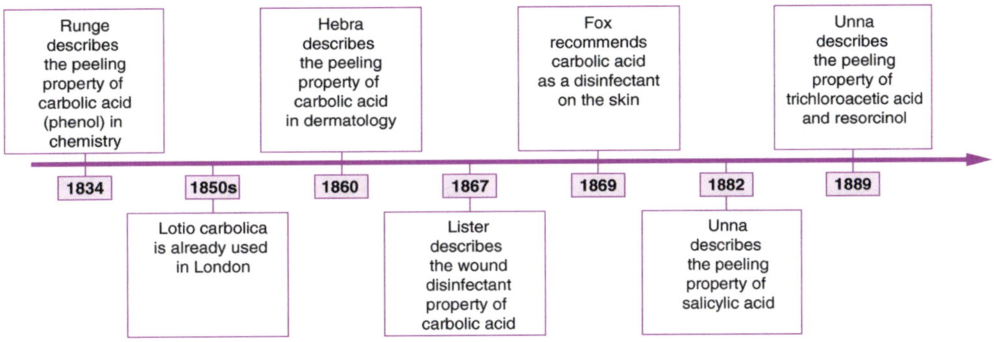

Figure 9.6. Timeline of the rise of chemical peeling in 19th-century European dermatology.

Source: https://onlinelibrary.wiley.com/cms/asset/1df198ed-2fb9-4c10-b38c-c31513669a98/jdv16307-fig-0005-m.jpg.

Test Your Knowledge

1. In which century did cryotherapy first gain medical interest?
2. What was the first chemical used in early chemical peels?

9.2. Mechanisms of Action

Learning Outcome

1. Explain how cryotherapy affects tissue.
2. Discuss the principles of electrosurgery.
3. Describe chemical processes involved in chemical peels.

The mechanisms of action of cryotherapy involve the application of extreme cold to the skin, resulting in localized cellular destruction. It begins with the freezing of the area to be treated and the formation of ice crystals. As temperature decreases, cell membranes become destabilized, leading to cellular lysis and death. The cryotherapy-induced tissue destruction not only effectively eliminates proliferating cells, such as those present in actinic keratoses abnormally, but also causes a localized inflammatory reaction. The healing and regeneration are promoted by the inflammation and result in the clearance of cellular debris. With the skin cell recovery, the cells can be made to appear more youthful. Therefore, cryotherapy can be not only a damaging therapy but also a rejuvenating and reparative agent, thereby increasing its efficacy as a dermatological treatment. Electrosurgery employs electrical currents in order to achieve multiple therapeutic goals, primarily through tissue destruction and coagulation. The action mechanism involves generating heat via high-frequency electrical currents to denature proteins and vaporize tissue. This result enables precise destruction of target lesions with minimal damage to surrounding normal tissue. In surgical interventions, electrosurgery effectively excises warts, moles, and other benign skin tumors, as well as cauterizes the blood vessels at the same time to curtail bleeding. Remarkably, recovery following electrosurgical procedures is shorter than that following traditional surgery, as the procedure is non-surgical and minimally invasive. As more physicians become adept at using this technology, the use of electrosurgery expands, treating a multitude of dermatologic conditions with great success. Chemical peels are another valuable modality in dermatology, based on the use of chemical agents to induce exfoliation and promote skin rejuvenation. The fundamental mode of action is controlled use of acids, such as alpha-hydroxy acids or trichloroacetic acid, that increase desquamation of the epidermis. On penetration, these agents produce a controlled destruction that activates the body's own healing mechanism. This not only results in the removal of the damaged superficial layers but also produces increased collagen synthesis, which leads to better skin texture and tone. Most commonly used to treat acne, sunspots, and fine lines, chemical peels can be adjusted in strength to achieve the desired depth of penetration. Mechanisms are guided by advancing research, with a focus placed on employing them for the treatment of benign as well as severe dermatoses, such as those contained in actinic keratoses, which have a high propensity for evolving into skin cancer (Berlin, 2010).

9.2.1. The Way Cryotherapy Affects Tissue

Cryotherapy, or cold therapy, is a treatment modality used to treat a wide range of dermatologic conditions by inducing controlled tissue necrosis. Severe cold can very simply lead to killing pathologic cells , such as warts and actinic keratoses. Following cryotherapy, the diseased tissue undergoes acute cooling, leading to vasoconstriction and eventual loss of blood supply. This action not only limits oxygen delivery to the target tissue but also induces a localized inflammatory response during rewarming, thereby recruiting immune cells to the area. Therefore, the involved tissue is rehabilitated with healthier cells, and an induced healing response can be particularly valuable in the treatment of superficial skin lesions and neoplastic diseases, effectively managing the biological potential of such skin involvement (Fang et al., 2022).

Analysis of the cellular reaction to cryotherapy reveals a multidimensional interaction of the physiological processes, which underscores its efficacy. At the cellular level, cryotherapy induces apoptosis—the regulated cell death that is responsible for the removal of deformed or abnormal cells. Simultaneously, the freezing process induces the formation of ice crystals in the tissue, which leads to cell lysis and necrosis in highly damaged tissue. The subsequent phase of thawing and rewarming induces angiogenesis, the formation of new blood vessels that drive tissue regeneration. This regenerative capacity not only accounts for the physical feel of skin but also underlies the overall process by which lesions heal. Such physiological alterations need to be explained since they reflect how cryotherapy is able to effectively re-establish normal tissue homeostasis, thereby achieving better clinical outcomes in dermatological treatment (Romero et al., 2023). In addition, cryotherapy's used not only for therapeutic purposes but also as a low-risk treatment for recalcitrant skin diseases. This effectiveness could be augmented with the application in combination with other treatment modalities chemical peels or electrosurgery, to enhance the overall therapeutic effect. Cryotherapy can pre-treat the skin for subsequent interventions by reducing inflammation and promoting an optimal healing environment. It has been particularly beneficial in the management of precancerous lesions, where its selective destruction of tissue minimizes the risk of malignant transformation. It is appropriate for use in conditions such as actinic keratosis, where regular follow-up and management are warranted to prevent the development of skin cancer. As research continues to uncover how cryotherapy alters tissue responses, its applications in dermatological practice remain relevant and are evolving (Fang et al., 2022) (Figure 9.7).

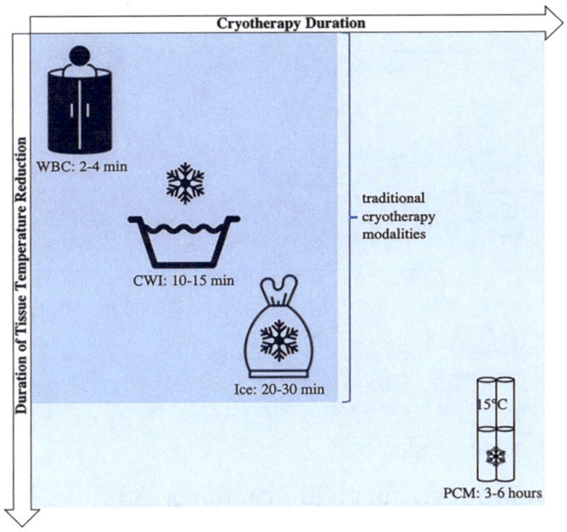

Figure 9.7. Cryotherapy duration and its effect on the duration of tissue temperature reduction.

Source: https://www.researchgate.net/profile/Susan-Kwiecien/publication/351005475/figure/fig2/AS:1143128111627746 3@1675220446025/Cryotherapy-duration-and-its-effect-on-duration-of-tissue-temperature-reduction-The.png.

9.2.2. Principles of Electrosurgery

Electrosurgery, a vital process applied in modern surgical procedures, employs high-frequency alternating current to excise or coagulate tissue. The technique differs from traditional surgical techniques in that it is more precise and entails less blood loss, thereby improving patient outcomes. Electrosurgery relies on the conversion of electrical energy into heat, which vaporizes tissue within the cell. Surgeons capitalize on this attribute for dissecting delicate tissues, allowing complicated procedures that call for an excellent level of control. As technology has improved, electrosurgical equipment has become more sophisticated and incorporates elements that enhance safety and efficacy, such as automatic current modulation and smoke evacuators, minimizing the risks of plume generation during surgery. Thus, electrosurgery became a basic instrument in the surgeon's armamentarium, paving the way to newer modalities for tissue manipulation. The basic applicability of electrosurgery extends beyond basic excision, encompassing several modes of application, such as cutting, coagulation, and fulguration. Each has a specific purpose: cutting is focused on incising tissues, coagulation on achieving hemostasis, and fulguration on destroying superficial lesions. Specifically, the ability of the electrosurgical technique to be tailored to the unique requirements of an array of procedures makes it more clinically relevant. Additionally, the ability to understand the laws governing the interaction between electrical and tissue currents is paramount for optimal benefit. The current frequency, electrode type, and tissue resistances can all significantly contribute to the success of the procedure. By controlling these variables, clinicians can adapt electrosurgical procedures to optimize patient safety and treatment effectiveness, thereby reaffirming the value of continuing education and training in this multifaceted discipline. Nevertheless, the practice of electrosurgery is not free from difficulties. Surgeons have to work around possible complications, such as thermal trauma to surrounding tissues and electrical system malfunctions. It is imperative to the practitioner's skills that they possess an expansive range of knowledge within safety protocols and the operation of equipment so that such risks can be prevented. Second, because electrosurgical technologies are continually evolving, surgeons must continually adapt to newer devices and techniques. Professional associations and health care organizations have a duty to provide education and training for surgeons to enable them to continue practicing in accordance with evolving methodologies. Books "Updates in Endoscopy" illustrate recent advancements and research directions in electrosurgery, providing professionals with the necessary information to refine their practice and provide effective, safe care (Amornyotin et al., 2022). Overcoming the challenges of electrosurgery will ultimately result in better delivery of surgeries for a variety of conditions, such as acute inflammatory illnesses and dermatological conditions (Peter et al., 2019) (Figure 9.8).

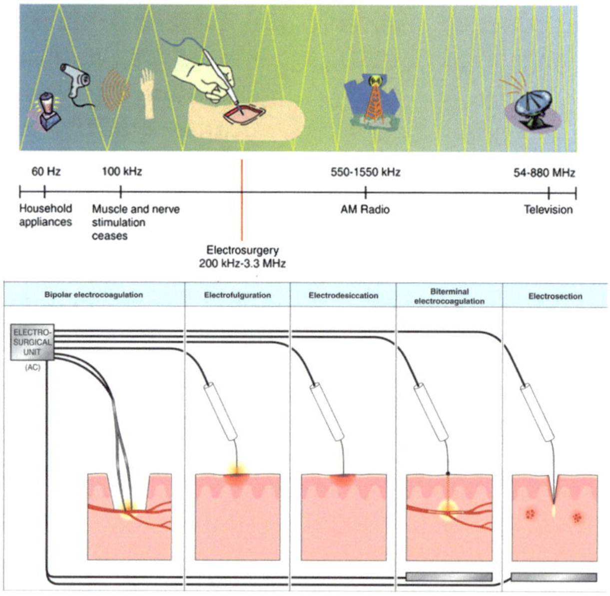

Figure 9.8. Electrosurgery, a critical technique utilized in modern surgical practices, employs high-frequency alternating current to excise or coagulate tissue.

Source: https://cdn.ymaws.com/www.aocd.org/resource/resmgr/meeting_resources/2019fall/syllabus/Shah.pdf.

9.2.3. Chemical Processes Involved in Chemical Peels

Chemical peels are a therapeutic technique applied to enhance the skin's appearance through controlled removal of its outer layers. The chemical reactions involved can be classified into superficial, medium, and deep peels based on a variety of agents , such as alpha-hydroxy acids (AHAs), beta-hydroxy acids (BHAs), and trichloroacetic acid (TCA). These agents facilitate the breakdown of intercellular bonds, leading to exfoliation of dead skin cells and promoting cellular turnover. Therefore, when these dead skin cells are removed, the underlying dermal layers are exposed, leading to improved skin texture and color. This action is particularly useful for acne scars, pigment disorders, and age spots, as it can stimulate collagen production and enhance overall skin health. In addition to enhancing cosmetic appearance, the biochemical reactions induced by chemical peels are a major factor in their therapeutic benefits. For example, AHAs, which are obtained from natural products fruits and milk, undergo a process of hydration and swelling, leading to a decrease in the visibility of fine lines and an increase in general skin hydration. Similarly, BHAs, such as salicylic acid, penetrate deeply into the pores of oily skin to break down sebum and prevent acne breakouts. Additionally, TCA functions via the process of coagulation necrosis, enabling precise destruction of epidermal tissue to achieve a rejuvenated appearance. This diversity of chemical activities vividly illustrates the richness and variability of chemical peels in dermatology. New technologies in dermatology have continued to shed light on the chemical processes that occur during peels. Hyperspectral imaging technology, for instance, has been explored to quantify skin states at the subclinical level and to provide better guidance for chemical agent application (Neittaanmäki-Perttu, 2015). The method enables practitioners to visualize underlying damage, thereby informing tailored treatment plans that support optimal healing and outcomes. Additionally, new medications, such as BF-200 ALA, are being investigated for use in conjunction with photodynamic therapy to improve treatment efficacy and reduce the side effects associated with chemical peels (Boshoff, 2016). With the development of such new treatments and formulations, the procedure for chemical peels is also improved, offering safer and more effective treatments for a wide range of skin conditions.

Test Your Knowledge

1. How does freezing in cryotherapy cause tissue destruction?
2. What is the basic principle that allows electrosurgery to cut or coagulate tissue?
3. What chemical reaction primarily occurs during a chemical peel to remove skin layers?

9.3. Applications in Medicine

Learning Outcome

1. Understand the uses of cryotherapy in dermatology.
2. Discuss about electrosurgery applications in surgical procedures.
3. Explain the indications for chemical peels in skin treatment.

The clinical application of cryotherapy extends beyond simple superficial treatment to include various therapeutic interventions for a range of skin disorders, such as warts and actinic keratosis. It is a technique that uses extreme cold to eliminate pathologic cells and is effective at reducing lesions with minimal harm to surrounding healthy tissue. This specificity not only shortens patients' recovery periods but also enables faster healing than conventional excision. The literature shows that cryotherapy significantly improves the quality of life of patients with dermatological conditions and, consequently, its value as an effective intervention in modern therapeutic management. The modality's versatility is further enhanced by its applicability to more complex conditions, enabling breakthrough research and clinical practice, thereby maximizing its contribution to evidence-based care. Electrosurgery is another major advance in the practice of medicine because it provides a versatile tool for tissue incision and blood vessel coagulation in surgical procedures. Precise excision and shrinkage of multiple neoplasms of the skin are accomplished with less bleeding and trauma using high-frequency electric currents. The immediate healing response in electrosurgery improves patient outcomes by reducing scarring and postoperative pain. Moreover, the integration of this technique in dermatologic surgery has made it possible for physicians to apply a more advanced technique in managing skin diseases, such as congenital melanocytic nevi, which are typically required to be well-thought-out due to their intricacy. Current evidence indicates that the addition of electrosurgery to adjunctive modalities can lead to greater efficacy in controlling such refractory lesions and thus address a significant gap in the use of evidence-based guidelines in dermatology (Lai, 2018).

Chemical peels are widely used in dermatology primarily for their ability to improve skin texture and treat disorders such as acne scars and photodamage. It involves the application of chemical substances to remove the top layers of the skin, inducing new life and revealing a healthier, smoother face beneath. The chemicals applied and the depth of penetration of the peel can be tailored to the individual's specific skin type and concern, making it a highly adaptable treatment. Current publications highlight the increased use of chemical peels to optimize the therapeutic potential for conditions such as melasma and post-inflammatory hyperpigmentation, reinforcing their position in contemporary medicine. Further, the incorporation of advanced diagnostic methods, such as dermatoscopy, can offer useful insights into skin conditions treated with chemical peels, facilitating better management, follow-up programs, and optimal evidence-based practices (Fang et al., 2022).

9.3.1. Uses of Cryotherapy in Dermatology

Among the various uses of cryotherapy in dermatology, its application for treating skin lesions and benign tumors has received considerable attention. The procedure entails the controlled use of extreme cold to induce cellular disruption, thereby causing tissue destruction. Common conditions treated with cryotherapy include warts, seborrheic keratosis, and keratoacanthomas. The freeze-thaw cycles rapidly destroy diseased tissue while minimizing damage to surrounding normal skin. For example, studies have shown that cryotherapy for the treatment of surface lesions achieves high rates of complete clearance and is therefore widely favored by dermatologists. Although this is well tolerated in most cases, side effects such as blistering or pigmentary changes can occur and thus require careful patient selection and adequate informed consent to optimize results. Cryotherapy also plays an essential role in the management of dermatologic diseases resulting from hyperkeratosis and inflammatory diseases. Such diseases as actinic keratosis, which can progress to squamous cell carcinoma, are responsive to cryotherapy. Therapy involves the application of cryogen, which induces cell apoptosis and inflammation, thereby promoting a healing response that can reduce keratinocyte proliferation. Experiments have proven that cryotherapy, when used as an adjunct to other treatments, for example, photodynamic therapy, can be effective in the treatment of patients with extensive actinic damage. The addition of these regimens has a synergistic effect by enhancing tolerability and effectiveness of dermatologic treatment, leading to increased patient satisfaction and therapeutic outcome. This synergy reflects the versatility and usefulness of cryotherapy in modern dermatology. Furthermore, cryotherapy has been used in expert protocols for refractory dermatologic disorders, as evidenced by its application in patients with tuberous sclerosis. A study demonstrated a triple laser protocol of therapy to manage facial angiofibroma's that are usually refractory to standard management. This is a new approach that combines various treatment modalities, with cryotherapy as a critical component, to achieve acceptable results with fewer complications. The study highlighted notable reductions in severity scores and reported high levels of satisfaction after treatment. Such findings attest to the adaptability of cryotherapy in systematic treatment regimens in dermatology, enabling experts to effectively treat complex dermatoses. Overall, the use of cryotherapy reflects the evolving landscape of dermatological therapy, equipping clinicians with tools to enhance patient care and improve therapeutic effectiveness in the management of diverse skin diseases (Figure 9.9).

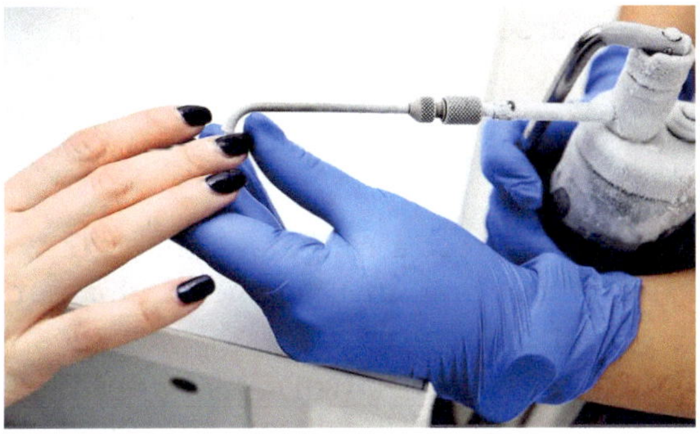

Figure 9.9. Dermatology treatments using cryotherapy.

Source: https://caloxinc.com/wp-content/uploads/2022/01/blog-dermatology-cryosurgery-wart-removal.webp.

9.3.2. Electrosurgery Applications in Surgical Procedures

Electrosurgery has become an important technique in various surgical procedures, using high-frequency electrical currents to achieve clear cuts and tissue coagulation. Electrosurgery has several advantages over traditional surgical techniques, including reduced blood loss, reduced postoperative pain, and shorter recovery times. Electrosurgery is particularly convenient in delicate surgeries, such as those encountered in dermatologic operations and minimal invasive surgeries, where precision is paramount. Surgeons have often employed electrosurgical units (ESUs) to create incisions with minimal thermal injury to adjacent tissues, thereby facilitating aesthetic outcomes and reducing complications related to scarring. The effectiveness of electrosurgery is evidenced by its use across numerous surgical disciplines, establishing it as a valuable resource in contemporary surgical therapy. Other than its function to cut and coagulate, electrosurgery also plays a significant role in the ablation and resection of tumors, especially malignant and benign. Using the technique, surgeons can readily target unwanted growth and simultaneously promote hemostasis to minimize the risk of excessive bleeding during and after the procedure. The use of electrosurgery in cancer surgery has been highly successful, with improved outcomes and patient satisfaction, owing to reduced recovery time and minimal complications. For example, it is widely used in the removal of dermatological tumors, where accuracy and non-invasiveness are paramount.

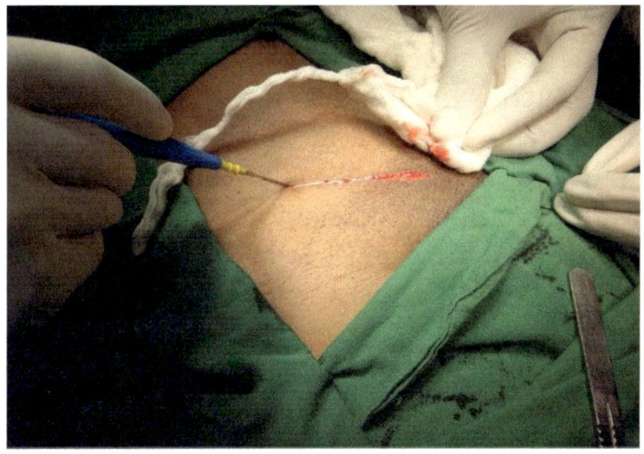

Figure 9.10. Skin incision by monopolar electrocautry.

Source: https://www.researchgate.net/publication/333255064/figure/fig2/AS:761184601006081@1558491959443/Skin-incision-by-monopolar-electrocautry.jpg.

The accuracy of tissue sculpting not only enables removal of the lesion but also preserves surrounding healthy tissue, underscoring the importance of the technique for achieving an optimal surgical result (Boshoff, 2016). Recent research also further expands the use of electrosurgery beyond its conventional uses, particularly its combination with other therapeutic modalities. The integration of electrosurgery with drug therapies, such as cryotherapy or photodynamic therapy, represents one hopeful path to improved patient care. For example, electrosurgical techniques may be used to precondition the operative field in anticipation of subsequent cryotherapy, thereby maximizing therapeutic effect on lesions. This therapeutic combination may not only maximize tissue responses but also aesthetic outcomes, as noted in treatment evaluations of cutaneous lesions. The ongoing research into these combined techniques, as well as the identification of predictors of optimum outcomes, will arguably continue to shape the course of surgical interventions in the future (Calzada et al., 2017) (Figure 9.10).

9.3.3. Indications for Chemical Peels in Skin Treatment

Chemical peels are a practical dermatologic treatment used to correct a range of skin conditions, from acne to signs of aging. Performed most often in the office, they involve the application of chemical solutions to induce controlled abrasion of the epidermis and dermis, cell turnover, and stimulation of collagen. Indications for chemical peeling include hyperpigmentation melasma and sun spots, and textural imperfections after photoaging. Chemical peeling can also be beneficial in the treatment of superficial scars and active acne by unclogging pores, improving overall complexion, and reducing inflammation. These markings highlight the role of chemical peels as a significant non-surgical intervention within the broader dermatologic therapeutic framework, particularly as patients increasingly favor procedures with minimal downtime and maximal cosmetic benefit. Although cosmetic indications remain significant, chemical peels can also be used to treat certain dermatologic disorders.

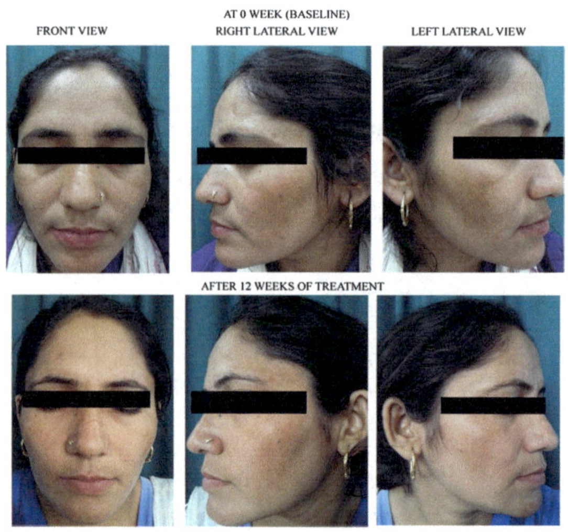

Figure 9.11. Photographs of patients undergoing 92% LA acid peel at 0 week and after 12 weeks.

Source: https://www.researchgate.net/publication/348043374/figure/fig3/AS:11431281173874872@1689056654178/Photographs-of-patients-on-92-LA-acid-peel-at-0-week-and-after-12weeks.png.

For instance, conditionally severe cutaneous patients, like those with actinic keratosis, can benefit from chemical peeling techniques through the removal of precancerous lesions. Triage of such cases is warranted, as untreated actinic keratosis can progress to squamous cell carcinoma and therefore requires active management. The choice of using various peel depths—superficial, medium, or deep—gives dermatologists the flexibility to tailor to the individual histological grading and clinical presentation of cutaneous lesions. This variability is complemented by advances in dermatologic technology and techniques, demonstrating the integration of these processes into the treatment of skin disease and patient satisfaction (Kololgi et al., 2023). This elevates the status of chemical peels not merely as a cosmetic adjunct but as part of an integrated dermatologic regimen. Patient considerations, including skin type and individual treatment goals, also influence the indications for chemical peels. These elements, such as the presence of comorbid underlying skin conditions, sensitivity to chemicals, and healing capacity, all play significant roles in determining the appropriateness of this form of treatment. For example, individuals with darker skin types will require specific protocols to prevent post-inflammatory hyperpigmentation. In this context, the integration of patient-centered care is imperative to ensure that patients receive tailored treatment plans that align with their concerns and needs. With non-invasive gaining popularity due to the increasing global prevalence of nonmelanoma skin cancers, there is a need for more stringent guidelines for chemical peeling (Baradarian, 2021). Evaluating the effectiveness and safety of such procedures indirectly fosters further advances in dermatological treatment (Figure 9.11).

Test Your Knowledge

1. What common skin lesions are treated using cryotherapy in dermatology?
2. In what types of surgical procedures is electrosurgery most commonly used?
3. What skin conditions are chemical peels commonly indicated for in cosmetic dermatology?

9.4. Benefits and Advantages

Learning Outcome

1. Explain the advantages of cryotherapy for skin health.
2. Understand the benefits of electrosurgery over traditional surgery.
3. Focus on positive outcomes of chemical peels for skin rejuvenation.

The benefits of cryotherapy, electrosurgery, and chemical peeling in dermabrasion extend beyond mere cosmetic correction; they also include significant enhancement of patient care. Cryotherapy, for instance, employs intense cold to destroy specific tissue, facilitating more effective removal of abnormal skin cells without harming adjacent healthy tissue. This method has the specific benefit of treating conditions such as warts and certain precancerous lesions, resulting in quicker healing with less scarring. These are not only results of enhanced patient satisfaction but also improved quality of life. As noted in recent literature, treatment modalities like cryotherapy could lead to evidence-based policy directions, in this case, pediatric applications, and a better understanding of its functional effects on children's overall health, as hinted by Lai (2018).

Electrosurgery, on the other hand, utilizes high-frequency electrical currents for both tissue incisions and coagulation to minimize bleeding during procedures. This technique is especially useful for the excision of skin lesions and tumors because it is efficient and accurate. The advantage of electrosurgery is that it heals rapidly, allowing patients to return to their daily routines sooner than with traditional surgery. Electrosurgery also reduces the rate of complications, such as infection, which is experienced in other surgical operations. The ability to perform procedures with less blood loss contributes to increased safety, further making electrosurgery a valuable asset in dermatologic practice. Continuous evaluation of the technique maintains its status as an ideal modality because it is part of a broader effort to enhance clinical outcomes and patient satisfaction (Neittaanmäki-Perttu, 2015). Chemical peels also offer many benefits in the area of skin revitalization, with great effectiveness in addressing many skin problems, such as acne scars and hyperpigmentation. The versatility of chemical peels makes it possible to treat an individual's skin type and condition. Not only does this maximize results, but it also reduces possible side effects, making chemical peels a versatile treatment for patients wishing to improve aesthetically. In addition, advances in formulation and application techniques have improved the overall tolerability of chemical peels, making them more acceptable to different patient populations. As additional research continues to support the effectiveness of these treatments, the promise of inexpensive and effective skin care further emphasizes the value of integrating chemical peels into everyday dermatological practice (Lai, 2018).

9.4.1. Advantages of Cryotherapy in Maintaining Skin Health

Cryotherapy, the local application of extreme cold to selectively damage tissues, offers significant advantages in promoting skin health.

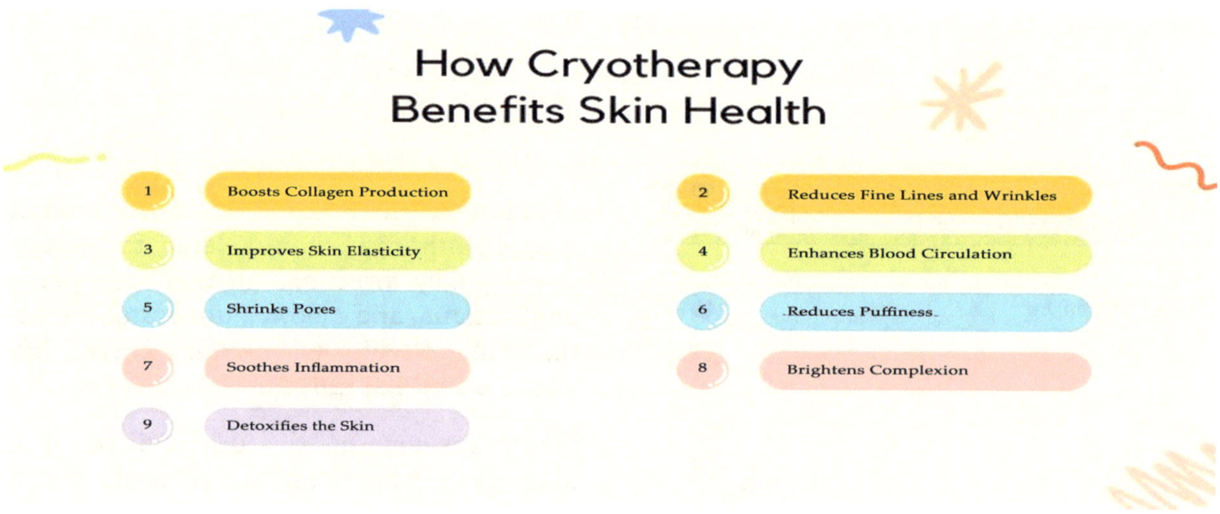

Figure 9.12. How cryotherapy benefits skin health.

Source: https://www.painflame.com/wp-content/uploads/2024/09/How-Cryotherapy-Benefits-Skin-Health-1.png.

A significant advantage is that it is effective against most skin lesions, including premalignant lesions such as actinic keratosis and squamous cell carcinoma in situ. Clinical research has shown that cryotherapy is effective in causing clearance of lesions, the success rates reported being as high as 100% when proper methods are used, such as the use of liquid nitrogen. This mode of treatment not only yields a high rate of clearance but is also an easily accessible, relatively simple intervention for medical practitioners, making it the first choice in outpatient settings. The rapid adoption of cryotherapy improves patient throughput and concordance, demonstrating its practical application in clinical practice (Arisi et al., 2022). In addition to managing precancerous lesions, cryotherapy is valuable for overall skin health by accelerating the healing of various dermatological lesions. The intense cold induces vasoconstriction, temporarily limiting blood flow to the area and reducing swelling and inflammation. Next, as the tissue gets heated, it causes vasodilation, resulting in a blood rush to the treated area. This blood flow delivers essential nutrients and proteins that accelerate the skin's natural repair mechanisms and enhance tissue repair. Additionally, cryotherapy has been shown to increase collagen production, a significant factor in maintaining skin flexibility and reducing signs of aging. The interaction of these physiological mechanisms reveals cryotherapy's multi-faceted role in skin health (Morton et al., 2013). Furthermore, the relatively low cost and noninvasive nature of cryotherapy make it an appealing option for patients seeking aesthetic improvement alongside medical treatment. Since the treatment is not surgical, cryotherapy tends to be less expensive than that of more invasive treatments, such as electrosurgery or chemical peels. They have minimal downtime, allowing them to return to their routine activities soon after treatment. The speed and convenience of cryotherapy are aligned with contemporary healthcare requirements for effective yet cost-effective therapeutic measures. As dermatologists further explore various therapeutic modalities, the merits of cryotherapy for skin health range from effective ablation of lesions to enhanced healing and cosmetic benefit—irrevocably establishing its position as a significant force among the treatment options in the field of skin therapy (Arisi et al., 2022) (Figure 9.12).

9.4.2. Benefits of Electrosurgery Over Traditional Surgery

The advent of electrosurgery has significantly transformed surgical interventions, yielding clear advantages over traditional surgery. The precision with which electrosurgical equipment operates is a primary benefit. By the employment of high-voltage electrical currents, electrosurgery can selectively modify tissue and cause minimal damage to neighboring structures. This is particularly advantageous in delicate surgeries where the structural integrity of adjacent tissue must be preserved. This is compared to more traditional surgical techniques, which create bigger fields of tissue destruction due to the fact that they are physically force-based. The greater accuracy of electrosurgery not only benefits the patient but also enables faster healing, as there is less trauma to the area. Electrosurgery also has widespread benefits for achieving hemostasis, the cessation of bleeding during surgery. Conventional surgery tends to require clamps or sutures to control bleeding, which may complicate the operating area and prolong operation time. Electrosurgery successfully coagulates blood vessels during cutting, thereby minimizing the need for additional procedures to control bleeding. Not only does this expedite the surgical process, but it also reduces the risk of postoperative complications related to excessive bleeding, such as hematoma formation or infection. In addition, the effectiveness of electrosurgery may lead to a reduction in the total time of surgery, therefore, the workload capacity of surgical teams during operations. Finally, postoperative benefits of electrosurgery further attest to the superiority of electrosurgery compared to traditional operations. Patients tend to experience less postoperative pain and take fewer analgesics following electrosurgical operations. Reduced tissue trauma results in a lower incidence of inflammatory reactions, with healing occurring more rapidly and shorter hospital stays. Furthermore, precision electrosurgery can reduce the incidence of scarring, a concern of paramount importance in cosmetic surgery. As patient satisfaction and quality of care become increasingly focused areas of healthcare practice, the advantages of electrosurgery over traditional methods grow ever more important. This shift in surgical techniques reflects a broader trend toward technologies aimed at optimizing patient outcomes, thereby rendering electrosurgery the method of choice in the majority of clinical scenarios.

9.4.3. Positive Outcomes of Chemical Peels for Skin Rejuvenation

The use of chemical peels has attracted considerable attention in dermatology, primarily because of their potential to enhance skin rejuvenation. In contrast to more aggressive treatments, chemical peels are a non-surgical technique for debriding the skin surface, thereby smoothing its texture and tone. Employing various agents, such as alphahydroxy acids, trichloroacetic acid, or salicylic acid, these procedures can address conditions as disparate as fine lines and age spots to severe acne scarring.

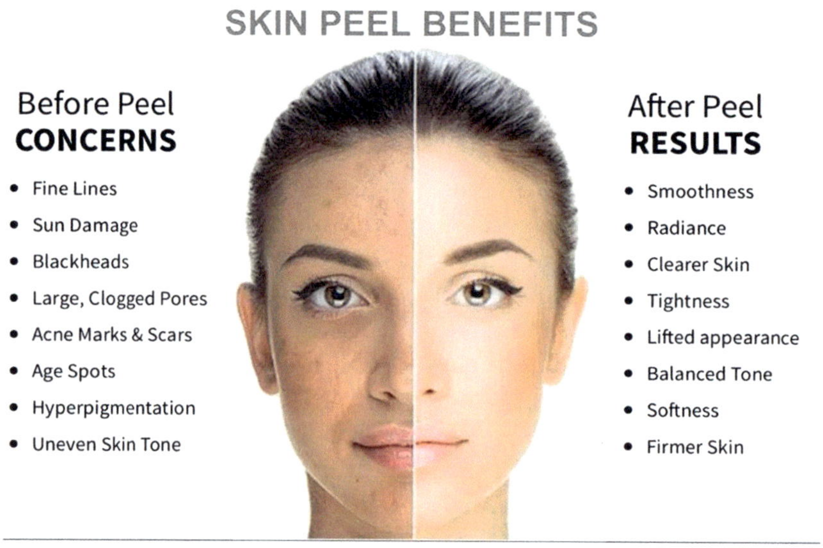
SKIN PEEL BENEFITS
Before Peel
CONCERNS
Fine Lines
Sun Damage
Blackheads
Large, Clogged Pores
Acne Marks & Scars
Age Spots
Hyperpigmentation
Uneven Skin Tone
After Peel
RESULTS
Smoothness
Radiance
Clearer Skin
Tightness
Lifted appearance
Balanced Tone
Softness
Firmer Skin

Figure 9.13. Skin peels benefits.

Source: https://radiantfr.com/wp-content/uploads/2024/12/WhatsApp-Image-2024-12-19-at-8.05.01-PM.jpeg.

Significantly, chemical peel-induced regenerative process involves stimulation of collagen production, which is essential in maintaining the elasticity of the skin as well as its youthful texture. The breakthrough in skin rejuvenation followed current dermatological practices, which emphasize non-invasive methods and holistic care within patients' treatment plans, a trend cited in the recent bulletin of dermatological breakthroughs and case studies (Kololgi et al., 2023). In addition to their cosmetic benefits, chemical peels are a promising alternative for a range of skin conditions, enhancing overall skin health. They are particularly useful for patients who are battling abnormal pigmentation and acne, not just leading to cosmetic enhancements but also psychological benefits acquired via boosted self-confidence. Patients have been reported to have more balanced skin and fewer breakouts following treatment, a significant positive effect. Moreover, chemical peels can be tailored to individual skin types and concerns, providing customized treatment protocols that minimize the risk of side effects. This modification is crucial for ensuring maximal benefits and maintaining a patient-centered practice in dermatology, which has increasingly been encouraged in the field (Kololgi et al., 2023).Beyond temporary cosmetic effects, chemical peels also promote long-term skin restoration. Follow-up treatments can yield more lasting effects, such as improved skin hydration and reduced signs of aging, because the peels effectively remove dead skin cells and stimulate new cell turnover. Such an ongoing effect not only enhances the appearance of the skin but also maintains overall skin health. Additionally, chemical peels can be less expensive than other dermatologic procedures and therefore may be a viable treatment option for more people. With a greater incidence of skin disease, the establishment and popularity of these non-surgical therapies become progressively more significant in promoting public skin health and shattering old treatment patterns, particularly as they pertain to benign skin diseases such as nonmelanoma skin cancer (Figure 9.13).

Test Your Knowledge

1. What are the main advantages of cryotherapy for treating superficial skin lesions?
2. What are the key benefits of electrosurgery compared to traditional scalpel surgery?
3. How do chemical peels improve skin texture and tone for rejuvenation?

9.5. Risks and Side Effects

Learning Outcome

1. Explain potential risks associated with cryotherapy.
2. Understand complications from electrosurgery.
3. Describe side effects of chemical peels.

The investigation into cryotherapy, electrosurgery, and chemical peels by necessity leads to an evaluation of their side effects and risks. Although generally recognized as beneficial for the management of many skin conditions, cryotherapy produces local side effects, such as erythema, edema, and pain at the site of treatment. More serious but rare complications include blistering and hyperpigmentation, particularly in patients with darker skin types. It is thus necessary for practitioners to be knowledgeable about such potential side effects so that patients can be well advised. The proper evaluation of a patient's health history and skin type should thus be done before treatment to prevent risks and achieve optimal results as clinically observed in the use of cryotherapy to dermatological diseases, where follow-up examinations have shown varying degrees of patient satisfaction. With electrosurgical selection, the scope of hazard extends to include complications both intra- and postprocedurally. Side effects of electrosurgery involve immediate manifestations , such as pain and redness, which are typically transient in nature. However, more severe hazards exist, including scarring, skin pigmentation changes, and damage to deeper tissues, if settings or instrumentation are used improperly. These side effects highlight the importance of employing trained practitioners with familiarity in the details of the procedure. The assessment of patient outcomes across studies highlights the importance of meticulous adherence to safety protocols to minimize complications and improve patient satisfaction, as evidenced by assessments conducted in clinical practice settings where electrosurgery was performed. Chemical peels are also associated with a range of potential side effects. Patients may experience temporary stinging or burning, and peeling of the outermost skin layer is a normal consequence of the procedure. However, it should be noted that deeper peels have a risk of more severe complications, such as prolonged erythema, scarring, or hyperpigmentation, especially in darker-skinned individuals. A prolonged preparatory phase, with adequate discussion of the risks, will enhance patient compliance and adherence to aftercare. Studies comparing patient reactions to chemical peels report varying degrees of satisfaction, underscoring the importance of appropriate patient selection and education to minimize undesirable side effects while optimizing the aesthetic outcome of the procedure.

9.5.1. Potential Risks Associated with Cryotherapy

Cryotherapy, which employs intense cold to treat a variety of medical conditions, has gained widespread popularity in both clinical and cosmetic uses. Nevertheless, despite its widespread adoption, certain potential risks of the treatment must be thoroughly assessed. Among such dangers is cryo-induced skin injury, which may manifest as frostbite or hypopigmentation. These side effects can lead to long-term dermatological complications, particularly when the cryogenic agent is applied incorrectly or the treatment duration exceeds the prescribed limits. Additionally, sensitive skin or inherent dermatological issues can exaggerate the side effects, which necessitate the use of an individualized treatment method. Proper patient evaluation is required to minimize the occurrence of such side effects and ensure safe application on a broad range of skin types. Apart from skin issues, the second concern of cryotherapy is the possibility of systemic effects, particularly among vulnerable groups. For instance, patients suffering from heart diseases will have adverse cardiovascular responses upon exposure to extremely cold temperatures. This is especially true during whole-body cryotherapy sessions, in which the entire body is cooled. Moreover, patients with certain medical backgrounds, such as neurological conditions, can experience unforeseen reactions to cryotherapy, leading to additional complications. It is necessary to conduct a comprehensive pre-treatment evaluation to identify contraindications that may be hazardous to the patient during treatment. Not only does this help ensure patient health, but it also maximizes the overall efficacy of cryotherapy. Finally, while some clinicians support the use of cryotherapy for conditions such as congenital melanocytic nevi (CMN), a balanced decision must be made between potential benefits and harms. Recent evaluations show that while cryotherapy can significantly reduce the visibility of CMN, it does not eliminate melanoma risk, which nonetheless remains a concern regardless of treatment. These aspects necessitate informed decision-making between clinicians and patients. These are the types of discussions that ought to involve potential outcomes, psychological impacts of treatment, and other treatment options. Additionally, the side effects of various treatments form the basis of not treating cryotherapy in solitude but with others, such as electrosurgery and chemical peels, all with unique risk profiles and therapeutic indices (Mia et al., 2024; Passeron et al., 2019).

9.5.2. Complications from Electrosurgery

The investigation into cryotherapy, electrosurgery, and chemical peels by necessity leads to an evaluation of their side effects and risks. Although generally recognized as beneficial for the management of many skin conditions, cryotherapy produces local side effects, such as erythema, edema, and pain at the site of treatment. More serious but rare complications include blistering and hyperpigmentation, particularly in patients with darker skin types. It is thus necessary for practitioners to be knowledgeable about such potential side effects so that patients can be well advised. The proper evaluation of a patient's health history and skin type should thus be conducted before treatment to minimize risks and achieve optimal results, as clinically observed in the use of cryotherapy for dermatological diseases, where follow-up examinations have shown varying degrees of patient satisfaction. With electrosurgical selection, the scope of hazard extends to include complications both intra- and postprocedurally. Side effects of electrosurgery include immediate manifestations such as pain and redness, which are typically transient. However, more severe hazards exist, including scarring, skin pigmentation changes, and damage to deeper tissues, if settings or instrumentation are used improperly. These side effects highlight the importance of employing trained practitioners with familiarity in the details of the procedure. The assessment of patient outcomes across studies highlights the importance of meticulous adherence to safety protocols to minimize complications and improve patient satisfaction, as evidenced by assessments conducted in clinical practice settings where electrosurgery was performed.

Chemical peels are also associated with a range of potential side effects. Patients may experience temporary stinging or burning, and peeling of the outermost skin layer is a normal consequence of the procedure. However, it should be noted that deeper peels have a risk of more severe complications, such as prolonged erythema, scarring, or hyperpigmentation, especially in darker-skinned individuals. A prolonged preparatory phase, with adequate discussion of the risks, will enhance patient compliance and adherence to aftercare. Studies comparing patient reactions to chemical peels report varying degrees of satisfaction, underscoring the importance of appropriate patient selection and education to minimize undesirable side effects while optimizing the aesthetic outcome of the procedure.

9.5.3. Side Effects of Chemical Peels

Chemical peels are better recognized to be useful for skin rejuvenation, but can cause a variety of side effects that require careful attention. Immediate responses in the shape of erythema and desquamation are usual, exhibiting the skin's inflammatory response to the chemical substances utilized. These effects can be distressing and cause temporary changes in pigmentation, typically referred to as post-inflammatory hyperpigmentation. While early restorative outcomes are rewarding, the risk of long-term side effects, especially for darker-skinned patients, necessitates a thorough pre-treatment consultation.

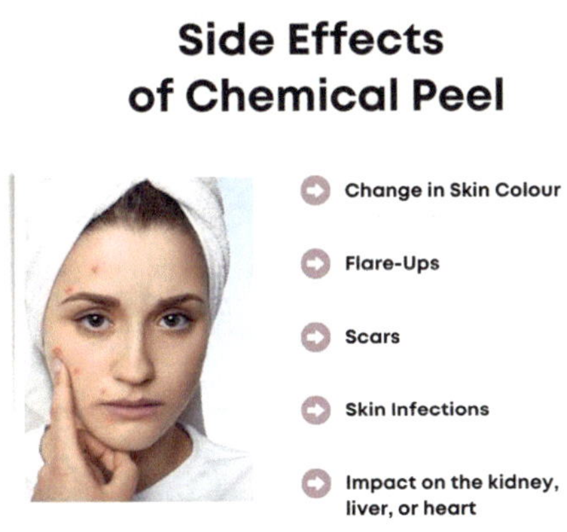

Figure 9.14. Side effects of chemical peel.

Source: https://www.kolorshealthcare.com/blog/wp-content/uploads/2023/09/Chemical-Peel-Side-Effects.jpg.

The risk of permanent pigmentation changes keeps many prospective candidates away, making informed consent and proper patient education all the more important in dermatology clinics. Along with acute reactions, chemical peels may also result in more severe complications. Infections may occur, primarily due to poor aftercare or unhygienic treatment conditions. These infections may present as superficial fungal or bacterial infections, complicate recovery, and, in severe cases, necessitate further medical intervention. Skin atrophy is also a common side effect, particularly for those who undergo medium- to deep-penetration peels. Atrophy may also result in thinning of the epidermis, which is weaker and more susceptible to additional injury, indicating the need to select the depth of peel according to the patient's skin type and condition. The risk of developing delayed side effects, such as scarring, is a valid concern in the practice of dermatology. In some patients, particularly those prone to keloid formation or other dermatoses, chemical peels can elicit a detrimental tissue reaction. The Koebner phenomenon, in which trauma to the skin causes new lesions, is of particular interest in this context. Also, one should urge people who need to go through such treatments to discuss their complete medical history, including past adverse reactions to dermatologic treatments like tattooing, which is discussed in reports describing cutaneous complications. Lastly, understanding the spectrum of potential chemical peel side effects is key to optimizing treatment benefit and ensuring patient safety, as it helps balance the benefits of skincare enhancement treatments against their risks (Beatrice et al., 2024; Neamonitou et al., 2024) (Figure 9.14).

Test Your Knowledge

1. What are the common side effects patients may experience after cryotherapy?
2. How can burns or tissue damage occur during electrosurgery procedures?
3. What are typical side effects of chemical peels, particularly with deeper peels?

9.6. Comparative Analysis

Learning Outcome

1. Compare the effectiveness between cryotherapy and electrosurgery.
2. Evaluate chemical peels against other skin treatments.
3. Deal with the cost-effectiveness of each treatment modality.

When evaluating the relative effectiveness of cryotherapy, electrosurgery, and chemical peeling, it is necessary to examine the unique clinical situations in which each has an advantage. Cryotherapy, in which tissue is destroyed by intense cold, is more commonly used as a first-line modality for treating warts and superficial skin lesions. Its simplicity of use and minimized recovery time also make it particularly well-suited for ambulatory settings. Despite this, clinical trials reveal that while cryotherapy may deliver partial responses, relapse is common, and treatments need to be repeated. Such findings suggest that a comparison study with alternatives such as electrosurgery, which ablates or coagulates tissue with high-frequency electric current, might yield more effective treatment for similarly benign dermatological lesions (Haddad et al., 2022). Electrosurgery stands apart for its ability to provide immediate tissue removal, with resultant clean margins that can be invaluable in preserving patient aesthetics and treating resident pathologies. The comparative analysis demonstrates that electrosurgery offers efficacy and safety, with evidence-based reductions in recurrence rates compared with cryotherapy for certain indications. While side effects scarring and pigmentation changes are noted, technical improvements have reduced their incidence. Further, examining electrosurgery as a factor in the removal of larger or multiple lesions allows comparison of its effectiveness with that of chemical peels, which address only textural surface improvements and pigmentation. However, the success of chemical peels largely depends on the formulation and concentration of the agents applied; therefore, standardizing treatment protocols in response to new evidence is questioned (Lai, 2018). Such critical comparisons between treatments highlight the need for personalized medicine—each modality's appropriateness may vary substantially depending on the individual patient's circumstances. For example, although chemical peels are highly effective in treating a broad spectrum of skin conditions, from acne to melasma, their results may lag behind those of electrosurgery for more invasive lesions. The spectrum of skin types and conditions requires a thorough investigation that encompasses patient-reported outcomes. Thus, inclusion of qualitative measures the Children's Dermatology Life Quality Index, can provide a more comprehensive picture of the broader effects of treatment decisions on quality of life in patients. Such a model of assessment is especially useful where the impact on child patients undergoing intervention is being considered, providing a superior overall impression of the efficacy and psychosocial consequences of each treatment modality (Lai ., 2018).

9.6.1. Comparison of Effectiveness Between Cryotherapy and Electrosurgery

As practice in dermatology evolves, the management of skin lesions requires an awareness of treatment options, particularly cryotherapy and electrosurgery. Cryotherapy uses intense cold to induce tissue damage, ultimately destroying lesions such as warts and keratoses. Electrosurgery, meanwhile, uses high-frequency electrical currents to excise or coagulate tissue, with a clear mechanism of action. Research has demonstrated that, although each may be effective, effectiveness varies with the site and nature of the lesion.

For genital warts, research has demonstrated that neither modality is superior; both have comparable recovery rates but differ in the number of sessions required, as reported in a randomized clinical trial comparing cryotherapy with carbon dioxide laser ablation (Godarzi et al., 2025). A comparison of the effectiveness of cryotherapy and electrosurgery reveals important differences that influence treatment selection.

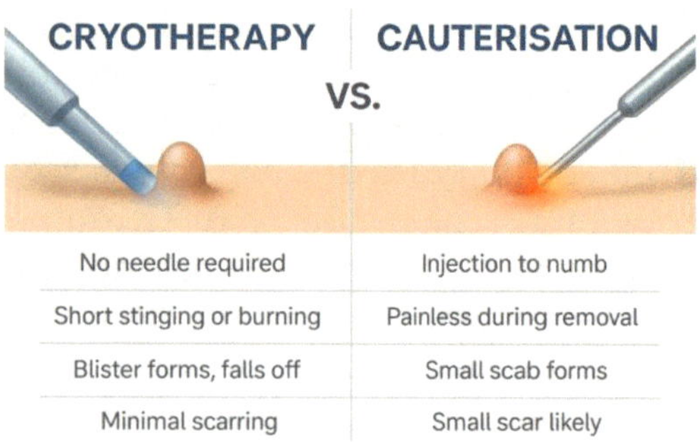

Figure 9.15. Cryotherapy vs. cauterization.

Source: https://www.perfectimageconsultants.co.uk/wp-content/uploads/2025/05/Cryotherapy-vs-Cauterisation-for-Skin-Tag-Removal.jpg.

Specifically, a comparison of the two treatment methods for cutaneous lesions such as sebaceous hyperplasia, seborrheic keratosis, and cherry angiomas reveals differences in the number of treatment sessions required, patient tolerance, and healing time. Electrosurgery may need less treatment to remove, but may also be more painful during the process compared to cryotherapy, which is generally well-tolerated. In addition, patient comments are likely to address the cosmetic outcome following treatment, emphasizing the importance of monitoring not only the efficacy of the method but also its effect on quality of life (Sadeghzadeh-Bazargan et al., 2024). Finally, the decision between cryotherapy and electrosurgery is not simply a matter of clinical efficacy but also patient factors. Patient preference, relative recurrence rates, and lesion type are all relevant factors in decision-making. While such reports do not represent an absolute advantage between them, they do imply the necessity of patient-tailored treatment programs to address individual patient needs. Long-term follow-up and continued research are warranted to more precisely determine the roles of electrosurgery and cryotherapy in dermatologic therapy, with a view toward optimal outcomes (Sadeghzadeh-Bazargan et al., 2024; Godarzi et al., 2025) (Figure 9.15).

9.6.2. Evaluating Chemical Peels Against Other Skin Treatments

Chemical peels are a universally accepted dermatologic modality identified by their characteristic of exfoliating and rejuvenating skin through the application of chemical solutions. There is a need to examine their efficacy relative to other therapies , such as cryotherapy and electrosurgery in terms of the targeted skin conditions at stake. Whereas chemical peels are effective in addressing very superficial issues such as fine lines, scarring from acne, and pigmentation, electrosurgery and cryotherapy may be indicated for deeper cutaneous lesions or precancerous lesions. Thus, an evaluation of the context in which these treatments are being conducted can significantly enhance patient results. Furthermore, the variable recovery time associated with each procedure is a significant factor in treatment selection, as patients may prefer less invasive procedures with a quicker return to regular activities. For a comparison of chemical peels with cryotherapy and electrosurgery, not only should their therapeutic effectiveness be compared, but also patient satisfaction and side effects. Cryotherapy, which uses extreme cold to destroy abnormal tissue, is an effective treatment for many dermatological conditions, including warts and superficial skin cancers. However, the procedure can cause significant pain during and following treatment, as well as risks of blistering or hyperpigmentation. Electrosurgery also offers an effective means of removing skin lesions but results in more severe scarring and longer recovery periods than chemical peels. Conversely, chemical peels are more likely to yield milder side effects, less pain, and fewer complications. Therefore, a choice among these treatments should balance effectiveness, healing time, and patient satisfaction. Increasing evidence supports combining chemical peels with other modalities to maximize treatment benefits. For instance, the comparative study contrasted the effectiveness of daylight photodynamic therapy (dl-PDT) and conventional photodynamic therapy (c-PDT) (Arisi et al., 2022). Despite similar effectiveness between the two modalities in treating actinic cheilitis, the minimally inflammatory reactions and lower pain scores observed with idl-PDT support the potential for combination protocols that leverage the strengths of multiple modalities. This blend could prove particularly helpful for individuals requiring effective and acceptable treatments for advanced dermatological conditions. As such, the ongoing research into treatment blends has the potential to make it possible to create personalized therapeutic regimens that take advantage of the value of chemical peels without being bound by the limitations of more invasive treatments (Amornyotin et al., 2022).

9.6.3. Cost-Effectiveness of Each Treatment Modality

In evaluating the cost-effectiveness of electrosurgery, chemical peels, and cryotherapy, it is necessary to consider not only costs but also outcomes. Cryotherapy, which is often utilized for dermatological lesions found superficially within the skin, tends to be less expensive than its counterparts, with lower operating costs and little apparatus needed. The modality's ability to provide treatment sessions relatively quickly enables both providers and patients to save money. Additionally, in measuring healing time and complication rates, cryotherapy has been shown to be a cost-effective intervention, reducing post-treatment resource allocation. However, the effectiveness of cryotherapy may be lesion-type dependent, prompting a differential treatment approach to maximize composite effect and utility. In contrast, electrosurgery, which is more expensive in most instances due to the capital-intensive nature of the required equipment and higher operator skill demands, has clear-cut advantages that offset its costs. It is particularly beneficial for other skin lesions, such as larger or more complex lesions, which, in turn, can significantly influence treatment success rates. The potential for lower recurrence rates of non-melanoma skin cancer (NMSC) with electrosurgery provides an economic rationale for its use, based on long-term healthcare cost savings from preventing subsequent complications of untreated malignant lesions. The introduction of newer electrosurgical methods has also helped achieve better procedures with quicker recovery and improved patient satisfaction, which, in turn, lead to better long-term economic outcomes (Timothy et al., 2022). Chemical peels provide a unique, cost-effective skin resurfacing and rejuvenation. Although treatment costs at the outset may appear to be a barrier, longer-term benefits typically outweigh the expenses in most cases for those patients wishing to improve skin quality and address conditions like photoaging. Recent developments in chemical peel formulations provide practitioners with enhanced capacity to treat complex types of skin and pathology in a suitable fashion, as described in new literature (Spandau et al., 2014). This versatility means that chemical peels are applicable to a broad patient population, facilitating more accessible healthcare and improved outcomes. In addition, the minimal need for extensive postoperative care contributes to cost savings in daily practice, allowing for patients and practitioners alike to reap the rewards of these treatments in an economically sustainable manner.

SUMMARY

The efficacy of cryotherapy, electrosurgery, and chemical peels in dermatologic treatments provides a wide perspective on the management of various cutaneous diseases. Each of these modalities has its specific mechanisms of action and indications, rates of success, and side effects, which need careful consideration by the operators and patients alike with all caution. Cryotherapy, for instance, has been successful in treating actinic keratosis and warts, whereas electrosurgery offers precision in excising skin lesions. Ultimately, the treatment is selected based on individual patient factors, including the specific skin condition being addressed and the desired cosmetic outcome. A relative comparison of the modalities shows that while cryotherapy and electrosurgery are beneficial in specific indications, chemical peels have a valuable role in skin rejuvenation and the treatment of acne scars. Interestingly, research shows that certain plant extracts, such as those from lemon and lime peels, possess antimicrobial properties that may be combined with curative effects through these methods (Nnebechukwu et al., 2025). Moreover, the selection among these dermatological treatments could also be based on the patient's history, personal preferences, and tolerance to various treatments. As evidenced by recent studies, including evaluations of photodynamic therapy, the comparative effectiveness of the treatments remains unclear (Aneesa, A., & Mohammed, T., 2024). While some have demonstrated photodynamic therapy's superiority in cosmetic outcomes, others have disagreed with the unequivocal effectiveness of cryotherapy for other conditions. Ultimately, advances in treatment modalities and research will be primarily responsible for further evolution in dermatological practice. Shared decision-making that integrates patient-related factors and clinical evidence will lead to optimal treatment outcomes in dermatology, emphasizing informed consent and tailored care plans.

Cryotherapy, electrosurgery, and chemical peels are individual modalities in dermatology used to treat a range of skin conditions. Cryotherapy, or cold therapy, is the use of cold temperatures to cause cell injury in defined areas of tissue, typically for the ablation of warts, skin tags, and lesions. This procedure is particularly favored for its high level of minimal invasiveness and rapid recovery, making it a popular option among the majority of patients receiving cosmetic enhancements. Of note, the efficacy of cryotherapy may depend on the practitioner's expertise and the specific condition targeted, underscoring the need for clinical competence to achieve optimal results. Consequently, complete familiarity with the mechanisms, benefits, and limitations of cryotherapy by both patients and practitioners is critical when they decide to pursue treatment. Electrosurgery uses high-frequency electrical currents to eliminate or destroy targeted tissue, providing a highly effective dermal correction tool. It is frequently used to remove benign tumors and precancerous lesions. Notably, electrosurgery not only enables precise tissue ablation but also minimizes bleeding by the coagulative effects. Notably, the procedure can be complicated by heat-induced damage to surrounding tissue and requires careful handling. Post-procedural outcomes and scarring potential are similar to those of other procedures, such as chemical peels, where the aesthetic outcome is a concern for patients. Practitioners should take into account variables such as potential complications documented in the literature to make informed decisions when choosing a patient's treatment. Chemical peels, one of this trinity's thirds, treat other dermatologic diseases, including acne and photoaging, and resurface the skin with the use of exfoliating agents. Peel depth can vary wider effects, affecting penetration into the skin and the resulting effects; greater depths yield more dramatic results but carry a greater risk of complications. Of interest, post-procedure care is absolutely vital to enhance healing and optimize results. As highlighted in observations of the efficacy of different modalities, each modality's potential harmful effect on cosmetic outcome scarring, must be considered. For instance, new technologies such as mesotherapy aim to reduce post-surgical scars, underscoring the ongoing pursuit of improving treatment options in dermatological procedures (Boshoff, 2016). In general, the distinct features of cryotherapy, electrosurgery, and chemical peels underscore their respective roles in skin therapy, providing clients and practitioners with different options for treating the skin (Romero et al., 2023).

KEY TERMS FROM THIS CHAPTER

Actinic keratosis
Blood vessels
Cellular debris
Chemical peel techniques
Chemical solutions
Congenital melanocytic nevi (CMN)
Cryotherapy
Customized therapy
Deep-penetration peels
Alpha hydroxy acids (AHAs)
Cell destruction
Cellular reaction
Chemical peels
Clinical efficacy
Contemporary surgical therapy
Cryotherapy-induced tissue destruction
Deeper peels
Dermatologic skin care

CRITICAL THINKING QUESTIONS

1. **What is the primary mechanism by which cryotherapy destroys tissue?**
   a. Coagulation of proteins
   b. Induction of oxidative stress
   c. Freezing intracellular water leading to cell rupture
   d. Heat denaturation of enzymes
2. **In electrosurgery, which mode is primarily used for cutting tissue?**
   a. Coagulation
   b. Fulguration
   c. Desiccation
   d. Pure cutting current
3. **Which of the following acids is most commonly used in superficial chemical peels?**
   a. Trichloroacetic acid (TCA)
   b. Salicylic acid
   c. Phenol
   d. Glycolic acid
4. **Which skin lesion is most commonly treated using cryotherapy?**
   a. Acne vulgaris
   b. Actinic keratosis
   c. Melanoma
   d. Psoriasis
5. **What is a key safety precaution when performing electrosurgery?**
   a. Ensure the patient is grounded properly
   b. Apply ice before the procedure
   c. Use antiseptic with alcohol base
   d. Avoid anesthesia

Short Answer Questions

1. What is the primary mechanism of tissue destruction in cryotherapy?
2. List three common dermatological conditions that are effectively treated with cryotherapy.
3. What are the potential side effects or complications associated with cryotherapy?
4. Differentiate between electrocoagulation and electrodessication in terms of mechanism and clinical use.
5. What safety precautions must be taken when performing electrosurgery in a patient with a pacemaker?
6. What is the difference between superficial, medium-depth, and deep chemical peels in terms of agents used and depth of skin penetration?
7. Name two commonly used agents in superficial chemical peels and their indications.
8. What are some contraindications or risks associated with chemical peeling procedures?

Answer to Critical Thinking Questions

1. (c); 2. (d); 3. (d); 4. (b); 5. (a)

REFERENCES

1. Amornyotin, S. (2022). Updates in endoscopy. In *IntechOpen eBooks*. https://doi.org/10.5772/intechopen.102227Aneesa, A., & Mohammed, T. (2024). The use of photodynamic therapy in actinic keratosis in comparison to cryotherapy and chemical peels. *Open Journal of Pharmacology and Pharmacotherapeutics*. https://www.semanticscholar.org/paper/a49c4613a6e21aa1abb81d655cd508cd80590bd1 (accessed on 21st July 2025).
2. Arisi, M., Gallì, B., Guasco Pisani, E., La Rosa, G., Licata, G., Rovaris, S., Tomasi, C., et al. (2022). Randomized clinical trial of conventional versus indoor daylight photodynamic therapy for treatment of actinic cheilitis. *Dermatology and Therapy, 12*, 2049–2061. https://doi.org/10.1007/s13555-022-00783-1 (accessed on 21st July 2025).
3. Bălăceanu-Gurău, B., Apostol, E., Caraivan, M., Ion, A., Tătar, R., Mihai, M. M., Popa, L. G., et al. (2024). Cutaneous adverse reactions associated with tattoos and permanent makeup pigments. *Journal of Clinical Medicine, 13*, 503–503. https://doi.org/10.3390/jcm13020503 (accessed on 21st July 2025).
4. Baradarian, S. (2021). Non-invasive strategies for the treatment of nonmelanoma skin cancers. https://repository.yu.edu/bitstream/20.500.12202/6904/1/Baradarian%20Sophia%20%20Honors%20Thesis%202021.pdf (accessed on 21st July 2025).
5. Berlin, J. M. (2010). Current and emerging treatment strategies for the treatment of actinic keratosis. https://core.ac.uk/download/pdf/8533577.pdf (accessed on 21st July 2025).
6. Boshoff, T. M. (2016). Mesotherapy Eporex treatments on post-operative mammary reduction scarring. https://core.ac.uk/download/222967500.pdf (accessed on 21st July 2025).
7. Fathi, R., Behan, J. W., & Julapalli, M. R. (2019). Special dermatologic surgery. https://doi.org/10.1002/9781118769836.ch16 (accessed on 21st July 2025).
8. Frommeyer, T. C., Rohan, C. A., Spandau, D. F., Kemp, M. G., Wanner, M., Tanzi, E. L., & Travers, J. B. (2022). Wounding therapies for prevention of photocarcinogenesis. *Frontiers in Oncology, 11*. https://doi.org/10.3389/fonc.2021.813132 (accessed on 21st July 2025).
9. Gilaberte Calzada, Y., Gracia Cazaña, T., & Juarranz De La Fuente, M. Á. (2017). Resistencias del carcinoma basocelular a la terapia fotodinámica con metil-aminolevulinato. https://core.ac.uk/download/289992120.pdf (accessed on 21st July 2025).
10. Godarzi, H., Nezhad, N. Z., Shahpar, A., Athar, M., & Ahramianpour, N. (2025). Comparison of the therapeutic effects of cryotherapy and carbon dioxide laser in the treatment of genital warts. *Egyptian Journal of Dermatology and Venereology*. https://www.semanticscholar.org/paper/2cb0228e616ab3a3b7400d91fcad0f7822c0632d (accessed on 21st July 2025).
11. Haddad, A., Hoyos Ramirez, J. L., Vila Claro, K. T., Gonzaga da Cunha, M., & Francischelli, M. (2022). Treatment of periorbital syringomas: Review of scientific literature in the last 5 years. https://core.ac.uk/download/547600138.pdf (accessed on 21st July 2025).
12. Hoeger, P. H., Kinsler, V. A., Yan, A. C., Harper, J., Oranje, A. P., Bodemer, C., Larralde, M., et al. (2019). Index. *Harper's Textbook of Pediatric Dermatology*. https://doi.org/10.1002/9781119142812.index (accessed on 21st July 2025).
13. Ianhez, M., Fróes Fleury, L. F., Miot, H. A., & Bagatin, E. (2013). Retinoids for prevention and treatment of actinic keratosis. *Anais Brasileiros de Dermatologia, 88*, 585–593. https://doi.org/10.1590/abd1806-4841.20131803 (accessed on 21st July 2025).

14. Kololgi, P., Hugar, M., Rathod, R., Nanjunda Swamy, B. L., Jagadish, P., Shruthi, H. N., Dyavannannavar, V. V., et al. (2023). *Yuvaderma E-Bulletin October 2023, Vol 8, Issue 2. Yuvaderma E-Bulletin, Vol 8, Issue 2.* http://prod-society-gallery-latest-v2.s3.amazonaws.com/files/Yuvaderma_Oct_2023_web_v3.pdf (accessed on 21st July 2025).

15. Lai, Y. (2018). Comparing congenital melanocytic nevus treatment effect on children's health-related quality of life. https://core.ac.uk/download/475688229.pdf (accessed on 21st July 2025).

16. Lin, J. Y., & Wan, M. T. (2014). Current evidence and applications of photodynamic therapy in dermatology. https://core.ac.uk/download/28949556.pdf (accessed on 21st July 2025).

17. Mologousis, M. A., Tsai, S. Y. C., Tissera, K. A., Levin, Y. S., & Hawryluk, E. B. (2024). Updates in the management of congenital melanocytic nevi. *Children, 11*, 62–62. https://doi.org/10.3390/children11010062 (accessed on 21st July 2025).

18. Morton, C. A., Birnie, A., Eedy, D. J., Hughes, J. R., Sahota, A., McDonagh, A. J. G., Buckley, D. A., et al. (2013). British Association of Dermatologists' guidelines for the management of squamous cell carcinoma *in situ* (Bowen's disease) 2014. *British Journal of Dermatology, 170*, 245–260. https://doi.org/10.1111/bjd.12766 (accessed on 21st July 2025).

19. Fang, Wei-Cheng; Chou, Pei-Chien; Chiu, Li-Wen; Ke, Chiao-Li2; Cheng, Shih-Tsun. Dermoscopy as a Diagnostic and Monitoring Tool for Recurrent Extramammary Paget's Disease. Indian Journal of Dermatology 67(6):p 819-820, Nov–Dec 2022. | DOI: 10.4103/ijd.ijd_771_22 (accessed on 21st July 2025).

20. Neamonitou, F., Neamonitos, K. K., Stavrianos, S., & Neamonitos, K. P. (2024). A triple laser combination treatment for facial angiofibromata management in tuberous sclerosis and literature review. *Archives of Plastic Surgery, 51*, 372–377. https://doi.org/10.1055/a-2306-0962 (accessed on 21st July 2025).

21. Neittaanmäki-Perttu, N. (2015). *Diagnosis and Treatment of Premalignant Changes of Photodamaged Skin: Novel Hyperspectral Imaging and New Therapeutical Aspects.* https://core.ac.uk/download/33734561.pdf (accessed on 21st July 2025).

22. Nguyen, V., Karimi, S., Rybiński, M., & Xing, Z. (2023). MedRedQA for medical consumer question answering: Dataset, tasks, and neural baselines. https://doi.org/10.18653/v1/2023.ijcnlp-main.42 (accessed on 21st July 2025).

23. Nnebechukwu, I. A., Ibrahim, J. H., & Nwogu, C. N. K., & Gloria, G. (2025). Comparative analysis of the phytochemical and antifungal properties of lemon and lime peels in preventing rot fungi in Irish and sweet potatoes. *Research Journal of Phytochemistry.* https://www.semanticscholar.org/paper/68633f591f3b0f740cd169ca1de29a5cfa538ac7 (accessed on 21st July 2025).

24. Passeron, T., Genedy, R. M., Salah, L. A., Fusade, T., Kositratna, G., Laubach, H. J., Marini, L., et al. (2019). Laser treatment of hyperpigmented lesions: Position statement of the European Society of Laser in Dermatology. *Journal of the European Academy of Dermatology and Venereology, 33*, 987–1005. https://doi.org/10.1111/jdv.15497 (accessed on 21st July 2025).

25. Ridha, I. M., & Sabir, H. J. (2019). Comparative study of cryotherapy versus trichloroacetic acid chemical peels in the treatment of actinic keratosis. https://core.ac.uk/download/229808794.pdf (accessed on 21st July 2025).

26. Sadeghzadeh-Bazargan, A., Shafiei, M., Atefi, N., Dehghani, A., Pashaei, A., Karimzadeh, M., & Goodarzi, A. (2024). Evaluation and comparison of the efficacy and safety of cryotherapy and electrosurgery in the treatment of sebaceous hyperplasia, seborrheic keratosis, cherry angioma, and skin tag: A blinded randomized clinical trial study. *Health Science Reports, 7.* https://www.semanticscholar.org/paper/226bc8a448d32c1475834ee4d1830460e2bca450 (accessed on 21st July 2025).
27. Seoane Romero, J. (2023). *Estudio Del Mecanismo De Cancerificación Y Opciones Terapéuticas En La Queilitis Actínica.* https://core.ac.uk/download/555990688.pdf (accessed on 21st July 2025).
28. Spandau, D., Loesch, M., Somani, A. K., Kingsley, M., & Travers, J. B. (2014). Skin resurfacing procedures: New and emerging options. *Clinical Cosmetic and Investigational Dermatology.* https://doi.org/10.2147/ccid.s50367 (accessed on 21st July 2025).
29. Usatine, R. P., Pfenninger, J. L., Stulberg, D. L., & Small, R. (2011). *Dermatologic and Cosmetic Procedures in Office Practice E-Book.* Elsevier Health Sciences. https://play.google.com/store/books/details?id=XFR7oNXY-NYC&source=gbs_api (accessed on 21st July 2025).

HAIR AND NAIL DISORDERS

10

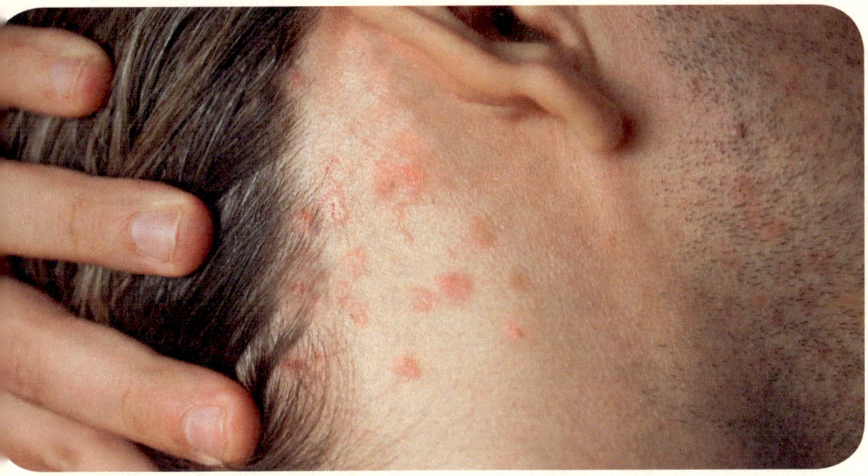

LEARNING OBJECTIVES

After studying this chapter, you will be able to:

1. Understand types of hair and nail disorders
2. Explain the causes of hair and nail disorders
3. Describe symptoms of hair and nail disorders

Introduction

The dermatology specialty encompasses a broad spectrum of hair and nail disorders, two anatomical structures that are not only of biological importance but also highly socially and psychologically relevant. The hair and nail disease spectrum ranges from simple complaints, such as dandruff and onychomycosis, to the more complex conditions, such as alopecia and psoriasis. These conditions all bear important implications for the social and self-esteem functioning of those afflicted, with implications for mental health and quality of life. Furthermore, many of these conditions are directly traceable to underlying medical conditions, so their inquiry is essential to dermatology practice and to the practice of integrative health fields. Understanding the complex etiology of hair and nail disorders facilitates improved diagnosis, treatment planning, and ultimately better patient outcomes. In recent years, new directions for therapeutic intervention have been opened by a better understanding of the biological processes that underpin hair and nail diseases. For example, immune-mediated mechanisms have been implicated in diseases such as psoriasis, which involves the nails as well as the skin (Raharja et al., 2021). The advent of targeted therapies is a step toward individualized medicine, aiming to tailor treatment options to the specific characteristics of a patient's disease. These developments underscore the necessity of interdisciplinary research by dermatologists, immunologists, and pharmaceutical scientists to optimize therapeutic strategies. Current work in the field acknowledges that skin health plays a vital role in overall systemic health, as the correlation between skin disease and conditions such as obesity and diabetes confirms. Moreover, greater knowledge of nail and hair disorders has led to increased interest in preventive and holistic approaches. Effective hair and nail care education, awareness of early-onset symptoms, and the importance of seeking early medical consultation are instrumental in managing such disorders. The more people know about their conditions, the better they are at advocating for themselves during clinical interactions, which is associated with better treatment outcomes. The ubiquity of stigma for visible skin disease throughout the ages highlights, all the more so, the imperatives to transform society, such as the imperative to get healthcare workers to adopt a humane, whole-person approach when dealing with patients suffering from hair and nail disorders. Conjoining psychosocial therapy with medical treatment will reinvigorate patients' resilience and address these ailments more effectively in the long term.

Definition of Hair and Nail Disorders

The term hair and nail disorders refers to a large collection of conditions that involve the structure and function of these appendages. Disorders of hair can present as changes in quality, quantity, or distribution of hair, such as alopecia, hypertrichosis, and several dermatitis types. Alopecia is defined by hair loss, which may be localized, such as alopecia areata, or diffuse, such as androgenetic alopecia. In addition, conditions telogen effluvium may cause diffuse hair loss in response to stressors. Understanding such illnesses is necessary for correct diagnosis and treatment because hair often has integral aesthetic and psychological roles in individuals' lives. On the other hand, nail diseases also pose particular challenges, typically arising from intrinsic pathologies or extrinsic factors. Some of the most common nail conditions are onychomycosis, or fungal disease of the nails, and psoriatic nails, which become pitted, discolored, or separated from the nail bed. Signs of these conditions should be recorded, as they may indicate the development of systemic diseases or infections. Nails are also significant indicators of overall health, as they serve as a gauge of nutritional status and potential internal complications. Successful treatment and management of nail diseases can render a wonderful difference in the quality of life of affected individuals, helping them achieve normalcy and self-confidence. Furthermore, it cannot be overstated that hair and nail disorders are associated with overall health conditions. For instance, illnesses chronic liver disease can trigger dramatic changes in the health of the nails and hair. It has been established through individual studies that mortality rates due to liver-related conditions, particularly in those suffering from substance use disorder, can be attributed to declining conditions of hair and nails, ultimately affecting patient outcomes (Kåberg et al., 2020). Therefore, a multidisciplinary approach to the diagnosis and treatment of hair and nail disorders, based on the patient's overall condition, is necessary. This perspective facilitates a deeper understanding of the significance of these disorders and their implications, enabling healthcare professionals to provide effective interventions that address the physiological and psychosocial aspects of patients' lives (Figure 10.1).

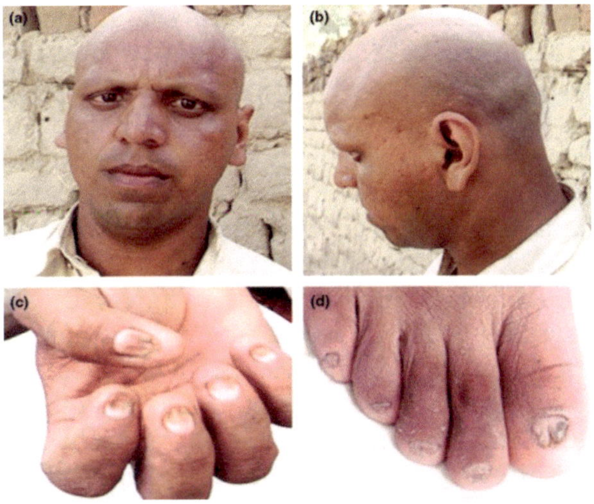

Figure 10.1. Clinical presentation of the hair and nails in the affected individual. (a) The eyebrows and eyelashes are completely missing; (b) complete absence of hair on the scalp; (c) fingernails; (d) dystrophic toenails.

Source: https://www.researchgate.net/profile/Dr-Ghazanfar-Ali/publication/6341871/figure/fig1/AS:280381816360965@1443859642140/Clinical-presentation-of-ED-of-the-hair-and-nails-in-the-affected-individual-IV-2-aThe.png.

Importance of Studying These Disorders

Understanding hair and nail disease is essential, not only for dermatologic health but also for social and psychological health. Hair and nail conditions can have a profound effect on individuals' self-esteem and overall quality of life because they often serve as external signals of identity. Because hair and nails are highly visible, their disease can lead to stigmatization and social isolation. By studying such disorders, clinicians and researchers can develop better treatments and diagnoses, so that individuals may receive the care and treatment they require. Additional knowledge in this discipline also supports preventive approaches, enabling individuals to maintain healthy hair and nails and potentially avoid more serious health problems associated with overlooked conditions. Therefore, an extended knowledge of these disorders goes beyond the province of mere clinical interest to social attitudes and individual psychosocial health. Beyond the psychosocial component, the study of hair and nail disorders is important for the detection of underlying systemic medical disorders. The majority of diseases of the hair and nails are indicative of other medical conditions, such as nutritional disturbances or endocrine disorders. For example, some dermatological findings, like alopecia, may be indicative of autoimmune disorders or thyroid disorders, and it is therefore important for health providers to identify these symptoms in early stages. By linking disorders of the hair and nails to overall health, clinicians can implement more comprehensive treatment strategies that consider the whole person rather than individual symptoms. These integrative approaches not only enhance patient outcomes but also foster a better appreciation of the interrelatedness of body systems, thereby supporting a model of health that values prevention as well as timely intervention.

Finally, further research into nail and hair disorders can help identify novel cures and therapeutic methods. There is substantial investment in this industry due to the global demand for beautiful hair and nails. The proper application of recent scientific progress, such as the research on biomaterials in regenerative medicine, reflects the potential benefits of ongoing research endeavors. As noted in the relevant literature, some studies identify novel applications of advanced materials that can significantly prolong treatment for such patients, thereby encouraging the design of improved solutions (He et al., 2023). Moreover, greater understanding of syndromes such as Complex Regional Pain Syndrome highlights the need for a science-driven treatment system in which ongoing research continues to generate beneficial knowledge, paving the way for landmark advances in the management of these once-intractable diseases (Harden et al., 2022). Lastly, the importance of hair and nail disorder study can never be overstated, as ongoing research not only responds to isolated questions regarding one's health, but also contributes towards further development of overall knowledge in dermatological science.

Overview of Common Types of Disorders

Among the various alopecia conditions that affect the hair and nails, alopecia areata is a prototype of a non-scarring autoimmune condition. Alopecia can present in varying degrees, ranging from small patches of hair loss to complete baldness of the scalp or body. The complex etiology of alopecia areata necessitates a thorough understanding of the pathogenetic mechanisms to improve treatment efficacy. Scientific studies have established that systemic pulse-dose corticosteroid therapy can induce hair regrowth; however, responses vary among patients, depending on numerous factors. Specifically, recent literature states that patients with shorter disease durations and younger ages will experience better rates of recovery, while others with histories of atopy or more severe forms of the condition will have less favorable outcomes. Hence, treatment approaches tailored to patients' characteristics and disease history are essential for effective management of alopecia areata (Rastaghi et al., 2023).

Diseases of the nails also have an important place within the general category of dermal diseases, with their presentation frequently mimicked by underlying systemic illnesses. Common types of nail disorders are onychomycosis, in which fungal infection leads to discoloration and brittleness, and koilonychia or spoon nails, which can be a sign of iron deficiency anemia. These can be due to a myriad of reasons ranging from nutritional deficiencies to long-term illnesses. For instance, patients with presentations of brittleness of the nails with overall weakness may require evaluation for probable causes , such as anaemia, a widespread concern globally. A clear understanding of the biological processes underlying such nail disorders can equip healthcare professionals with the information necessary for accurate diagnosis and effective treatment strategies (Hurley, 2007). This integrated model of management enhances patient outcomes and addresses both the cosmetic and physiological aspects of nail disorders. Recognition of the interrelationship between hair and nail disease underscores the importance of a comprehensive clinical evaluation. Both diseases can serve as markers of overall well-being, with underlying complications that require prompt intervention. For instance, dermatologists must not only examine the hair and nails but also consider factors such as diet, lifestyle, and other health conditions that may precipitate these disorders. Detailed histories and symptomatic questioning are critical, with some presentations, including brittle nails or hair, being pointers to more severe underlying conditions, such as autoimmune disease or nutritional deficiency. Incorporating a collaborative care model with multidisciplinary input can optimize treatment modalities and patient adherence. Overall, there needs to be a focus on combined approaches that not only restore appearance but also induce overall well-being and quality of life (Hurley, 2007).

10.1. Types of Hair Disorders

Learning Outcome

1. Describe androgenetic alopecia.
2. Define alopecia areata.
3. Understand telogen effluvium.

The landscape of hair disease is diverse in terms of manifestations and etiology. Genetic hair diseases are among the significant groups that are associated with mutations implicated in the development of hair shafts and density.

Conditions ectodermal dysplasias, a group of genetic disorders, illustrate the intricate relationship between genes and hair growth. These patients often exhibit hypotrichosis (thinned hair growth), among other features, such as dental abnormalities and facial dysmorphism. These genomic alterations, including the novel TSPEAR variant, attest to the ongoing contributions of genomic studies in elucidating hair disorders and their complex modulations. Genetic sequencing technological advances provide evidence of the etiology of these disorders that reveal directions for potentially useful approaches to targeted intervention and individualized therapeutic interventions that have the potential to enhance the quality of life of people with these conditions (Akçahan Akalın et al., 2025). Environmental factors contribute significantly to the health and cosmetic appearance of hair, alongside genetic determinants. Increasing amounts of evidence have made a connection between exposure to environmental toxins and various hair disorders, including hair loss and texture alterations. Studies have shown that pollutants disrupt the growth cycle of hair and are implicated in inflammatory diseases that worsen the scalp's health. The role of biomarkers in assessing exposure to these environmental toxins has taken center stage in research, enabling researchers to track the health risks of pollution. Analysis of hair and nail samples for biomarkers can be an effective approach to understanding the broader public health significance of external exposure, as well as its impact on individual health. Combining environmental assessments with clinical outcomes may help better control hair disorders resulting from external factors. Psychosocial considerations also play a dominant part in disorders of hair, particularly those resulting in alopecia areata. This autoimmune condition can cause rapid, patchy loss of hair and has a great emotional effect on the person. The psychoemotional impact transcends appearances, predisposing to anxiety and depression as pressures arising from physical appearance due to society's growth. With greater awareness of the psychosocial impact of hair conditions, there is an increased need for holistic treatment approaches that address both the medical and psychological components. Treatment modalities may include counseling, especially cognitive behavior therapy, engaging with the emotional suffering of hair loss. Interventions like this have stressed the necessity for an integrated strategy in addressing hair disorders as a manifestation of the interaction of genetic, environmental, and psychological elements in management and treatment (Akçahan Akalın et al., 2025).

10.1.1. Androgenetic Alopecia

Androgenetic alopecia (AGA), also known as male and female pattern baldness, is a prevalent form of hair loss due to hormonal and genetic factors. It is a gradual, progressive thinning of the hair according to predictable patterns. In males, it starts at the temples and top of the head; in females, it starts at the temples and top of the head and then spreads to the crown. This condition can not only impact physical appearance but also psychological health, with issues including low self-esteem and depression. AGA is estimated to occur in more than 50% of men and a high percentage of women by the age of 50 years, indicating its expansive prevalence and impact on beauty and masculinity attitudes in society. Through continued research, it is important to recognize the implications for AGA in both clinical management and psychosocial impacts. The pathophysiology of androgenetic alopecia is a complex interaction between genetic predisposition and hormonal action, specifically dihydrotestosterone (DHT) action. DHT is a strong androgenic steroid produced from the conversion of testosterone. It binds to androgen receptors on hair follicles and contributes to miniaturization, shortening hair cycles, and promoting hair loss. Genetic differences associated with the androgen receptor gene also contribute to increased susceptibility to AGA. New studies have also begun to look at the potential connection between AGA and systemic diseases, suggesting that individuals with hair loss might be more susceptible to certain metabolic or cardiovascular diseases. As the condition progresses, understanding such correlations is necessary to develop comprehensive treatment modalities, particularly those that account for aesthetic impact as well as overall health. Moreover, recent evidence indicates that systemic conditions such as COVID-19 can influence hair diseases and exacerbate underlying conditions such as AGA. More notably, telogen effluvium and high incidences of alopecia areata have been noted in patients after COVID infection, which is of concern to those who have a propensity towards androgenetic alopecia.

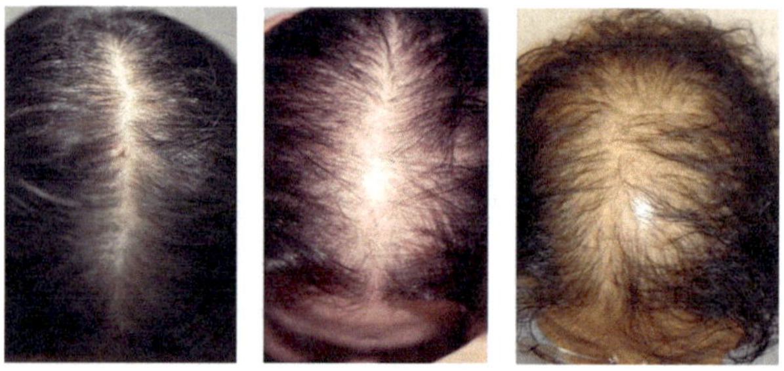

Figure 10.2. Androgenetic alopecia in women.

Source: https://www.researchgate.net/publication/313792549/figure/fig2/AS:462445513842689@1487267010518/Androgenetic-Alopecia-in-Women-Ludwig-Classification.png.

The pandemic's stress also adds more challenges to individuals with hair loss conditions, further enhancing the psychological load of AGA. There is evidence showing a high correlation between the emotional disturbance resulting from AGA and psychosocial dimensions of large-scale diseases, such as COVID-19, which have been shown to impact the condition of hair. Treatment strategies in the future should be guided by the resolution of these issues, allowing the care delivered to be holistic in nature and considering physical as well as psychological aspects of health, as viewed in studies of alopecia's psychological impact and more generalized health effects (Wollina et al., 2022; Muntyanu et al., 2023) (Figure 10.2).

10.1.2. Alopecia Areata

Alopecia areata is a common, nonscarring disease characterized by sudden, patchy hair loss that can involve any region of the body. The condition is an autoimmune phenomenon characterized by targeting of hair follicles, resulting in unsightly patches of baldness that can significantly affect a person's self-esteem and psychological well-being. The condition arises from a misplaced immune response that attacks hair follicles in error, disrupting the cycle of hair growth without in any way destroying the follicles themselves. The temporary nature makes it feasible that there can be regrowth, a glimmer of hope in an otherwise agonizing process of losing one's hair. Despite its comparatively harmless pathophysiology, its psychosocial effect is considerable in that patients undergo stigmatization or anxiety due to how they look, as noted by research that listed the psychological outcomes of alopecia areata. Epidemiological figures indicate that the lifetime risk of developing alopecia areata is approximately 2%, with age groups primarily undergoing onset in their third or fourth decades. The condition shows no significant difference in incidence across races, suggesting shared susceptibility. There have been genetic predispositions, and therefore, it is of high priority for research into its etiology and management. Moreover, alopecia areata tends to appear with psychiatric comorbidities like anxiety and depression that could further accentuate the emotional stress of hair loss. The connection underscores the need for comprehensive management strategies that address both the physical manifestations of the disorder and its psychological complications, supporting an integrative approach to managing patients with alopecia areata. Alopecia areata therapies remain limited; thus, there is a need for innovative measures to combat its effects. Although a few patients may respond to therapies with corticosteroids, minoxidil, or immunotherapy, the availability and effectiveness of these drugs vary significantly from individual to individual. The majority of patients resort to cosmetic therapies such as wigs or hairpieces, particularly when traditional therapies prove disappointing. This wigmaker dependence underscores one facet of social fairness in healthcare—the differential access to care materials across regions and healthcare systems, as evidenced by ongoing controversy over NHS provision of wigs (Ross et al., 2024). As awareness increases, there is a greater need for standardized treatment protocol implementation and for greater resource availability for alopecia areata, in line with best-practice recommendations for comprehensive care and support within psychological and dermatological frameworks (Ross et al., 2024) (Figure 10.3).

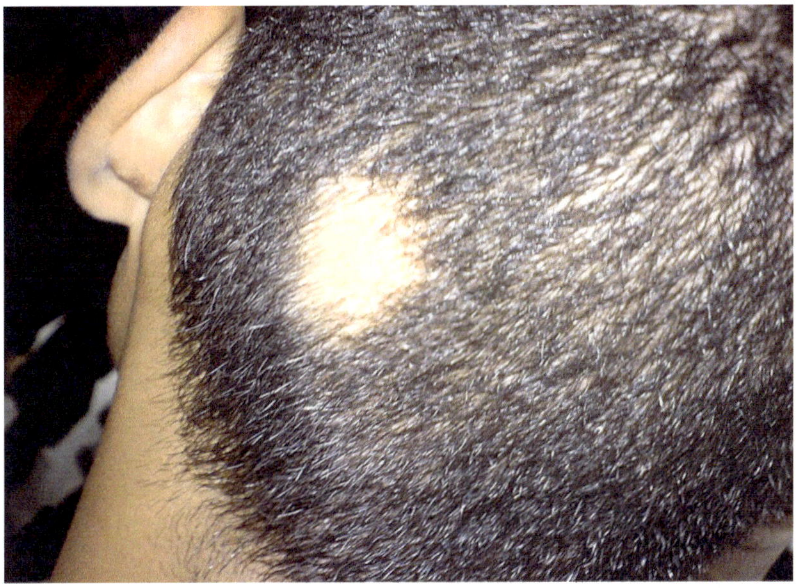

Figure 10.3. Alopecia areata seen on the back of the scalp.

Source: https://upload.wikimedia.org/wikipedia/commons/thumb/3/38/Allopecia_areata.JPG/800px-Allopecia_areata.JPG.

10.1.3. Telogen Effluvium

Telogen effluvium is characterized by diffuse shedding of hair because of disruptions in the cycle of hair growth, particularly during the telogen stage. Telogen effluvium is induced by multiple causes, including stress, endocrine disturbances, and malnutrition. For instance, stressful events giving birth or serious illness can induce a sudden acceleration of hair loss, which typically occurs two to three months after the event. The physiological response to such stressors is seen by an increased number of hair follicles entering the telogen phase, resulting in visible thinning. Understanding the pathophysiology of telogen effluvium is most valuable because it facilitates recognition of causative factors and, consequently, targeted treatment designed to address the cause of baldness rather than merely its symptoms. Recent research has underscored the role of micronutrients in normal hair, suggesting that deficiency might play a major role in the pathogenesis of telogen effluvium. The essential vitamins and minerals , such as iron, zinc, and the B vitamins are required to provide for normal hair follicle function and for normal hair growth. Nutrient-dependent levels can disrupt the continuation of the hair cycles and increase hair shedding. As highlighted in recent literature, correction of such deficiencies can be a reversible risk factor for the management of the condition. With a better understanding of the interplay among diet, micronutrient status, and hair health, health professionals are now in a more favorable position to intervene with a more holistic approach to treating patients with telogen effluvium, thereby achieving improved outcomes in hair restoration and overall well-being (Hind et al., 2018). Diagnosis of telogen effluvium requires a thorough evaluation of the clinical history of the patient and potential underlying disease, since the symptomatology overlaps with other conditions of hair loss. This is typically achieved by evaluating variables like stress levels, hormonal status, and nutritional status that influence hair growth. Current research has theorized that conditions such as thyroid abnormalities and iron deficiency may lead to abnormal hair shedding (Wolff et al., 2016). Management of telogen effluvium is typically conservative but may, if necessary, include lifestyle modifications, nutritional supplementation, and stress-management measures. While hair loss can be distressing for patients, telogen effluvium is, to a significant extent, reversible with appropriate management, and hair growth tends to recur within months. This underscores the importance of early diagnosis and treatment of the condition to improve patients' quality of life (Figure 10.4).

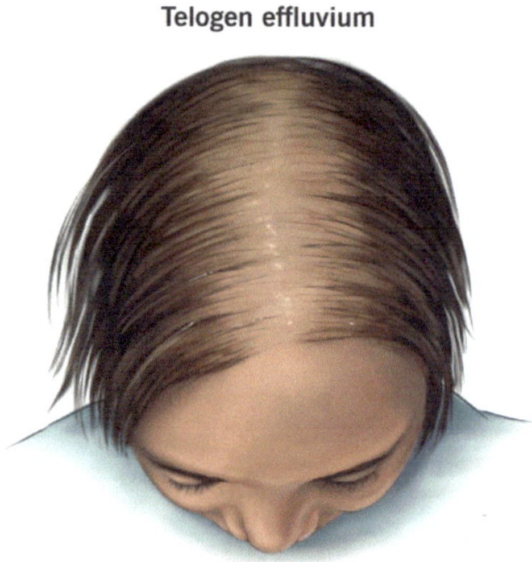

Figure 10.4. Illustration of telogen effluvium.

Source: https://my.clevelandclinic.org/-/scassets/images/org/health/articles/24486-telogen-effluvium.

Test Your Knowledge

1. What is the main cause of androgenetic alopecia?
2. How does alopecia areata typically present on the scalp?
3. What triggers telogen effluvium, and how does it affect hair growth?

10.2. Types of Nail Disorders

Learning Outcome

1. Describe onychomycosis, a fungal nail infection.
2. Define ingrown nails.
3. Understand nail psoriasis.

Nail disease can be an expression of more widespread systemic disease, and a number of types of nail disorders with varying clinical features and significance exist. Perhaps the most frequent is fungal infection of the nails, or onychomycosis, affecting the nail bed primarily and presenting with discoloration, thickening, and nail loss. Fungal infections are classified by etiology, with the most common pathogens being dermatophytes, particularly Trichophyton rubrum, which has previously been documented to account for a high percentage of such infections in patients (Powell et al., 2022). The epidemiology of onychomycosis shows a higher prevalence among older age groups, possibly secondary to age-related changes in nail architecture and decreased immune status. It is therefore critical to understand the incidence and characteristics of these causative organisms to inform effective management and treatment strategies.

Another prominent class of nail disorders includes those caused by trauma, which may present as ridges, splits, or complete avulsion of the nail. Trauma may be acute due to accidents or injury, or chronic due to repetitive excess pressure from footwear or repetitive motion. The response of the nail matrix to trauma is likely to lead to apparent alterations that have the potential to impact a person's lifestyle, like pain and cosmetic concerns. Complications can manifest in terms of infections, which may exacerbate the original trauma, thereby making protective strategies and early intervention all the more important. It has been found through research that awareness about nail health and potential threats can reduce the incidence of trauma-induced disorders, promoting better overall nail care and preventive practices in those who have a history of such damage. Aside from infections and trauma, systemic disorders account for the majority of nail disorders, with evidence indicating a link between overall well-being and nail health. Conditions eczema and psoriasis can cause several forms of nail alteration, including ridging, pitting, and discoloration. Such observations can provide valuable diagnostic clues to underlying systemic illness, guiding clinicians toward appropriate treatment modalities. Certain patients with CRPS, for example, exhibit alterations in hair, skin, and nails, indicating broader pathophysiologic implications (Antonia et al., 2020). Awareness of the types of nail diseases and their associations with systemic health is essential for clinicians, as it enables an integrated approach to the diagnosis, care, and treatment of both nail disease and chronic illness.

10.2.1. Onychomycosis

Onychomycosis, a fungal infection of the nails, is a significant clinical issue in hair and nail disease. It is characterized by the invasion of dermatophytes, yeasts, or non-dermatophyte molds of the nail plate and surrounding tissues, and it is often associated with discolored, thickened, and brittle nails. The prevalence of onychomycosis is demographically heterogeneous, with a greater proportion of older persons bearing the brunt of age-related changes in nail morphology and immune function. Onychomycosis is not merely a cosmetic issue but also carries related major morbidity in the form of pain and secondary infections. Common modes of infection are driven by an imbalance in the skin microbiome, with opportunistic fungi invading and displacing normal flora, a process similar to that described for *Candida* species by Talapko et al. (2021). Also involved are concomitant environmental factors, such as moisture and trauma, in exacerbating the onset and development of the conditions. Diagnosis of onychomycosis is a multidisciplinary procedure, typically initiated by a thorough clinical assessment and followed by laboratory confirmation. Clinicians typically use potassium hydroxide (KOH) preparations or cultures to identify the specific etiologic pathogens, which is the most important factor in developing effective treatment protocols. Furthermore, advances in the technological diagnostics available in dermatology, such as machine learning algorithms, are being explored in order to enhance diagnosis validity and provide more opportunity for early intervention, implying greater convergence between technology and dermatology (Chan et al., 2020). Determination of which type of fungus is present is also important, since dermatophytes typically must be treated differently from yeasts or molds. This multifaceted system of diagnosis highlights the complexity of onychomycosis therapy, which is primarily based upon an understanding of fungal pathophysiology and host immunity. Treatment of onychomycosis is based on the severity of infection and the etiological fungi. Antifungal therapy is both systemic and topical, and systemic drugs such as terbinafine and itraconazole are effective for more extensive infections. On the other hand, local agents may be sufficient for localized infections, but with minimal impact due to insufficient penetration through nails. There is a need for consideration of patient comorbidities and tolerance to drugs when choosing the treatment to provide a patient-specific approach to treating the disease. Additionally, technological innovations provide new avenues for treating onychomycosis. For instance, laser treatment has been explored for its ability to target fungal cells specifically without affecting adjacent tissue. With further research and development, the use of these varying treatment modalities can increasingly rely on evidence-based outcomes and improved therapeutic protocols, thereby favorably advancing patient outcomes within the framework of hair and nail disease (Figure 10.5).

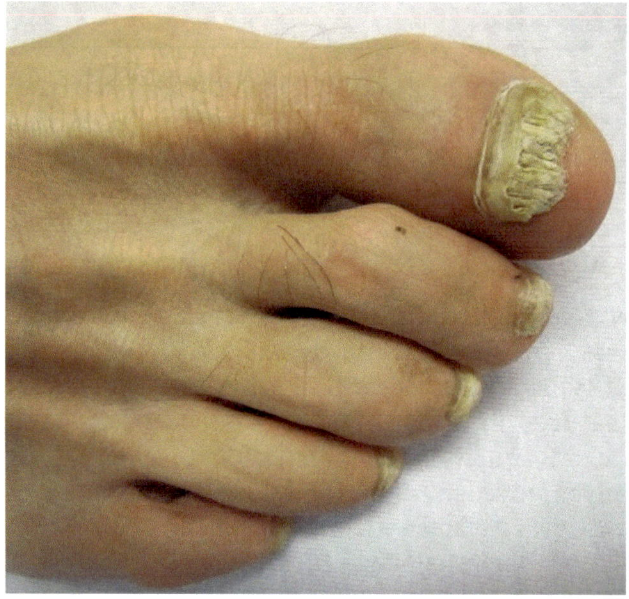

Figure 10.5. Onychomycosis of the toenails.

Source: https://upload.wikimedia.org/wikipedia/commons/thumb/a/a4/Oncymycosis.JPG/800px-Oncymycosis.JPG.

10.2.2. Ingrown Nails

Ingrown nails, or clinically onychogryphosis, is a common nail disease involving the migration of the nail into the skin. The toes, the great toe especially, can be presented in diverse ways, such as redness, swelling, and tenderness. Ingrown nails typically occur due to improper methods of nail cutting, such as cutting the nails short or cutting the nails to their tips, thereby placing the nail in a position to grow into the soft tissues. Subsequently, this displacement can lead to secondary infections, with the exposed skin becoming inflamed and irritated. In some cases, ingrown nails can progress to more complex dermatologic disorders, particularly in individuals with pre-existing conditions such as diabetes mellitus, where infection and delayed healing are significantly heightened and necessitate appropriate management regimens. Treatments for ingrown nails range from conservative to surgical, depending on the severity and duration of the disorder. Primary therapy typically involves soaking the infected foot in warm water to reduce inflammation and alleviate pain, and applying antiseptic ointment to prevent infection. Over-the-counter painkillers are also effective in managing sudden pain that arises with the condition. When conservative management fails, a physician may recommend more advanced operations , such as partial nail avulsion or application of phenol to prevent recurrence. These treatments are made to correct the etiology of the ingrown nail with a low risk of recurrence. Early treatment cannot be stressed too much because untreated conditions may lead to complications, such as abscess formation and chronic pain, adversely impacting the patients quality of life. The relationship between ingrown nails and other nail disorders underscores the need to raise awareness of proper nail care and management practices. Etiologic knowledge of ingrown nails may deter individuals from engaging in dangerous nail-grooming techniques, thereby promoting better individual outcomes. Moreover, conditions affecting the integrity of the nails, such as those caused by untoward dermatologic events surrounding targeted therapies, can exacerbate ingrown nails. For instance, drugs that induce nail bed alteration can lead to a greater incidence of conditions like paronychia, which predisposes patients to ingrown nails (Mario et al., 2018). Emollients and keratolytics, such as urea, have also proven effective therapies for treating secondary conditions and promoting nail health, underscoring the importance of overall management of dermatologic treatment (Pan et al., 2013). Since ingrown nails are a recurring but controllable disorder, knowledge of their causative conditions is crucial in ensuring improved nail health in general (Figure 10.6).

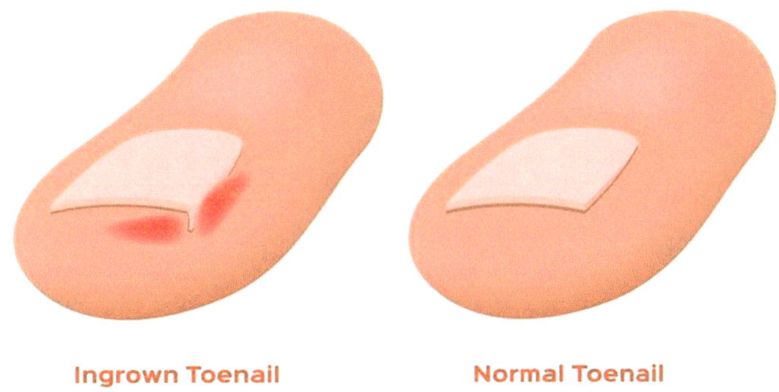

Figure 10.6. Diagram showing ingrown nails and a normal toenail.

Source: https://sa1s3optim.patientpop.com/assets/images/provider/photos/2352619.jpg.

10.2.3. Nail Psoriasis

Nail psoriasis, which is among the manifestations of psoriasis that affect the nails, is difficult both to diagnose and manage. Nail psoriasis is normally manifested by alterations in the appearance of the nails, including pitting, coloration, and thickening of the nails. Such signs and symptoms are painful physically and cause distress psychologically because they can affect self-esteem as well as social life. The pathophysiology of nail psoriasis is characterized by an abnormal immune response that perpetuates overproduction of skin cells and inflammation. As with other dermatologic presentations of psoriasis, involvement of the nails is generally continuous and can truly affect daily functioning. Identification of the distinctive features of nail psoriasis is essential for proper management, as it may require treatments distinct from those used for plaque psoriasis. The treatment of psoriasis of the nails tends to be both systemic and topical in nature. Mild cases can often be managed with topicals, such as corticosteroids or vitamin D analogs, while more severe cases often necessitate the use of systemic medications. Systemic therapies, including biologics, such as proinflammatory cytokine-directed agents , such as interleukin 17 (IL-17), have emerged to prominence due to their efficacy and potency in immune system modulation. New descriptions of the role of IL-17 in psoriasis pathogenesis and the promise of treatments targeting this cytokine to help patients with nail disease. As our understanding of IL-17 grows, so too does the promise of tailored treatment plans that may enhance patient health and outcomes (José et al., 2019).

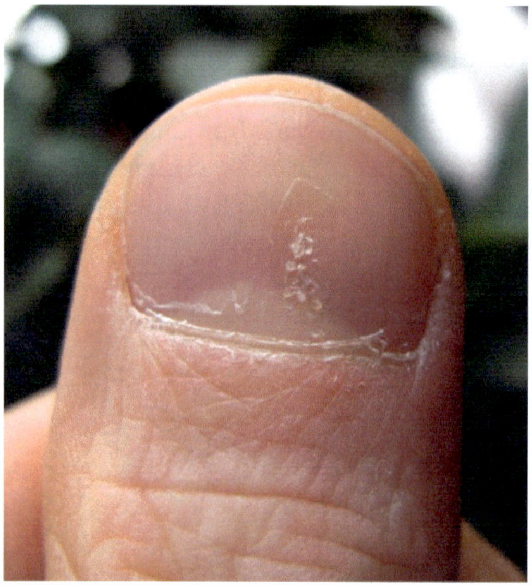

Figure 10.7. Psoriasis of a fingernail, with visible pitting.

Source: https://upload.wikimedia.org/wikipedia/commons/thumb/b/b3/Luszczyca_paznokcia.jpg/800px-Luszczyca_paznokcia.jpg.

In addition to pharmacological treatment, addressing the psychosocial aspects of nail psoriasis is necessary for integrated care. Patients can become stigmatized or embarrassed due to visible nail changes and withdraw from social activity and possess an inferior quality of life. Supportive treatment, including counseling and education, can empower patients suffering from these consequences. Moreover, a multidisciplinary system that includes dermatologists, rheumatologists, and mental health professionals can facilitate integrative treatment. By understanding the interface between physical symptoms and mental well-being, the treatment model can be optimized, enabling patients to be treated not only for the physical symptoms of nail psoriasis but also to overcome psychosocial barriers (Figure 10.7).

Test Your Knowledge

1. What is onychomycosis? Explain.
2. How does nail psoriasis differ from regular psoriasis on the skin?

10.3. Causes of Hair Disorders

Learning Outcome

1. Explain how genetic factors play a pivotal role in the development and manifestation of various hair disorders.
2. Describe how hormones , such as estrogen and testosterone lead to various hair disorders.
3. Understand environmental influences for hair disorders.

Conditions of the hair can be caused by a number of factors genetic, environmental, and psychological factors. Genetic predilection plays a significant role in most hair conditions, such as androgenetic alopecia, also known as male or female pattern baldness. In other cases, one inherits the susceptibility to thinning or loss of hair, which occurs over several years because of the hormones that govern hair follicle biology. Environmental reasons, including exposure to powerful chemicals found in hair products, excessive heat from styling tools, and air pollution, may exacerbate underlying conditions or create new ones. Furthermore, lifestyle components, such as nutrition or stress, are involved with hair health. Identifying these multifactorial causes can assist in the proper treatment and prevention of individuals with hair disorders. Endocrine system imbalances, and particularly hormonal imbalances, are the focus in the pathogenesis of hair pathology. Polycystic ovary syndrome (PCOS) in women is a disorder that leads to elevated androgenic levels, which can result in signs of hirsutism and androgenic alopecia. Alternatively, thyroid disorders, hypothyroidism, and hyperthyroidism can cause alterations in hair texture and density. Additionally, certain medications, like those used in chemotherapy or hormonal therapy, can result in hair loss as a secondary effect. Psychological factors, in turn, including stress and depression, have been reported as contributing causes of hair disorders by research, which also tend to impact phases of hair growth. Management of endocrine status and determination of the hormonal basis of hair disorders are required for comprehensive care of patients. Inflammatory and infectious conditions are also etiologies of hair disease, often complicating diagnosis and treatment. Scaly scalp infections , such as tinea capitis (scalp fungus) can result in patchy loss of hair and require antifungal therapy to resolve. Inflammatory diseases like alopecia areata, an autoimmune disease, result in sudden patchy hair loss and have been linked to other autoimmune diseases, highlighting the complex interaction between immune status and hair health. Moreover, skin disorders psoriasis or seborrheic dermatitis are capable of producing flaking and inflammation, which adversely affect the vitality of hair. Effective management of hair disorders often necessitates treating early infections or inflammatory conditions, and current investigations are uncovering genetic and environmental factors that contribute to these diseases, potentially enabling improved therapeutic approaches in the future.

10.3.1. Genetic Factors

Genetic factors play a significant part in the etiology and clinical manifestation of most hair and nail diseases. Numerous studies have identified genetic loci that influence hair density and quality and may contribute to conditions such as alopecia or male pattern baldness. Genome-wide association studies (GWAS) have indicated that traits such as follicular unit density (FUD) and hairs per follicular unit (HFU) are significantly influenced by genetic factors. For instance, the analysis identified strong associations with loci implicated in hair follicle morphogenesis, suggesting a genetic component in hair pathologies. These findings not only enhance our insight into these disorders but also suggest potential directions for individualized treatment modalities, as knowing the genetic background can assist in identifying targeted medications or prophylactic measures for at-risk individuals for hair disorders, including the therapeutic effectiveness of drugs like finasteride (Qian et al., 2025). Hair disease is not unique in its genetic determinants; it is characterized by multidimensional interactions with environmental factors. Investigations have established the way genetic tendencies interact with lifestyle factors, such as diet and environmental toxins, to influence hair growth and quality. For example, body mass index, gender, and age are demographic factors that have been associated with variation in hair density traits. This multifaceted relationship suggests that while genetic determinants beget a basal risk profile, environmental determinants may either amplify or attenuate such genetic vulnerabilities. Sophisticated phenotyping methods and statistical techniques allow researchers to examine such interactions more rigorously. Appreciation of the synergy between genetics and the environment is imperative for healthcare clinicians, with the aim of treating hair disorders holistically, thereby enabling tailored patient care and management (Qian et al., 2025). Nail disorders, like their hair counterparts, also have extensive genetic components. Genetic mutations have been associated with many nail pathologies, such as onychodystrophy and nail-patella syndrome, which may lead to abnormal nail patterns and growth. For instance, mutations in genes involved in keratin synthesis can cause brittle nails, a common disorder that may present with symptoms attributable to genetic predisposition. Building on knowledge of nail disorders, recent research on oculocutaneous albinism has shown that defects in genes responsible for melanin synthesis influence the visual properties of hair and nails, highlighting a complex network of genes that regulate these features. By exploring these genetic relationships, researchers can move toward a more profound understanding of nail illnesses and create molecular diagnostic tests that enable the identification and management of such diseases in clinics (Figure 10.8).

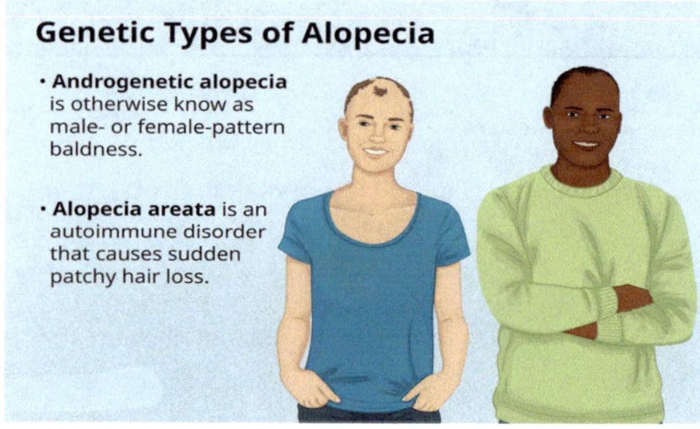

Figure 10.8. Genetic types of alopecia.

Source: https://www.verywellhealth.com/thmb/Bfe3XwYNKZ8-gp3QYXx51yhh1OY=/1500x0/filters:no_upscale():max_bytes(150000):strip_icc()/IsAlopeciaGenetic-d2c01ba95869447a8db87f088c14e241.jpg.

10.3.2. Hormonal Changes

Hormonal changes are key to the health and maintenance of hair and nails, including their growth and overall appearance. Hormonal alterations in estrogen and testosterone, for instance, lead to a variety of hair diseases , such as excessive thinning or hair loss. Estrogen has been found to enhance hair growth, and the decrease in its levels at menopause leads to increased hair loss among women. In addition, conditions polycystic ovary syndrome (PCOS) accompany elevated levels of testosterone, which can cause androgenic alopecia, where hair thins out, and bald patches begin to appear. An understanding of these hormonal dynamics is essential for diagnosing and treating hair diseases, as these conditions typically require interventions targeting the underlying hormonal imbalance.

The influences of these hormonal changes are not limited to the scalp; they also play a significant role in nail health. Hormonal imbalance may lead to alterations in the growth patterns of nails, resulting in symptoms like slow nail growth or brittle nails. An example is thyroid hormones, which are vital for regulating keratin metabolism, the protein used in nail formation. Underactive thyroid or hypothyroidism may lead to brittle, peeling, or slow-growing nails. Hyperthyroidism, in turn, may lead to rapid nail growth but with brittleness. In addition, hormonal changes caused by stress or nutritional deficiencies can exacerbate the aforementioned conditions to create a complex interrelationship between nail disease and systemic conditions that demands clinical evaluation and management as a whole.

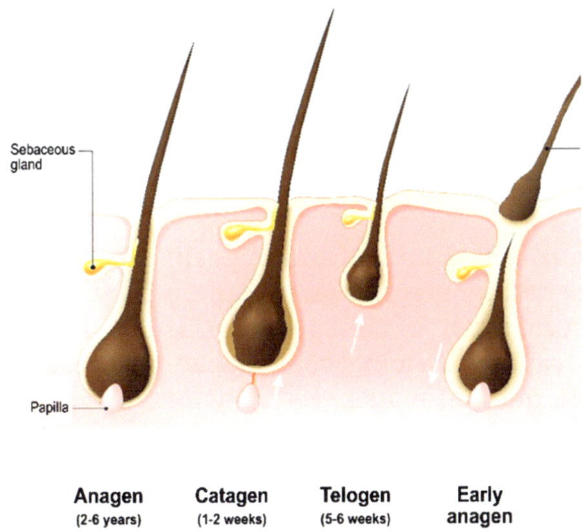

Figure 10.9. Hormones and hair loss.

Source: https://www.zrtlab.com/media/2196/hormones-and-hair-loss.png.

Research indicates that dermatologic presentation is often a sign of intrinsic hormonal pathology and a useful clue to the patient's overall condition. For instance, eating disorders are generally associated with hormonal imbalances that can result in severe hair and nail disorders. Patients may experience hair loss and brittle nails due to inadequate intake of essential nutrients resulting from abnormal eating patterns. The deficiencies lead to abnormal hormone levels, which further exacerbate dermatologic manifestations. Multidisciplinary management that incorporates dermatological evaluations, nutritional assessments, and psychiatric treatment is necessary to optimally address these health concerns. By identifying the link between hormonal imbalance and hair and nail diseases, healthcare providers can develop targeted treatments to restore both cosmetic appearance and overall well-being in affected individuals (Alsatti et al., 2024; Rallis et al., 2024) (Figure 10.9).

10.3.3. Environmental Influences

Environmental factors assume a crucial role in the etiology and exacerbation of nail and hair diseases. Exposure to pollutants, chemicals in cosmeceuticals, and water quality can have a profound impact on hair and nail health. For example, heavy metals in certain cosmetic products and in water supplies may cause chemical damage to hair, rendering it brittle and prone to breakage. Moreover, exposure to harmful chemicals, such as phthalates and parabens that are widely used in cosmetics, may disrupt hormone balance and potentially lead to hair growth and texture disorders. Understanding such environmental factors is not only essential in risk reduction but also in the development of treatment and prevention strategies that seriously consider consumer safety and health. The use patterns of beauty products further complicate how environmental concerns affect hair and nail health, particularly among targeted groups. African American and other women of color are found to use more hair and beauty products, including dangerous substances, in response to social ideals and standards of beauty. Increased exposure within an environment where the regulation of harmful substances in cosmetics is lacking only serves to worsen the issue. The significant racial and ethnic disparities in product use emphasize the important need for health interventions that are specific. Notably, marginalized women tend to have more negative health consequences due to social and environmental determinants, highlighting the important need for incorporating environmental justice into beauty product-related health practice (Ami et al., 2017). Moreover, systemic issues, such as socioeconomic disparities and discriminatory advertising, exacerbate environmental forces that influence hair and nail disease. The vast majority of individuals who reside in impoverished communities have zero exposure to secure beauty products and are regularly subjected to advertisements that promote potentially dangerous products. This situation is an overlap of beauty ideals, environmental exposure, and health disparities. Thus, scientists and medical practitioners are called to action to address these disparities by advocating for greater control over and knowledge of the harmful chemicals in beauty products. By adopting an environmental justice framework, it is possible to promote healthier beauty practices to improve outcomes for individuals with hair and nail disorders while advancing equity across populations (Mataix et al., 2023).

Test Your Knowledge

1. How do genetic factors contribute to hair disorders like androgenetic alopecia?
2. What hormonal changes are commonly linked to hair loss or thinning?

10.4. Causes of Nail Disorders

Learning Outcome

1. Describe fungal infections.
2. Focus on trauma to the nail.
3. Define systemic diseases in the manifestation of various nail disorders.

Nail disease can be caused by a variety of intrinsic and extrinsic factors that disrupt the process of keratinization and normal nail plate health. Among the characteristic causes is systemic diseases of health, such as autoimmune diseases, that can lead to changes in the appearance and texture of the nail. Psoriasis and lichen planus, for instance, are known to cause pitting, ridging, and discoloration of the nail as a result of inherent inflammatory processes. In addition, nutrient deficiencies, particularly biotin, zinc, and iron, may be responsible for growth impairment and nail brittleness, underscoring the role of nutrition in nail integrity. Another interesting aspect is the impact of environmental exposure, such as chemicals or excessive moisture, which tends to soften the nail plate and gives rise to a range of disorders in the form of peeling or splitting. Chemotherapeutic agents can be pivotal in the development of nail disorders, as they are toxic to rapidly dividing cells, including those that line the nail matrix. Hydroxyurea, a cytostatic medication commonly used to treat specific blood disorders, has been reported to cause melanonychia, characterized by brown-black discoloration of the nails, particularly with prolonged administration (Sun et al., 2022). The pigmentation results from the cytotoxic effect of the drug on the nail matrix, a seal on the intricate relationship between medication and the integrity of the nail. Furthermore, nail disease resulting from medications underscores the need to understand the potential side effects of seemingly harmless treatments. By monitoring such responses, medical professionals are better positioned to counsel and treat patients who experience these side effects. In addition, personal care and cosmetic products have a notable impact on nail health, often causing adverse reactions that undermine nail strength. Most nail products, including treatments and polishes, use harsh chemicals that tend to enhance results, such as dermatitis or allergic reactions. As established in studies, allergic reactions to certain cosmetic products used in nail care typically present as redness, itching, and swelling, which may ultimately lead to nail dystrophy (Medhi et al., 2017). Moreover, improper use of nail enhancement products like acrylics and gels can form deformities as well as infections that affect the internal composition of the nail. Attention to ingredient safety and application procedures is important in averting these hazards and maintaining nail health, underscoring the significant role of beauty regimens in nail condition.

10.4.1. Fungal Infections

Fungal infections, particularly those affecting the hair and nails, constitute a large subgroup of dermatoses that pose diagnostic challenges. Tinea capitis, or ringworm of the scalp, is a typical fungal infection that primarily affects the scalp hair follicles. The causative agents of this infection are most commonly dermatophytes, a type of fungus that obtain their energy by breaking down keratin, a vital structural protein in hair and nails. The infection is marked by symptoms of hair loss, scaling, and inflammation, which are known to severely affect the patient's quality of life. Early diagnosis is vital, as the disease, when left untreated, can result in chronic infection and complications like secondary bacterial infection.

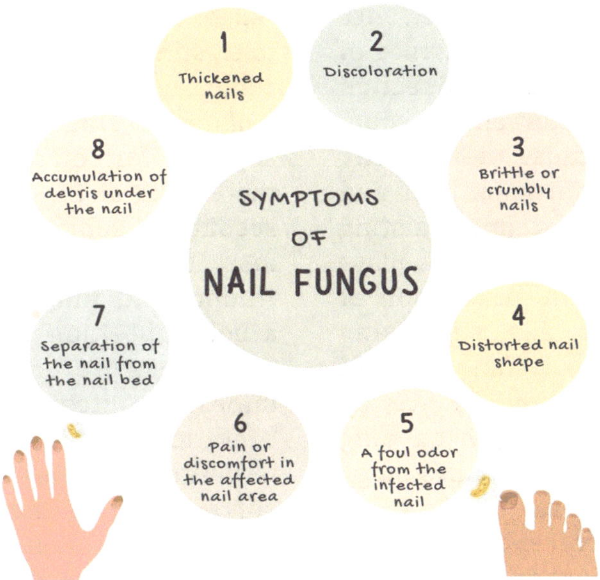

Figure 10.10. Symptoms of nail fungus.

Source: https://continentalhospitals.com/uploads/mceu_83904277117014273958800.jpg.

The relationship of fungal infection to underlying disease, such as immune deficiencies, makes treatment more complicated, emphasizing the need for detailed awareness of the etiologic agent causing such infection (Bobonich, M., & Nolen, M. E., 2021). Diseases of the nail, including onychomycosis, constitute a high majority of those that cause fungal infection of the nail plate, the characteristic of fungal invasion leading to discoloration of the nail, thickening, and ultimate destruction. The most common causative agents of onychomycosis are dermatophytes, yeasts, and non-dermatophyte molds, each with distinct virulence characteristics that influence the severity and chronicity of the infection. For instance, *Candida albicans*, a normally commensal organism of the skin and mucosal surfaces, can cause opportunistic infections when host or environmental factors disrupt the equilibrium of the normal flora (Talapko et al., 2021). All share common risk factors of age, diabetes, and immunosuppression, which predispose to the development of more virulent onychomycosis presentations. Nail fungal infections are often treated with a combination of therapeutic modalities, including topical antifungals and, in resistant disease, systemic treatment to achieve satisfactory control (Bobonich, M., & Nolen, M. E., 2021). Prevention and control strategies for fungal infections of the hair and nails focus on developing good hygiene habits and monitoring risk factors. Applying precautions such as keeping the skin dry, avoiding sharing personal grooming devices, and antifungal dusting of high-risk sites is a sound strategy to reduce the incidence of these infections. Additionally, public education on the importance of early intervention could lead to better outcomes because the majority of individuals wait for treatment for hair and nail diseases due to disease stigma. Existing studies also indicate that the microbiome plays a crucial role in managing the population of fungal communities on the skin, suggesting that a balanced microbial environment might avoid the risk of fungal infections. Hence, by combining prevention practices with ongoing education and research of the pathophysiology of the infections, medical practitioners can enhance the treatment and prevention of fungal hair and nail infections (Talapko et al., 2021) (Figure 10.10).

10.4.2. Trauma to the Nail

Nail trauma is also an overlooked, ubiquitous characteristic of nail disorders that can significantly impair an individual's quality of life. Trauma in various forms, such as crushing injuries, hemangiomas, and even repetitive stress injury, can lead to varying nail abnormalities and pain. If the nail matrix is damaged, its impact can manifest itself in an infinite number of ways, including ridging, discoloration, or even nail separation. This kind of trauma can not only be local but also suggest more general health problems, as the health of the nails is a general health indicator. Hence, it is important to understand the importance of nail trauma so that proper diagnosis and treatment can be made, since practitioners must be sensitive to the physical and psychological consequences of such trauma to patients. In addition to physical damage, fungal infections can complicate nail pathologies by introducing an additional layer of complexity in diagnosis and treatment. Fungal infections can exacerbate initial nail trauma, leading to chronic nail dystrophies and necessitating extensive management procedures. As noted in the literature, advanced fungal infections of the nails can be secondary to existing conditions, considerably altering the clinical management strategy required to restore nail health. Traumatic injury to a nail can create a portal for infection, potentially amplifying the effects of the initial injury and leading to secondary sequelae, such as permanent nail loss. By knowing the interaction between trauma and fungal disease, clinicians are in a better position to develop better treatment strategies, preventing long-term issues and improving outcomes for patients in nail-related conditions. Clinical management of nail injury is multidisciplinary, with both protective and corrective treatments at times. Protective management alone, in some cases, is critical in preventing permanent damage and usually consists of covering the broken nail with gauze or a bandage to allow healing. In addition to immediate first aid for traumatic injury, other interventions may be necessary depending on the severity of the injury. This can include surgery to close extensive lacerations or aesthetic surgery to enhance deformity from disfiguring nail repair. Education regarding proper nail care can reduce risk of future trauma, particularly in high-risk populations for nail injury. By raising awareness of the potential consequences of nail trauma, patients and healthcare professionals can work together to improve nail health and overall well-being, particularly in relation to hair and nail disease, as the cosmetic impact on patients can be considerable (Figure 10.11).

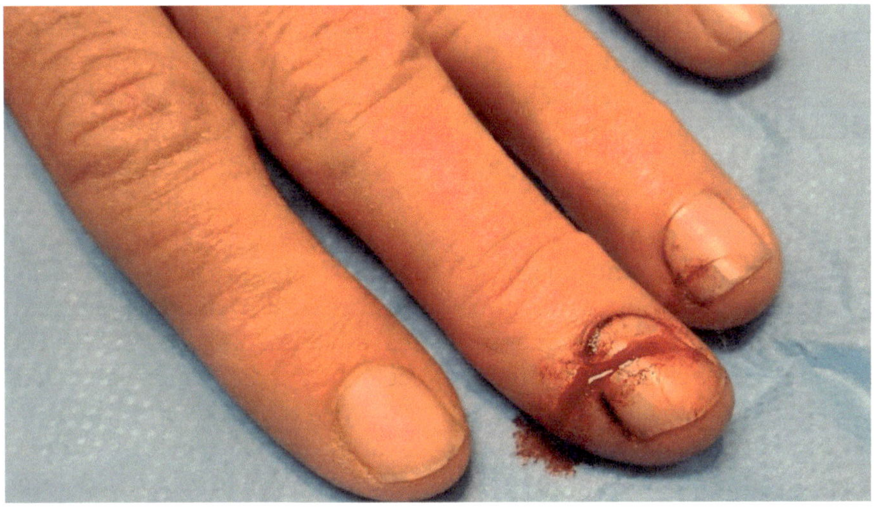

Figure 10.11. Example of nail trauma in a woman.

Source: https://www.researchgate.net/publication/335037952/figure/fig3/AS:789613811605510@1565270011513/Example-of-nail-trauma-in-a-woman.ppm.

10.4.3. Systemic Diseases

Systemic illness is the major etiology of many hair and nail diseases and is often used as a sign of disease in general health. As an example, autoimmune diseases , such as alopecia areata not only affect the scalp but also cause significant nail changes, such as pitting and ridging.

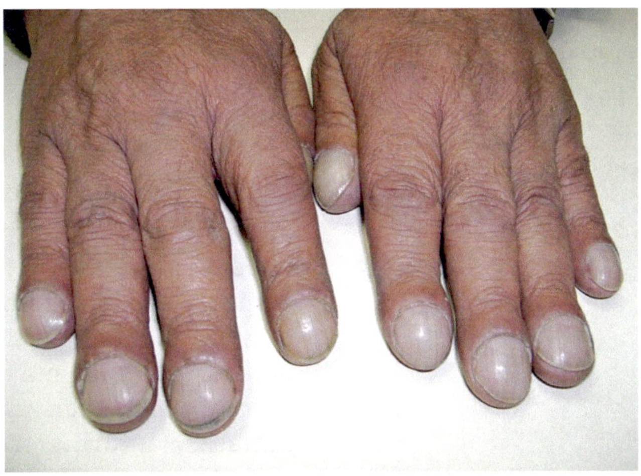

Figure 10.12. Clubbing fingers.

Source: https://upload.wikimedia.org/wikipedia/commons/thumb/b/bb/Dedos_con_acropaquia.jpg/800px-Dedos_con_acropaquia.jpg.

It has been demonstrated that the extent and nature of alopecia areata may correlate directly with patients' histories of other systemic illnesses, suggesting a multifaceted relationship between hair follicle health and immune responses. (Rastaghi et al., 2023) points out that diseases atopy, thyroid disease history, and severe forms of alopecia can play an important role in treatment, highlighting the need for an exhaustive appraisal of a patient's health when diagnosing and treating hair diseases. The synergy between systemic illness and hair and nail illness extends to the skin conditions that can accompany them. Chronic inflammatory diseases, such as lichen planus, depict this relationship vividly. Lichen planus has also been linked with various systemic diseases, including viral hepatitis and autoimmune illnesses. (Bardazzi et al., 2020) claims that the pigmentosus form of lichen planus demonstrates an altered immune system reaction, resulting in hyperpigmentation and changes in hair and nail condition as sequelae. These systemic associations mandate that health care professionals recognize evidence of systemic disease in the face of what appears to be an isolated dermatologic process, so that a coordinated treatment plan can be instituted. Treatment of hair and nail conditions also requires familiarity with systemic side effects of therapeutic agents, particularly when corticosteroids and other immunosuppressants are used. Systemic illnesses, as for instance ulcerative colitis, may lead to hair and nail alterations as drug side effects of medication in the form of drugs like infliximab. The patient case in Bardazzi et al. (2020) illustrates that continuous therapies can disrupt dermatological health, thereby complicating diagnosis and management options. Doctors need to be cautious in evaluating such interferences, without worsening systemic illnesses, while treating disorders of nails and hair. A multidimensional strategy that encompasses both local and systemic aspects is necessary for optimal patient outcomes in hair and nail health (Figure 10.12).

Test Your Knowledge

1. How do fungal infections lead to nail disorders like onychomycosis?
2. What types of trauma can cause damage to the nails and affect their growth?
3. Which systemic diseases are commonly associated with changes in nail appearance or health?

10.5. Symptoms of Hair Disorders

Learning Outcome

1. Describe hair thinning and loss.
2. Understand the symptoms of changes in hair texture.
3. Discuss scalp irritation.

Hair disease presents with a range of symptoms that significantly affect both physiological health and mental well-being. Loss of hair is one of the most frequent symptoms and may appear in various patterns and types , such as alopecia areata or androgenetic alopecia. Not only do these conditions lead to reduced hair density, but they may also result in changes in hair texture, such as thinning or brittleness. Patients suffering from disorders related to the function of the thyroid will develop some symptoms, including dry and brittle hair, which are products of hormonal imbalances affecting the follicles' health. These hair disorders may be accompanied by fatigue, weight fluctuations, and skin changes, necessitating a thorough evaluation to assess hair health. The multidimensional etiology of such signs is important to recognize when formulating appropriate treatment plans, as they are typically associated with general health conditions (Charan, 2025).

Hair illnesses will, in some cases, be reflective of characteristic signs of certain underlying conditions. Individuals with Cronkhite-Canada syndrome, for instance, have prominent loss of hair alongside other ectodermal abnormalities. This condition illustrates the intersection of systemic diseases and hair health, and how gastrointestinal health can directly affect hair follicle function. Symptoms may include not only hair loss but also gastrointestinal distress, cutaneous hyperpigmentation, and taste alterations, suggesting broader ectodermal involvement. The correlative nature of hair conditions with other systemic symptoms requires an integrative approach to diagnosis, in which practitioners must consider the reciprocal relationships among the skin, hair, and the patient's overall well-being. As evidenced by medical outcomes, managing these interlinked symptoms often results in noticeable improvements in both hair and overall health (Nin et al., 2024). It is essential to recognize all symptoms associated with hair disorders to ensure effective diagnosis and treatment. Thinning of the hair, changes in growth patterns, and changes in texture are some symptoms that also act as important indicators for the clinician. Additionally, the psychological impact of hair loss cannot be overlooked since it has a tendency to induce anxiety and depression in patients. The complementarity between the physical manifestations of hair disorders and their emotional effects underscores the need for an integrated approach to treatment. Total management can be a combination of medical treatment, lifestyle modifications, and psychological therapy, with the aim of healing both the physical and emotional effects of these disorders. Early detection and intervention are crucial to improving outcomes, as many people may remain silent, unaware of the underlying causes of hair conditions (Charan, 2025).

10.5.1. Hair Thinning and Loss

The state of hair loss and thinning is complex and affects a significant majority of the global population across age and gender. The disorder normally presents itself in the thickening of hair or alterations in hair texture, both of which are the source of mental disturbance and a decrease in self-esteem. Factors underlying hair thinning and loss include genetic predisposition, hormonal imbalances, and environmental factors. Interestingly, androgens play a key role in conditions like androgenetic alopecia, in which a genetic predisposition leads to hair follicles becoming miniaturized over time. In addition, insufficient intake of adequate nutrition, particularly vitamins and minerals required for hair growth, also assists in thinning of the hair. Thus, awareness of the actual reason behind hair loss is essential for proper diagnosis and treatment, allowing individuals to address both the physical and psychological issues related to this condition. The clinical presentation of hair loss and balding may also be a manifestation of systemic diseases. In some cases, excessive hair shedding may be a presentation of an inflammatory or autoimmune process, for example, alopecia areata, where the body's immune system attacks hair follicles in error. Environmental stress and exposure to toxins may also enhance these conditions. For instance, cadmium toxicity is now an emerging issue associated with other medical disorders aside from alopecia, that is, organ damage and other system failure, which shows that monitoring exposure in the environment is of utmost importance (Rahimzadeh et al., 2017). A full assessment, including medical history and scalp examination, is essential in establishing the type of alopecia and its potential causes. It is only with a full understanding of these underlying reasons that health professionals can design effective management plans, which may include lifestyle changes or specific medications. Integrative treatment plans for the management of thinning and hair loss may include medical interventions and preventive options. Topical substances , such as minoxidil have been in the limelight to stimulate hair growth, while anti-androgens , such as finasteride are utilized to inhibit the hormonal mechanisms underlying hair thinning. Besides, the treatment of nutritional deficiencies with a balanced diet supplemented with iron, zinc, and vitamins could improve the general health of the hair and also halt further loss. Secondly, advances in genetics could aid the identification of genetic markers of hair thinning, as seen with the discovery of chromatin-remodeling factors such as SMARCC2, which point to more universal genetic interactions in hair disease (Machol et al., 2018). Therefore, patient education on hair care routines and the psychological impact of hair loss is imperative, focusing not only on restoring hair density but also on overall well-being (Figure 10.13).

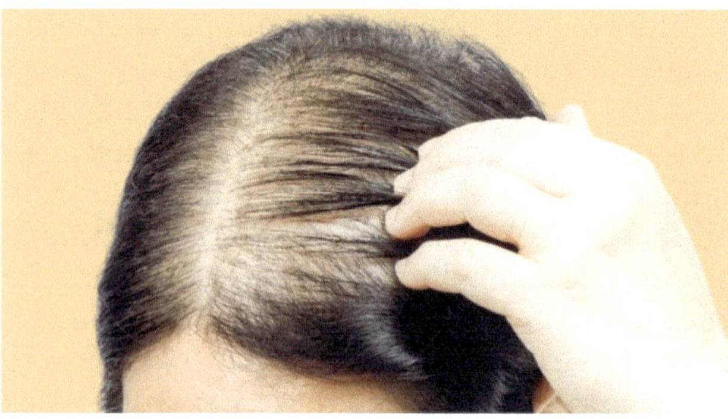

Figure 10.13. Thinning hair in women.

Source: https://cdn.shopify.com/s/files/1/2270/9565/t/32/assets/reason-for-hair-thinning-and-loss-1669787237662.jpg?v=1669787238.

10.5.2. Changes in Hair Texture

Changes in hair texture are a which is a prominent feature of hair and nail disorders and often signals underlying health conditions or environmental influences. Changes in hair texture result from multiple factors, including nutritional deficiencies, endocrine alterations, and environmental influences. For instance, direct effects of vitamin and mineral deficiencies on the hair result in textures, such as dryness, brittleness, or oiliness. Research indicates that a balanced diet is essential not only for maintaining overall health but also for hair health, influencing parameters such as elasticity and strength to support healthy hair growth (Michalak et al., 2021). Thus, awareness of these changes is critical for addressing the root causes of hair-texture changes. In addition to nutritional influences, hormonal fluctuations can cause marked changes in hair texture. Any condition , such as hormonal imbalances, usually experienced at puberty, pregnancy, or menopause, can lead to a change in the properties of the hair, affecting its thickness and wave pattern. For example, increased levels of androgens can lead to a thicker texture or a change from straight to wavy hair. These changes in hormones can affect not only the aesthetic appearance of hair, but also its flexibility and health. Furthermore, the emotional and psychological implications of these changes can induce heightened stress that, in turn, creates a cycle in which tension also induces issues with hair texture. By analyzing these factors, we can more clearly see the broader significance of hair-texture alteration in relation to health and self-perception. Finally, external factors, such as chemical processing and environmental conditions, determine changes in hair texture. Long-term application of hair dyes, relaxers, or heat products may penetrate the hair cuticle, resulting in altered texture in the nature of frizz, split ends, or limpness. Furthermore, long-term exposure to harsh weather, pollution, and sunlight can degrade the quality of natural hair, further resulting in texture loss. Recent research has shown that certain biocompatible ingredients added to cosmeceuticals, such as chitin and chitosans, can mitigate these adverse effects by conditioning hair and promoting healing (Casadidio et al., 2019). Understanding how these external factors interact and influence hair texture is vital for formulating effective treatments and preventive therapies for hair and nail diseases (Figure 10.14).

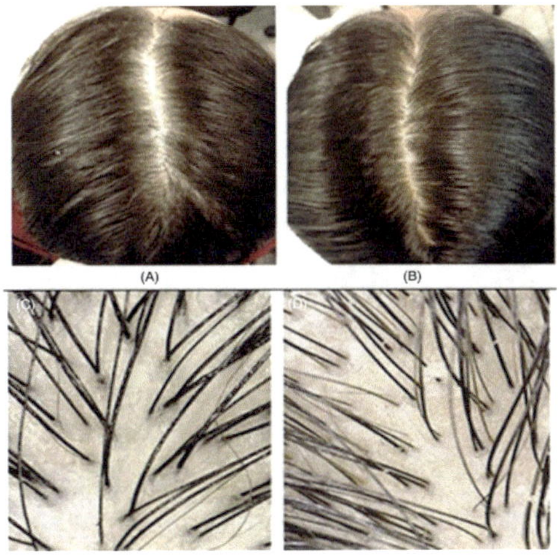

Figure 10.14. (A) The female patient with telogen effluvium shows decreased hair density and widening of the central part before treatment. (B) Shows marked improvement in hair growth and narrowing of the central part after mesotherapy injection. (C) Trichoscopy for the same patient before treatment, shows decreased total hair count and increased single hair follicular unit. (D) After treatment, shows an increased number of total hair count, appearance of new hair, and an increased number of multiple hair follicular units.

Source: https://www.researchgate.net/publication/362099996/figure/fig2/AS:11431281173879526@1689067305422/A-Female-patient-with-telogen-effluvium-shows-decreased-hair-density-and-widening-of.png.

10.5.3. Scalp Irritation

Scalp irritation is a multifactorial disorder that significantly impairs individuals' quality of life. It can take the form of redness, itching, flaking, or burning and, in general, leads to discomfort and embarrassment. The causes of scalp irritation are multifactorial and include dermatological disorders, allergic contact dermatitis to shampoos, and environmental factors such as pollution and overexposure to the sun. Chronic scalp inflammation may also be associated with underlying systemic disease or lifestyle factors such as stress and dietary imbalance, which may increase the risk of symptoms. Awareness of these causes is crucial for effective management, as therapy often requires developing a tailored strategy that addresses both symptoms and etiology. Relief of scalp inflammation involves a range of therapeutic interventions from topical therapy to alteration of personal care. Hydrocortisone creams and antihistamines can reduce allergic symptoms and itching, and medicated shampoos containing agents such as salicylic acid or ketoconazole can minimize dandruff and seborrheic dermatitis. Additionally, lifestyle modifications, like the use of gentler shampooing products that are free of sulfates and fragrances, are also recommended to decrease exposure to irritants. However, it is also important to realize that the effectiveness of the interventions could vary from one person to another, and therefore, the necessity for personalized treatment protocols as recommended by medical practitioners. This holistic approach not only affords symptomatic relief but also more effectively maintains scalp health. Furthermore, new approaches to scalp wellbeing, including the development of novel delivery systems for therapeutic drugs, have shown potential towards the treatment of scalp conditions. Among these advancements is the use of dissolving microneedles, which have been described as capable of delivering medications through the skin barrier, thereby enhancing therapeutic outcomes in scalp disease. These microneedles have the potential to deliver active ingredients with targeted specificity, thereby enhancing the treatment of scalp irritation through deeper penetration and prolonged release of tailored compounds. With ongoing investigation into their applications, including in medical areas such as hair and scalp disease, integration of such technology might prove to be a treatment paradigm shift that offers new hope to patients with chronic scalp irritation (Sartawi et al., 2022). As advances in understanding the molecular underpinnings of irritation continue to emerge, opportunities for individualized, targeted therapies grow, with a corresponding impact in other areas, such as oncology (Anand et al., 2022) (Figure 10.15).

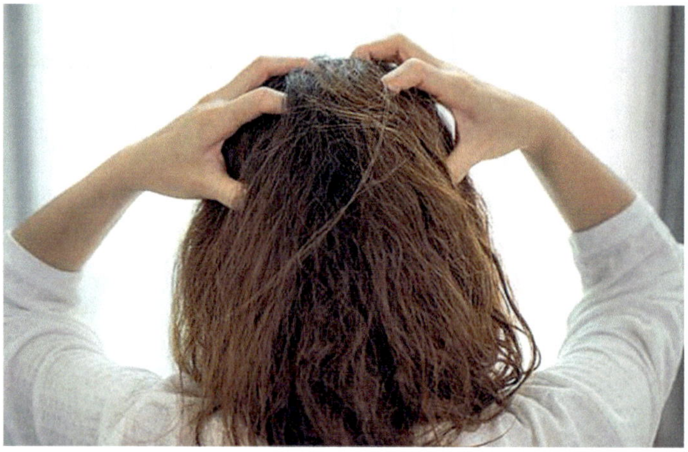

Figure 10.15. Scalp irritation is a multifaceted condition that can significantly affect an individual's quality of life.

Source: https://domf5oio6qrcr.cloudfront.net/medialibrary/16130/conversions/gettyimages-2067234535-thumb.jpg.

Test Your Knowledge

1. What are the early signs of hair thinning that might indicate a disorder?
2. How can changes in hair texture, like increased dryness or brittleness, signal a hair disorder?

10.6. Symptoms of Nail Disorders

Learning Outcome

1. Understand the discoloration of nails.
2. Define nail brittleness and splitting.
3. Understand pain and inflammation associated with nail disorders.

Nail disorders can present in various ways, typically as signs of underlying conditions rather than purely aesthetic concerns. Nail coloration changes, texture, and growth habits are some of the typical symptoms, which are significant pointers to an individual's overall health condition. For instance, a pale or white nail may indicate anemia, whereas discoloration may indicate fungal infection, such as onychomycosis. In addition, illnesses like hypothyroidism, present in Ayurvedic texts as Anukta Vhadhies, can lead to nail growth retardation alongside other systemic manifestations like fatigue and loss of weight (Charan, 2025). Understanding the symptoms is crucial for early detection and treatment, as untreated nail disorders can lead to severe underlying diseases. Another important feature is the formation of ridging, pitting, or brittleness, which is typically associated with a range of nail disorders, including eczema and psoriasis. Nails' strength and integrity can be compromised by various factors, including nutritional deficiencies, infections, and hormonal disorders. In particular, brittle nails are a sign of hypothyroidism, in which low thyroid hormone levels reduce keratin production and thereby nail strength and resistance (Charan, 2025). More importantly, individuals with nail atrophy, as seen in some rare conditions like Cronkhite-Canada syndrome, will also have additional signs and symptoms like gastrointestinal symptoms and alopecia. These complex interactions underscore the necessity of a balanced approach to assessing nail health. The psychological and emotional impact that is related to nail disease should be addressed because these conditions will have an enormous influence on those persons' self-esteem, mood, and overall mental state. Social withdrawal or appearance anxiety may occur in response to changes in nail coloration, brittleness, or deformity. To others, nails serve as a reflection of personal hygiene and grooming; therefore, overt defects may provoke feelings of inadequacy. Healthcare providers must take these psychosocial components into consideration when managing nail disorders so that a holistic approach can treat both physical and emotional issues. By understanding the nuances of nail disease, practitioners can improve patient outcomes and quality of life in patients with nail disease.

10.6.1. Nail Discoloration

Discoloration of the nails is a grave indicator of internal health issues, which may be an outward manifestation of systemic and local diseases. If the nails appear abnormal in color, such as yellow, green, or blue, this is primarily suggestive of dermatological or systemic disease. For instance, a yellowish hue may indicate fungal infections or respiratory disorders, whereas a bluish hue due to hypoxia can indicate more severe cardiovascular disease. Therefore, practitioners will use variations in nail color for diagnostic purposes, prompting further investigation of the patient's overall condition. Understanding these associations is critical to intervention and early diagnosis, making awareness of changes in nail color not only a cosmetic concern but part of medical assessment. Although systemic illness is a common etiology, nail color change can also be induced by various exogenous factors, including trauma, chemical exposure, or inadequate nail hygiene. Damage to the nail matrix, most often due to physical trauma, can cause streaks or spots that alter the color of the nails. Likewise, certain chemical substances found in nail polish or cleaning solutions can cause discoloration later on in life. Regular manicures involving soaking nails in toxic solutions can exacerbate these conditions, leading to chronic discoloration. To resist these conditions, proper nail hygiene is essential. These include avoiding the use of harsh chemicals, maintaining nail moisture, and maintaining a well-balanced diet, as nutrient deficiencies can also affect nail health. Maintenance of these areas can ensure not just the aesthetic value of the nails but their structural integrity as well. Various medical conditions can cause nail discoloration, and in some cases, this discoloration may indicate serious health problems. For example, color change can occur from CRPS, with one having a number of symptoms , such as swelling and color changes in the skin, including the nails. Autonomic dysregulation in CRPS may cause nails with discoloration due to altered blood flow or other trophic changes in the affected area. Additionally, conditions psoriasis and infection diseases, such as onychomycosis, significantly alter nail color and texture. Therefore, determining the broader context of nail color change is a critical component of accurate diagnosis and management. With awareness of such conditions, health workers can develop targeted interventions that address the underlying conditions and the cosmetic problems associated with nail color change, thereby enhancing patient outcomes and well-being (Emmelot, 2022; Anand et al., 2022) (Figure 10.16).

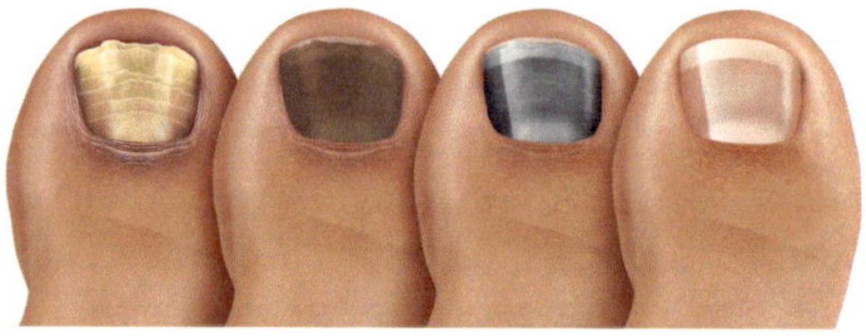

Figure 10.16. Toenail discoloration.

Source: https://andersonpodiatrycenter.com/wp-content/uploads/2022/10/toenail-discoloration-anderson-podiatry.webp.

10.6.2. Nail Brittleness and Splitting

Splitting and brittleness of the nails are emergent conditions in the overall category of hair and nail disease that affect not only the presentation of the nails but also their structure. Nail splitting and brittleness can result from a range of causes, including environmental factors, nutritional deficiencies, and systemic diseases. For instance, excessive exposure to water, exposure to harsh chemicals, and repetitive use of nail polish may weaken the nail structure and thus increase susceptibility to brittleness. Moreover, malnourishment, particularly of crucial vitamins and minerals, has been reported as a probable cause for nail affliction. Experiments have shown that a deficiency in biotin, iron, and proteins can have adverse effects on the production of keratin, the chief structural component of nails, which makes them appear brittle and split. Understanding the etiology of these conditions is crucial for effective prevention and treatment planning. Nail brittleness is more than superficial and typically serves as a marker for systemic disease. Psoriasis or hypothyroidism might be manifested through alterations in nail morphology, alerting healthcare providers to more serious health issues. In addition, some skin disorders, such as eczema and lichen planus, may directly affect nail integrity, leading to brittleness and splitting. When nail brittleness is associated with internal disorders, treatment protocols must address both the presenting symptoms and the underlying disease states responsible for the nail condition. Therefore, dermatologists are well positioned to diagnose the underlying causes of nail brittleness, ranging from basic lifestyle modifications to more complex medical treatments, to restore nail health. Successful treatment of nail brittleness and splitting often requires a multimodal approach that combines topical and systemic agents. Topical treatments, including moisturizing oils and strengthening preparations, can forestall further damage and encourage growth and resistance. Moreover, a diet rich in vitamins, particularly biotin and silica, is beneficial for strengthening the nails. Systemically, adjustment of hormonal imbalance or treatment of the underlying medical condition may be necessary to achieve long-term results. Additionally, understanding proper nail hygiene and care practices enables individuals to make informed choices to protect their nail health. With an extensive understanding of nail brittleness and splitting, people can improve not only the appearance of their nails but also their overall well-being, affirming the connection between health in the body and the aesthetic outcome (Figure 10.17).

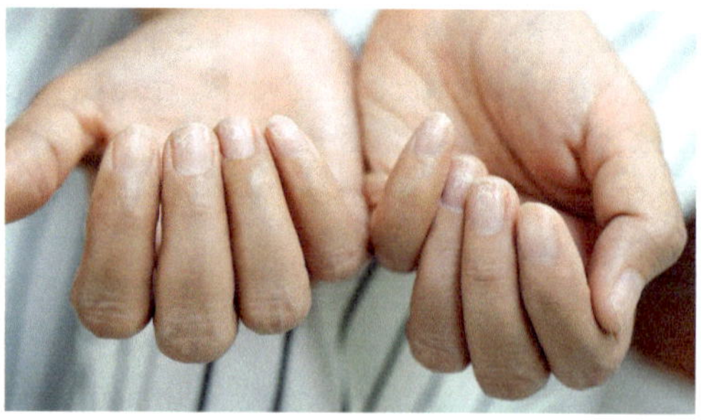

Figure 10.17. Too little moisture is a possible cause of brittle nails.

Source: https://www.medicalnewstoday.com/articles/brittle-nails#causes.

10.6.3. Pain and Inflammation

Pain and inflammation are significant body responses that often present in conditions affecting the hair and nails in a negative way. The physiological responses can manifest in a number of disorders leading to pain and disability in everyday living. For instance, conditions such as alopecia areata or nail fungal infection can trigger significant inflammatory responses. This pain, redness, swelling, and inflammation affect not only local tissue but may also intrude on general emotional functioning. Clinicians must know how inflammation and pain interplay in these illnesses so they can design targeted therapeutic regimens to alleviate symptoms and regain the patients' quality of life. Therefore, understanding the pathophysiological mechanisms underlying such reactions may improve diagnosis and treatment planning for hair and nail disorders. In addition, the biopsychosocial model of chronic pain further emphasizes that pain can outlast its initial biological etiology and lead to chronic primary pain (CPP) in some patients. When there is pain for prolonged periods of time, especially in those cases linked with nail and hair disorders , such as chronic nail dystrophy, the resulting emotional distress may significantly impact the mental health of the patient. The psychosocial nature of pain emphasizes the need for multi-faceted treatment encompassing not only the physical but also the emotional components of care. For this purpose, an interdisciplinary team comprising dermatologists, psychologists, and pain medicine specialists can provide a more comprehensive treatment regimen for patients with such conditions. Treating pain and psychosocial factors simultaneously will yield better outcomes and increase patient satisfaction. Evidence highlights the necessity of individualized treatment regimens that integrate pharmacological and non-pharmacological strategies for managing pain associated with hair and nail disorders. Inflammatory processes linked to such conditions can also be manifestations of underlying immunological derangement since new findings in the nosology of immunological disorders (Bousfiha et al., 2020) would suggest. associations enable more effective treatment pathways that consider not only pain management but also cellular-level inflammation. This multifactorial approach promotes the development of specific treatment plans that can be adjusted based on a patient's unique symptoms and biological factors. As studies continue to elucidate the complexity of pain and inflammation in nail and hair diseases, it is important for medical professionals to remain up to date and attuned to these emerging findings to deliver better patient care and outcomes (Michael et al., 2018).

Test Your Knowledge

1. What causes discoloration of nails, and how can it indicate an underlying disorder?
2. What are the common signs of pain and inflammation in the nails, and what might they suggest?

SUMMARY

Management and diagnosis of hair and nail disorders require a comprehensive approach that integrates clinical expertise with advanced diagnostic methods. Proof of the increase in the incidence of the conditions indicates that practitioners are increasingly having to be equipped with up-to-date information and methodology for the diagnosis and treatment of hair and nail disorders. It has been highly beneficial with the advent of high-frequency ultrasonography (HFUS), which facilitates visualization of hair follicles and nail units with great detail. In addition to enhancing diagnostic accuracy, this imaging method provides critical information on the course and response to treatment of various disorders, which directly bears on patient outcomes (Polańska et al., 2025). It is imperative that practitioners engage with these emerging technologies to remain at the forefront of dermatological practice. In addition, the structural dynamics and best practices of nail clinics play a key role in specifying the therapeutic context for nail disorders. Research on nail clinics, particularly by practitioners who are members of the Council for Nail Disorders, generates important insights into the working paradigms that underpin effective diagnosis and treatment. The findings reveal that most clinics are new and predominantly located within teaching institutions, which offer diverse learning experiences for medical trainees (Soliman et al., 2025). The combination of academic training and exposure aids in delivering an improved quality of care to ensure new clinicians are appropriately equipped to manage complex nail disorders. As such clinics expand, the sharing of knowledge and innovations in the field will be instrumental in disseminating best practices that meet patients' needs. Finally, fostering a culture of cooperation among healthcare providers interested in hair and nail conditions will be essential to promoting evidence-based care practices. Networking and knowledge-sharing forums can better equip clinicians with an understanding of complex conditions affecting hair and nails. By highlighting the value of a multidisciplinary approach, clinicians can integrate evidence from technology, pathology, and dermatology to achieve integrated patient care. With the widespread use of clinical images and dermoscopy in nail clinics, the value of integrated examination tools in clinical practice is increasingly recognized (Soliman et al., 2025). In the years to come, sustained investment in research and education will ensure that healthcare practitioners remain up to date with novel developments in nail and hair disease, resulting in improved patient outcomes and satisfaction.

In disorders of hair and nails, one must understand the multi-dimensional character of the disease in order to attain a correct diagnosis and treatment. Alopecia, onychomycosis, and psoriasis, for instance, illustrate the complexity of hair and nail disorders, with genetic, environmental, and lifestyle factors influencing them. For instance, alopecia can be due to autoimmune processes, genetics, or endocrine conditions, and onychomycosis is basically due to fungal infections that affect the look and integrity of nails. Moreover, illnesses like psoriasis not only affect the skin but can also affect nail beds to a significant degree, leading to physical and emotional distress for individuals suffering from such disorders. Identifying these etiologies is the first step toward tailored pharmacologic and non-pharmacologic treatment regimens designed to enhance the quality of life of those affected. Furthermore, the cosmetic use of beauty products significantly contributes to the causation and exacerbation of disorders of the hair and nails, particularly among certain demographic groups. Certain hair products containing risky chemicals, such as straighteners and relaxers, disproportionately hurt women of color and are connected with a variety of health issues, from scalp conditions to possible links with reproductive health issues. In addition, the impact of ingredients in beauty products extends beyond the individual's own immediate health and results in broader public health issues. Exposure gaps in beauty products containing hazardous chemicals underscore the need for regulation to ensure safety and improve health equity. This is made possible by specifying how environmental factors interact to affect hair and nail diseases, thereby enabling them to address the varying challenges that different populations face in medical practice (Ami et al., 2017). Lastly, the management of nail and hair disorders requires an inter-disciplinary strategy, with the expertise from all sectors encompassing dermatology, environmental science, and public health. Professionals need to consider not only the individual symptom presented but also the broader social and environmental determinants that contribute to the development of such conditions. For instance, health disparities experienced by marginalized groups point to the extreme urgency for targeted research and policy action toward limiting exposure to toxic chemicals in cosmetics. Furthermore, educating patients on the correct application of cosmetics and the potential side effects of their beauty regimen can empower them to make healthier choices. It is important that healthcare professionals, researchers, and policymakers work together to frame a comprehensive framework incorporating individual well-being and community wellness regarding nail and hair disorders, with an emphasis on continuous advocacy, regulation, and education practice enhancement (Lakshmi et al., 2018).

KEY TERMS FROM THIS CHAPTER

- Alopecia
- Androgenetic alopecia (AGA)
- Autonomic dysregulation
- Chronic scalp inflammation
- Chronic scalp irritation
- Dermatological science
- Dermatology specialty
- Dihydrotestosterone (DHT) action
- Disease stigma
- Ectodermal dysplasias
- Environmental assessments
- Environmental factors
- Environmental influences
- Environmental toxins
- Etiologic knowledge
- Follicle biology
- Fungal communities
- Fungal infection

CRITICAL THINKING QUESTIONS

1. **Which of the following is the most common cause of alopecia areata (a hair loss disorder)?**
   a. Fungal infection
   b. Autoimmune response
   c. Genetic mutation
   d. Nutritional deficiency
2. **Which of the following is a symptom of onychomycosis (fungal nail infection)?**
   a. Yellowing and thickening of nails
   b. Painful red rash on the nail bed
   c. Sudden hair thinning
   d. White spots on the nails
3. **Which of the following nail disorders is characterized by nails that are spoon-shaped (concave)?**
   a. Beau's lines
   b. Onychocryptosis
   c. Koilonychia
   d. Paronychia
4. What is the main cause of traction alopecia?
   a. Severe heat exposure
   b. Physical trauma or tension from hairstyles
   c. Hormonal imbalance
   d. Bacterial infection
5. **Psoriasis can affect the nails, leading to which of the following symptoms?**
   a. Dark spots under the nail
   b. Pitting or small depressions on the nail surface
   c. Thickening of the nail cuticle
   d. Complete loss of nail growth

Short Answer Questions

1. What are the primary types of hair disorders, and how do they differ in terms of causes and symptoms?
2. How does androgenetic alopecia affect both men and women differently?
3. What are the most common causes of nail disorders like fungal infections and trauma to the nails?
4. How do hormonal changes, such as during pregnancy or menopause, contribute to hair disorders?
5. What environmental influences, like diet or exposure to toxins, can lead to both hair and nail disorders?
6. What are the common symptoms of nail disorders, such as nail discoloration or brittleness?
7. How can stress and systemic diseases, like diabetes or thyroid disorders, cause hair or nail issues?
8. What treatments are available for hair disorders like alopecia areata or telogen effluvium?

Answer to Critical Thinking Questions

1. (b); 2. (a); 3. (c); 4. (b); 5. (d)

REFERENCES

1. Ahmed, A., Almohanna, H., Griggs, J., & Tosti, A. (2019). Genetic Hair Disorders: A review. *Dermatology and Therapy, 9*(3), 421–448. https://doi.org/10.1007/s13555-019-0313-2Akalın, A., Koç, N., Özşin-Özler, C., Karaosmanoğlu, B., Ürel-Demir, G., Taşkıran, E., Utine, G., et al. (2025). A novel pathogenic TSPEAR variant in a family with clinical variability: Definition of dental anomalies and review of the literature. *Molecular Syndromology*. https://www.semanticscholar.org/paper/9bfa1ab97b586cd84a9fda682a3fd95cbddd8b23 (accessed on 21st July 2025).
2. Almohanna, H. M., Ahmed, A., Tsatalis, J. P., & Tosti, A. (2018). The role of vitamins and minerals in hair loss: A review. *Dermatology and Therapy, 9*, 51–70. https://doi.org/10.1007/s13555-018-0278-6 (accessed on 21st July 2025).
3. Alsatti, H., Almalki, B., & Alghamdi, Y. (2024). Abemaciclib-associated skin, hair, and nail toxicities: A case report. *Cureus, 16*. https://www.semanticscholar.org/paper/2495ac08d2f672c81d523b11db5e9991a9415d30 (accessed on 21st July 2025).
4. Anand, U., Dey, A., Singh Chandel, A. K., Sanyal, R., Mishra, A., Pandey, D. K., De Falco, V., et al. (2022). Cancer chemotherapy and beyond: Current status, drug candidates, associated risks and progress in targeted therapeutics. *Genes & Diseases, 10*, 1367–1401. https://doi.org/10.1016/j.gendis.2022.02.007 (accessed on 21st July 2025).
5. Bardazzi, F., Misciali, C., Evangelista, V., & Loi, C. (2020). Ulcerative colitis and progressive acquired hyperpigmentation on the face and neck. A case of infliximab-related lichen planus pigmentosus. *Dermatologic Therapy, 33*. https://www.semanticscholar.org/paper/737beb37af00a349891b4e9ffe357d03c7ccd1eb (accessed on 21st July 2025).
6. Bastidas Torres, D. M., Cantos Pesántez, M. P., Espinoza Calle, J. E., Yascaribay González, J. P., Holguin Cagua, D. J., Bravo Vinces, K. L., Gómez González, R. C., et al. (2023). The pattern and clinical profile of alopecia areata. Panoramic review: Update and advances on etiopathogenesis, associated factors, diagnosis, complications, management and prognosis in treatment 2023. *EPRA International Journal of Multidisciplinary Research (IJMR)*. https://www.semanticscholar.org/paper/069d514f90e0b4f3ec7715066d52d3b250e95cda (accessed on 21st July 2025).
7. Bobonich, M., & Nolen, M. E. (2021). *Dermatology for Advanced Practice Clinicians*.
8. Bongomin, F., Gago, S., Oladele, R., & Denning, D. W. (2017). Global and multi-national prevalence of fungal diseases—Estimate precision. *Journal of Fungi, 3*, 57–57. https://doi.org/10.3390/jof3040057 (accessed on 21st July 2025).
9. Bousfiha, A., Jeddane, L., Pïcard, C., Al-Herz, W., Ailal, F., Chatila, T. A., Cunningham-Rundles, C., et al. (2020). Human inborn errors of immunity: 2019 update of the IUIS phenotypical classification. *Journal of Clinical Immunology, 40*, 66–81. https://doi.org/10.1007/s10875-020-00758-x (accessed on 21st July 2025).
10. Casadidio, C., Vargas Peregrina, D., Gigliobianco, M. R., Deng, S., Censi, R., & Di Martino, P. (2019). Chitin and chitosans: Characteristics, eco-friendly processes, and applications in cosmetic science. *Marine Drugs, 17*, 369. https://doi.org/10.3390/md17060369 (accessed on 21st July 2025).
11. Chan, S., Reddy, V., Myers, B., Thibodeaux, Q., Brownstone, N., & Liao, W. (2020). Machine learning in dermatology: Current applications, opportunities, and limitations. *Dermatology*

and Therapy, 10, 365–386. https://doi.org/10.1007/s13555-020-00372-0 (accessed on 21st July 2025).

12. Charan, D. S. (2025). Hypothyroidism treated through Ayurveda: A clinical case study. *International Journal of Scientific Research in Engineering and Management*. https://www.semanticscholar.org/paper/5fd99f9e8dcc4fe217b368d1d26be509f2d3441d (accessed on 21st July 2025).
13. Docherty, A., Mullins, N., Ashley-Koch, A. E., Qin, X. J., Coleman, J. R. I., Shabalin, A., Kang, J., et al. (2023). GWAS meta-analysis of suicide attempt: Identification of 12 genome-wide significant loci and implication of genetic risks for specific health factors. *The American Journal of Psychiatry, 180*(10), 723–738. https://www.semanticscholar.org/paper/e2af2e2393a481739871006e584dd931898c7fe3 (accessed on 21st July 2025).
14. Emmelot, C. H. (2022). *Complex Regional Pain Syndrome Type I*. CRC Press eBooks. https://doi.org/10.1201/9781003313540-16 (accessed on 21st July 2025).
15. Fiorenzano, A., Storm, P., Sozzi, E., Bruzelius, A., Corsi, S., Kajtez, J., Mudannayake, J., et al. (2024). TARGET-seq: Linking single-cell transcriptomics of human dopaminergic neurons with their target specificity. *Proceedings of the National Academy of Sciences of the United States of America, 121*. https://www.semanticscholar.org/paper/a0e1fc3d60291f4731ae0a66afe1bf759c15d27d (accessed on 21st July 2025).
16. García Ruiz de Morales, J. M., Puig, L., Daudén, E., Cañete, J. D., Pablos, J. L., Olveira, A., González Juanatey, C., et al. (2019). Critical role of interleukin (IL)-17 in inflammatory and immune disorders: An updated review of the evidence focusing in controversies. *Autoimmunity Reviews, 19*, 102429–102429. https://doi.org/10.1016/j.autrev.2019.102429 (accessed on 21st July 2025).
17. Harden, R. N., McCabe, C., Göebel, A., Massey, M., Suvar, T., Grieve, S., & Bruehl, S. (2022). Complex regional pain syndrome: Practical diagnostic and treatment guidelines, 5th edition. *Pain Medicine, 23*, S1–S53. https://doi.org/10.1093/pm/pnac046 (accessed on 21st July 2025).
18. He, H., Zhang, R., Zhang, P., Wang, P., Chen, N., Qian, B., Zhang, L., et al. (2023). Functional carbon from nature: Biomass-derived carbon materials and the recent progress of their applications. *Advanced Science, 10*. https://doi.org/10.1002/advs.202205557 (accessed on 21st July 2025).
19. Hurley, G. (2007). Anemia: Overview and management. https://www.semanticscholar.org/paper/dd3e0c07c2ba7b762ffff34c585d5627271e21ee (accessed on 21st July 2025).
20. Jagasia, M., Greinix, H., Arora, M., Williams, K. M., Wolff, D., Cowen, E. W., Palmer, J., et al. (2014). National Institutes of Health consensus development project on criteria for clinical trials in chronic graft-versus-host disease: I. The 2014 diagnosis and staging working group report. *Biology of Blood and Marrow Transplantation, 21*, 389–401.e1. https://doi.org/10.1016/j.bbmt.2014.12.001 (accessed on 21st July 2025).
21. Kåberg, M., Larsson, S., Jerkeman, A., Nystedt, A., Duberg, A. S., Kövamees, J., Ydreborg, M., et al. (2020). High risk of non-alcoholic liver disease mortality in patients with chronic hepatitis C with illicit substance use disorder. *Scandinavian Journal of Gastroenterology, 55*, 574–580. https://www.semanticscholar.org/paper/966de08b760d79fc87bb044d1cd5117d3b09abfb (accessed on 21st July 2025).

22. Kimbrel, N., Ashley-Koch, A., Qin, X., Lindquist, J., Garrett, M., Dennis, M. F., Hair, L. P., et al. (2022). Identification of novel, replicable genetic risk loci for suicidal thoughts and behaviors among US military veterans. *JAMA Psychiatry.* https://www.semanticscholar.org/paper/852c2e89a9f507fd131eb50d7af52f0b7deba4a3 (accessed on 21st July 2025).

23. Lacouture, M. E., & Sibaud, V. (2018). Toxic side effects of targeted therapies and immunotherapies affecting the skin, oral mucosa, hair, and nails. *American Journal of Clinical Dermatology, 19*, 31–39. https://doi.org/10.1007/s40257-018-0384-3 (accessed on 21st July 2025).

24. Machol, K., Rousseau, J., Ehresmann, S., Garcia, T. X., Nguyen, T. T. M., Spillmann, R. C., Sullivan, J. A., et al. (2018). Expanding the spectrum of BAF-related disorders: De novo variants in *SMARCC2* cause a syndrome with intellectual disability and developmental delay. *The American Journal of Human Genetics, 104*, 164–178. https://doi.org/10.1016/j.ajhg.2018.11.007 (accessed on 21st July 2025).

25. Mataix-Cols, D., Fernández de la Cruz, L., de Schipper, E., Kuja-Halkola, R., Bulik, C. M., Crowley, J. J., Neufeld, J., et al. (2023). In search of environmental risk factors for obsessive-compulsive disorder: Study protocol for the OCDTWIN project. *BMC Psychiatry, 23*. https://doi.org/10.1186/s12888-023-04897-4 (accessed on 21st July 2025).

26. Medhi, B., Sarma, P., & Kumar, H. (2017). Cosmetovigilance in India: Need of the day. *Indian Journal of Pharmacology, 49*, 341. https://doi.org/10.4103/ijp.ijp_45_18 (accessed on 21st July 2025).

27. Michalak, M., Pierzak, M., Kręcisz, B., & Suliga, E. (2021). Bioactive compounds for skin health: A review. *Nutrients, 13*, 203–203. https://doi.org/10.3390/nu13010203 (accessed on 21st July 2025).

28. Muntyanu, A., Gabrielli, S., Donovan, J., Gooderham, M., Guenther, L., Hanna, S., Lynde, C., et al. (2023). The burden of alopecia areata: A scoping review focusing on quality of life, mental health and work productivity. *Journal of the European Academy of Dermatology and Venereology, 37*, 1490–1520. https://doi.org/10.1111/jdv.18926 (accessed on 21st July 2025).

29. Nicholas, M. K., Vlaeyen, J. W. S., Rief, W., Barke, A., Aziz, Q., Benoliel, R., Cohen, M., et al. (2018). The IASP classification of chronic pain for ICD-11: Chronic primary pain. *Pain, 160*, 28–37. https://doi.org/10.1097/j.pain.0000000000001390 (accessed on 21st July 2025).

30. Nin, T., Kamikozuru, K., Takagawa, T., Shinzaki, S., & Tsuzuki, K. (2024). Clinical features of taste disorders in Cronkhite-Canada syndrome: A report of 10 cases. *Chemical Senses.* https://www.semanticscholar.org/paper/c2f73b860e8458c49d9d4190630d6ad59999ad1b (accessed on 21st July 2025).

31. Pan, M., Heinecke, G., Bernardo, S., Tsui, C., & Levitt, J. (2013). Urea: A comprehensive review of the clinical literature. *Dermatology Online Journal, 19*. https://doi.org/10.5070/d31911020392 (accessed on 21st July 2025).

32. Polańska, A., Mikiel, D., SzymoniakLipska, M., Olszewska, B., & DańczakPazdrowska, A. (2025). High-frequency ultrasonography in hair and nail disorders—How it may be helpful. *Diagnostics, 15*. https://www.semanticscholar.org/paper/cc6194dbbc0ca9c51c01602de7558c606570b25d (accessed on 21st July 2025).

33. Powell, J., Porter, E., Field, S., O'Connell, N. H., Carty, K., & Dunne, C. (2022). Epidemiology of dermatomycoses and onychomycoses in Ireland (2001–2020): A single-institution review.

Mycoses, 65, 770–779. https://doi.org/10.1111/myc.13473 (accessed on 21st July 2025).

34. Qian, Q., Gu, Y., Luo, J., Wu, S., Li, J., Li, J., Peng, Q., et al. (2025). Genetic and environmental factors affecting hair density in East Asian populations. *The British Journal of Dermatology.* https://www.semanticscholar.org/paper/72e060e1bda639f647a92d59a8107dbe71dbc7bc (accessed on 21st July 2025).
35. Raharja, A., Mahil, S. K., & Barker, J. N. (2021). Psoriasis: A brief overview. *Clinical Medicine, 21*, 170–173. https://doi.org/10.7861/clinmed.2021-0257 (accessed on 21st July 2025).
36. Rahimzadeh, M. R., Rahimzadeh, M. R., Kazemi, S., & Moghadamnia, A. A. (2017). Cadmium toxicity and treatment: An update. *DOAJ (Directory of Open Access Journals), 8*, 135–145. https://doi.org/10.22088/cjim.8.3.135 (accessed on 21st July 2025).
37. Rallis, E., Lotsaris, K., Grech, V., Tertipi, N., Sfyri, E., & Kefala, V. (2024). The nutrient–skin connection: Diagnosing eating disorders through dermatologic signs. *Nutrients, 16*. https://www.semanticscholar.org/paper/2c3d4f4e717d5534cf52015813e8c19f404daa9a (accessed on 21st July 2025).
38. Rastaghi, F., Kaveh, R., Yazdanpanah, N., Sahaf, A., & Ahramyanpour, N. (2023). The efficacy and adverse effects of corticosteroid pulse therapy in alopecia areata: A review article. *Dermatology Practical & Conceptual, 13*. https://www.semanticscholar.org/paper/c232b1af60c308a7c4f2a450d7cef1ce2395ee4d (accessed on 21st July 2025).
39. Rodrigues, K. S., Oliveira-Ribeiro, C., de Abreu Fiuza Gomes, S., & Knobler, R. (2017). Cutaneous graft-versus-host disease: Diagnosis and treatment. *American Journal of Clinical Dermatology, 19*, 33–50. https://doi.org/10.1007/s40257-017-0306-9 (accessed on 21st July 2025).
40. Ross, H., Ong, X. H., Harries, M., & Asfour, L. (2024). BH13 Current wig prescribing practices and financial evaluation in a National Health Service foundation trust: Lessons learnt and future challenges. *British Journal of Dermatology*. https://www.semanticscholar.org/paper/76e710b980f3bd6651aeaef332803730c5e01ede (accessed on 21st July 2025).
41. Sartawi, Z., Blackshields, C., & Faisal, W. (2022). Dissolving microneedles: Applications and growing therapeutic potential. *Journal of Controlled Release, 348*, 186–205. https://doi.org/10.1016/j.jconrel.2022.05.045 (accessed on 21st July 2025).
42. Soliman, S., Rich, P., & Hinshaw, M. A. (2025). Current practices of subspecialty nail clinics: Results of a survey of the members of the Council for Nail Disorders. *Skin Appendage Disorders.* https://www.semanticscholar.org/paper/ad38b4960339b19dbfb3c5aaa6833f78b72d1313 (accessed on 21st July 2025).
43. Sun, Y., Xu, Z., & Ding, X. (2022). Recurrent melanonychia on multiple nails and alopecia induced by hydroxyurea therapy. *Chinese Medical Journal, 135*, 2142–2142. https://doi.org/10.1097/cm9.0000000000002141 (accessed on 21st July 2025).
44. Talapko, J., Juzbašić, M., Matijević, T., Pustijanac, E., Bekić, S., Kotris, I., & Škrlec, I. (2021). *Candida albicans*—The virulence factors and clinical manifestations of infection. *Journal of Fungi, 7*, 79–79. https://doi.org/10.3390/jof7020079 (accessed on 21st July 2025).
45. Ten Brink, A. F., Peters, L., Kompouli, P. I., Jordan, A., McCabe, C., Göebel, A., & Bultitude, J. H. (2020). Bodily changes and sensory sensitivity in complex regional pain syndrome and fibromyalgia. *Pain, 161*, 1361–1370. https://doi.org/10.1097/j.pain.0000000000001830 (accessed on 21st July 2025).

46. Wang, Y., Chang, Y., Gao, M., Zang, W., & Liu, X. (2024). Genetic analysis of albinism caused by compound heterozygous mutations of the *OCA2* gene in a Chinese family. *Hereditas, 161.* https://www.semanticscholar.org/paper/e0ebbb8735b2fe38e90de1f3c538b235bdf308b5 (accessed on 21st July 2025).

47. Wolff, H., Fischer, T. W., & Blume-Peytavi, U. (2016). The diagnosis and treatment of hair and scalp diseases. *Deutsches Ärzteblatt International.* https://doi.org/10.3238/arztebl.2016.0377 (accessed on 21st July 2025).

48. Wollina, U., Abdelmaksoud, A., Chiriac, A., Brzeziński, P., & Temiz, S. A. (2022). Symptomatology and treatment of COVID-19 affecting skin appendages: A narrative review beyond COVID-toes. *PubMed.* https://www.semanticscholar.org/paper/1a917d9d7f36ac72f214071bc1133c3903f6dc5a (accessed on 21st July 2025).

49. Yatham, L. N., Kennedy, S. H., Parikh, S. V., Schaffer, A., Bond, D. J., Frey, B. N., Sharma, V., et al. (2018). Canadian Network for Mood and Anxiety Treatments (CANMAT) and International Society for Bipolar Disorders (ISBD) 2018 guidelines for the management of patients with bipolar disorder. *Bipolar Disorders, 20,* 97–170. https://doi.org/10.1111/bdi.12609 (accessed on 21st July 2025).

50. Zota, A. R., & Shamasunder, B. (2017). The environmental injustice of beauty: Framing chemical exposures from beauty products as a health disparities concern. *American Journal of Obstetrics and Gynecology, 217,* 418.e1–418.e6. https://doi.org/10.1016/j.ajog.2017.07.020 (accessed on 21st July 2025).

PSYCHODERMATOLOGY AND PSYCHOCUTANEOUS DISORDERS

11

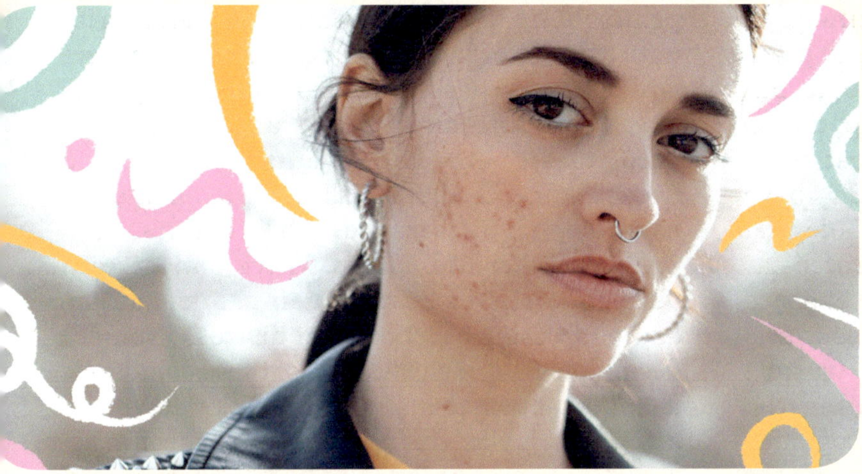

LEARNING OBJECTIVES

After studying this chapter, you will be able to:

1. Understand historical background of psychodermatology and psychocutaneous disorders
2. Discuss the biological basis underlying psychodermatology
3. Describe common psychocutaneous disorders
4. Define diagnosis and assessment of the complexity of psychodermatology
5. Explain treatment modalities in psychodermatology

Introduction

The intersection of psychological issues and dermatological conditions has gained prominence in the medical literature, leading to the development of psychodermatology as a significant area of study. Psychodermatology examines how mental states can influence dermatological conditions, and how these conditions can, in turn, affect psychological states. A knowledge of the intricate interactions between psyche and skin is of crucial significance, as the majority of skin diseases, such as psoriasis and eczema, have been shown to possess significant psychosocial burdens attached to them. In explaining these dynamics, psychodermatology seeks not only to treat dermatological conditions effectively but also to address the concurrent psychological anguish associated with these conditions, highlighting the interrelatedness of the body and mind in disease and health. The role of childhood trauma in the etiology of skin disorders and the timing and degree of their onset is a rationale for an integrated approach to psychodermatology. Research has shown that traumatic experiences in childhood play a crucial role in the pathogenesis of varied disorders, like chronic inflammatory conditions, including psoriasis. For instance, emotional, physical, and sexual abuse, and emotional neglect have been linked to heightened severity of psoriasis and development of depressive symptoms in traumatized individuals. The discovery brings to focus the significance of screening and treating not only the physical manifestations but also the psychological effects of trauma. With this understanding of the connections, clinicians can develop more integrated treatment plans that address not only the dermatologic but also the psychological elements of patients' health (Erfanian, 2018). Moreover, treatments like Cognitive Behavioral Therapy (CBT) have been effective in alleviating the psychological morbidity of chronic skin diseases. Research has demonstrated that CBT can significantly enhance the quality of life for individuals with psoriasis through processes such as establishing a trusting patient-clinician relationship, validating the legitimacy of suffering, and influencing cognitive restructuring. Not only do these interventions aim to improve emotional functioning, but they may also lead to better clinical outcomes for dermatologic conditions. Therefore, ongoing research into psychodermatology and psychocutaneous disorders is vital for refining patient care and outcomes and for ensuring that the psychological and dermatological aspects of health are treated holistically (Laoudi, 2017).

Definition of Psychodermatology

Psychodermatology is a cross-disciplinary field that is essentially the intersection of dermatology and psychology and addresses the subtle nexus between psychological states and cutaneous conditions. It recognizes that dermatologic illnesses might often be precipitated or exacerbated by psychological stressors, a mechanism that creates a vicious cycle perpetuating mental and physical misery. This area is especially important because most patients with skin conditions present with underlying psychological factors that often go unaddressed in traditional dermatology practice. Thus, an inclusive method that takes into account emotional and psychological considerations in addition to physical symptoms becomes pivotal. Involving dermatologists and mental health professionals in tandem can radically improve treatment outcomes by enabling holistic care that encompasses both mind and body in healing procedures, a unifying principle of psychodermatology. Familiarity with the different psychocutaneous disorders encompassed within psychodermatology also needs to be acquired. These are self-inflicted dermatoses, such as dermatitis artefacta and trichotillomania, that usually stem from internal psychological disturbances. Such conditions can present as harmful habits where patients can develop habits to worsen their skin condition, adding to their psychological distress. Notably, dermatologists' identification of these conditions is important since many patients can downplay any psychological disturbances in the beginning, resulting in poor treatment. Psychodermatology thus seeks to bridge the gap between the dermatological and psychological equivalents of symptoms, providing a point of access for effective intervention that treats both aspects of patients' experience, emphasizing the necessity of collaboration between dermatologists and mental health professionals (Gupta et al., 1987).

To practice psychodermatology effectively, there is a prerequisite of elementary knowledge of dermatology as well as psychological principles. Dermatologists must learn therapeutic communication techniques to deal with the emotional histories behind skin ailments, which contain intrinsic themes of loss and anxiety. Training involves not only feeling out the psychosomatic origins of most illnesses but shaping treatment plans that incorporate psychological therapy. This can range from basic counseling techniques to more intricate psychotherapeutic approaches, ideally accomplished by a combination of dermatologists and psychotherapists. The intermingling of psychological and dermatological therapy is a reflection of an increasing awareness of the profound mind-body connection, as argued by researches that elicit the psychological characteristics which are typically prevalent in psychodermatological patients. In addition, as the European Academy of Dermatology and Venereology points out, a paradigm shift to the integration of psychological training in dermatology is essential in recognizing and therefore managing such complex cases (Poot et al., 2007) (Figure 11.1).

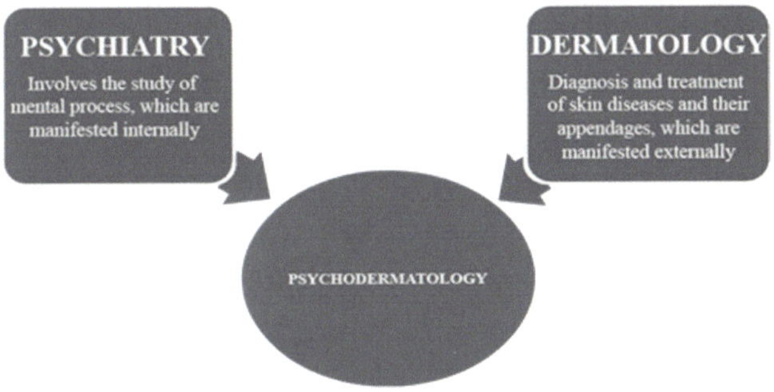

Figure 11.1. Psychodermatology.

Source: https://www.medicaljournals.se/acta/content_files/files/web/4665-web-resources/image/9936.png.

Importance of the Mind-Skin Connection

The interplay between psychological functions and cutaneous illnesses underscores the importance of the mind-skin interface, particularly in psychodermatology.

Research shows that an aggressive proportion of patients with skin illnesses, such as psoriasis or eczema, acquire concomitant psychiatric disorders, which aggravate their clinical presentation. The unique bond between the skin and the brain must be traced to their shared embryological origin, which means that psychological stressors manifest as dermatological disease, thereby creating a vicious cycle of distress (Rostenberg, 1960). The intricate mesh of intercommunication emphasizes the need for an integrated treatment regimen, one that addresses both the psychological and the physiological aspects of skin disorders as a unified entity. Understanding the mechanisms of this mind-skin interface allows practitioners to design more effective treatment plans. For instance, cognitive behavioral therapy (CBT) is a prominent therapeutic method in coping with the psychological distress of diseases like psoriasis, whose visual appearance greatly influences the quality of life of a patient. In practice, the evidence is that successful CBT will produce reductions in emotional distress, and as it does so will have an impact not only on the mental health of the patient but also on the severity of the skin problem. Having this two-way impact provides new avenues for recovery and further evidence that managing stress and maintaining emotional balance are central to optimal dermatological health (Laoudi, 2017).

Furthermore, the social consequences of the mind-skin connection cannot be overlooked. Skin disorders have a strong stigma associated with them, one which can lead to the continuation of embarrassment and isolation among sufferers. Physical visibility of skin disorders makes the situation even worse since individuals will undergo social penalties, which lead to psychological suffering. Psychosomatic responses to such stigmatization testify to the profound effect environmental and social forces have upon mental health, reflecting expressions in classical literature that equate external perceptions with internal feelings (Balasubramani, 2011). To this extent, enhancing understanding of the mind-skin interface thus not only supports treatment strategies but also encourages a social shift toward compassion and care for persons experiencing psychocutaneous disorders (Figure 11.2).

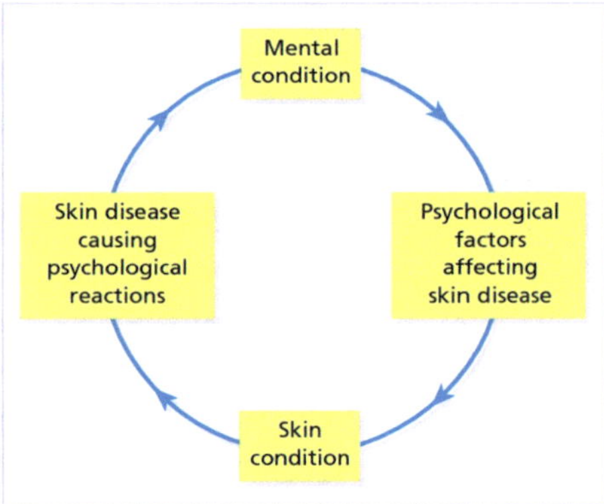

Figure 11.2. Mind–skin interactions.

Source: https://plasticsurgerykey.com/wp-content/uploads/2016/04/c23f0011.jpg.

Overview of Psychocutaneous Disorders

Psychocutaneous disorders constitute a separate overlap of psychological and dermatological health that mirrors the psychosomatic relationship between mental states and dermatologic illness. This category consists of some dermatologic conditions that are either aggravated or triggered by psychological states , such as depression, anxiety, and stress. Of these, one of the best recognized is psoriasis, an autoimmune condition both marked by its physical manifestations and the psychological impact with which it besets its victims. Many patients with psoriasis report extreme emotional distress, which itself can then exacerbate their skin lesions and so create a vicious cycle that makes treatment more difficult. An understanding of the psychology of such disorders is necessary, as this allows more effective treatment programs that address not only the skin but also the mental health issues involved in the patient, resulting in a better quality of life and outcome. Furthermore, diseases like atopic dermatitis (AD) bring out the emotional suffering typically felt by adolescents, particularly at ages of development when body image and social acceptance are paramount. AD is characterized by severe pruritus and compromised function of the skin's barrier, which interferes with socialization and access to education. With augmented responsibility for self-control by teenagers, psychological tension levels increase, possibly leading to erosion of self-esteem and overall quality of life. Topical corticosteroids and emollients are primarily the treatment protocols applied; however, failure in control leads to relapse, exacerbating psychological issues. Educational interventions to increase disease knowledge and self-management skills in this age group have been helpful adjuncts to standard treatments, emphasizing the importance of addressing both physical and mental health factors in treatment regimens (Hwang, 2017).

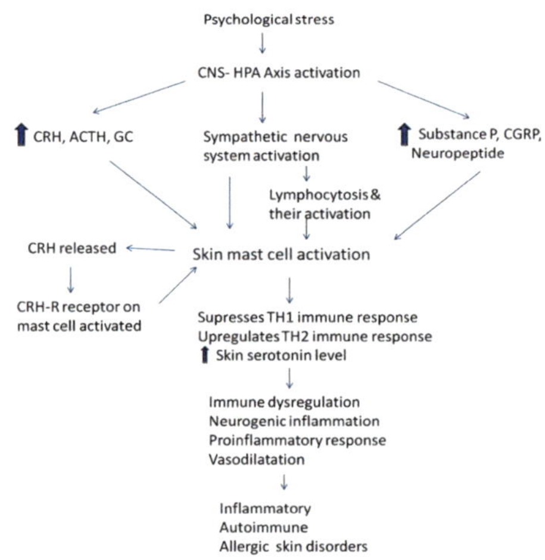

Figure 11.3. Flow-chart describing interplay of various factors leading to skin disorders originating from psychological stress.

Source: https://ijdvl.com/content/126/2013/79/2/Images/ijdvl_2013_79_2_176_107632_f10.jpg.

The concurrence between psychological health and cutaneous diseases underscores the value of incorporating psychotherapeutic techniques, such as Cognitive Behavioral Therapy (CBT), into dermatological treatment regimens. Research has established that CBT helps to significantly alleviate the mental distress of skin disorders like psoriasis. Central to the process of therapy are factors , such as patient involvement, development of a trusting relationship with therapists, and cognitive restructuring of thoughts regarding the condition. These factors facilitate a positive environment that not only reduces emotional suffering but also helps patients better cope with their conditions using self-kindness. The development of models such as "Guided Therapeutic Growth" illustrates how mental health treatments can revitalize the patient experience, enhance therapeutic effectiveness, and promote resilience despite chronic skin disorders (Laoudi, 2017). A holistic treatment approach is essential for optimal treatment outcomes in psychocutaneous disorders (Figure 11.3).

11.1. Historical Background

Learning Outcome

1. Understand early theories of skin and mental health.
2. Discuss the development of psychodermatology as a field.
3. Focus on milestones in psychodermatology and psychocutaneous disorders research and treatment.

Historical research into the intricate relationship between psychiatric status and skin diseases discovers a centuries-long understanding of stress's effects on the health of the skin. The Egyptians and Greeks identified a connection between psychological distress and skin disease, but it was not until many years later that the rudimentary foundation of psychodermatology was established. With the beginning of the modern era, the academic perspective shifted, incorporating biopsychosocial models that gave a significant focus on the psychological processes involved in the dermatologic conditions. For instance, recent studies have found that high perceived levels of psychological stress are significantly correlated with most skin symptoms among non-healthcare-seeking groups, thereby lending validity to ancient accounts through scientific means (Stewart, 2019). This historical context highlights a sustained evolution in insight, in which the overlap between mind and skin disease is increasingly recognized within medical paradigms. Alopecia offers the par excellence illustration of how those earlier perceptions have shaped modern practices in psychodermatological diagnosis. In the past, alopecia has been seen largely as a cosmetic issue, the profound psychological and social connotations of which were frequently ignored by practitioners. However, recent studies illustrate that alopecia patients experience profound identity transformations, emotional suffering, and social isolation, hence undermining its current place in the medical arena. Patients have been discovered to experience drastic identity transformations on numerous occasions, leading to increased psychological suffering (McCarthy, 2024). Consequently, the previously historical downgrade of alopecia to a cosmetic sole issue is increasingly eroded by this evidence, requiring enhanced understanding among clinicians to appreciate the deep psychological consequences at risk. The emergence of psychodermatology has created an increasing literature requiring holism in the management of skin disease. This approach prioritizes treating both psychological phenomena and cutaneous symptoms as a single set of phenomena. Criticism of dermatological practice in the past was primarily directed towards deficiencies in grasping the psychological loads of patients with skin disease. These debates have been a foundation of the development of professional therapeutic models that confront this point of contact, on the assumption that cutaneous health cannot be fully understood without consideration of the patient's psychological health. The continuing research into the interconnections of stress and dermatological disorders, as exemplified by robust correlations documented in recent studies, reinforces the call for an integrated understanding that brings together emotional, psychological, and dermatological practice

(Stewar, 2019; McCarthy, 2024). This innovative strategy not only enhances patient treatment outcomes but also redefines the scope of practice in dermatology.

11.1.1. Early Theories of Skin and Mental Health

In the evolution of dermatological science, early hypotheses linking mental disease to skin disease laid the groundwork for a broader conception of psychodermatology. Historically, skin ailments were viewed mostly in physical terms with little concern for the psychological factors that can hasten or contribute to such afflictions. Pioneering physicians began to hypothesize that emotional distress can manifest itself as dermatological presentation and thus came to appreciate the role of mind-body interaction in skin disease management. This new paradigm recognized that patients will commonly present with underlying emotional issues, and hence treatment professionals must not only address surface presentations but also establish a therapeutic environment that embraces and accommodates psychological factors (Poot et al., 2007). These were the findings that resulted in a shift towards an integrated treatment approach, where mental health assumed the status of an important aspect of effective dermatological care. Further, as the research went on, some psychodermatological disorders began to be characterized by their own unique emotional and psychological factors. Conditions like psoriasis and eczema were getting better known not only for the cutaneous manifestation but also for the pain that these inflict on the patients emotionally. For instance, psoriasis has been associated with significant psychological impairment that affects overall well-being and exacerbates underlying mental illness—diseases that regularly are overlooked in standard dermatologic treatment (Laoudi, 2017). This recognition of emotional effects opened new avenues for intervention, emphasizing the use of cognitive-behavioral therapy (CBT) and other therapy models that address the psychological underpinnings of skin disease. Early theorists thus laid the groundwork for integrative treatment modalities that address the complex interrelationship between mental health and skin health. As psychodermatology has evolved, early theory has been further elucidated, leading to advanced clinical practices. Dermatologists realized that the patient with skin disease feels shame, anxiety, and social isolation, behaviors that reinforce or worsen their disease. In recognizing that a majority of these patients possess alexithymic traits—struggling to express and recognize emotions—psychodermatological specialized training was necessary (Poot et al., 2007). The training was multidisciplinary and emphasized the need for improved communication skills to better identify and manage patients' emotional distress. With the inclusion of psychological assessment instruments in dermatology practice, clinicians can provide more individualized treatments, ultimately leading to better patient outcomes and a more holistic healing process that addresses both the mind and body in psychodermatology.

11.1.2. Development of Psychodermatology as a Field

Psychodermatology has emerged as a specific clinical specialty to address the complex relationship between skin illness and emotional health. Historically, dermatology has operated largely in the biomedical model, even to the extent of dismissing the mind's contribution to skin illness. Yet, with the growing recognition of the body-mind relationship, the necessity for holism has become clear. Psychodermatology seeks to bridge the gap by addressing both the psychological and dermatological dimensions of patient care. This innovation is particularly noteworthy against the backdrop of growing evidence of the efficacy of psychodermatological interventions, which are increasingly considered cost-effective and beneficial for patients with skin disorders. As outlined by Altunay et al.

(2023), the establishment of specialist psychodermatology services across Europe is uneven, and greater organizational support and resource allocation are needed to ensure optimal utilization of this subspecialty's potential. As psychodermatology continues to develop, the environment in which practitioners work is also evolving. The specialty recognizes the importance of dermatological and psychological expertise in treating patients with psychocutaneous illness. Practitioners are encouraged to engage in so-called dermatology psychology, that is, the therapeutic potential of dermatological consultations. Moreover, more awareness of patients with emotional issues, such as alexithymia, is essential during the treatment process. According to Poot et al. (2007), extended education is necessary, including both dermatologic and psychotherapeutic skills. This dual training allows clinicians to consider patients' affective histories and adapt their therapeutic style, offering a comprehensive practice that acknowledges the psychological origins of dermatologic complaints. While promising, psychodermatology is faced with primary barriers to access and standardization of treatments. The majority of countries still do not have organized psychodermatology services, while in others, the growth rate of this subspecialty is slow. The absence of full services can lead to gaps in treatment for patients, as not all regions are equipped with the necessary staff who specialize in dermatology and psychology. Coordination between mental health workers and dermatologists has never been more critical, as the multifactorial nature of psychodermatological illnesses requires multidisciplinary practice. As mentioned in Altunay et al. (2023), further efforts to establish and institutionalize such specialist services across Europe are necessary, to raise awareness and encourage the integration of psychosocial considerations into standard dermatological practice. Without these developments, patients can be expected to continue receiving substandard treatment that is not entirely suited to their needs (Figure 11.4).

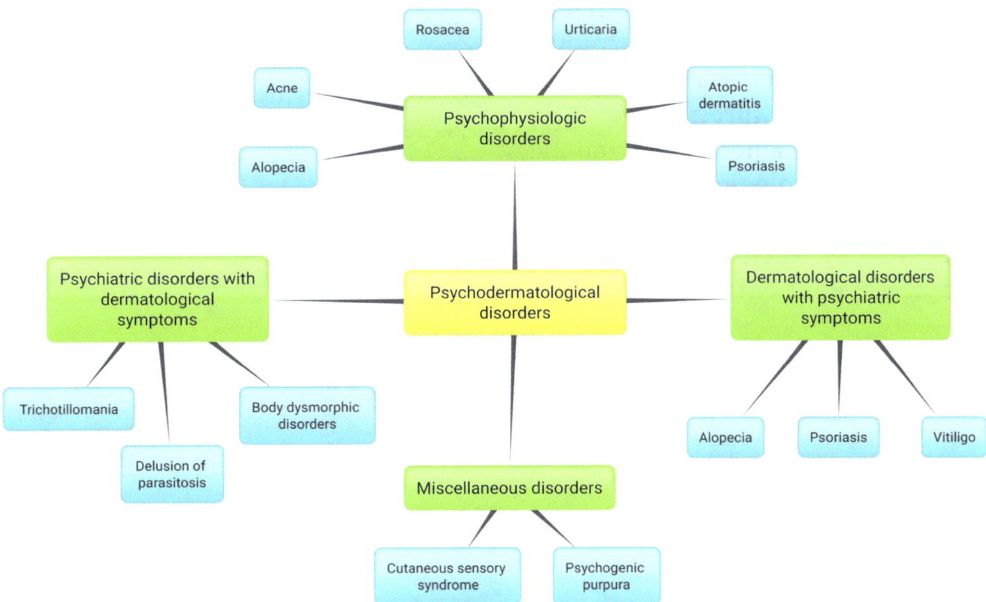

Figure 11.4. Classification of psychodermatology.

Source: https://www.researchgate.net/profile/Mohamed-Elsaie/publication/343956213/figure/fig1/AS:11431281173834041@1689052914895/Classification-of-psychodermatology.png.

11.1.3. Key Milestones in Research and Treatment

The interaction of psychosocial components and dermatological disorders has provided significant advancements in psychodermatology and studies on psychocutaneous disorders. From the early stages, the identification of the relationship between mental health and dermatological disorders gave a platform to develop further studies and treatments. Initial studies indicated that stress, anxiety, and depression can aggravate some already present skin diseases, such as eczema and psoriasis. This understanding encouraged investigators to pursue a therapy that integrates psychological treatment with dermatologic intervention. The development of psychodermatological models has therefore become a basis for understanding the influence of psychosocial processes on the appearance and course of skin disorders, representing a turning point toward integrated care in dermatology. Further advancements in this field were facilitated by the establishment of multidisciplinary clinics, which brought together dermatologists, psychologists, and psychiatrists to provide comprehensive care. The clinics have shed more light on the dynamic interactions between psychological distress and cutaneous presentations, with patients yielding benefits in the process. Including evidence-based psychological treatments, such as CBT, within treatment plans has been beneficial. Studies have shown that patients undergoing psychotherapy experienced reduced severity of their skin condition and improved mental well-being. The observation that the evidence pointed to addressing both physical and mental health in treating psychocutaneous disorders was a paradigm shift in clinical practice, as it recognized the importance of multilateral care pathways. Recent research further builds on these initial milestones, charting the neurobiological mechanisms underlying the skin-psyche connection. For instance, research on the role of cytokines in emotional and physical states has revealed that inflammation serves to integrate these two spheres. This information has strengthened the case for individualized therapeutic treatment aimed at the dermatologic manifestation and the psychological state of the disease. Besides, public campaigns for education and awareness among health workers emphasize the need for training in psychodermatology to equip practitioners with the ability to detect and treat comorbid psychiatric disorders better. According to the existing literature, failure to address related issues can lead to undertreatment and worse outcomes for patients, underscoring the importance of recent research and treatment advances (Program TURO et al., 2023).

Test Your Knowledge

1. What were some early theories linking skin conditions to mental health in ancient or pre-modern medicine?
2. When and how did psychodermatology emerge as a recognized medical subspecialty?

11.2. The Biological Basis

Learning Outcome

1. Discuss neuroimmunology and skin health.
2. Understand the role of stress in skin disorders.
3. Describe hormonal influences on skin conditions.

The interplay between dermatologic and psychological disease necessitates an understanding of the biological basis of psychodermatology. Chronodermatoses often come as a solution to an acute stressor by a complex neuro-endocrine system interrelating emotional health and skin integrity. Such cases of skin disease often exacerbate psychological morbidity, forming a vicious cycle in which skin disease heightens anxiety and anxiety in turn worsens skin disease. The critical role of cytokines in mediating inflammatory responses further underscores this connection, as both mood disorders and immune regulation are affected by these signaling molecules. Therefore, patients with chronic skin disease can develop symptoms of depression and anxiety, complicating their treatment and necessitating an integrated treatment approach that considers the psychological and physiological aspects. The threefold subdivision of psychodermatological disorders into psychophysiological disorders, secondary psychiatric disorders, and primary psychiatric disorders provides a model of inspection of the biological mechanisms of skin and mind. Psychophysiological disorders are characterized by skin disorders triggered by stress that present the immediate impact of psychological stressors on biological functioning. Conversely, secondary psychiatric disorders emerge as psychiatric responses to cutaneous lesions and, in doing so, illustrate how chronic illness is able to produce altered mental states. Last, primary psychiatric disorders, with resulting skin alteration due to underlying psychiatric illness, illustrate the complexity of biological interactions. Familiarity with these classifications helps clinicians understand the disease process and develop appropriate therapeutic interventions that target the biological pathways involved in these conditions (Petek et al., 2009). Moreover, the chronicity of dermatologic conditions tends to lead to long-standing psychological morbidity, emphasizing the need for a comprehensive treatment approach. The biological basis of this relationship is underscored by the phenomenon of sickness behavior, wherein biological responses to dermatologic issues may be expressed in the form of depression and anxiety symptoms. Stress also adds to these disorders, such that they pose a cyclical pattern of suffering and emotional tension. Therapeutic approaches that incorporate consultative-liaison psychiatry perspectives facilitate comprehensive treatment by bridging the gap between the physical manifestation of cutaneous disorders and their psychological implications. By facilitating cooperation between dermatologists and mental health practitioners, healthcare providers can optimize patient outcomes and address the intricate interplay among skin health, psychological functioning, and biological functioning (Georgieva, 2017).

11.2.1. Neuroimmunology and Skin Health

Neuroimmunology explores the intricate relationship between the nervous system, immune system, and skin health, emphasizing the role psychological disorders play in influencing dermatoses. Chronic skin disorders often have a significant psychological load, which makes inflammation worse and disrupts the healing process of the skin. The role of stress in neuroendocrine mechanisms that control skin illness is well documented, suggesting that emotional well-being is intricately linked to dermatological health. This affirms the fact that patients suffering from chronic skin conditions often find themselves experiencing increased anxiety and tension levels, possibly impeding their recuperation and quality of life at large. The fact that psychological states can affect immune responses adds to research on psychodermatology, further underscoring the need for more holistic treatment approaches to skin diseases (Georgieva, 2017). Moreover, the connection between skin well-being and stress reflects biochemical processes in the body, particularly in conditions such as acne. There is evidence that heightened emotional stress can trigger the release of hormones and cytokines, thereby altering skin conditions. Specifically, acne patients have altered concentrations of substance P, a neuropeptide in inflammatory responses, which rise during stressful episodes (Cybulski et al., 2016). While the severity of acne is not directly related to stress, the effects of psychological states reveal how tolerance and coping styles to stress may influence the course of skin conditions. The findings show the considerable value added in the integration of psychological assessment and management into dermatology, such that stress relief could potentially lower the incidence of skin diseases. Lastly, keeping neuroimmunology in mind while practicing psychodermatology necessitates deviating from classical treatment models and advocating a multidisciplinary approach. Practitioners have to not only address the somatic presentation of skin illness but also incorporate mental health care as a central component of patient management. Convergence allows for an in-depth understanding of how mental health influences somatic symptoms in a bid to provide bespoke therapeutic interventions addressing both psychological and dermatological needs. This approach can encourage patients to develop healthier coping mechanisms and increase resistance to psychological stressors that could trigger skin disease. By recognizing the interdependence of body and mind, neuroimmunology has the potential to improve treatment efficacy in dermatologic health, consistent with the emerging recognition of psychodermatology (Georgieva, 2017) (Figure 11.5).

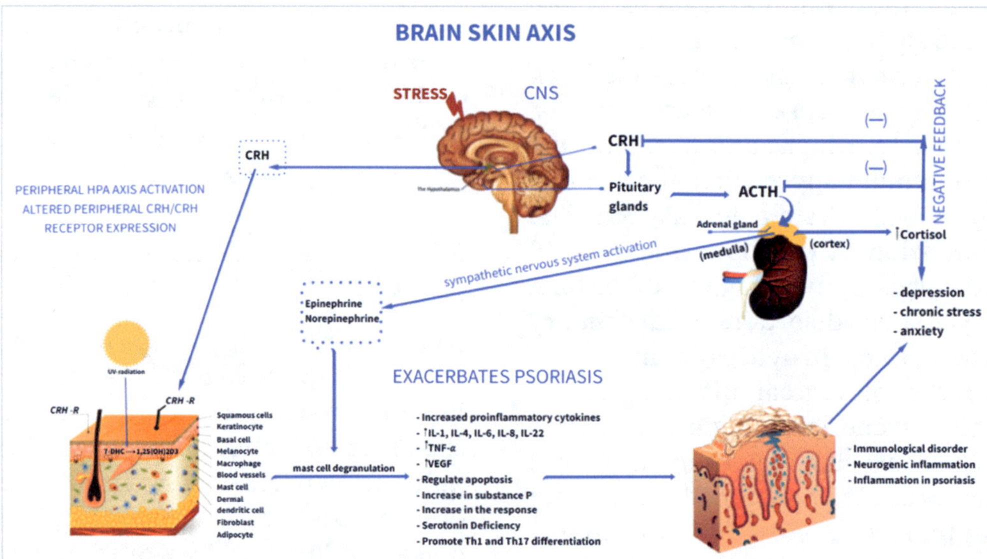

Figure 11.5. Brain–skin axis: association between psoriasis and depression. Stress acts via several pathways to exacerbate psoriasis, via the central and peripheral HPA axes, regulation of cytokine production, and activation of the sympathetic nervous system.

Source: https://www.mdpi.com/ijms/ijms-23-00669/article_deploy/html/images/ijms-23-00669-g001.png.

11.2.2. The Role of Stress in Skin Disorders

Stress profoundly affects the onset and exacerbation of most skin diseases, generating complex interactions between psychological states and dermatological well-being. Activation of the hypothalamic-pituitary-adrenal (HPA) axis triggers the stress response, leading to increased cortisol and other stress hormones. Such biochemical changes are capable of causing inflammation and immune dysfunction, which play roles in skin diseases such as eczema, psoriasis, and acne. This connection underscores the importance of considering psychological factors in dermatological practice, as stress management may help resolve underlying skin disorders. Moreover, patients with chronic skin illnesses are also more likely to experience heightened emotional distress, therefore creating a vicious cycle of experiencing stress aggravating skin symptomatology and worsening of skin ailments aggravating stress, further making it difficult for dermatologists to treat patients. The pathological skin picking disorder also illustrates the pathogenetic role of stress in skin disease. Patients with this condition are characterized by compulsive skin picking, which is typically a maladaptive coping mechanism for the resolution of internal tension and stress. Skin treatments in the majority of cases are not sufficient by themselves if the psychiatric aspect of skin picking, such as obsessive-compulsive disorder, and anxiety disorders is not resolved. Experiments have established that the psychological distress associated with skin disease can manifest as somatic symptoms, and that an interdisciplinary approach to treatment, such as dermatological and psychiatric interventions, becomes crucial. An understanding of the psycho-emotional factors underlying skin impairment is essential for developing effective therapeutic interventions and improving patient adherence to management regimens. A multidisciplinary model that brings together dermatological and psychiatric interventions is thus central to combating this pernicious disease. The biopsychosocial model offers a robust framework for explaining the interaction between stress and skin disease, emphasizing the need for multidisciplinary management in psychodermatology. Stress-related skin diseases frequently require intervention procedures that not only comprise medical and dermatologic treatment but also mental health management. The combination of psychological therapy, such as cognitive-behavioral therapy, with dermatologic procedures can enhance patient resistance to stress-related exacerbations of skin disease. Furthermore, effective psychiatric comorbidity management can significantly improve patient outcomes by reducing the psychological weight of visible skin diseases. As pointed out in recent literature, collaboration between dermatologists and mental health professionals is most essential in treating the dermatological and psychiatric aspects of such diseases with a better quality of life for patients (Benea et al., 2015; Barham et al., 2025) (Figure 11.6).

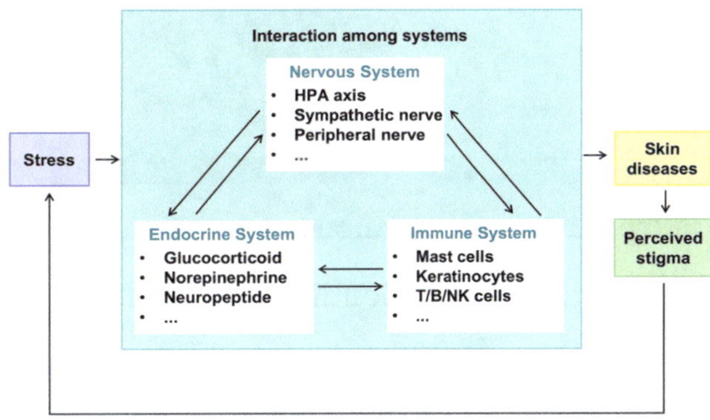

Figure 11.6. The vicious cycle between psychological stress and skin diseases.

Source: https://ars.els-cdn.com/content/image/1-s2.0-S0889159123003768-gr1_lrg.jpg.

11.2.3. Hormonal Influences on Skin Conditions

The relationship between hormonal effects and skin disease is a significant area of inquiry for psychodermatology. Hormones, particularly stress hormones cortisol, also play a key role in maintaining healthy skin. An increase in levels of stress hormones can lead to exacerbation of inflammatory cutaneous diseases, such as eczema and psoriasis, and is implicated in alterations of the immunological status of the skin. These disruptions are typically complemented by psychological disorders, which emphasize the connection between mental health and skin presentations. Effectively, patients with chronic dermatitis can also simultaneously develop heightened anxiety and depression, creating a cycle that complicates the psychological as well as the dermatological treatment process. These comorbidities underscore the need for interdisciplinary management that addresses both emotional and physical skin health concurrently in collaborative psychodermatology practices (Petek et al., 2009). In addition to stress hormones, sex hormones , such as estrogen and testosterone also contribute to skin disorders.

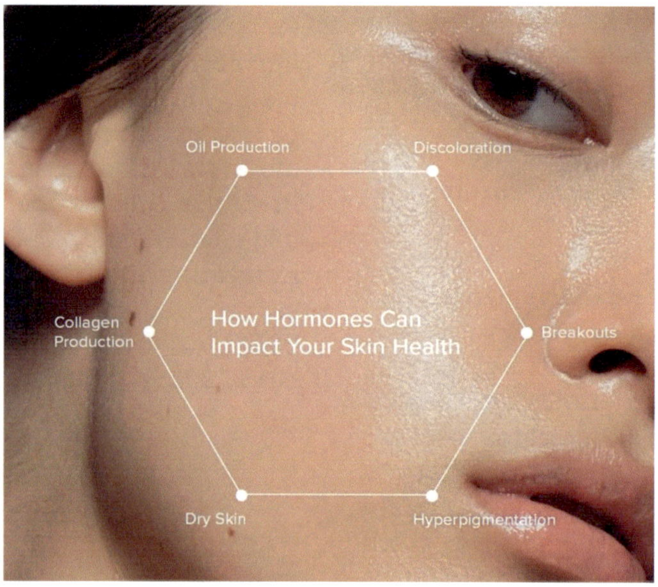

Figure 11.7. How hormones can impact skin health.

Source: https://www.southfaceskin.com/wp-content/uploads/2024/10/SOUTHFACE-59.jpg.

Alterations in these hormones bring about and initiate most dermatoses, particularly at significant periods , such as puberty, menstruation, or menopause. Hormonal fluctuations may affect sebum secretion, leading to acne or changes in skin hydration that might give rise to conditions such as atopic dermatitis. The intricacy of the interactions is further emphasized by the fact that skin diseases can induce psychological distress, which in turn results in a feedback loop where both illnesses perpetuate each other. Therefore, knowledge of the hormonal underpinnings of skin changes is of immediate utility for their treatment, necessitating an integration of dermatologic and psychiatric principles capable of influencing both aspects of patients' welfare (Ferreira et al., 2009). Furthermore, the interplay between the neuroendocrine system and skin health is an exciting area of investigation in psychodermatology. The hypothalamic-pituitary-adrenal axis regulates inflammation and the stress response, significantly affecting skin function and healing. Disregulation of the axis leads to malfunction of tissue regeneration and exacerbation of skin conditions, which may, in turn, affect the state of mind. Such inflammatory cytokines are mediators and thus fall under the control of dermal inflammation as well as mood disorders. This means that advances in the neuro-immune-endocrine physiology of the skin may enable new therapeutic strategies that simultaneously address psychocutaneous disorders and hormonal influences on cutaneous disorders. The better scientists understand associations, the more probable integrative therapies that consider both psychological and dermatological treatments are (Petek et al., 2009) (Figure 11.7).

Test Your Knowledge

1. How does neuroimmunology explain the connection between the nervous system and skin health?
2. What role does stress play in triggering or worsening skin disorders?

11.3. Common Psychocutaneous Disorders

Learning Outcome

1. Define psoriasis and its psychological impact.
2. Describe acne and body image issues.
3. Deal with eczema and emotional triggers.

The crossing of psychological states and dermatological conditions has given rise to psychocutaneous disorders, a group that comprises most conditions in which the mind and skin intersect. Amongst these, conditions , such as psoriasis, eczema, and acne are often complicated by psychological stressors, making for a management problem. Psoriasis, for example, is an archetypal case in point, given the fact that triggering is most commonly linked to stress, anxiety, and depression. This bidirectional interaction underscores the necessity of an interdisciplinary treatment plan, with dermatologists collaborating with mental health professionals to address both cutaneous and underlying psychological conditions. As the literature emphasizes, understanding this interaction is crucial for effectively managing it and improving outcomes in patients with common psychodermatological diseases (Souza et al., 2019). Another significant region of concern between psychocutaneous disorders is delusion inversus, in which a patient with a relatively trivial dermatological condition has an exaggerated sense of the gravity of their disease. This illness confounds psychiatric and dermatologic diagnosis, posing difficulties to medical professionals who may be seeing patients who come in with distress regarding perceived risks not substantiated by medical evidence. These patients are responsible for inappropriate intervention and an extended therapeutic process, emphasizing the need for healthcare professionals, particularly dermatologists, to recognize these patients and properly treat their psychological conditions. As there is hardly any literature concerning delusion inversus specifically, clinicians are compelled to make inferences from more generic categories of delusional disorder, an approach that poses clear gaps in knowledge and management in this regard (Souza et al., 2019). Finally, the development of expert psychodermatology services plays a significant role in enhancing the care of patients afflicted with psychocutaneous disorders. Such services are either lacking or poorly developed in most regions, leading to worse treatment outcomes and deteriorated quality of life among people who carry the disease. Research has shown that adding psychological support to dermatological management can yield better outcomes and cost savings, further attesting to the value of a multidisciplinary approach. Despite growing recognition of psychodermatology as an essential subspecialty within dermatology, significant barriers remain, including unequal service availability across Europe and a slow pace of progress toward comprehensive care options. It is critical to diminish these disparities in order to provide patients with the integrative, informed care they need to properly manage their skin disorder and mental health (Figure 11.8).

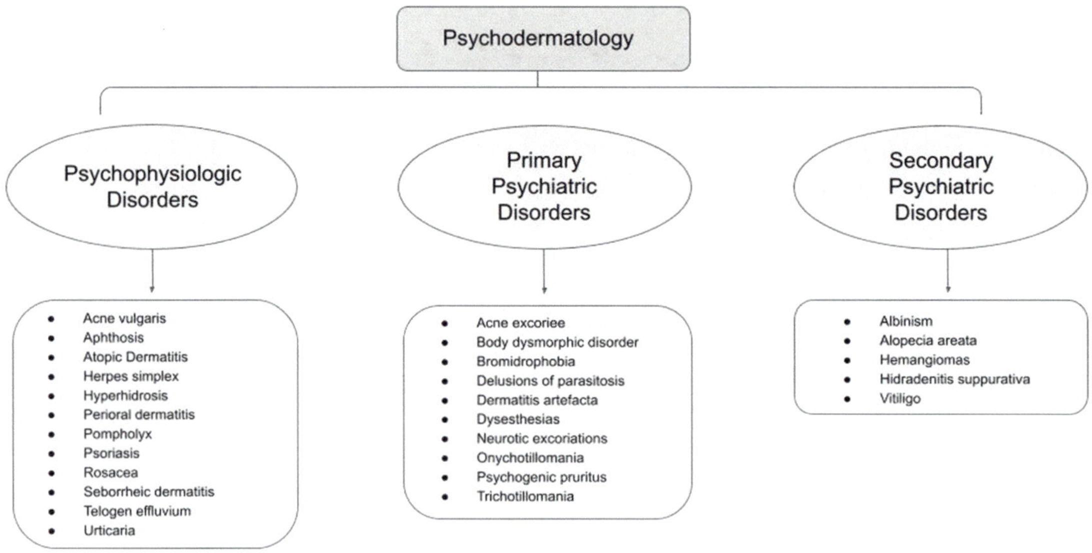

Figure 11.8. Psychodermatology disorders. Psoriasis, trichotillomania, and vitiligo are among the most common psychodermatologic conditions.

Source: https://www.researchgate.net/publication/375081544/figure/fig1/AS:11431281215788444@1704388610864/Psychodermatology-disorders-psoriasis-trichotillomania-and-vitiligo-are-just-a-few.png.

11.3.1. Psoriasis and Its Psychological Impact

Psoriasis, being an inflammatory skin disease, impacts not just physical symptoms; psychologically, it is severe and, in most instances, debilitating. Isolation, anxiety, and depression due to externally evident lesions are experienced by patients most commonly. Such emotional distress can impact their quality of life significantly, with heightened perception of stigma and self-consciousness. According to psychodermatology research, there exists a proven strong association between mental health and skin diseases, and there is an emphasis on offering combined mechanisms for care that address the dermatological as well as psychological components of psoriasis. These findings endorse the fact that treatment of psychiatric comorbidities among psoriasis patients can optimize treatment outcome and general quality of life, highlighting the importance of a universal, multidisciplinary approach to treatment in the field of psychodermatology and psychocutaneous disorders (Altunay et al., 2023).

Psoriasis's psychological distress overflows into many areas of daily functioning, bordering on relationships, work performance, and self-esteem. Research indicates that individuals with psoriasis are at increased risk of anxiety disorders, particularly due to the chronic nature of their condition and the observable impact on their skin. The observable characteristic of psoriasis might lead to negative body image that aggravates feelings of inadequacy in addition to social withdrawal. Notably, patients develop alexithymia, a condition of being unable to identify and express emotional feelings, which complicates their recovery on a psychological level (Poot et al., 2007). It is necessary for dermatologists and mental health professionals to be made aware of this interplay between emotional and somatic signs due to the fact that it may inform more efficient treatment modalities that are tailored based on the individual needs of psoriasis patients. Advances in psychodermatology emphasize the necessity of multidisciplinary interventions to bring dermatology and psychotherapy together. By enabling dermatologists to develop improved communication skills, alongside psychotherapy training, the medical system can create an environment ready for well-rounded patient care. The evolving focus on psychodermatology emphasizes the recognition of the psychological elements of skin disorders, particularly when emotional disturbance associated with conditions, such as psoriasis reflects physical disturbances. Having dedicated psychodermatology services can alleviate some of the mental distress experienced by patients, providing earlier access to appropriate mental health services. Finally, these advances are necessary in an effort to develop a more effective care system for individuals affected by psychocutaneous conditions (Altunay et al., 2023) (Figure 11.9).

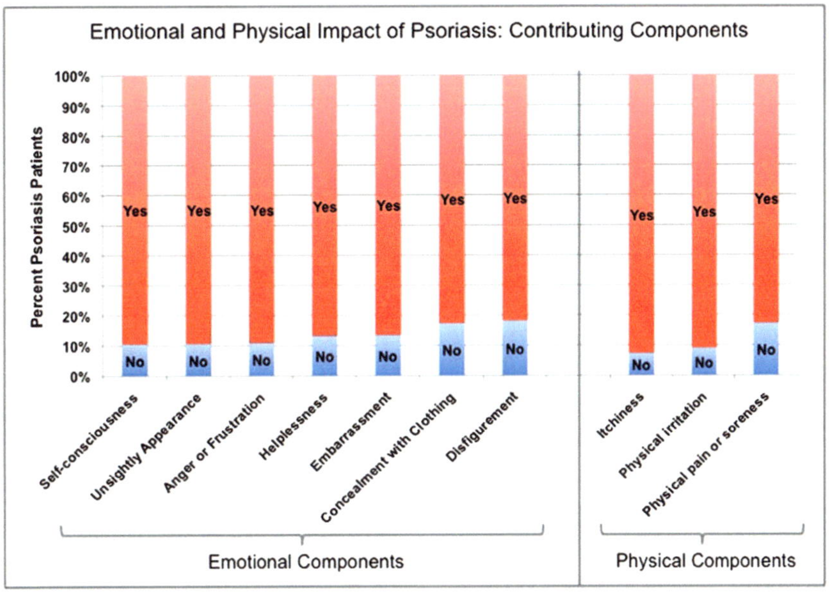

Figure 11.9. Emotional and physical impact of psoriasis: contributing components.

Source: https://www.researchgate.net/profile/Bruce-Bebo/publication/234041065/figure/fig5/AS:669665588166661@1536672126336/Emotional-and-Physical-Impact-of-Psoriasis-Contributing-Components.ppm.

11.3.2. Acne and Body Image Issues

The connection between body image disturbance and acne is a critical concern in psychodermatology. Acne, a common dermatologic disease, does not only affect the body but also the psyche of the person itself, causing fear and self-consciousness. The disfiguring nature of acne might lead to most having a negative self-concept, often exacerbating distress over how they look. The patients of visible skin illnesses generally have issues with social stigmatization, which only adds to their psychological problems and influences their quality of life. Literature suggests that the psyche has a profound effect on the body image of a person, suggesting that dermatologists need to value the psychological implications involved in illnesses like acne in order to provide comprehensive care (Marron, S. E., & Tomas-Aragones, L., 2016). Therefore, addressing body image concerns is essential as part of an integral treatment process, underscoring the importance of psychological and dermatological interventions. Moreover, the social implications of acne are not only for the individual but also for interpersonal relationships and social interactions. The shame associated with visible acne can lead to social withdrawal, enhancing mental health implications even further. In evading potentially critical confrontations, people can become ever more alone, developing higher levels of anxiety and depression. The communication of concerns of body image among victims of acne underscores the reciprocal interaction between physical and emotional health. It is crucial to note that such emotional distress may be caused not only by the physical quality of the skin condition itself but also by cultural and societal pressures to conform to a specific beauty ideal. Fostering a healthier body image can significantly contribute to the well-being of acne sufferers, underscoring the need to address both mental resilience and dermatological conditions (Basta-Juzbašić, A., & Bukvić Mokos, Z., 2015).

Finally, adequate attention for the psychological impact of acne ought to be a multidisciplinary approach involving dermatologists, psychologists, and counselors. This joint action is key towards comprehending the interaction between acne, body image, and mental health. Dermatologists need to recognize signs of body image dissatisfaction while taking a helpful and compassionate stance towards patients. It is essential for such experts to create a friendly environment in which individuals feel free to articulate concerns regarding appearance, therefore reducing feelings of embarrassment or shame. Positive body image interventions can foster self-esteem and personal empowerment, thereby improving the quality of life for acne patients. Through closing the interface between dermatology and psychological care, practitioners can devise comprehensive treatment strategies that treat both the visible symptoms of acne and the underlying psychological issues (Marron, S. E., & Tomas-Aragones, L., 2016) (Figure 11.10).

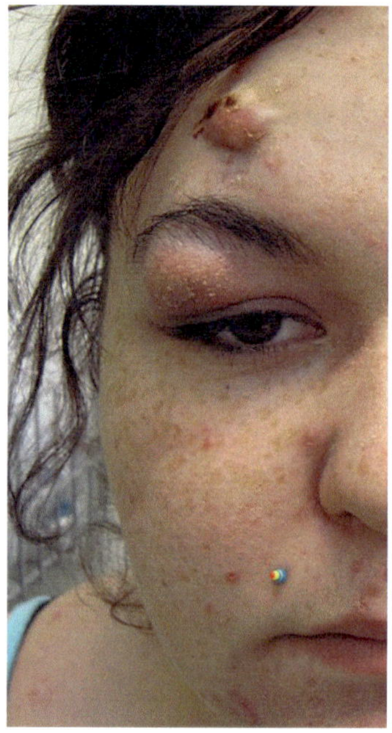

Figure 11.10. Close-up photo of a severe case of cystic acne.

Source: https://upload.wikimedia.org/wikipedia/commons/thumb/1/1f/Cysticacne-cropped.jpg/320px-Cysticacne-cropped.jpg.

11.3.3. Eczema and Emotional Triggers

Eczema, particularly atopic dermatitis, is a poignant example of the way dermatological disorders are so intimately entwined with emotional health, a pervasive theme of psychodermatology. The disease is a long-standing inflammatory disorder of the skin that typically becomes more severe with emotional stress, one of several examples of how psychological factors affect physical symptoms immediately. Eczema sufferers are frequently plagued by heightened anxiety, especially during the onset of attacks or the visible manifestations of their condition. The psychosocial effect cannot be overstated; patients complain of embarrassment and self-consciousness, most notably among adolescents. At this stage of life, when body image and social acceptance become central, the impact of eczema can lead to a significant decline in self-esteem and well-being, highlighting the intersection of emotional stimuli and body states in psychodermatological conditions (Georgieva, 2017). The role of emotional stimuli in eczema development is further enhanced in periods of psychological distress, which is a common phenomenon among both youth and adult populations. Stress and anxiety are classic precipitants of acute eczema flare-up, suggesting that the mind-skin relationship is not merely utilitarian but profound. As emotional tension is experienced, the stress response can trigger inflammatory mechanisms that worsen eczema. This vicious cycle creates the kind of situation where worsening of the condition of the skin further intensifies emotional distress, leading to a cycle of anxiety and flare-ups of the skin. Awareness of this process becomes critical for clinicians, who must include both psychological and dermatological interventions to engage whole-person care (Hwang, 2017). Recent research points to the necessity of treating psychological disturbances along with the traditional dermatologic therapy for eczema. The effectiveness of educational therapy in adolescents offers a promising way to manage the disease overall. By providing young patients with knowledge about their condition and coping strategies, medical doctors can facilitate self-regulation and reduce stress related to eczema. Counselling and support groups have also proved effective in reducing feelings of loneliness and anxiety, and fostering a sense of community and empathy among sufferers. Lastly, these measures show that a treatment plan must account for the psychological dynamics of eczema to improve overall disease outcomes and quality of life for patients (Hwang, 2017) (Figure 11.11).

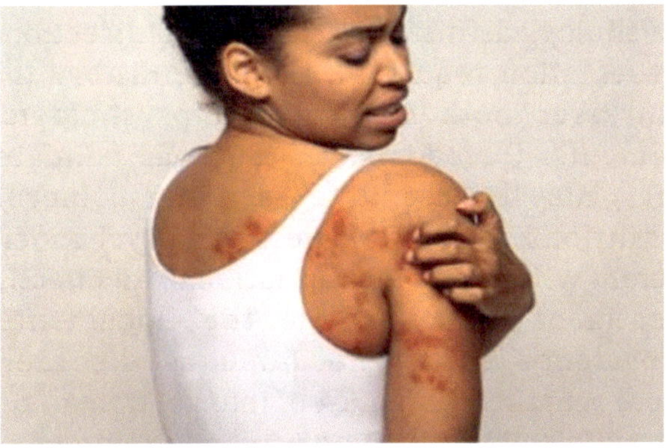

Figure 11.11. Eczema serves as a poignant example of the intricate relationship between dermatological conditions and emotional health.

Source: https://www.datelinehealthafrica.org/ckfinder/userfiles/files/Black%20lady%20with%20contact%20dermatitis.jpg.

Test Your Knowledge

1. How does psoriasis affect a patient's psychological well-being?
2. What body image issues are commonly associated with acne?
3. In what ways can emotional stress trigger or worsen eczema?

11.4. Diagnosis and Assessment

Learning Outcome

1. Understand clinical evaluation techniques in psychodermatology.
2. Explain the importance of psychological assessments in dermatology.
3. Discuss the significance of a multidisciplinary approach in psychodermatology.

The nuance of psychodermatology requires a high-level diagnostic and evaluation process that recognizes the interplay between psychological and dermatological disorders. The clinician can see patients whose psychiatric symptoms exist through dermatologic presentation, or whose dermatologic diseases are exacerbated by psychological disturbance. This bidirectional presentation requires a thorough history that addresses both medical and psychological elements. Questionnaires, such as validated ones, may be useful to ascertain comorbid conditions, but awareness of psychosocial factors will lead to the formation of an effective treatment plan. Despite the documented prevalence of psychocutaneous disorders, there remains a vast lack of information among dermatologists regarding psychodermatological disorders, as only 13.75% of them are aware of psychocutaneous disorders (Hashmi et al., 2022). Therefore, an interdisciplinary assessment plan that encourages communication between mental health practitioners and dermatologists is crucial for optimal patient management. Accurate diagnosis of psychodermatological disorders relies on a multidisciplinary team-based approach. The optimal model involves a team of dermatologists, psychiatrists, and psychologists who can collectively evaluate the patient's physical and psychological symptoms. By working together, the team can develop a systematic evaluation plan, including both clinical interviews and standardized psychological testing. This collaborative effort assists in distinguishing between primary cutaneous illnesses, which may have symptoms of underlying psychiatric disturbance, and primary psychiatric disorders that produce evident skin signs, such as delusional parasitosis or body dysmorphic disorder. The availability of specialist clinics that handle psychodermatology can enhance service provision and address the particular needs of patients with such multifactorial diseases (Bewley, A., & Taylor, R., 2016). Telehealth technology is increasingly used to diagnose and evaluate psychodermatological diseases. The integration of Artificial Intelligence (AI) into medical practice has the potential to standardize the assessment process, support remote consultations, and enhance patient access. AI can facilitate detailed data collection from patient surveys and visual inspections of skin lesions, providing clinicians with significant context that informs diagnosis (Hashmi et al., 2022). Furthermore, electronic health records generated from telehealth consultations may serve as valuable historical information for ongoing treatment and management of psychocutaneous disorders. Telepsychiatry has found wider applications, but in psychodermatology, it remains evolving. Emerging evidence shows the effectiveness of this approach, particularly when symptom self-rating and observation are incorporated into an overall treatment program, which can lead to improved patient outcomes for patients with complicated psychological and dermatologic complications.

11.4.1. Clinical Evaluation Techniques

Clinical assessment techniques in psychodermatology are necessary to accurately diagnose and treat psychocutaneous disorders, as these inevitably interweave the dermatologic and psychological aspects. These techniques typically begin with a comprehensive clinical interview, in which therapists assess not only the physical manifestations of skin diseases but also the psychological factors that can exacerbate or even cause these dermatologic conditions. The integration of standardized tools like depression and anxiety rating scales can introduce quantitative data, which can be utilized to detect intrinsic psychosocial stressors. Such a comprehensive assessment system thus presents a complete picture of the patient, aligning treatment interventions that address skin wellness and psychiatric well-being concurrently, and improved intervention outcomes as highlighted in recent reports on complex cases , such as dermatitis artefacta (Mariah et al., 2024). Moreover, applying multidisciplinary approaches to clinical evaluation is important given the complex interplay between skin conditions and mental states. Collaboration among dermatologists, psychiatrists, and psychologists allows for the formulation of customized treatment plans that combine dermatologic treatment with psychological therapy. For example, patients with chronic skin diseases, such as psoriasis, are prone to develop comorbid psychiatric disorders that need integrated care to address these related conditions. Evidence indicates that patients receiving psychodermatology services, delivered through multidisciplinary teams, have improved outcomes compared with patients receiving fragmented care (Mariah et al., 2024). The strategies underscore the importance of holistic clinical assessment approaches in delivering effective management of psychocutaneous disorders. In addition to traditional evaluation methods, innovative therapeutic strategies, such as mindfulness-based stress reduction (MBSR) interventions, have been found to be useful in the cultivation of psychological resilience among skin disease patients. Clinical studies have established that patients who received MBSR programs experienced significant anxiety score decreases and thereby could be useful as an adjunct therapy to standard dermatological care. The long-term sustainability of such psychological advantage depends on ongoing evaluation, so psychodermatology practitioners can adjust their practice based on ongoing patient feedback. As the outcomes of mindfulness practice demonstrate, integrating psychological techniques into clinical assessment not only promotes greater patient engagement but also deepens understanding of the complexities of psychocutaneous disorders, ultimately improving holistic care.

11.4.2. Psychological Tests in Dermatology

The necessity of psychiatric assessment in dermatology is underscored by the complex interplay of mental and skin disorders. Patients with dermatologic diseases , such as psoriasis and atopic dermatitis are prone to serious emotional morbidity, causing them to endure more suffering from their physical symptomatology. A skin disease is not merely a physical disease; it can impact one's psychological well-being, giving rise to anxiety, depression, and social exclusion. To this end, providing comprehensive psychological assessments enables medical personnel to assess patients' status of mental health so treatment programs are set not just in response to the dermatological but to the psychological components of their condition as well. Such an integrated approach enhances the level of care and significantly improves patient outcomes. For a given set of dermatological conditions, targeted psychological assessments can inform treatment protocols that include both dermatological and psychological interventions. For instance, cognitive behavioral therapy (CBT) has succeeded in reducing the psychological distress associated with skin conditions like psoriasis. Research evidence indicates that patients who receive CBT not only show improved emotional well-being but also experience reduced clinical severity of their dermatological conditions (Laoudi, 2017). Psychological assessments in these models determine the causes of patient distress and enable more individualized treatment. Through determining the connection between psychological factors and dermatologic presentation, practitioners can use holistic care strategies that go beyond symptom relief. Additionally, the adolescent group is the most difficult group to handle while addressing psychological aspects of dermatologic conditions. Atopic dermatitis, for example, can severely affect youth during their formative years, interfering with their social competence and self-esteem (Hwang, 2017). Psychological functioning may be assessed using tests applicable to this age category to determine the specific stressors adolescents experience while learning to live with their condition. By integrating education-based interventions based on these tests, healthcare providers can empower their patients, encouraging self-management and resilience. Thus, psychological exams not only serve as diagnostic tools but also as impetuses for the establishment of effective therapeutic and educational interventions, which amplify the management of psychodermatological conditions among younger populations (Figure 11.12).

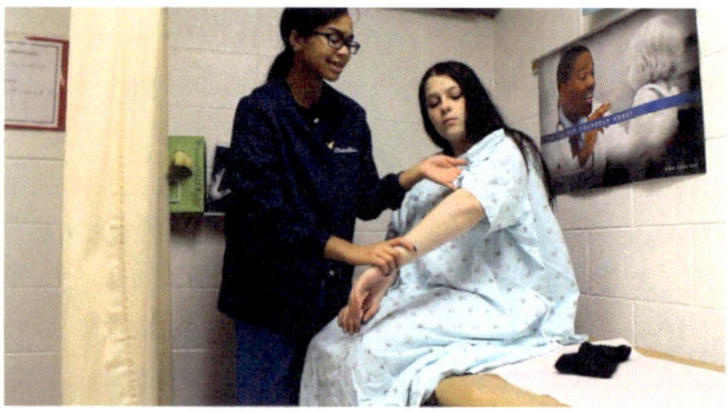

Figure 11.12. The importance of psychological assessments in dermatology is underscored by the complex interplay between skin conditions and mental health.

Source: https://i.ytimg.com/vi/zoCUDGclcDk/maxresdefault.jpg.

11.4.3. Importance of a Multidisciplinary Approach

The relevance of multidisciplinary psychodermatology ultimately stems from the intricate interplay between psychiatric and dermatological disorders. That interaction illustrates how some psychological disorders manifest in dermatological expression, necessitating an integrative strategy for effective treatment. Disorders , such as trichotillomania, for example, present patients whose behaviors have a direct impact upon their skin health on a lasting basis, posing a dual challenge to treating clinicians. Thus, interaction between mental health practitioners and dermatologists is paramount in the treatment of these disorders as a whole. By working together, healthcare professionals can optimize patient outcomes by addressing both psychological and dermatological needs through an integrated approach. In the long term, this is not only useful for maximizing the effectiveness of treatments but also for addressing the overall biopsychosocial foundations of patients' morbidity (Barham et al., 2025). Treatment of psychocutaneous disease presents unique challenges due to the fact that skin and mental well-being are closely connected. There is a significant comorbidity between depression and dermatological conditions, and research has demonstrated that nearly 30% of those afflicted with skin disease also have depression symptoms (Petek et al., 2009). This dual aspect of skin and mental well-being makes it imperative that treatment be a combined approach using both dermatological and psychological intervention. Through the integration of services across disciplines, clinicians can construct individualized interventions that account for the multidimensional characteristics of these disorders. Not only does collaboration guarantee efficient symptom management, but it also treats the psychosocial stressors that can worsen both psychiatric and dermatologic conditions. In this sense, the multidisciplinary model is not only beneficial but also imperative for promoting whole-patient care in psychodermatology. Besides, the multidisciplinary system encourages further understanding of how psychosocial factors influence the management and development of skin disorders. The system enables healthcare professionals to have increased interaction among them, and a greater comprehension of every patient's unique case is obtained. For instance, patients having severe stressors may learn that their skin disorders become intensified, thereby forming a vicious cycle of physical symptoms and psychological conditions. Through an integrated framework, healthcare teams will be better able to treat these problems by employing comprehensive strategies for both the symptoms of dermatological disorders and the underlying psychological factors. Thus, multidisciplinary management not only enhances clinical effectiveness but also improves overall quality of life for individuals with psychodermatological conditions, thereby bridging the gap between physical and psychological welfare in clinical practice (Petek et al., 2009; Barham et al., 2025).

Test Your Knowledge

1. What clinical evaluation techniques are used to assess psychodermatological conditions?
2. How are psychological assessments integrated into the diagnosis of skin disorders?
3. Why is a multidisciplinary approach important in managing psychodermatology patients?

11.5. Treatment Modalities

Learning Outcome

1. Understand the integration of psychotherapeutic interventions in the management of psychodermatological conditions.
2. Discuss the intersection of psychodermatology and pharmacological treatments.
3. Focus on integrative approaches and lifestyle modifications in the realm of psychodermatology.

Treatment in psychodermatology involves a multidisciplinary approach, in which dermatological and psychiatric treatment is synergistically merged in order to cure the complex correlation between skin ailments and psychological factors. Because stress and anxiety usually aggravate most of the skin diseases , such as atopic dermatitis or psoriasis, consideration of psychological treatment as opposed to standard dermatologic treatment is crucial. Successful management is sometimes supplemented with cognitive-behavioral therapy (CBT) to enable the patients to change inappropriate thoughts and behaviors related to their skin disorders. This model of therapy has been proven to be useful, especially in pathological skin picking, where the correlation between dermatological symptoms and states of mind is most evident. These therapies can significantly enhance the patient's quality of life by addressing both overt symptoms as well as inner psychological distress, creating a holistic model of treatment addressing both psychosocial and biological dimensions of the disorder (Benea et al., 2015).

Psychotherapy is also supplemented with pharmacological therapies, which form a cornerstone of the therapeutic environment in psychodermatology. Medications , such as selective serotonin reuptake inhibitors (SSRIs) are usually recommended for individuals with anxiety or obsessive-compulsive signs as a result of dermatological diseases. A study stresses that these drugs should be used to alleviate comorbid psychological symptoms, thus enhancing compliance with dermatologic therapy. Moreover, when these pharmacotherapies are complemented by counseling, a synergistic effect is achieved, enabling patients to manage the emotional consequences of cutaneous disease.

The need for this combined strategy is evident, as neglect of psychiatric aspects can lead to partial resolution of dermatological treatment and, occasionally, worsening patient outcomes (Albert et al., 2023). Use of a multidisciplinary approach is essential to optimize treatment modalities in psychodermatology. Through collaborative care among dermatologists, psychologists, and other healthcare providers, a unified support system emerges that can better diagnose and treat the many challenges faced by patients with psychodermatological disorders. Future clinical practice and research call for standardized treatment systems and classification systems to ensure procedural consistency across fields. This partnership not only enhances understanding of the biopsychosocial model that guides skin disease but also facilitates the development of innovative interventions tailored to distinct needs. As therapies continue to develop, the use of psychosocial assessments and integrative treatments will likely lead to improved outcomes for patients with these complex and often incapacitating illnesses (Benea et al., 2015; Albert et al., 2023) (Figure 11.13).

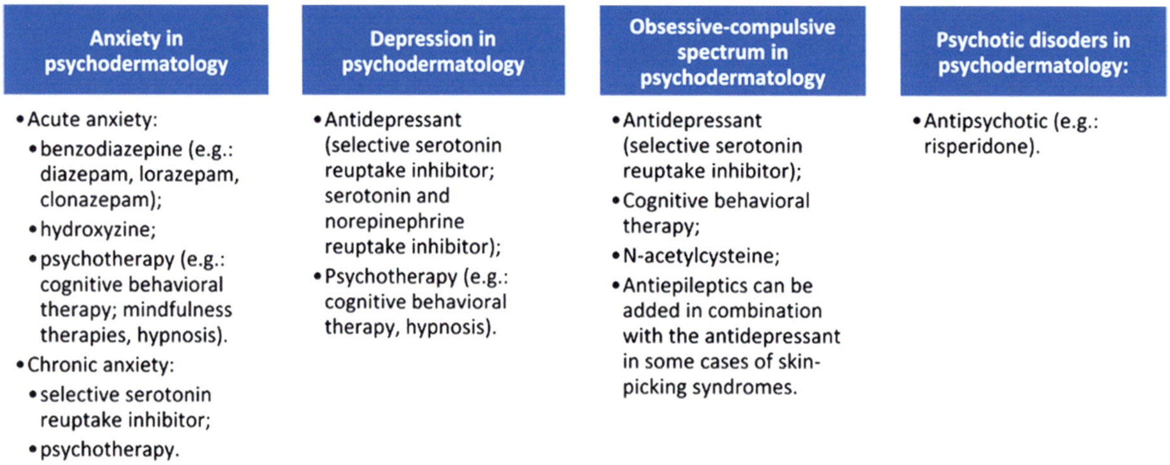

Figure 11.13. Common treatments in psychodermatology, considering the main psychopathologies observed in clinical practice.

Source: https://www.researchgate.net/publication/342694305/figure/fig2/AS:11431281173876136@1689060083624/Common-treatments-in-psychodermatology-considering-the-main-psychopathologies-observed.png.

11.5.1. Psychotherapeutic Interventions

The inclusion of psychotherapeutic interventions in the management of psychodermatological disorders has a significant effect on patient outcomes. In particular, the psychological aspect of skin conditions underscores the need for a multimodal treatment approach that integrates dermatological and mental health interventions. Participation with emotional state conditions, such as anxiety, depression, and stress, is necessary because these elements typically aggravate skin conditions. Using the methods of brief therapy, clinicians can significantly alleviate the psychological burden of such disorders. For instance, it has been proven that short-term psychotherapy led to a considerable reduction in the rates of anxiety and depression among military personnel experiencing stress disorders, once again testifying to the effectiveness of psychotherapy in strengthening emotional well-being as well as resistance to stress (Klymenko et al., 2025). Greater emphasis on tailored psychotherapeutic interventions underscores their appropriateness and validity to treat psychocutaneous disorders. New research has introduced gender-differentiated psychoeducational interventions, which modify the therapeutic approach based on the unique demands of individuals who have been affected by traumatic incidents. The personalized approach has greatly enhanced the efficacy of treatment, underscoring how individualized treatment can enhance the quality of life for combat-induced depression-related disorders. The benefits of personalized treatment extend beyond symptom relief to include a return of self-image and improved coping responses to stressors, essential factors in managing the interaction between psychological distress and dermatological symptoms (Kozhyna, N., & Nemchenko, A., 2025). In psychodermatology, effective psychotherapeutic intervention plays a core role not only in stabilization of mental health but also in improving dermatological results. When psychotherapists work with dermatologists, they can develop comprehensive treatment plans addressing skin as well as psychic issues. This coordinated care implies that the psychological factors underlying or exacerbating skin conditions can be appropriately managed. As evidenced by notable improvement observed in patients treated with psychotherapeutic management, this coordinated care can lead to greater emotional stability, enhanced interpersonal relationships, and a healthier coping style to stress. Hence, the addition of psychotherapeutic intervention to dermatological practice not only meets immediate distress but also creates long-lasting emotional resistance in dermatological patients with psychocutaneous disorders, clearing the way for subsequent therapeutic advances.

11.5.2. Pharmacological Treatments

The overlap of psychodermatology with drug therapies emphasizes the need to address both psychiatric and dermatological symptoms of patients. Pharmacological treatment is crucial in the context of patients suffering from conditions pathological skin picking that typically occur with psychiatric disorders such as obsessive-compulsive disorder (OCD). In one of the notable cases, a 17-year-old female patient was accompanied by dermatological symptoms to her psychological well-being, also proving the twofold nature of such illnesses (Benea et al., 2015). Pharmacological treatments not only alleviate skin symptoms but also address underlying psychological disorders. A variety of drug classes, like the selective serotonin reuptake inhibitors (SSRIs), are promising in mitigating compulsive behaviors of such disorders, thereby complementing an integrative approach to treatment. On a broader scale, the categorization of psychodermatological disorders helps gain insights into individualized pharmacologic management. Current classification systems group these disorders by psychiatric etiology, enabling clinicians to use more effective treatment regimens. For instance, disorders , such as delusional parasitosis and neurotic excoriations require finely tuned approaches based on pharmacotherapy for the underlying psychiatric symptomatology (Bramono et al., 2020). By integrating dermatology and psychiatry, clinicians can optimize treatment efficacy. Coordination allows a comprehensive assessment of patient needs, facilitating the development of individualized pharmacologic treatment protocols that address skin disorders and their psychogenic etiology. Moreover, effective management of psychodermatologic diseases through pharmacologic approaches needs continuous monitoring and patient compliance. Because patients with dermal diseases present with a high comorbidity of psychiatric diseases, maintaining open communication channels for treating patients is crucial (Bramono et al., 2020). Complacency to psychiatric therapy can exacerbate dermatological symptoms, complicating overall treatment. Therefore, therapists must cultivate a strong therapeutic alliance to encourage compliance, acknowledge patientspatterns of their symptoms, and provide ongoing support.

Prioritizing treatment compliance to pharmacotherapy has the potential to greatly enhance patient outcomes by managing both psychosocial and dermatological components of such complex disorders (Figure 11.14).

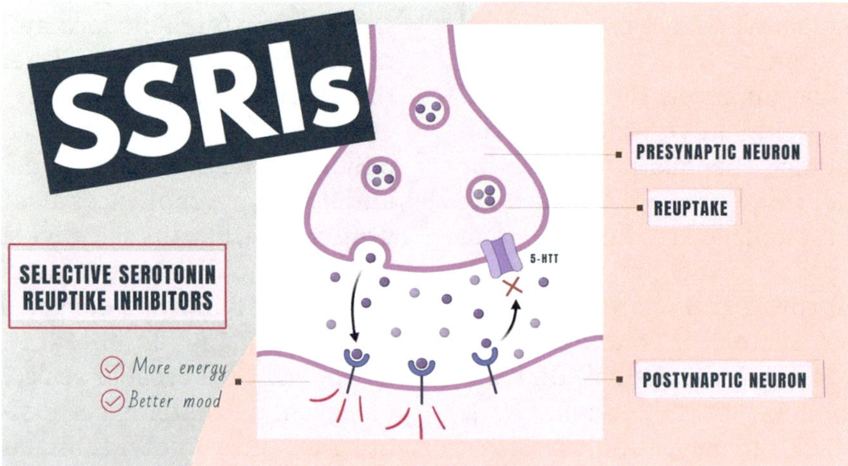

Figure 11.14. Selective serotonin reuptake inhibitors (SSRIs).

Source: https://i.ytimg.com/vi/SwsWkTWJMTw/maxresdefault.jpg.

11.5.3. Integrative Approaches and Lifestyle Modifications

In the field of psychodermatology, holistic strategies are important in managing skin disorders with predominantly psychological determinants. These strategies are intended to resolve the interrelatedness of body and mind, addressing both the corporeal manifestations and also the emotional and cognitive underpinnings of skin disorders. For instance, therapies that incorporate the application of mindfulness, meditation, and cognitive-behavioral strategies have reported positive outcomes for individuals with psychosomatic skin disorders. By enhancing personal awareness and reducing stress levels, such therapies have the ability to improve the provocation of conditions like eczema and psoriasis, which have powerful psychological etiologies. An integrated treatment model that combines psychological and dermatological interventions improves understanding of the patient's experience and healing. Lifestyle modification is also vital in integrative management of psychocutaneous conditions. Dietary modifications, such as the avoidance of offending foods and supplementing with anti-inflammatory nutrients, have been shown to have a positive impact on the skin. Additionally, routine physical activity, known to reduce stress and improve mood, may also have beneficial effects on skin outcomes. The establishment of healthy sleep habits is another crucial factor, as poor quality sleep can exacerbate both mental illness and skin conditions. In addition, social support and therapeutic relationships within therapeutic environments can significantly contribute to treatment adherence and overall patient well-being. When these lifestyle changes are incorporated with traditional dermatological therapies, there is a synergistic outcome that can be life-changing for both the psychological coping and integrity of the skin. The success of integrative therapies and lifestyle changes ultimately depends on their ability to empower patients. By involving patients themselves in their treatment, practitioners instill a sense of control that can optimize therapeutic benefit. This patient-centered approach encourages individuals to take responsibility for their physical and mental health, thereby improving adherence to treatment protocols. Patient education regarding the two-way relationship between mental health and skin diseases makes it simpler for the patient to comprehend the impact of their lifestyle on their condition. Therefore, they are encouraged to adopt sustainable practices that can facilitate healing and promote long-term skin wellness. The inclusion of traditional and complementary practices is a paradigmatic example of an innovative approach to more integrated health consideration in psychodermatology, providing a gateway to innovative and effective treatment methods.

Test Your Knowledge

1. What types of psychotherapeutic interventions are commonly used in psychodermatology?
2. How do pharmacological treatments address both skin symptoms and psychological factors?
3. What are some examples of integrative approaches in managing psychocutaneous disorders?

SUMMARY

The integration of psychodermatology as a component of mental health and dermatology is essential in tackling psychocutaneous disorders in general. The new specialty emphasizes the importance of understanding how psychological factors influence dermatological conditions and, conversely, how skin conditions influence mental health. As evidenced by the numerous accounts of conditions , such as lichen planus, with which patients are now presenting heightened psychological upset, the nexus of psychological well-being and skin disease cannot be overlooked. Multidisciplinary management by mental health professionals and dermatologists can optimize patient outcomes and quality of life. Evidence supporting the organized delivery of psychodermatology care is provided, as is evidence of the need for specialized clinics that offer both physical and mental management of skin disease. A stepped level of care is used by most clinics, with patients tiered based on the severity of psychological distress, progressing to specialists. These models not only clarify patient treatment but also enhance communication and interprofessional collaboration among health care providers. By continuously assessing the psychological and emotional impact of skin diseases, professionals can better identify patients who require additional psychological treatment, thereby promoting care continuity and patient satisfaction (Zhou et al., 2017).

In addition, the relation between conditions like lichen planus and associated mental disorders, that is, depression, highlights that there is a necessity for additional research in this regard. Evidence indicated that psychological disturbances in patients who presented with the aforementioned observable manifestations of skin disease presented a notable decline in quality of life, with a high prevalence of depression (Sawant et al., 2015). The finding highlights the importance of incorporating routine psychological disturbance screenings within the practice of dermatology as a precursor to implementing early intervention strategies. These procedures not only help identify psychological disorders but also help develop overall treatment plans that minimize the long-term impact of these diseases on patients' lives. With an emphasis on psychological well-being and dermatology, psychodermatology can significantly improve overall patient health and treatment outcomes.

Psychodermatology is an interdisciplinary field that integrates dermatologic and psychological concerns, elucidating the complex relationship between mental and skin health. One must understand such a connection to adequately address patient care, as diseases like eczema, psoriasis, and acne are prone to stimulate significant psychological disturbance in a person. The effect of such cutaneous diseases on people's self-perception and management of interpersonal relationships speaks volumes about the need to employ an integrated approach towards treating such diseases. There has been a recent focus on the lack of well-evidenced treatments based on high-standard evidence, thus impacting the ability of healthcare practitioners to treat such psychodermatological disorders to the fullest. The European Society of Dermatology and Psychiatry has taken the initial steps towards classifying psychodermatological terms more rationally, thereby enabling better communication among mental health professionals and dermatologists (Jemec et al., 2014). This evolution benefits both specialties, enabling interdisciplinary collaboration that ultimately improves patient care. The psychological effect of skin disease runs deep, with significant implications for psychosocial adjustment. In those with chronic diseases psoriasis, the psychological impact can be catastrophically disabling, not only affecting the self-esteem of the patient but also interpersonal relationships and overall sense of well-being. A recent body of evidence shows that Cognitive Behavioral Therapy (CBT) is useful in reducing the psychological suffering of having psoriasis. By modifying cognitive distortions and increasing coping capacity, CBT alleviates emotional distress and promotes self-compassion, enabling individuals to manage their condition in a positive way (Laoudi, 2017). This therapeutic model points to the necessity of the integration of psychological care into dermatologic therapy, paving the way for more integrated treatment models that treat physical as well as emotional dimensions of skin diseases. There is a need to develop a conceptual framework that encompasses the therapeutic processes in psychodermatology to inform future interventions. Results of contemporary qualitative studies offer a model, Guided Therapeutic Growth, that identifies essential elements associated with effective CBT outcomes in patients with psoriasis. These include engagement in the therapeutic process, the creation of a trusting therapeutic relationship, and the validation of affect related to the skin condition (Laoudi, 2017). Conversely, the presence of factors negative preconceptions about therapy or absence of appropriate guidance on the part of the therapist can hinder the course of treatment. Emphasis on such co-related factors not only proves useful for clinicians in a bid to modify their therapeutic interventions but also allows individuals to manage better with their experiences of distress, thus paving the way for better psychosocial adaptation and overall well-being among the victims of psychocutaneous disorders.

KEY TERMS FROM THIS CHAPTER

- Biopsychosocial model
- Chronic skin disorders
- Cognitive Behavioral Therapy (CBT)
- Dermatological treatment regimens
- Emotional health
- Inflammatory cutaneous diseases
- Integrated treatment plans
- Mindfulness-based stress reduction (MBSR)
- Multidisciplinary clinics
- Body-mind relationship
- Chronodermatose
- Dermatological disorders
- Eczema
- Holistic care
- Inflammatory cytokines
- Mental health professionals
- Mind-skin interface
- Neuroendocrine system

CRITICAL THINKING QUESTIONS

1. **Which of the following best describes psychodermatology?**
   a. Study of skin infections caused by bacteria
   b. The relationship between psychological factors and skin disorders
   c. The treatment of skin cancer
   d. The role of diet in skin health
2. **What is the biological basis most commonly implicated in psychodermatology?**
   a. Autoimmune dysfunction
   b. Bacterial infection
   c. Genetic mutation
   d. Neuroimmunocutaneous endocrine system interactions
3. **Which of the following is a common psychocutaneous disorder?**
   a. Psoriasis
   b. Acne vulgaris
   c. Trichotillomania
   d. Melanoma
4. **What is the first step in diagnosing psychocutaneous disorders?**
   a. Psychological evaluation and patient history
   b. Skin biopsy
   c. Blood tests
   d. Allergy testing
5. **Which treatment modality is commonly used in psychodermatology?**
   a. Antibiotics alone
   b. Cognitive-behavioral therapy combined with dermatologic treatment
   c. Surgery
   d. Radiation therapy

Short Answer Questions

1. What were some early beliefs or theories about the relationship between the mind and skin health in the history of psychodermatology?
2. How did psychodermatology develop into a distinct field combining dermatology and psychiatry?
3. What biological mechanisms link psychological stress to skin disorders according to neuroimmunology?
4. Which hormones play a significant role in psychodermatological conditions, and how do they affect the skin?
5. What are some common psychocutaneous disorders, and how do psychological factors influence their presentation?
6. What clinical and psychological assessment tools are used to diagnose psychodermatological conditions?

Answer to Critical Thinking Questions

1. (b); 2. (d); 3. (c); 4. (a); 5. (b)

REFERENCES

1. Német, B., Sárdy, M., Magyar, A., Albert, D., Kohutics, K., & Rigó, A. (2023). A krónikus bőrgyógyászati betegségek pszichológiai megközelítése – a pszichodermatológia szerepe, fő kihívásai és feladatai. *Mentálhigiéné És Pszichoszomatika, 24*(4), 253–267. https://doi.org/10.1556/0406.2023.00045Altunay, I. K., Balieva, F. N., Bewley, A., Bobko, S., et al. (2023). White paper on psychodermatology in Europe: A position paper from the EADV Psychodermatology Task Force and the European Society for Dermatology and Psychiatry (ESDaP). https://core.ac.uk/download/617933586.pdf (accessed on 21st July 2025).

2. Atienza, M. A. D., Capiroso, M. R., Batac, M., et al. (2024). Knowledge, attitude, and practice patterns on psychodermatology among Filipino dermatologists: A cross-sectional study. *Acta Medica Philippina, 58*, 50–59. https://www.semanticscholar.org/paper/23f5d06a974c40de827d704d735ae33420b59426 (accessed on 21st July 2025).

3. Balasubramani, N. (2011). A study of psychiatric morbidity and stressful life events in psoriasis. https://core.ac.uk/download/235655696.pdf (accessed on 21st July 2025).

4. Barham, W. T., Castine, A. M., Dorius, B., Edinoff, A., et al. (2025). Exploring the relationship between psychiatric illness and dermatological disorders: A narrative review. https://core.ac.uk/download/659397631.pdf (accessed on 21st July 2025).

5. Basta-Juzbašić, A., & Bukvić Mokos, Z. (2015). Skin changes in primary psychiatric disorders. https://core.ac.uk/download/33281974.pdf (accessed on 21st July 2025).

6. Benea, V., Georgescu, S. R., Leahu, D., Raileanu, M., et al. (2015). Pathological skin picking: Case presentation and review of the literature. https://core.ac.uk/download/144552337.pdf (accessed on 21st July 2025).

7. Bewley, A., & Taylor, R. (2016). Psychodermatology and psychocutaneous disease. https://www.semanticscholar.org/paper/da706dc410cb0dbe93b4cf2200cf92fbab38d131 (accessed on 21st July 2025).

8. Bramono, K., Lusiana, L., Prayogo, R. L., Sitohang, B., et al. (2020). Case series of primary psychiatric skin disorders with multi-disciplinary approach. https://core.ac.uk/download/639382340.pdf (accessed on 21st July 2025).

9. Broderick, C., Wilson-O'Raghallaigh, J., Murphy, L., Moran, E., Power, L., Cannon, M., O'Kane, M., et al. (2018). Psychodermatology U.K. *British Journal of Dermatology, 179.* https://www.semanticscholar.org/paper/20fa7659d4c174d3f8d7b3220ac338613783ee42 (accessed on 21st July 2025).

10. Bucan, J. I., Braut, T., Kršek, A., Sotošek, V., & Batičić, L. (2025). Updates in gastroesophageal reflux disease management: From proton pump inhibitors to dietary and lifestyle modifications. *Gastrointestinal Disorders.* https://www.semanticscholar.org/paper/a5ad244b16a71a2aecc0725d60b8efabb4a823a2 (accessed on 21st July 2025).

11. Cybulski, M., Kaczmarek, M., Michalak, M., Mojs, E., et al. (2016). Stressful events and serum concentration of substance P in acne patients. https://core.ac.uk/download/635527932.pdf (accessed on 21st July 2025).

12. De Souza, B., & McMichael, A. (2019). A new somatic-type delusional disorder subtype: Delusion inversus. https://core.ac.uk/download/237711092.pdf (accessed on 21st July 2025).

13. Erfanian, M. (2018). Childhood trauma: A risk for major depression in patients with psoriasis. https://core.ac.uk/download/227338375.pdf (accessed on 21st July 2025).
14. Estill, M. C., & Jafferany, M. (2024). Treatment of dermatitis artefacta: A systematic review. *European Medical Journal.* https://www.semanticscholar.org/paper/9ab4cc5ad4f7603d7c3dc4c8d2c0ffbe9d076dc1 (accessed on 21st July 2025).
15. Ferreira, L. M., Furtado, F., Gragnani, A., Hochman, B., et al. (2009). Control of the skin scarring response. https://core.ac.uk/download/37708563.pdf (accessed on 21st July 2025).
16. Georgieva, F. (2017). Psychoneuroimmunology and impact of stress in chronic skin conditions. https://core.ac.uk/download/389004340.pdf (accessed on 21st July 2025).
17. Goldstein, L. B. (2024). Pediatric psychodermatology and trichotillomania: Update on strategies for effective treatment. *International Journal of Clinical Case Reports and Reviews.* https://www.semanticscholar.org/paper/07040a950125165cf0cf1ff9f0823e224cfe4201 (accessed on 21st July 2025).
18. Gómez García, L. A. (2020). Psychodermatologic pathology in adolescents: Findings from the Colombian National Mental Health Survey. https://core.ac.uk/download/517318916.pdf (accessed on 21st July 2025).
19. Gupta, A. K., Gupta, M. A., & Haberman, H. F. (1987). The self-inflicted dermatoses: A critical review. http://deepblue.lib.umich.edu/bitstream/2027.42/26860/1/0000425.pdf (accessed on 21st July 2025).
20. Hashmi, N., Noorani, M., Ventriglio, A., Berardis, D. D., Ullah, I., Askari, S., & Goldust, M. (2022). Integrating artificial intelligence and telehealth services in psychodermatology. *Journal of Cosmetic Dermatology, 22.* https://www.semanticscholar.org/paper/2e453bcd74899334466104b772c8010ad22986cb (accessed on 21st July 2025).
21. Hwang, B. (2017). Educational interventions targeting adolescents with atopic dermatitis. https://open.bu.edu/bitstream/2144/26735/5/Hwang_bu_0017N_13190.pdf (accessed on 21st July 2025).
22. Jemec, G. B. E., Ring, H. C., & Smith, M. N. (2014). Self-inflicted skin lesions: A review of the terminology. https://core.ac.uk/download/33262710.pdf (accessed on 21st July 2025).
23. Klymenko, I. S., Haladza, M., & Pysarenko, T. V. (2025). Evidence-based practice in short-term psychotherapeutic interventions. *Psychiatry Neurology and Medical Psychology.* https://www.semanticscholar.org/paper/d2105a48f4f3816565802fe13f1ececf7acef300 (accessed on 21st July 2025).
24. Kozhyna, N., & Nemchenko, A. (2025). Psychoeducational interventions in personalized therapy of depressive disorders in persons affected by combat actions. *Ukrains'kyi Visnyk Psykhonevrolohii.* https://www.semanticscholar.org/paper/7f12b39008b318981dd7158e607771ad0725126e (accessed on 21st July 2025).
25. Laoudi, M. (2017). Understanding the factors that contribute to the outcome of cognitive behavioral therapy as adjunct to medical treatment in a sample of individuals with psoriasis: A constructivist grounded theory study. https://core.ac.uk/download/82968840.pdf (accessed on 21st July 2025).
26. Marron, S. E., & Tomas-Aragones, L. (2016). Body image and body dysmorphic concerns. https://core.ac.uk/download/289983952.pdf (accessed on 21st July 2025).

27. McCarthy, A. (2024). A qualitative exploration of alopecia: Impact, coping and interactions with professionals. https://core.ac.uk/download/624085167.pdf (accessed on 21st July 2025).

28. Fang, Wei-Cheng; Chou, Pei-Chien; Chiu, Li-Wen; Ke, Chiao-Li2; Cheng, Shih-Tsun. Dermoscopy as a Diagnostic and Monitoring Tool for Recurrent Extramammary Paget's Disease. Indian Journal of Dermatology 67(6):p 819-820, Nov–Dec 2022. | DOI: 10.4103/ijd.ijd_771_22 (accessed on 21st July 2025).

29. Petek, A., Degmečić, D., Radanović-Grgurić, L., Koić, O., & Filaković, P. (2009). Comorbidity of depressive and dermatologic disorders–Therapeutic aspects. https://core.ac.uk/download/14420569.pdf (accessed on 21st July 2025).

30. Poot, F., Sampogna, F., & Onnis, L. (2007). Basic knowledge in psychodermatology. https://core.ac.uk/download/54284589.pdf (accessed on 21st July 2025).

31. Sawant, N., Vanjari, N. A., Khopkar, U., & Adulkar, S. (2015). A study of depression and quality of life in patients of lichen planus. *The Scientific World Journal, 2015.* https://doi.org/10.1155/2015/817481 (accessed on 21st July 2025).

32. Singh, J. (2025). Integrative Ayurvedic approaches in the clinical management of osteoporosis: A transdisciplinary perspective on bone health and regeneration. *International Journal for Multidisciplinary Research.* https://www.semanticscholar.org/paper/5bc96d3838c6cfbe4047627e6fa9dc27096b8612 (accessed on 21st July 2025).

33. Snaychuk, L. A., Pejic, S. R., Ornstein, T., & Basedow, C. A. (2024). Addiction treatment outcomes: Examining the impact of an inpatient program for substance use disorders and concurrent mental distress. *Alcoholism Treatment Quarterly, 42*, 210–225. https://www.semanticscholar.org/paper/3aebe7c9adbacb9a3d851eecc277e1e1c5ca39da (accessed on 21st July 2025).

34. Stewart, T. (2019). Stress and the skin: Exploring the associations between perceived stress and self-reported skin symptoms and signs. https://unsworks.unsw.edu.au/bitstreams/45c59b93-cb81-4a28-aaa4-7bad9b9e6b61/download (accessed on 21st July 2025).

35. The Undergraduate Research Opportunities Program, Boston University. (2023). *The 26th Annual Boston University Undergraduate Research (UROP) Abstracts.* https://open.bu.edu/bitstream/2144/46942/7/2023_UROP_Abstract_Booklet_Final_10-19-2023.pdf (accessed on 21st July 2025).

36. Torales, J., Barrios, I., Echagüe, A., Paredes, X., Torres-Romero, A., Malvido, K., Vázquez, M. A., et al. (2025). Knowledge and awareness in psychodermatology: Findings from a survey among Ibero-Latin American dermatologists. *Industrial Psychiatry Journal, 34*, 16–24. https://www.semanticscholar.org/paper/d2e5b636614c29faeee54ae445b51a6b86506548 (accessed on 21st July 2025).

37. Vanjari, N. A., Sawant, N. S., Adulkar, S., & Khopkar, U. (2015). A study of depression and quality of life in patients of lichen planus. https://core.ac.uk/download/192708067.pdf (accessed on 21st July 2025).

38. Zhou, S., Mukovozov, I., & Chan, A. W. (2017). What is known about the psychodermatology clinic model of care? A systematic scoping review. *Journal of Cutaneous Medicine and Surgery, 22*, 44–50. https://doi.org/10.1177/1203475417719045 (accessed on 21st July 2025).

DERMATOLOGIC EMERGENCIES AND TREATMENT

12

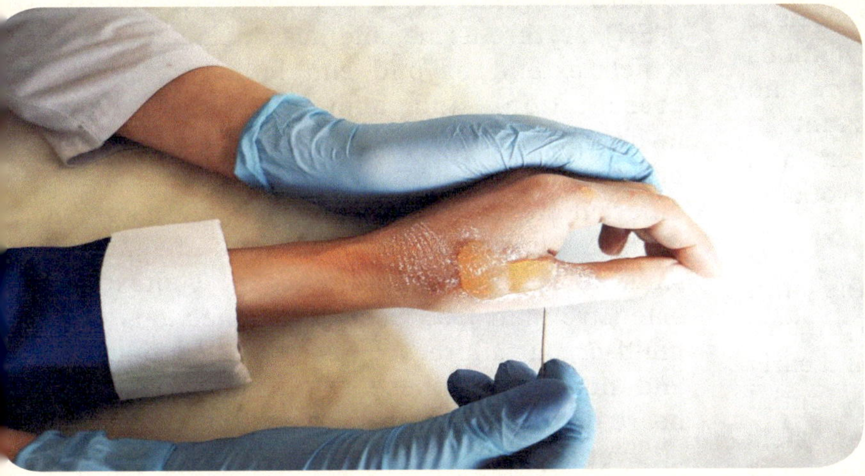

Introduction

Cutaneous diseases often progress rapidly, overwhelming patients and physicians when they present as emergencies. Such cases need to be identified and treated quickly since delays can result in severe morbidity or death. Cutaneous emergencies are a variety of acute cutaneous illnesses that are characterized by massive systemic effects or diffuse destruction of the skin. Among these, Stevens-Johnson Syndrome (SJS) and Toxic Epidermal Necrolysis (TEN) are life-threatening conditions that most commonly result from medication, whereas erythroderma and necrotizing fasciitis are generalized skin inflammation and infection that require immediate medical attention. Understanding the pathophysiology, initial clinical presentation, and treatment priority sequence is essential for effective treatment of such cases. Emergency and primary care physicians should thus be equipped to recognize such conditions early so that they can implement life-saving measures and arrange specialty care. The presentation of cutaneous emergencies tends to overlap with that of other systemic diseases, so it is not easy

LEARNING OBJECTIVES

After studying this chapter, you will be able to:

1. Describe Stevens-Johnson syndrome (SJS)
2. Explain Toxic Epidermal Necrolysis (TEN)
3. Define erythroderma, generalized exfoliative dermatitis
4. Understand necrotizing fasciitis, a flesh-eating disease
5. Discuss about diagnostic approaches for Stevens-Johnson syndrome (SJS), Toxic Epidermal Necrolysis (TEN), Toxic Epidermal Necrolysis (TEN), necrotizing fasciitis
6. Deal with effective management of dermatologic emergencies

to diagnose. SJS and TEN, for example, present with epidermal necrolysis and detachment, resulting in large areas of denuded skin that leave the patient vulnerable to infection and fluid loss. Erythroderma is generalized erythema and scaling that may be due to exacerbations of chronic dermatoses or drug reactions. Necrotizing fasciitis presents as a severe soft tissue infection with out-of-proportion pain and severe systemic toxicity. Accurate differentiation depends on careful history-taking, physical exam, and laboratory workup. Early diagnosis is essential because the therapeutic interventions vary significantly; while supportive care and immunomodulation are very important in SJS/TEN, extensive surgical debridement and antibiotic treatment are essential in necrotizing fasciitis (Alfuraih et al., 2023).

The roles of family physicians and emergency personnel extend beyond primary diagnosis to include coordinated care and early referral. Because of the rarity but potential severity of dermatologic emergencies, their diagnosis typically requires consideration of unusual clinical presentations and red flags for deterioration. Beyond prompt stabilization fluid management and infection prevention, coordination by multidisciplinary teams, including dermatology, surgery, and intensive care services, optimizes outcomes. Additionally, teaching frontline workers about risk factors, common precipitants individual medications or infections, and prevention improves early intervention capacity. The integration of a systematic musculoskeletal and systemic evaluation, as advocated in rheumatological clinical practice, can also be used to elucidate complex presentations and systemic involvement of certain dermatologic emergencies (Almoalli& Cheikh, 2021). Increased clinical expertise and structured methods remain the keystones for effective management of these acute life-threatening dermatologic emergencies.

Definition and Importance of Dermatologic Emergencies

The practice of clinical medicine is frequently characterized by conditions that require immediate intervention to prevent irreversible harm or death. Added to these are the dermatologic emergencies, a series of acute skin disorders with swift progression and potentially life-threatening course. Some of these emergencies include Stevens-Johnson Syndrome (SJS), Toxic Epidermal Necrolysis (TEN), erythroderma, and necrotizing fasciitis, which extend beyond simple dermatologic presentations and demonstrate systemic involvement and complex pathophysiology. Their presentation requires urgent identification to differentiate them from less urgent dermatoses because delay in treatment and diagnosis leads to serious morbidity in the context of extensive skin loss, secondary infection, and multi-organ failure. A grasp of the definition and nuances of these conditions is at the heart of both generalists and dermatologists, and yet is paramount to inter-disciplinary care and emergency management. This street-level information is the foundation for effective therapeutic strategies that have the potential to transform patient outcomes (Almoalli & Cheikh, 2021).

In addition, the relevance of dermatologic emergencies is accentuated by their high fatality and the complicated medical management entailed. For instance, SJS and TEN are catastrophic mucocutaneous reactions primarily due to the application of drugs, triggering extensive epidermal necrolysis and detachment evocative of severe burns. The severity of such syndromes is not only acute cutaneous damage but also systemic compromise in the form of dehydration, electrolyte imbalance, and sepsis, which needs to be managed with utmost attention to fluids and infection in intensive care units. Erythroderma, as an expression of a chronic dermatologic disease, assumes an emergency dimension when it results in extreme disruption of thermoregulation and barrier functions. Thus, they demand immediate, multidisciplinary intervention in the form of etiological treatment, symptomatic care, and intensive monitoring, whose severity is exacerbated in practice by their instability and early diagnostic challenges, thereby supporting specialist alertness and intervention (Almoalli & Cheikh, 2021). The value of early diagnosis and treatment of dermatological emergencies extends beyond the tangible, immediate clinical benefits to encompass the overall quality of healthcare systems and patients' quality of life. Such acute dermatologic conditions, if inadequately managed, are at risk of causing long-term physical disfigurement, psychological damage, and excessive utilization of healthcare resources, including lengthy in-hospital stays and intensive care. Also, the variable presentations and heterogeneous etiologies of such disorders as necrotizing fasciitis—aside from being an extremely aggressive, spreading soft tissue infection with high mortality—demand aggressive surgical and medical therapy with a high index of suspicion to avert progression. Education and awareness of dermatologic emergencies facilitate early referral to specialized centers and coordination with multidisciplinary teams, including dermatologists, critical care physicians, and infectious disease specialists, which are vital for optimizing survival and functional recovery. This emphasizes the subtle synergy between timely clinical decision-making and comprehensive treatment, emphasizing the irreplaceable role of knowledge of dermatologic emergencies in modern practice (Almoalli & Cheikh, 2021).

Overview of the Most Prevalent Conditions: SJS, TEN, Erythroderma, and Necrotizing Fasciitis

Among dermatologic emergencies, several conditions pose a particular risk because they can rapidly progress and may be life-threatening. Stevens-Johnson Syndrome (SJS) and Toxic Epidermal Necrolysis (TEN) are two of the most severe mucocutaneous reactions, most frequently induced by medications or infections. Both diseases share extensive epidermal necrosis and detachment but differ in severity; SJS affects less than 10% of the body's surface area, while TEN affects over 30%. Clinically, they present as painful rashes, blisters, and mucosal disease that can impair vital functions such as vision and respiration. Rapid diagnosis and treatment of the syndromes are required, with supportive therapy in intensive care and often withdrawal of offending agents. Their pathogenesis involves a complex, immune-mediated process that leads to keratinocyte apoptosis, underscoring the applicability of immunological principles to management. In contrast to SJS and TEN, erythroderma is a diffuse inflammatory dermatosis characterized by erythema and scaling on more than 90% of the body surface. It usually occurs as an exacerbation of underlying dermatoses, drug eruption, or malignancy, and can cause systemic complications , such as fluid loss, impairment of thermoregulation, and secondary infection. Generalized redness, exfoliation, and edema characterize erythroderma, which requires a full assessment to establish the underlying cause. Management. is to stabilize the patient, treat the cause, and prevent complications with close skin care and observation. Because of its potential to mimic or coexist with other life-threatening cutaneous emergencies, erythroderma demands differential diagnostic acumen. Its recognized morbidity promotes early treatment to prevent the evolution and systemic dissemination that typically follow in this condition. Necrotizing fasciitis is an aggressively progressive soft tissue infection with widespread necrosis of the fascia and subcutaneous tissue. The fulminant bacterial disease, typically polymicrobial, necessitates urgent surgical debridement with broad-spectrum antibiotics to prevent death. Inadvertent clinical presentations may be initially inappropriate, with out-of-proportion swelling and pain, progressing to rapid systemic toxicity, septic shock, and multi-organ failure. Underlying diabetes or immunosuppression increases susceptibility. Compared with the predominantly immunologic epidermal necrosis of SJS and TEN, necrotizing fasciitis is characterized by direct microbial invasion and toxin-mediated tissue damage, with markedly contrasting therapeutic emphases. Prompt diagnosis and aggressive multidisciplinary therapy are essential, with delay causing irreparable damage to prognosis. Coordination of clinical vigilance and surgical readiness is pivotal to properly managing this dire dermatologic catastrophe (Almoalli & Cheikh, 2021).

Importance of Timely Diagnosis and Treatment

Accurate clinical diagnosis often is the key initial step toward optimal results in patients with severe dermatologic emergencies , such as Stevens-Johnson Syndrome (SJS) and Toxic Epidermal Necrolysis (TEN). Both conditions initially present with subtle yet characteristic mucocutaneous symptoms that are readily misdiagnosed, thereby delaying treatment. Early discrimination by less severe cutaneous reactions or by infectious etiology enables early action and the removal of offending agents, thereby preventing further progression. Moreover, the implementation of supportive care within intensive care environments minimizes complications such as sepsis and multi-organ failure.

Early diagnosis by frontline emergency and primary care clinicians is important, as these practitioners are the initial point of contact for acute presentations (Alfuraih et al., 2023). With aggravating epidermal detachment, the window of opportunity for therapeutic response becomes dramatically restricted, with a need for early diagnosis and management with complex interventional treatment to reduce morbidity and mortality rates. Treatment of necrotizing fasciitis and erythroderma also hinges on quick and timely clinical intervention. Necrotizing fasciitis is very fast, within hours, and kills skin, fat, and fascia, and requires immediate surgical debridement and broad-spectrum antimicrobial drugs. Delayed treatment can lead to permanent tissue loss and systemic toxicity and thus early suspicion and diagnosis are important.

Similarly, erythroderma with diffuse erythema and scaling requires early evaluation to identify inciting causes such as drug reactions, malignancies, or psoriasis flares. Delayed identification of these acute dermatoses can initiate systemic complications, including fluid imbalance and infection, that lengthen the hospital stay and result in healthcare costs. Therefore, early diagnosis not only directly affects patient survival but also optimizes the utilization of healthcare resources within healthcare systems, emphasizing clinician vigilance and immediate treatment (Alfuraih et al., 2023).

In addition to immediate life-saving treatments, early diagnosis and therapy are important for preventing long-term sequelae and improving patients' quality of life in such dermatologic emergencies. For instance, SJS/TEN patients typically experience irreversible ocular sequelae, scarring, or psychosocial distress that can be minimized by the use of early ophthalmologic assessments and rehabilitation protocols conducted in the acute environment. Application of multidisciplinary approaches, including rheumatologists and dermatologists, in combination with conventional ophthalmologists optimizes diagnostic yield and therapeutic specificity, particularly when comorbidities obscure presentations. Furthermore, early intervention strategies enable timely initiation of immunomodulatory or biologic therapy when necessary, thereby preventing disease progression. Overall, the combination of early diagnosis and individually tailored treatment regimens is integral to optimal clinical results, highlighting the catalytic role of early diagnosis in the dermatologic emergency management protocol.

12.1. Stevens-Johnson Syndrome (SJS)

Learning Outcome

1. Explain the definition and pathophysiology of SJS.
2. Describe common triggers and risk factors associated with SJS.
3. Focus on clinical presentation and symptoms of SJS.

The onset of life-threatening dermatoses in emergency situations mandates prompt recognition and management to prevent high morbidity and mortality. These include Stevens-Johnson Syndrome (SJS), a catastrophic medical condition characterized by acute mucocutaneous necrosis and epidermal sloughing, usually secondary to drug adverse effects. SJS is clinically characterized by an antecedent prodrome of flu-like illness, evolution into a painful blistering skin rash and mucositis, distinguishing it from benign dermatoses. The widespread epidermal involvement leads to disruption of the barrier such that patients are at heightened risk for secondary infection, fluid imbalances, and sepsis. Management is aimed at early identification and removal of the offending agent, in addition to support in intensive care units. Understanding the pathophysiology of SJS, particularly its immunologic nature and predisposing factors, helps clinicians individualize treatment protocols to prevent disease progression and improve outcomes in critically ill patients. Hospitalization rates and clinical severity indicators point to the emergent nature of SJS among dermatologic emergencies. Retrospective analyses from urban tertiary-care hospitals suggest that SJS accounts for a significant proportion of cutaneous diseases requiring inpatient care. Unlike milder dermatoses, SJS patients tend to present with extensive, painful blistering eruptions accompanied by mucosal ulcers, which render outpatient management unsuitable. These traits are directly related to the need for advanced wound care, pain management, and multidisciplinary treatment to address systemic complications. The acute presentation and rapid course of SJS also necessitate that emergency physicians be more attentive to earlier dermatology assessment and the initiation of appropriate systemic therapy. This evidence highlights how clinical factors may be distinguished in order to guide triage, and ultimately provide timely specialist treatment for SJS patients to reduce morbidity (Chong et al., 2011).

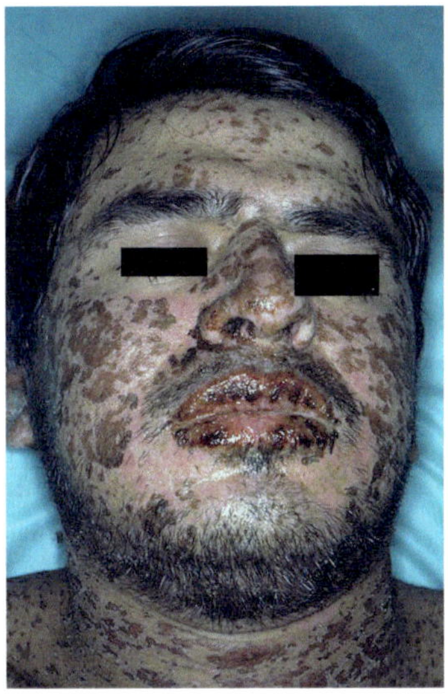

Figure 12.1. Man with characteristic skin lesions of Stevens–Johnson syndrome.

Source: https://upload.wikimedia.org/wikipedia/commons/5/58/Stevens-johnson-syndrome.jpg.

Therapeutic approaches to Stevens-Johnson Syndrome have been advanced by the advent of immunomodulatory therapies aimed at preventing immune-mediated epidermal damage. Immunotherapy, including checkpoint inhibitors, has revolutionized the practice of oncology but emphasizes the risk of immune-related adverse effects, one of which is severe cutaneous reactions like SJS. Management of such immune-related toxicity includes early identification and withdrawal of offending agents, as well as immunosuppressive therapeutic interventions such as corticosteroids or intravenous immunoglobulin. The interface of these therapies with dermatologic emergencies also requires earnest supportive care and interdisciplinary coordination to optimize results. Emergency physicians must thus remain vigilant for evolving treatment landscapes and associated cutaneous side effects to effectively address the complex clinical scenarios of SJS and to utilize evidence-based, multidisciplinary management approaches (Brém et al., 2020) (Figure 12.1).

12.1.1. Definition and Pathophysiology of SJS

The complex interaction between the immune mechanisms is the cause of most of the fulminant cutaneous emergencies, necessitating in-depth knowledge about their pathophysiology to optimize treatment regimens. Stevens-Johnson Syndrome (SJS) is a rare but severe mucocutaneous reaction, usually due to drug-induced adverse effects. It includes widespread epidermal necrolysis and detachment, with mucous membrane erosion. The immunopathogenesis is mediated by granulysin and other cytotoxic proteins secreted by natural killer cells and cytotoxic T cells, leading to keratinocyte apoptosis. This process results in the characteristic epidermal slough and systemic inflammation of SJS. Although drugs such as antibiotics and anticonvulsants are common inducers, SJS pathophysiology mechanistically overlaps with immune-mediated effects observed with checkpoint inhibitor therapy, demonstrating the evolving immunologic paradigms relevant to dermatological emergencies (Brém et al., 2020). Clinical manifestations of SJS reflect its pathophysiology, with systemic involvement that is difficult to predict and treat. Following an inciting drug or infection, stimulated cytotoxic lymphocytes recognize drug-associated peptides presented by keratinocytes and trigger widespread apoptosis.

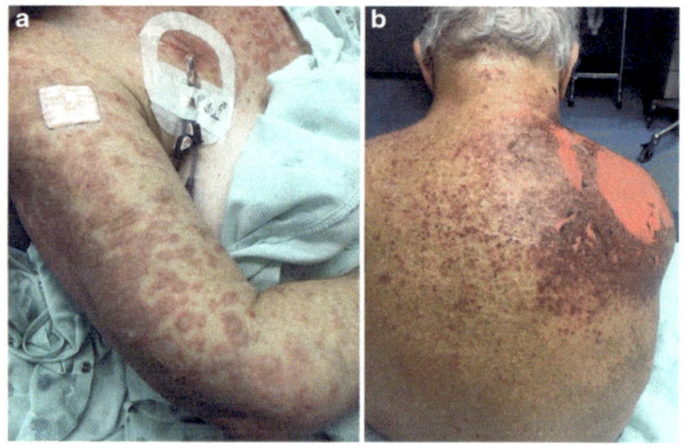

Figure 12.2. (a) Stevens-Johnson syndrome with blisters developing in atypical targetoid papules. (b) Erosion and denuded skin in fully evolved Stevens-Johnson syndrome.

Source: https://www.researchgate.net/publication/326352370/figure/fig2/AS:1145677576978432@1650162228255/a-Stevens-Johnson-syndrome-with-blisters-developing-in-atypical-targetoid-papules-b.png.

This immunologic assault ravages the integrity of the skin, renders it susceptible to secondary infection, and leads to a systemic inflammatory response syndrome. Complicating the process further, patients become vulnerable to developing severe complications sepsis, multiorgan failure, and sequela in the long term, including scarring and eye damage. Understanding these cellular and molecular processes is essential for early diagnosis and treatment to prevent morbidity, and is aligned with the importance of comprehensive clinical evaluation techniques in autoimmune and inflammatory diseases, which share common overlapping pathology (Almoalli & Cheikh, 2021). Pathophysiologically, epidermal necrosis in SJS reflects the catastrophic consequences of immune dysregulation, distinguishing it from other cutaneous emergencies in both course and management. Unlike in erythroderma or necrotizing fasciitis, SJS is predominantly due to apoptotic pathways through a hypersensitivity reaction, hence the urgency of instantaneous causative agent removal. In SJS, immune-mediated mechanisms, in particular, also affect several molecular pathways, including Fas-FasL interactions and the perforin-granzyme system, which offer promising targets for targeted therapy as research continues to evolve. The abundant immunologic insight drawn from SJS clarifies the total understanding of dermatologic urgencies, making the worth of multidisciplinary treatment to address cutaneous as well as systemic presentations reasonable (Brém et al., 2020; Almoalli & Cheikh, 2021) (Figure 12.2).

12.1.2. Common Triggers and Risk Factors

Identification of the underlying causes of dermatologic emergencies is central to effective management and diagnosis. Drug reactions, primarily to antibiotics, anticonvulsants, and nonsteroidal anti-inflammatory drugs, are among the primary offenders of Stevens-Johnson Syndrome (SJS) and Toxic Epidermal Necrolysis (TEN). These are prone to induce abnormal immunity, resulting in widespread epidermal necrosis. Infections like Mycoplasma pneumoniae are just as guilty, especially in younger populations. The complex mechanisms of such triggers make early identification difficult, underscoring the importance of clinicians carefully noting patient history and medication exposure. Furthermore, genetic factors, including certain HLA alleles, have been shown to increase the risk of these adverse reactions. Identifying these factors enables early detection and intervention, which is critical given the rapid course and high mortality of these conditions (Alfuraih et al., 2023). Erythroderma with extensive erythema and scaling involving large areas of the body surface is largely due to underlying dermatoses, such as pre-existing psoriasis or drug hypersensitivity reactions. The chronicity or abruptness of such precipitating factors determines the intensity of the eruption. Systemic medications like sulfonamides and antiepileptics have been frequently involved in erythrodermic eruptions. Furthermore, underlying malignancy and immune dysregulation contribute to skin susceptibility. Environmental stimuli, such as exposure to allergens or irritants, can worsen the dermal inflammation of erythroderma. This identification of such risk factors is not only helpful for early diagnosis but also for guiding therapeutic management of both the cutaneous and systemic components of this potentially lethal condition (Castello et al., 2020). Necrotizing fasciitis is an aggressive soft tissue infection that follows trauma, surgery, or compromise of skin integrity as a portal site for pathogen invasion. Risks are elevated in immunocompromised states of diabetes mellitus, malignancy, and chronic kidney disease. Bacterial pathogens, especially Group A *Streptococcus* and polymicrobial flora, produce toxins that accelerate tissue destruction. Delayed diagnosis owing to the nonspecific presentation of early signs commonly leads to added morbidity and mortality. The interaction of these risk factors highlights the importance of increased clinical suspicion in high-risk populations, particularly those with a past history of recent invasive interventions or chronic diseases. Preventive interventions and early treatment rely on identifying these predisposing factors to mitigate the destruction caused by this surgical emergency (Castello et al., 2020; Alfuraih et al., 2023).

12.1.3. Clinical Presentation and Symptoms

The cutaneous presentation of dermatologic emergencies is usually nonspecific and often complicated by a rapid course, making early diagnosis challenging. The patients of Stevens-Johnson Syndrome (SJS) and Toxic Epidermal

Necrolysis (TEN) typically develop characteristic mucocutaneous lesions following prodromal flu-like illness , such as sore throat, malaise, and fever. The lesions begin as erythematous macules, followed by painful blisters, and finally widespread epidermal shedding. The extensive necrosis of the skin in TEN, greater than 30% of body surface area, is a more severe manifestation than SJS, in which less than 10% is involved. Manifestations of the mucosae, specifically the oral, ocular, and genital mucosae, are the hallmarks of these disorders and are the expression of systemic severity of the disease. This process requires early recognition and treatment to prevent sequelae, such as secondary infection and multi-organ failure (Alfuraih et al., 2023). Erythroderma is a severe skin emergency characterized by a typical clinical presentation of diffuse scaling and erythema involving more than 90% of the body surface area. The patients have systemic symptoms, including fever, chills, and malaise, indicating the disorder's pronounced inflammatory nature. The skin appears diffusely red and inflamed and may exhibit edema or lichenification in chronic lesions. Generalized skin involvement undermines the skin's barrier function, and the patient is at risk of fluid and electrolyte imbalance, thermoregulatory disturbances, and secondary infection. Identification of underlying causes—ranging from drug eruptions to cutaneous T-cell lymphoma—dictates targeted treatment. Prompt recognition of erythroderma's typical presentations can be life-saving since postponed treatment may result in immense morbidity (Castello et al., 2020). Necrotizing fasciitis, on the other hand, offers a protracted infection with an initial presentation of local pain out of proportion to physical examination. Erythema, warmth, swelling, and tenderness in the affected area, along with early signs, are followed by systemic toxicity, including fever, tachycardia, and hypotension. As the infection progresses, the skin changes to blistering, ecchymosis, and terminal necrosis with crepitus, which may be palpable due to subcutaneous gas production. The most typical observation of necrotizing fasciitis is the destruction of the acute fascia and subcutaneous tissue, followed by systemic inflammatory response syndrome and multiorgan failure in the case of no treatment. The subtlety of early clinical signs requires clinicians to maintain heightened suspicion to enable prompt surgical debridement and antimicrobial therapy (Alfuraih et al., 2023) (Figure 12.3).

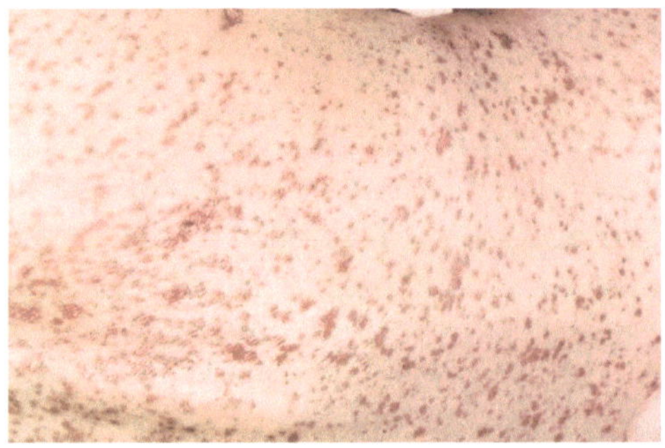

Figure 12.3. Typical pattern of Stevens-Johnson syndrome. Blisters develop on widespread purpuric macules.

Source: https://www.researchgate.net/profile/Luigi-Naldi/publication/15722296/figure/fig1/AS:601651597557767@1520456327157/Typical-Pattern-of-Stevens-Johnson-Syndrome-Blisters-develop-on-widespread-purpuric.png.

Test Your Knowledge

1. What is Stevens-Johnson Syndrome, and how does it affect the skin and mucous membranes?
2. What is the underlying pathophysiology of Stevens-Johnson Syndrome?
3. What are the most common triggers or risk factors associated with SJS?

12.2. Toxic Epidermal Necrolysis (TEN)

Learning Outcome

1. Understand the definition of TEN and differentiation from SJS.
2. Describe etiology and associated medications for TEN.
3. Discuss clinical features and progression of the disease.

The clinical picture of dermatologic emergencies includes illnesses that are highly acute in their course and require emergent treatment to avoid major morbidity and mortality. Among these, one of the most severe manifestations is Toxic Epidermal Necrolysis (TEN), characterized by extensive epidermal peeling and mucous membrane involvement. The pathophysiology of TEN typically involves an immunologically mediated process triggered by therapeutic drugs, leading to widespread keratinocyte apoptosis. Prodromal manifestations of fever and malaise are succeeded by an abrupt onset of painful, erythematous macules that become confluent and create large bullous lesions. Early identification by clinicians is required to avoid such severe complications as sepsis and multi-organ failure by starting supportive care in specialized units. The immediacy inherent in TEN management aligns with universal principles of dermatologic emergencies, underscoring the value of rapid diagnosis to optimize patient outcomes (Falodun, O., & Ogunbiyi, A., 2010).

The diagnostic approach to TEN is the integration of clinical diagnosis and histopathological establishment with skin biopsy. Differential diagnosis is employed to rule out other blistering illnesses with an overlapping presentation that can masquerade as TEN, such as staphylococcal scalded skin syndrome or autoimmune blistering disease. Physical exam is significant, with the positive Nikolsky's sign—gentle skin rubbing leading to exfoliation—a characteristic finding. Of interest, the pathogenesis of TEN is most commonly drug-induced, with common culprits being anticonvulsants, sulfonamides, and nonsteroidal anti-inflammatory agents. Idiopathic TEN or TEN due to trivial trauma burns, has been described; however, with reference to the diverse possible causation and the need for detailed patient history assessment. Early identification of atypical presentations is potentially lifesaving, as delays in diagnosis significantly increase the risk of mortality (Berkeley et al., 2010).

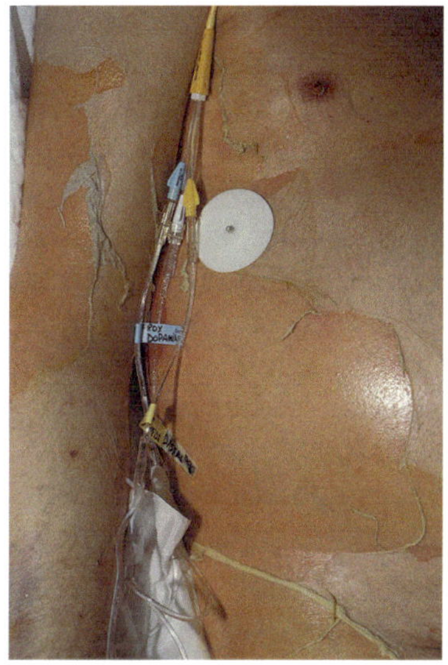

Figure 12.4. Toxic epidermal necrolysis.

Source: https://upload.wikimedia.org/wikipedia/commons/a/ae/Toxic-epidermal-necrolysis.jpg.

Therapy for TEN is, by its nature, multidisciplinary, aimed at withdrawal of offending agents and vigorous supportive therapy to restore fluid and electrolyte balance, provide wound care, and prevent secondary infection. Admission to a burn or intensive care unit is often warranted on the basis of the severity of epidermal loss and its systemic impact. Adjunctive therapeutic strategies, including immunomodulation with intravenous immunoglobulin or corticosteroids, remain the subject of ongoing debate but may benefit in certain cases. The potential for complications, especially sepsis and respiratory failure, mandates close observation and infection control measures. Lastly, early diagnosis and vigorous management protocols are in line with standard emergency protocols for dermatalogical conditions, which demand quick action to reduce skin failure and improve patient survival rates in TEN (Falodun, O., & Ogunbiyi, A. . 2010) (Figure 12.4).

12.2.1. Definition and Differentiation from SJS

The clinical setting of severe cutaneous adverse reactions is complex, and definitions are needed to influence effective treatment strategies. Stevens-Johnson Syndrome (SJS) has been described as a potentially life-threatening hypersensitivity reaction induced primarily by drugs or infection. It is characterized by epidermal necrosis and mucocutaneous disease and typically involves less than 10% of body surface area (BSA). This distinction is essential since the degree of skin separation directly correlates with diagnosis and treatment. SJS is distinguished from its more malignant counterpart, Toxic Epidermal Necrolysis (TEN), by the extent of epidermal separation to a great degree—more than 30% BSA in TEN. These conditions are more a continuum of severity than discrete categories, underscoring the importance of careful clinical assessment to detect early signs and anticipate worsening. Differentiating SJS from other cutaneous emergencies, such as erythroderma or necrotizing fasciitis, is critical due to their difference in pathophysiology and therapeutic needs. Erythroderma, or exfoliative dermatitis, classically presents as diffuse erythema covering more than 90% BSA with scaling and potential systemic signs but without SJS's epidermal full-thickness necrosis. On the other hand, necrotizing fasciitis is a virulent bacterial infection characterized by uncontrolled soft-tissue necrosis, systemic toxicity, and a distinct etiology compared with the immune-mediated pathology of SJS. A delicate clinical evaluation, complemented by histopathological examination, can distinguish SJS, thereby enabling appropriate intervention; misdiagnosis may delay necessary therapy and worsen outcomes in patients with skin emergencies.

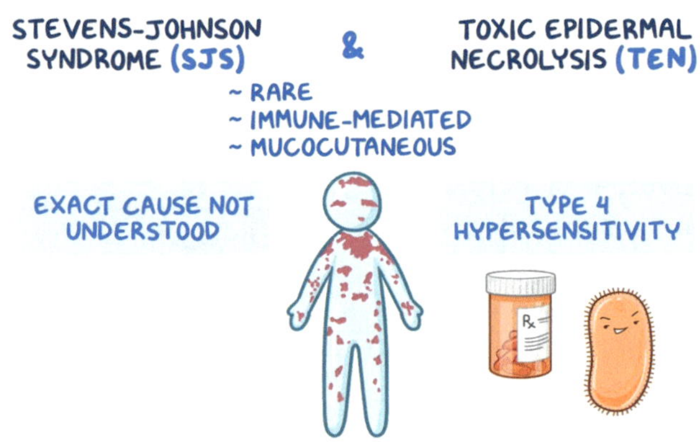

Figure 12.5. Stevens-Johnson syndrome (sjs) and toxic epidermal necrolysis (TEN).

Source: https://d16qt3wv6xm098.cloudfront.net/o-aPNPQzR0aLpBMC5GNKiaCmRASyAIH3/_.jpg.

The subtle recognition of SJS and its differential diagnosis with other dermatological disorders frequently depends on histopathology and clinical appearance. While skin biopsy remains the optimal way to secure a diagnosis, clinical presentation, such as extent of mucosal involvement, target lesions, and systemic signs, provides valuable pointers towards diagnosis. Notably, SJS is largely an immune-mediated phenomenon involving cytotoxic T-cell-induced keratinocyte apoptosis, whereas erythroderma frequently results from chronic neoplastic or inflammatory processes. Understanding this pathophysiologic difference is crucial to management, which may involve immunosuppressive therapy, which differs markedly from the antimicrobial and surgical treatments required for necrotizing fasciitis. The integration of multidisciplinary experience, through the facilitation of comprehensive patient assessment protocols, optimizes diagnostic specificity and sharpens paradigms of care for these interplaying dermatologic emergencies (Almoalli & Cheikh, 2021) (Figure 12.5).

12.2.2. Etiology and Associated Medications

The pathogenesis of life-threatening dermatologic emergencies typically involves complex immunologic and environmental interactions; therefore, careful scrutiny of potential etiologic factors is necessary. Stevens-Johnson Syndrome (SJS) and Toxic Epidermal Necrolysis (TEN), for example, predominantly present as idiosyncratic drug reactions, and in particular pharmacologic agents have the prime role in creating such fatal conditions. Medications , such as sulfonamides, antiepileptic agents , such as carbamazepine and phenytoin, and nonsteroidal anti-inflammatory drugs (NSAIDs) have known associations with these syndromes.

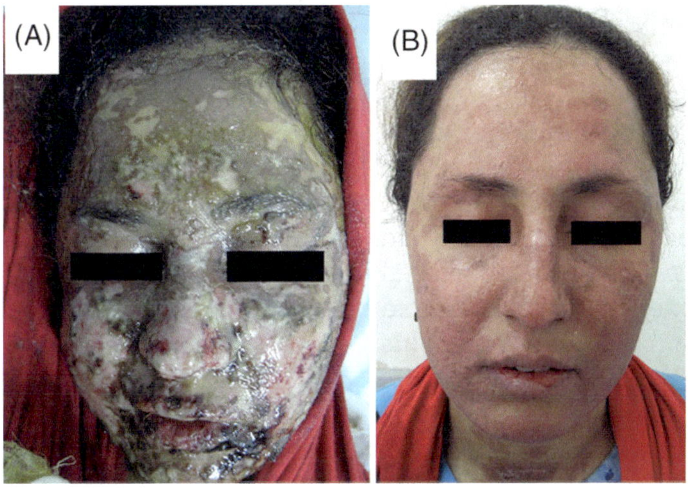

Figure 12.6. A case of toxic epidermal necrolysis (TEN). (A) Before treatment. (B) Excellent improvement after symptomatic treatment only.

Source: https://www.researchgate.net/profile/Doaa-Aboutaleb/publication/343580322/figure/fig1/AS:11431281173800304@1689045731981/A-case-of-toxic-epidermal-necrolysis-TEN-A-Before-treatment-B-Excellent-improvement.png.

The underlying immunologic process is usually a T-cell-mediated cytotoxic reaction against keratinocytes bearing drug-related antigens with extensive epidermal necrosis. It is crucial to identify the offending drug so that early withdrawal can be done to avoid more disease. This complex interplay of drug exposure and immune response justifies the clinical imperative of having ongoing awareness when prescribing established high-risk drugs in order to prevent sudden dermatologic emergencies.

In addition to drug-induced immunologic responses, erythroderma encompasses a broader spectrum of etiologies that involve both primary cutaneous diseases and systemic diseases. Classic stimuli include exacerbation of underlying dermatoses , such as psoriasis and atopic dermatitis, drug hypersensitivity syndromes, and even neoplasias , such as cutaneous T-cell lymphoma. Erythroderma-inducing drugs closely overlap with SJS/TEN drugs, particularly anticonvulsants and antibiotics, thereby establishing pharmacologic agents as a significant etiologic factor. Unlike the predominantly immune-cytotoxic pathophysiology of SJS/TEN, erythroderma's pathophysiology usually involves generalized inflammation and perturbation of skin barrier function with consequent diffuse erythema and scaling. Establishing the etiology of the drug is still important for effective management, as withdrawal of the offending agent will usually lead to clinical improvement. Thus, meticulous medication histories and knowledge of probable drug culprits continue to be fundamental to the care of erythroderma and the prevention of worse outcomes (Almoalli & Cheikh, 2021). Necrotizing fasciitis, being predominantly an infectious etiology, also exhibits a multifactorial etiology secondary to patient comorbidities and occasionally by immunomodulating drugs. This rapidly progressive soft-tissue infection is most commonly caused by polymicrobial invasion, including Group A Streptococcus, anaerobes, and Gram-negative rods, entering via breaches in skin integrity. Immunosuppressive therapy, such as the use of corticosteroids or chemotherapy medications, can predispose individuals to invasive infections by compromising host defenses. In addition, recent trauma or surgery creates windows of opportunity for the invasion of bacteria, further enhancing susceptibility. Although antibiotics remain the primary determinant of treatment, prior administration of certain drugs inadvertently increases risk by blunting immunity or masking early warning signs. Awareness of this etiologic complexity, keeping in mind both microbial and drug considerations, guides appropriate therapeutic measures and prevents death in necrotizing fasciitis (Figure 12.6).

12.2.3. Clinical Features and Progression of the Disease

The onset of Stevens-Johnson Syndrome (SJS) and Toxic Epidermal Necrolysis (TEN) typically begins with nonspecific prodromal manifestations, including fever, malaise, and pharyngitis, before the characteristic mucocutaneous findings. The initial clinical appearance is painful erythematous macules that rapidly progress to become blisters and epidermal loss over a large percentage of the skin, simulating severe burns. These cutaneous emergencies target the skin and various mucosal surfaces the oral, ocular, and genital mucosa, and cause intense pain and secondary complications. Histopathologically, typical features such as necrotic keratinocytes and lymphocytic exocytosis are strongly represented in major cutaneous adverse reactions, whereas minor forms such as maculopapular exanthema are less frequently associated with these features. Elevated serum granulysin levels, particularly in SJS/TEN patients, are directly correlated with disease severity, underscoring its role as a biomarker for monitoring disease progression (Jacquline et al., 2018). Such molecular markers illuminate the immunopathogenesis and may direct early therapeutic measures. For erythroderma, the clinical course is one of diffuse erythema and scaling of greater than 90% of the body surface area, with marked systemic effects. The patients may present with limited dermatitis that rapidly progresses to generalized erythema, marked edema, and desquamation. Such extensive dermal involvement disrupts the skin's barrier function, predisposing patients to electrolyte imbalance, infections, and impaired temperature regulation. Although erythroderma can result from underlying dermatoses, drug reactions, or neoplasms, its rapid progression warrants immediate identification and management to prevent morbidity. Clinical presentation is typically characterized by distinctive anatomical locations scrotum and labium majora, common to nonvenereal genital dermatoses, for which differentiation from infection is essential in order not to miss the diagnosis (Maalik Babu, 2015). Prompt dermatologic assessment is called for, in view of the potential systemic implications. Necrotizing fasciitis is characterized by aggressive soft-tissue destruction that profoundly affects deeper subcutaneous tissue and fascial planes. The disease characteristically follows with painful and out-of-proportion pain to apparent cutaneous alterations in the initial course, followed by rapidly increasing edema, erythema, and skin necrosis. Systemic toxicity is a common occurrence in the form of fever, hypotension, and multi-organ dysfunction, and usually mandates immediate surgery. Clinically, necrotizing fasciitis's fulminant course is clinically replicated by other dermatologic emergencies but requires immediate differentiation due to its distinctive pathophysiology and immediate requirement for treatment. Unlike its presentation in erythroderma or SJS/TEN, wherein peeling of the epidermis predominates, necrotizing fasciitis is made up of extensive fascia destruction involving multidisciplinary management. Identification of these clinical presentations and stages in all dermatologic emergencies is essential to optimize early diagnosis and improve patient outcomes.

Test Your Knowledge

1. What is Toxic Epidermal Necrolysis, and how is it different from Stevens-Johnson Syndrome?
2. Which medications are most commonly associated with triggering TEN?
3. What are the typical clinical features seen in patients with TEN?

12.3. Erythroderma

Learning Outcome

1. Explain definition and classification of erythroderma.
2. Understand causes and underlying conditions.
3. Discuss about symptoms and systemic effects.

Evidence of generalized skin involvement in acute dermatologic emergencies can complicate clinical diagnosis and treatment, requiring immediate attention to clinical details that distinguish it from mimicking serious diseases. Erythroderma with generalized erythema and scaling over greater than 90% body surface area is an urgent dermatologic problem due to its potential for systemic complications via fluid imbalance, thermoregulatory derangement, and secondary infection. Unlike Stevens-Johnson Syndrome (SJS) and Toxic Epidermal Necrolysis (TEN), which are predominantly epidermal detachment and mucous membrane diseases, erythroderma typically arises from exacerbations of underlying dermatoses, drug reactions, or malignancy. Early recognition is vital because it is a highly morbid and fatal condition and requires careful evaluation, including patient history, laboratory investigations, and skin biopsy when necessary, in order to exclude it compared to other blistering disorders. Prompt stabilization of the patient's systemic condition, alongside targeted dermatologic treatment, is called for in the prevention of progression and secondary complications (Alfuraih et al., 2023). Clinical treatment of erythroderma must extend beyond the dermatological presentation to address systemic effects resulting from impaired skin barrier function. Disseminated inflammation and exfoliation induce increased insensible water loss, extensive protein loss, and increased susceptibility to infection, collectively contributing to patient morbidity. Therefore, treatment guidelines emphasize supportive therapy, such as fluid and electrolyte maintenance, temperature control, and nutritional support, as in burn management. Identification and elimination of precipitating cause, that is, stopping offending drug or managing underlying dermatoses , such as psoriasis or atopic dermatitis, are paramount for clinical resolution. In addition, erythroderma is often managed in a multidisciplinary manner, with referral to dermatology, infectious disease, and critical care specialists to optimize outcomes. This interdisciplinary intervention underscores the urgency of early recognition and treatment of erythroderma as a dermatologic emergency (Alfuraih et al., 2023). Despite advancements in its understanding and treatment, erythroderma remains a challenging condition in clinical practice due to heterogeneity and risk of sudden worsening if improperly treated. Erythroderma needs to be distinguished from overlapping presenting disorders , such as SJS/TEN and necrotizing fasciitis since therapeutic modality and prognosis vary vastly. Recent studies prove the value of complete musculoskeletal and systemic evaluation in the presence of erythroderma in patients harboring underlying rheumatologic disease, with acknowledgment of the potential for worsening cutaneous manifestations and complications due to systemic inflammation. Continued research regarding biomarkers and novel therapeutics will be necessary to further improve diagnostic precision and patient outcomes. Combining supportive initial therapy with targeted interventions remains essential for successful treatment of erythroderma, a general skin emergency (Figure 12.7).

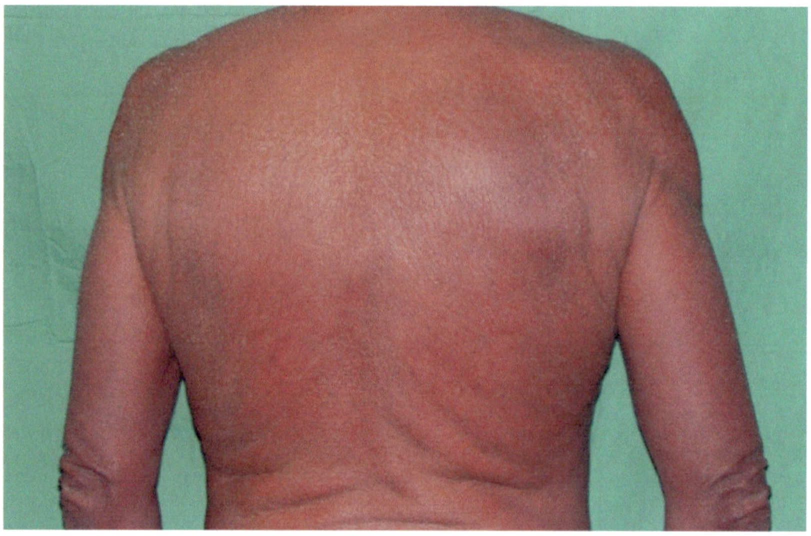

Figure 12.7. Erythroderma.

Source: https://www.thedermspecs.com/wp-content/uploads/2013/04/Erythroderma.png.

12.3.1. Definition and Classification of Erythroderma

The emergencies of dermatology are complicated and thus must be comprehensively understood as far as conditions with widespread skin manifestation, like erythroderma, are concerned. The majority of erythroderma cases present as diffuse erythema and scaling, manifesting as a severe cutaneous reaction involving more than 90% of the body surface area. It lacks an effect on localized dermatoses, with respect to systemic implications, including fluid and electrolyte derangements and susceptibility to infection. Because of its extensive skin involvement, erythroderma requires prompt clinical diagnosis and management, independent of other dermatologic emergencies such as Stevens-Johnson Syndrome (SJS) or Toxic Epidermal Necrolysis (TEN), which are primarily confined to epidermal detachment. Understanding the definition of erythroderma among dermatologic emergencies aids clinicians in prioritizing differential diagnoses and employing applicable interventions, thereby highlighting its distinctive pathophysiology relative to necrotizing fasciitis and other skin diseases (Almoalli & Cheikh, 2021). Etiological classification of erythroderma drives therapeutic management and prognosis. It is arbitrarily classified as primary or secondary erythroderma. Primary erythroderma arises from pre-existing cutaneous dermatoses , such as psoriasis, atopic dermatitis, or cutaneous T-cell lymphoma, indicating exacerbation of chronic skin conditions. Secondary erythroderma is often drug-induced, resulting from systemic drugs or toxins. Infectious causes and idiopathic conditions are also etiological contributors to the classification. This etiologic stratification is significant because, in addition to guiding patient management, it identifies potential systemic complications associated with the underlying etiology. The classification also helps distinguish erythroderma from other severe cutaneous eruptions, such as SJS/TEN, which are predominantly immunologically mediated hypersensitivity reactions rather than chronic inflammatory processes. Clinically, erythroderma is a dermatological emergency owing to its systemic implications, but it has heterogeneity that necessitates an advanced method of classification and treatment. It is important to note the extent and cause of erythroderma, as its clinical appearance tends to overlap with other dermatological emergencies, to avoid immediate diagnosis. The condition's classification is determined through a multidisciplinary evaluation that may include biopsy, serologic testing, and detailed drug history. Such a comprehensive assessment differentiates erythroderma from other syndromes, making for targeted therapies and care support plans that address cutaneous injury alongside systemic danger. On this basis, erythroderma is classified alongside SJS, TEN, and necrotizing fasciitis as a severe disease that warrants rapid treatment due to its potential to cause life-threatening consequences (Almoalli & Cheikh, 2021).

12.3.2. Causes and Underlying Conditions

The precipitating causes of dermatologic emergencies , such as Stevens-Johnson Syndrome (SJS) and Toxic Epidermal Necrolysis (TEN) are also multifactorial, typically involving immune-mediated processes started primarily by drugs. Drugs , such as anticonvulsants, sulfonamides, and allopurinol have been frequent offenders, but drug hypersensitivity has emerged as an etiologic factor in these severe cutaneous adverse drug reactions. Apart from drugs, infections , such as Mycoplasma pneumoniae have also been reported as precipitants, predominantly in the pediatric population. The pathophysiology involves an abnormal immune reaction in which cytotoxic T cells induce widespread keratinocyte apoptosis, leading to extensive epidermal separation. Besides environmental stimuli, host predispositions, particularly certain HLA alleles, also dictate susceptibility, displaying a balance between environmental and host determinants. An understanding of these causes is instrumental in developing early detection and prevention strategies to reduce the morbidity and mortality associated with SJS and TEN. Underlying systemic illness is an important contributory factor in the pathogenesis of erythroderma and has a propensity to complicate the course of the disease. Chronic dermatoses like eczema and psoriasis are capable of advancing to erythroderma when propagated by infections, drug eruptions, or withdrawal from therapy. Hematologic neoplasias like cutaneous T-cell lymphoma also have a penchant to develop erythroderma as their first sign, suggesting neoplastic skin invasion. Diffuse inflammation and epidermal hyperproliferation cause widespread disruption of the cutaneous barrier, leaving patients at risk of secondary infection and metabolic consequences. Immune dysregulation, which may be linked to cytokine imbalances, underlies these alterations, underscoring the need for rigorous diagnostic evaluation to identify causative factors. The multifactorial etiology of erythroderma requires a multidisciplinary treatment approach that addresses the primary etiology and systemic involvement to optimize patient outcomes. Necrotizing fasciitis is a rapidly progressive soft-tissue infection that typically results from polymicrobial invasion following trauma, surgery, or comorbidities such as diabetes mellitus and immunosuppression. Infection leads to widespread necrosis of fascia and subcutaneous tissue, driven by bacterial exotoxins and an agonal host inflammatory response. While a predominant pathogen is Group A *Streptococcus*, anaerobic and facultative organism synergy frequently complicates the infectious field. Invasive infections are characterized by local predisposing conditions (i.e., disruption of the skin) coupled with systemic susceptibilities (i.e., peripheral vascular disease), thereby heightening risk. The pathogenesis is microvascular thrombosis and consequent tissue ischemia, which enhances tissue destruction. Prompt identification of such predisposed conditions is very important, as delays in diagnosis drive mortality rates dramatically. Treatment is based on early surgical debridement combined with empirical, broad-spectrum antimicrobial therapy directed at the identified pathogens, reflecting the severity of this cutaneous emergency (Almoalli & Cheikh, 2021) (Figure 12.8).

Causes	Frequency (%)
Psoriasis	11 (36.6)
Eczema	8 (26.7)
Drug-induced erythroderma	5 (16.7)
Colloidan baby	1 (3.3)
Pityriasis rubra pilaris	1 (3.3)
Idiopathic	4 (13.3)

Figure 12.8. Causes of erythroderma.

Source: https://www.researchgate.net/publication/342442514/figure/tbl1/AS:906294873579521@1593088944278/Causes-of-erythroderma-n30.png.

12.3.3. Symptoms and Systemic Effects

The dermatologic emergency cutaneous manifestations typically extend deep into the underlying systemic manifestations, with dramatic effects on patient outcomes. For instance, in Toxic Epidermal Necrolysis (TEN) and Stevens-Johnson Syndrome (SJS), patients experience a prodromal flu-like illness characterized by fever, malaise, and sore throat before the typical mucocutaneous erosions. These systemic prodromal signs are indicative of generalized immune activation and are often associated with tender erythematous macules and generalized epidermal shedding. Involvement is not limited to the skin; mucous membranes—the oral, ocular, and genital areas—are frequently affected, leading to serious complications such as conjunctivitis and respiratory compromise. These emergent syndromes require early recognition and treatment, as the systemic immune response drives the high morbidity and mortality associated with these conditions (Jacquline et al., 2018). In erythroderma, a cutaneous emergency characterized by widespread erythema and scaling of the skin exceeding 90% of body surface area, both severe cutaneous inflammation and the physiologic demands imposed by an abnormal skin barrier contribute to systemic effects. The patient typically presents with features of high fever, chills, lymphadenopathy, and hemodynamic instability, manifesting a systemic inflammatory response. The compromised skin barrier renders these patients prone to increased transepidermal water loss, thermoregulatory failure, and secondary infections, contributing to systemic complications. Metabolic requirements are also increased due to the skin's heightened turnover and inflammatory state, resulting in subsequent hypoproteinemia and nutritional insufficiency. Thus, erythroderma emerges as a multisystem disorder requiring urgent management with multidisciplinary intervention to address cutaneous instability in addition to systemic derangements (Jacquline et al., 2018). Necrotizing fasciitis does have severe progressive soft tissue destruction and systemic toxicity that emphasizes the extensive systemic ramifications, all too often superseding the presenting local infection. Early presentation includes painful out-of-proportion-to-visual skin changes, fever, tachycardia, and hypotension foretelling impending septic shock. The infection advances aggressively along fascial planes, leading to widespread tissue necrosis and severe inflammatory responses that may culminate in multi-organ failure. Laboratory abnormalities, including leukocytosis, elevated C-reactive protein, and metabolic acidosis, are common and correlate with the degree of systemic disease. If not treated with aggressive surgical measures and aggressive supportive care, mortality is considerable. This virulence underscores the need for early diagnosis and multidisciplinary treatment regimens that address not only the cutaneous devastation but also the systemic inflammatory cascade (Castello et al., 2020).

Test Your Knowledge

1. What is erythroderma, and how is it classified?
2. What are the common causes and underlying conditions that lead to erythroderma?
3. What are the main symptoms observed in patients with erythroderma?

12.4. Necrotizing Fasciitis

Learning Outcome

1. Understand the definition and types of necrotizing fasciitis.
2. Describe risk factors and common pathogens associated with necrotizing fasciitis.
3. Discuss clinical signs and urgency of treatment.

Understanding the emergent nature of certain dermatologic diseases is central to clinical practice, as subtle early findings can rapidly progress to life-threatening manifestations. Necrotizing fasciitis is an example of such an emergency, a rapidly progressive infection that results in necrosis of skin, fat, and tissue overlying the muscle. Its early presentations may resemble benign cellulitis or even mild soft-tissue infection, with the risk of misdiagnosis. But the swift course, so characteristically with undue pain, systemic toxicity, and skin discoloration, should alert clinicians to a deeper, invasive process. Prompt recognition in primary care or emergency clinics is critical because delay greatly aggravates morbidity and mortality. Emergency room physicians and family medicine physicians, therefore, need to be adept at detecting necrotizing fasciitis from less acute skin infections in order to initiate timely intervention (Alsudairy et al., 2023). Alertness may be the difference between life and catastrophe. The pathophysiology of necrotizing fasciitis is polymicrobial infection, usually by

Group A *Streptococcus, Staphylococcus aureus*, and anaerobes, with extension to contiguous muscles, leading to extensive tissue necrosis within a short period through exotoxin production and ischemia. The clinical path can run a course of hours, with systemic inflammatory response syndrome and multi-organ failure if left untreated. Diagnosis is dependent on a high level of suspicion supplemented by the clinical picture and laboratory findings , such as elevated white blood cell count, hyponatremia, and lactic acidosis. Imaging modalities such as MRI or CT scans may delineate fascial involvement, but surgical exploration remains the diagnostic and therapeutic gold standard. Management requires emergent surgical debridement, broad-spectrum antibiotics, and supportive critical care. Multidisciplinary care must be coordinated, and intensive monitoring may be required alongside multiple operative interventions, underscoring the severity of this dermatologic emergency (Kellen, R., & Berlin, J. M., 2018).

Necrotizing fasciitis is especially noteworthy among dermatologic emergencies due to its aggressive nature and the need for urgent intervention. Compared with more severe dermatologic conditions, such as Stevens-Johnson Syndrome or erythroderma, necrotizing fasciitis poses a challenge for clinicians because it often presents in the early stages as a milder infection, delaying treatment. Education and awareness are most critical for healthcare practitioners to improve rates of early detection and treatment. Referral for surgery and intensive care at specialized centers is generally warranted. In addition, advances in wound care, reconstructive surgery, and supportive therapies such as intravenous immunoglobulin have contributed to improved outcomes but cannot compensate for the need for early diagnosis. Overall, necrotizing fasciitis is a critical intersection of dermatology and emergency medicine that underscores the importance of rapid, aggressive intervention to preserve life and limb (Alsudairy et al., 2023; Kellen, R., & Berlin, J. M., 2018) (Figure 12.9).

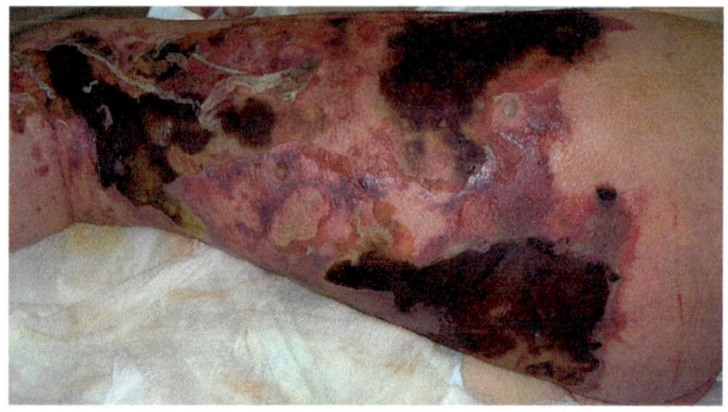

Figure 12.9. Person with necrotizing fasciitis. The left leg shows extensive redness and tissue death.

Source: https://upload.wikimedia.org/wikipedia/commons/thumb/6/6a/Necrotizing_fasciitis_left_leg.JPEG/1024px-Necrotizing_fasciitis_left_leg.JPEG.

12.4.1. Definition and Types of Necrotizing Fasciitis

The dermatologic emergency spectrum encompasses a range of severe conditions that should be identified and managed early. Among them, necrotizing fasciitis is one of the most virulent soft-tissue infections, with destruction of subcutaneous tissue and fascial planes occurring within minutes. It is typically underdiagnosed in its early stages due to its nonspecific presentation, but rapidly advances to lead to systemic toxicity and death if not urgently treated. Necrotizing fasciitis is clinically defined by widespread necrosis of the fascia and cover tissues with disproportionate pain out of proportion to the extent of visible skin alterations. Knowledge of the pathophysiology and presentation will help distinguish it from other cutaneous emergencies, such as SJS or TEN, which are characterized by nearly entirely epidermal detachment rather than deep tissue necrosis. These distinctions emphasize the importance of recognizing necrotizing fasciitis among dermatologic emergencies to initiate immediate medical and surgical intervention (Almoalli & Cheikh, 2021).

Necrotizing fasciitis is typically classified into types based on microbial etiology and clinical presentation. Type I, the most common, involves a polymicrobial infection typically comprising aerobic and anaerobic bacteria, such as *Bacteroides* species and Enterobacteriaceae, which synergistically contribute to tissue destruction. Type II is caused predominantly by monomicrobial infections, frequently by Group A *Streptococcus*, which is responsible for rapid disease progression and systemic toxicity. Less commonly, Type III necrotizing fasciitis results from marine organisms like *Vibrio vulnificus*, while Type IV is fungal in origin. Both forms of MD pose unique challenges in diagnosis and management, including the use of pathogen-specific knowledge to guide antibiotic therapy and surgical debridement. Delineation of these forms is critical on the basis of variation in clinical presentation, risk factors, and patient prognosis, which reflects the importance of correct classification within the paradigm of emergency dermatology (Almoalli & Cheikh, 2021). In the clinical setting, recognition of the diverse presentations of necrotizing fasciitis requires a multidisciplinary approach, with clinical suspicion informed by laboratory findings and imaging results.

The patient may initially present with erythema, edema, and intense pain, often accompanied by systemic signs , such as fever and hypotension. The rapid progression to skin color alteration, bullae, and necrosis typically signifies advanced disease and warrants emergent surgical consultation. Earlier laboratory indicators, such as elevated white blood cell count, C-reactive protein, and serum creatinine, help gauge severity but are not specific. Studies on imaging like MRI and CT scans provide crucial information about the extent of involvement of the fascia and guide therapeutic planning. Adding this wide-ranging diagnostic strategy enhances early identification and management of necrotizing fasciitis, distinguishing it from other skin emergencies such as SJS, TEN, and erythroderma, which have characteristic clinical and pathological presentations (Almoalli & Cheikh, 2021) (Figure 12.10).

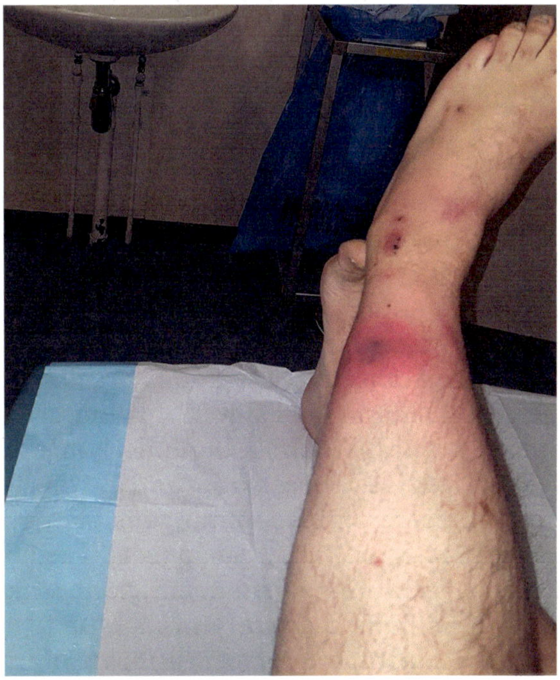

Figure 12.10. Early symptoms of necrotizing fasciitis. The darker red center is going black.

Source: https://upload.wikimedia.org/wikipedia/commons/thumb/b/bd/Early_symptoms_of_NF.jpg/800px-Early_symptoms_of_NF.jpg.

12.4.2. Risk Factors and Common Pathogens

Several predisposing conditions underlie the progression of dermatologic emergencies, which typically increase their severity and complicate their clinical course in most cases. Immunocompromised states from HIV infection, malignancy, or secondary to iatrogenic causes , such as chemotherapy and immunosuppressive therapy significantly predispose to life-threatening cutaneous adverse drug reactions

, such as Stevens-Johnson Syndrome (SJS) and Toxic Epidermal Necrolysis (TEN). Genetic predispositions, as defined by specific human leukocyte antigen (HLA) alleles, have been associated with an increased risk of these disorders following exposure to certain drugs, including anticonvulsants, sulfonamides, and nonsteroidal anti-inflammatory drugs. Additionally, underlying systemic diseases, including autoimmune disease, can enhance skin disease through dysregulated immune mechanisms. Clinicians can tailor prevention and early therapy to reduce progression and mortality in these acute dermatologic syndromes by understanding these factors. In contrast, necrotizing fasciitis has a distinct risk factor profile, characterized by alterations in cutaneous integrity and heightened systemic vulnerability. Trauma, surgical wounds, or underlying skin disease provide portals of entry for soft tissue plane-colonizing pathogens. Patients with diabetes mellitus, peripheral vascular disease, or chronic renal insufficiency have impaired immune defense and altered tissue perfusion, constituting the ideal environment for rapid infection spread. Predominant pathogens implicated are group A *Streptococcus* (*Streptococcus pyogenes*), *Staphylococcus aureus*, with or without methicillin resistance, and polymicrobial synergisms with facultative and anaerobic bacteria. Such pathogens are likely to release virulence factors that contribute to deep-tissue necrosis and systemic toxin production, thereby necessitating prompt surgical and antimicrobial intervention. Understanding these risk factors enables early detection and aggressive management, which are necessary to prevent excessive mortality from necrotizing fasciitis. Erythroderma, characterized by widespread erythema and scaling involving more than 90% of the body surface area, is often multifactorial in etiology, with specific pathogenetic associations. Precipitating causes usually involve flare-ups of pre-existing dermatoses, such as psoriasis or atopic dermatitis, drug reactions, and neoplasms, such as cutaneous T-cell lymphoma. Infectious etiologies could also be present, particularly where secondary bacterial overgrowth or viral infections are introduced into the clinical picture. Whereas *Staphylococcus aureus* commonly colonizes erythrodermic skin and causes superinfection, the pathogenesis of this condition is often accompanied by multifaceted immune dysregulation, causing epidermal barrier compromise. Their identification as risk factors and the contribution of microbial pathogens to the process are paramount in driving supportive treatment and specific antimicrobial therapies with a view to optimizing clinical outcomes in a condition that often entails systemic complications. (Almoalli & Cheikh, 2021).

12.4.3. Clinical Signs and Urgency of Treatment

Early identification of cutaneous signs in cutaneous emergencies is necessary because of the threat of quick systemic deterioration and death. For conditions Stevens-Johnson Syndrome (SJS) and Toxic Epidermal Necrolysis (TEN), early signs and symptoms are typically flu-like and progress rapidly to a painful blistering dermatitis with mucous membrane involvement. The epidermal peeling and diffuse erythema, which are characteristic, describe widespread disruption of the cutaneous barrier leading to fluid loss and infection risk requiring emergency intervention. Similarly, the cessation of fever, alteration in mentation, and hypotension in these patients are indicators of deterioration to systemic inflammatory response syndrome (SIRS) and the need for emergency intensive care treatment. Recognition of these initial clinical features is crucial for early discontinuation of offending drugs, symptomatic management, and referral to specialists, underscoring the importance of maintaining a high level of suspicion in high-risk patients (Adaskevich, 2016). Clinical presentation, such as generalized erythema covering more than 90% of the body surface area and scaling and pruritus accompanying it, needs to be properly assessed while treating erythroderma because the syndrome can complicate into life-threatening conditions. The thermoregulatory and protective functions of the skin are disrupted in erythroderma, thus increasing the risk of infection, fluid, and electrolyte imbalance. Urgent treatment priorities aim to identify the primary causes—drug reactions, malignancies, and everything in between—and to initiate supportive treatments such as fluid balance, nutrition, and infection management. The severity of epidermal growth in erythroderma makes it necessary to carefully monitor for systemic complications , such as sepsis or cardiac failure, thereby emphasizing the need for early diagnosis and treatment (Adaskevich, 2016). Necrotizing fasciitis presents one of the most acute dermatologic uses thereof can be sufficiently disturbed to alter its normal function, and one of the most miserable of diseases. There are several precipitating conditions that may be involved in the pathogenesis of necrotizing fasciitis, including fever, tachycardia, hypotension, and severe sepsis or septic shock, which necessitate immediate surgical debridement and broad-spectrum antibiotics. The window of opportunity for successful intervention in necrotizing fasciitis is brief; delays exponentially increase mortality. Early diagnosis is facilitated by the initial presentation being cellulitic, a factor emphasizing the need for diagnostic vigilance and aggressive management to prevent massive tissue loss and multi-organ failure.

Test Your Knowledge

1. What is necrotizing fasciitis, and what are its main types?
2. What risk factors increase the likelihood of developing necrotizing fasciitis?

12.5. Diagnostic Approaches

Learning Outcome

1. Discuss about clinical evaluation and history taking for managing dermatologic emergencies.
2. Understand laboratory tests and imaging studies.
3. Focus on differential diagnosis considerations.

Early detection of dermatologic emergencies requires a nuanced approach that integrates clinical expertise with rapid assessment tools. Patients coming in for emergency treatment are likely to present with cumulating signs like diffuse erythema, blistering, or necrosis, which can obscure the diagnosis if carefully separated. Patient history of recent drug use and prior infections makes up the foundation of differentiation of Stevens-Johnson Syndrome (SJS) and Toxic Epidermal Necrolysis (TEN) from other acute dermatoses. For instance, mucosal involvement and acute epidermal detachment are traditional features which require immediate recognition. Invasive skin biopsies, though disruptive, provide definitive diagnosis by revealing characteristic histopathologic features , such as epidermal necrosis of the entire thickness in TEN. Emergency and family physicians should maintain a heightened index of suspicion and initiate early intervention, as delay is strongly associated with morbidity and mortality in cases such as SJS/TEN (Alfuraih et al., 2023).

Erythroderma, meanwhile, requires a systematic diagnostic approach since it has diverse etiologies ranging from drug reactions to secondary systemic illness. Diagnosticians should give primary consideration to distinguishing erythroderma from other generalized skin inflammation by detailed clinical examination and specific laboratory investigations. Complete blood counts and inflammatory markers in blood studies allow one to differentiate between systemic involvement, while skin biopsies reveal minute findings , such as lymphocytic infiltration, which result in certain diagnoses. The diagnostic strategy is also aided by the inclusion of imaging investigations in the case of suspected systemic complications, that is, infections or malignancies, which usually accompany widespread involvement of the skin. Given the high complexity of erythroderma, a multidisciplinary assessment is essential to ensure accurate diagnosis of the underlying cause and timely treatment (Almoalli & Cheikh, 2021).

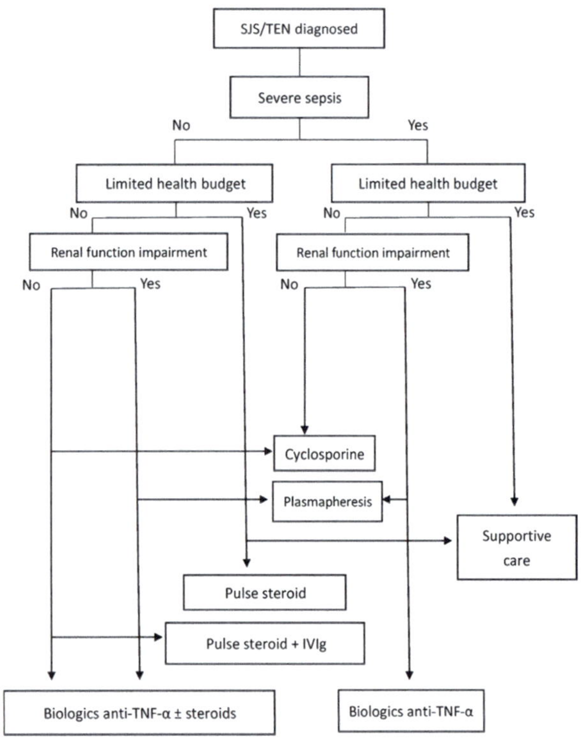

Figure 12.11. Algorithm for choosing systemic treatments for SJS/TEN.

Source: https://www.researchgate.net/publication/363063523/figure/fig1/AS:11431281210349294@1702045667502/Algorithm-for-choosing-systemic-treatments-for-SJS-TEN.tif.

Necrotizing fasciitis also poses a clearly emergent diagnostic challenge owing to the acute progression and potentially life-threatening nature. Early clinical suspicion is critical, often triggered by disproportionate pain, swelling, erythema, and systemic signs , such as fever or sepsis. Diagnostic imaging, for example, magnetic resonance imaging (MRI) and computed tomography (CT), facilitates early diagnosis by delineating fascial plane involvement; however, confirmation depends on surgical exposure. Laboratory indicators, such as elevated white blood cell count and C-reactive protein levels, signal inflammatory activity but lack specificity. Prompt biopsy and microbiologic cultures guide definitive antimicrobial treatment and surgical debridement. Consultation with dermatology and surgical experts helps encourage a holistic diagnostic strategy, optimizing patient outcomes for this high-stakes emergency (Alfuraih et al., 2023) (Figure 12.11).

12.5.1. Clinical Evaluation and History Taking

Appropriate clinical evaluation is the backbone in the treatment of dermatologic emergencies , such as Stevens-Johnson Syndrome (SJS), Toxic Epidermal Necrolysis (TEN), erythroderma, and necrotizing fasciitis. Because of their acute presentation and severe morbidity, patients require meticulous and thorough history taking and physical examination. Obtaining the history of onset and progression of symptoms, recent drug intake, infection, or systemic symptoms can lead to early diagnosis and management. Particularly, a careful assessment of recent drug exposure is required because certain drugs may be habitual culprits of SJS and TEN. At the same time, the evaluation must emphasize the presence of systemic features of sepsis and multi-organ failure, which are commonly observed in these severe skin conditions. This broad clinical environment allows the providers to distinguish such emergencies from other cutaneous or systemic conditions that may mimic their presentation, and thus receive on-time, appropriate treatment. While taking history, a complete evaluation of the patient's past medical history, such as prior skin conditions, immune status, and associated illnesses, is crucial. For example, it may be secondary to underlying dermatoses or hematologic neoplasms, and the discovery of these associations not only affects diagnosis but also therapeutic management. Attention to chronology of symptoms, such as skin detachment sequence, distribution pattern of lesions, and mucosal involvement, also assists in refining the differential diagnosis. The clinician should note whether it is accompanied by systemic symptoms such as fever, malaise, and respiratory compromise to identify potential complications. Meticulous drug timeline and history of recent infection are important to ascertain, as evidence accumulates supporting a drug hypersensitivity reaction as the basic mechanism for most cutaneous emergencies like SJS and TEN. Moreover, assessment for possible risk factors, such as genetic predisposition or pre-existing immunosuppression, raises clinical suspicion and guides further testing. Physical examination complements history-taking by providing important visual and tactile information about the distribution and intensity of cutaneous disease. Cornerstone clinical findings such as epidermal detachment, a positive Nikolsky sign, and necrotic tissue help establish some diagnoses and guide immediate management. In necrotizing fasciitis, identification of evidence of out-of-proportion pain, edema, and erythema with aggressive extension can require emergent surgery. A comprehensive, systemic evaluation is also needed to assess airway patency, hydration, and organ function, as these conditions often present with multisystem involvement. Such extensive assessment calls for a multidisciplinary approach and synthesis of clinical skills, with the importance of directed examination techniques emphasized in rheumatology and dermatology literature (Almoalli & Cheikh, 2021). Hence, the integration of comprehensive history-taking and deliberate physical examination is the basis for accurate diagnosis and successful treatment planning in dermatological emergencies.

12.5.2. Laboratory Tests and Imaging Studies

The diagnosis of threatening skin diseases, such as Stevens-Johnson Syndrome (SJS) and Toxic Epidermal Necrolysis (TEN), essentially relies on the following particular laboratory tests to confirm clinical impressions and gauge the severity of system involvement. The initial evaluations typically include complete blood counts (CBCs) to assess for leukocytosis or anemia, which may indicate infection or systemic inflammation. Serum electrolyte panels are also necessary to identify electrolyte imbalances secondary to fluid loss from extensive skin denudation. Liver and kidney function tests are routinely monitored because these organs are frequently subjected to secondary insult from diffuse body involvement in these diseases. Furthermore, skin biopsies, although not technically laboratory tests, provide histopathologic evidence of necrotic keratinocytes and subepidermal bullae consistent with SJS/TEN, thereby informing appropriate treatment and diagnostic planning. For erythroderma, a comprehensive laboratory workup is critical in differentiating it from other dermatologic and systemic illnesses. Because of the polymorphous etiology of erythroderma-like drug reactions, malignancies, or exacerbation of underlying dermatoses, lab work tries to identify the overall systemic status and etiology of the patient. Anemia or eosinophilia may be proven by a CBC to substantiate an allergic or neoplastic etiology. Inflammatory markers, such as erythrocyte sedimentation rate (ESR) and C-reactive protein (CRP), are used to determine the degree of systemic inflammation. Liver function tests and renal function tests screen for organ impairment commonly associated with severe erythroderma. These tests determine the urgency and type of intervention required, enabling clinicians to tailor therapies to achieve optimal patient outcomes. Necrotizing fasciitis is a surgical emergency that requires immediate imaging to complement clinical examination for early diagnosis and therapy. Although laboratory results showing elevated white blood cell count and C-reactive protein indicate the severity of infection, imaging modalities provide important anatomical information. Sonography may quickly reveal fluid accumulation or gas within soft tissues, suggesting necrotizing processes. Computed tomography (CT) scans provide higher-resolution images that delineate fascial plane involvement and the extent of tissue destruction, thereby guiding surgical debridement planning. Magnetic resonance imaging (MRI) is particularly valuable in cases of uncertainty due to its excellent soft-tissue contrast. These laboratory and imaging techniques together ensure prompt, accurate diagnosis of necrotizing fasciitis, thereby improving the likelihood of successful treatment and survival (Almoalli & Cheikh, 2021) (Figure 12.12).

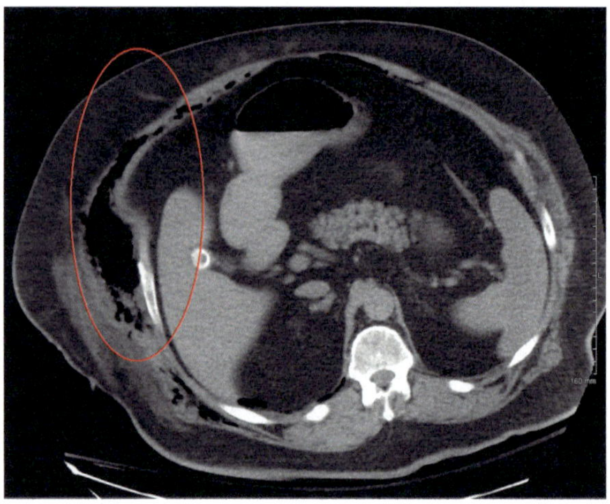

Figure 12.12. Necrotizing fasciitis producing gas in the soft tissues as seen on CT scan.

Source: https://upload.wikimedia.org/wikipedia/commons/thumb/f/fb/Pnecrotisingfasc.png./800px-Pnecrotisingfasc.png.

12.5.3. Differential Diagnosis Considerations

Accurate assessment in cutaneous emergencies requires the ability to distinguish among conditions that present similarly. Stevens-Johnson Syndrome (SJS) and Toxic Epidermal Necrolysis (TEN), for instance, both have mucocutaneous blistering and epidermal sloughing, but differentiating is based on the extent of cutaneous and systemic involvement. Also important is the discrimination of these disorders from life-threatening drug reactions , such as erythroderma, which presents with generalized erythema and scaling but frequently lacks the necrotic epidermal detachment of SJS/TEN. Inappropriate failure to diagnose the underlying disease can render timely interventions useless, so the role of total clinical examination in conjunction with histopathological correlation, where available, cannot be overemphasized. Differential diagnosis, therefore, depends on correlating clinical presentation with history in the patient, including recent exposure to drugs, infection, or systemic illnesses, to tailor proper management plans. Differential diagnosis of necrotizing fasciitis from other dermatological emergencies is also more challenging because of its fulminant soft-tissue extension and virulence. Unlike SJS, TEN, or erythroderma, necrotizing fasciitis with deeper fascial plane and subcutaneous tissue involvement is preceded by out-of-proportion pain and systemic toxicity. The initial presentation may imitate cellulitis or acute soft tissue infection so that diagnosis is delayed. Radiological modalities MRI or CT may be helpful in cases of clinical suspicion by demonstrating gas in soft tissues or fascial edema, whereas definitive diagnosis relies on surgical exploration and tissue biopsy. Differentiation is needed, since necrotizing fasciitis necessitates emergent surgical debridement with concomitant broad-spectrum antibiotics, as opposed to the mainly supportive or immunomodulatory treatments employed for

SJS, TEN, or erythroderma (Almoalli & Cheikh, 2021). Interdisciplinary investigation optimizes diagnostic accuracy, especially in ambiguous cases. Attention to mimicking conditions is important, since autoimmune blistering diseases, drug reaction with eosinophilia and systemic symptoms, severe cutaneous adverse reactions, and infectious etiologies can present similarly to SJS, TEN, erythroderma, or necrotizing fasciitis. *Pemphigus vulgaris* and bullous pemphigoid involve blistering and erosions but typically have more indolent courses and usual immunopathologic findings. Similarly, staphylococcal scalded skin syndrome (SSSS) may present with SJS/TEN-like epidermal peeling, with a predilection for infants and young children and mucous membrane sparing. Exclusion of concurrent dermatoses, such as exacerbated psoriasis or cutaneous lymphoma, influences therapeutic decisions in erythroderma. A multidisciplinary diagnostic strategy with input from dermatopathology, microbiology, and laboratory markers remains invaluable in the appropriate differentiation of these entities and optimizing patient outcomes.

Test Your Knowledge

1. Why is a thorough clinical evaluation and patient history essential in diagnosing dermatologic emergencies?
2. What laboratory tests are commonly used to support the diagnosis of severe skin conditions?
3. How can imaging studies aid in the assessment of dermatologic emergencies like necrotizing fasciitis?

12.6. Treatment Strategies

Learning Outcome

1. Understand general management principles for dermatologic emergencies.
2. Focus on specific treatments for SJS and TEN.
3. Manage erythroderma and necrotizing fasciitis.

Effective management of dermatologic emergencies , such as Stevens-Johnson Syndrome (SJS) and Toxic Epidermal Necrolysis (TEN) involves early identification and supportive treatment to avoid morbidity and mortality. Stabilization, in most cases, includes fluid resuscitation and wound care identical to burn therapy, with emphasis on preventing secondary infection and correcting electrolytes. Termination of the offending agent also forms a top priority since these conditions are most often drug-induced. Adjunctive therapies, including systemic corticosteroids and intravenous immunoglobulins, remain controversial but are applied in some clinical settings to modulate the immune response. Improved treatment outcomes result from multidisciplinary coordination with dermatology, intensive care, and infectious diseases specialists. Early recognition and individualized supportive treatment are of utmost importance, emphasizing prompt diagnosis and appropriate referral pathways through primary care given the rapid progression of these syndromes and the risk of systemic complications (Alfuraih et al., 2023).

Necrotizing fasciitis requires aggressive, multimodal treatment due to its violent progression and high mortality. Surgical debridement of the necrotic tissue is the treatment of choice and should be performed urgently to cut off the spread of infection. Empiric intravenous broad-spectrum antibiotics are administered before culture results guide specific therapy to a polymicrobial infection characteristic of the disease. Supportive treatment in an intensive care unit setting is aimed at hemodynamic stability, pain management, and sepsis or organ failure.

Adjunctive treatment, including hyperbaric oxygen therapy, has been explored but remains adjunctive rather than active. Early diagnosis and intervention beginning at the primary level play a significant role in prognosis, emphasizing the importance of attention to dermatologic emergencies by family physicians (Alfuraih et al., 2023). Erythroderma presents unique treatment challenges that emphasize the identification and management of underlying etiologies, which in most cases are exacerbations of pre-existing dermatoses, infections, or drug reactions. Supportive therapy is aimed at restoring skin barrier integrity and managing symptoms such as pruritus, desquamation, and fluid imbalance. Severe illness may occasionally require hospitalization for optimization of observation and implementation of systemic therapy in the form of corticosteroids or immunosuppressants once the etiology has been established. Because of the diverse clinical presentation and possibly lethal complications , such as thermoregulatory instability or secondary infection, accurate diagnosis followed by targeted therapy is essential. Family physicians and dermatologists must collaborate to adhere to guidelines and ensure continuity of care, ultimately resulting in improved outcomes in this high-risk patient population (Alfuraih et al., 2023).

12.6.1. General Principles of Management of Dermatologic Emergencies

Management of dermatologic emergencies requires an all-encompassing approach that prioritizes prompt diagnosis and patient stabilization. The primary assessment should be addressed in the sequence of airway, breathing, and circulation because in serious skin conditions , such as Stevens-Johnson Syndrome (SJS) and Toxic Epidermal Necrolysis (TEN), Sepsis, acute respiratory distress, or fluid imbalance is a common complication. Prompt identification of the precipitant, usually drug-related, and causative agent removal are crucial actions to prevent aggravation of the course. Supportive care is central, particularly in fluid and electrolyte management, infection prevention, and maintenance of skin integrity through wound care, in a manner akin to burn techniques. Multidisciplinary care, with the active involvement of dermatologists, intensivists, and infectious disease specialists, enhances outcomes through integrated management that prevents and corrects systemic complications most frequently associated with these illnesses (Almoalli & Cheikh, 2021).

Once the acute phase is stabilized, attention shifts to individualized therapy to modulate the underlying infectious or inflammatory process specific to the dermatologic emergency. With conditions like necrotizing fasciitis, aggressive surgical debridement and broad-spectrum intravenous antibiotics are needed to prevent rapid loss of tissue and systemic toxicity. With erythroderma, however, careful evaluation of the causative agent—drug, infection, or related to malignancy—is necessary to control the choice of treatment, such as corticosteroids or immunosuppressive agents. Careful monitoring for complications such as secondary infection, metabolic disturbances, and organ system failure is essential throughout the course of care. Treatment guidelines emphasize careful attention to pain control and nutritional supplementation, both of which are important aspects of healing and patient comfort (Almoalli & Cheikh, 2021). In conjunction with clinical management, effective general principles emphasize early communication and documentation, patient education, and psychosocial support, since dermatologic emergencies are highly stressful and have sequelae beyond the initial presentation. Having clear lines of communication between medical staff ensures timely data and coordinated care plans, which can mean the difference between life and death in fast-evolving conditions like SJS/TEN and necrotizing fasciitis. Documentation of the medication history, clinical presentation, and response to therapy enables continuous assessment and the development of secondary prevention strategies. Moreover, patient and family education on disease status, complications, and warning signs of recurrence is crucial for improving prognosis and adherence to follow-up management. The inclusion of psychological support centers also addresses the psychological trauma of visible loss of skin and disfigurement, a characteristic indicative of an all-around approach to management of dermatologic emergencies (Almoalli & Cheikh, 2021).

12.6.2. Specific Treatments for SJS and TEN

Treatment of Stevens-Johnson Syndrome (SJS) and Toxic Epidermal Necrolysis (TEN) is complex and aimed at halting disease progression while maintaining vital organ function. Treatment begins with the discontinuation of the offending drug at the earliest, which is necessary to prevent inducing additional epidermal damage. Supportive care is still the mainstay and may involve intensive care or a burn unit due to extensive loss of skin. Fluid resuscitation, electrolyte management, and infection prevention are optimized to maintain homeostasis and minimize the risk of mortality. Wound management methods incorporate approaches similar to those used in burn management, including the use of non-adherent dressings and close observation to prevent secondary infection. Management of pain and nutrition also significantly affects patient outcomes, informing an intensive treatment protocol tailored to patient requirements and the extent of epidermal detachment. These initial measures set the stage for adjunctive therapies aimed at modulating the immune response. Immunomodulatory therapies aim to counteract the uncontrolled inflammatory cascade in SJS and TEN. Systemic corticosteroids have been the traditional option due to their potent anti-inflammatory effect. Their use remains controversial, however, due to conflicting evidence regarding efficacy and infection risk. Intravenous immunoglobulin (IVIG) therapy is a second adjunct, working through neutralization of Fas ligand-induced keratinocyte apoptosis, which plays a key role in disease pathogenesis. While evidence of benefit in arresting epidermal detachment and promoting healing has been noted in some studies, heterogeneity in clinical trial outcomes has precluded widespread approval.

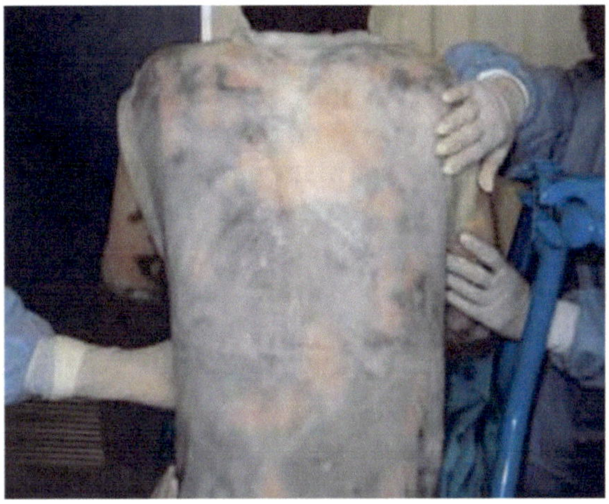

Figure 12.13. Care of the skin in SJS/TEN.

Source: https://www.researchgate.net/profile/Rannakoe-Lehloenya/publication/281003632_Management_of_Steven-Joh nson_s yndrome_and_toxic_epide rmal_necrolysis/links/59a8ae2baca27202ed5f53c2/Management-of-Steven-Johnso n-syndrome-and-toxic-epidermal-necrolysis.pdf?_tp=eyJjb250ZXh0I jp7ImZpcnN0UGFnZSI6Il9kaXJlY3QiLCJwYWdlIjoicHVibGljYXRpb24ifX0.

Other immunosuppressants, such as cyclosporine, are promising by inhibiting T-cell mediated cytotoxicity, potentially reducing mortality. Nonetheless, no single immunotherapy has definitively demonstrated sustained superiority, underscoring the need for personalized treatment within multidisciplinary teams. Newly developed insights into immune-related toxicities that arise from cancer therapy offer valuable lessons that can be applied to SJS and TEN care. Immune checkpoint inhibitors (ICIs), while revolutionizing oncologic treatment, can potentially trigger severe dermatologic immune-related adverse events mimicking or exacerbating conditions like SJS/TEN. The dynamic nature of pharmacovigilance data underscores the importance of early detection and intervention to minimize such complications (Brém et al., 2020; Ardizzoni et al., 2020). This strategy underscores the overarching principle that immune modulation can be a double-edged sword, requiring fine adjustment. What has been learned from immune-oncology informs probable future directions, including targeted biologic therapy against specific inflammatory mediators implicated in epidermal necrolysis. Such precision medicine approaches might maximize treatment benefit through diminishing toxigenic immune activation while preserving vital host defense and thus enhance treatment for such fulminant dermatologic emergencies (Figure 12.13).

12.6.3. Management of Erythroderma and Necrotizing Fasciitis

Effective management of erythroderma depends on an early and exhaustive diagnostic approach because erythroderma normally precedes a systemic or cutaneous disease. The patient should first be stabilized by the clinician by addressing fluid and electrolyte imbalances, given the extensive cutaneous involvement, which predisposes to transepidermal water loss and infection. Supportive care entails meticulous monitoring for signs of secondary infection that may lead to septicemia, especially in a patient with predisposing comorbidities , such as diabetes mellitus and anemia. The treatment plan typically involves detection and cessation of the offending agent, particularly in drug-induced etiologies, and administration of systemic corticosteroids or immunosuppressants, depending on the underlying etiology. Multidisciplinary care integration with dermatology, infectious disease, and critical care services enhances outcomes because specialist wards are better equipped to manage the complexity of this life-threatening emergency (Skayem et al., 2024). A multidisciplinary effort is needed because erythroderma has a tendency to cause generalized skin barrier disturbance, which needs to be tightly controlled through infection control scrutiny (Adriana-Ionela et al., 2024). Necrotizing fasciitis is an aggressively progressive soft-tissue infection that requires early recognition and treatment to reduce mortality. Therapy involves aggressive surgical debridement of necrotic tissue and empiric broad-spectrum antibiotic therapy to cover polymicrobial pathogens, including *Staphylococcus aureus, Pseudomonas aeruginosa*, and Gram-negative bacilli. Early diagnosis typically relies on the presence of clinical markers , such as severe pain disproportionate to physical exam, systemic toxicity, and progressive erythema and edema. Adjunct therapy includes hemodynamic stabilization and close monitoring for emerging septic shock. Presence of comorbid conditions like chronic heart failure or immune suppression can exacerbate the disease course, underlining the importance of individualized care plans. Multimodal therapy also includes wound care modalities and may be supplemented by hyperbaric oxygen, although this is adjunctive. The requirement for early surgery, coupled with aggressive antimicrobial and supportive care, is the cornerstone of optimal necrotizing fasciitis treatment (Skayem et al., 2024; Adriana-Ionela et al., 2024).

Erythroderma and necrotizing fasciitis underscore the significance of dermatologic emergency skill based on networked care and innovative models for delivering care. Teledermatology initiatives, particularly urgent store-and-forward systems, have emerged as a means of optimizing patient triage and enabling rapid expert consultation without in-person referral to specialized dermatologic emergency departments. The model has been found to be beneficial in the management of serious cutaneous emergencies, including erythroderma and necrotizing fasciitis, by enabling rapid diagnosis and initiation of therapy. Besides, these telemedicine systems are useful in conserving limited healthcare resources and cutting down preventable hospitalizations, especially crucial at times of high patient flow and thinning manpower (Skayem et al., 2024). The measures underscore the importance of developing innovative dermatological emergency care systems that integrate technology with specialty expertise to further enhance patient care while addressing the workforce challenge of managing complex skin conditions (Adriana-Ionela et al., 2024) (Figure 12.14).

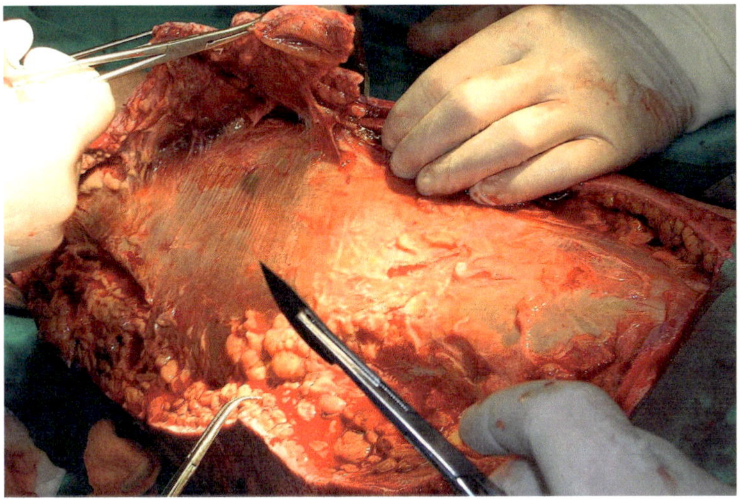

Figure 12.14. Necrotic tissue from the left leg was surgically removed.

Source: https://upload.wikimedia.org/wikipedia/commons/thumb/7/73/Necrotizing_fasciitis_left_leg_debridement.JPEG/1024px-Necrotizing_fasciitis_left_leg_debridement.JPEG.

Test Your Knowledge

1. What are the general management principles for handling dermatologic emergencies?
2. What specific treatments are recommended for patients with Stevens-Johnson Syndrome (SJS) and Toxic Epidermal Necrolysis (TEN)?

SUMMARY

The complexities associated with the management of skin emergencies, such as Stevens-Johnson Syndrome (SJS), Toxic Epidermal Necrolysis (TEN), erythroderma, and necrotizing fasciitis, require a multidisciplinary approach to optimize patient outcomes. These conditions often have overlapping clinical presentations that may complicate early diagnosis and intervention, underscoring the need for early recognition. Primary care physicians and emergency medicine physicians play a crucial role in detecting subtle skin manifestations before life-threatening deterioration. Implementation of evidence-based treatment protocols and supportive care interventions significantly contributes to survival and long-term morbidity. Furthermore, knowledge of the pathophysiological mechanisms that underlie these emergencies enhances clinical acumen and therapeutic precision. A combination of early diagnosis, withdrawal of causative drugs, and intravenous fluid replacement is the cornerstone of effective treatment and emphasizes the role of enhanced vigilance in clinical practice (Alfuraih et al., 2023). Despite enhanced diagnostic techniques and therapeutic regimens, mortality and morbidity with such life-threatening skin emergencies remain high, necessitating continued research and education. The rarity of conditions such as SJS and TEN predisposes to delayed referrals and inadequate management, highlighting the need for increased awareness among clinicians. Integrating recent literature with practice guidelines facilitates earlier diagnosis and tailored interventions, reducing the burden of complications. Multidisciplinary treatment, for example, by intensivists, rheumatologists, infectious disease specialists, and dermatologists, plays a vital role in successful overall management, especially in complex cases with systemic spread. Enhanced training and capacity in emergency departments can improve initial assessment, while ongoing educational initiatives ensure that frontline doctors remain aware of emerging treatment trends (Almoalli & Cheikh, 2021). In short, management of dermatologic emergencies, such as SJS, TEN, erythroderma, and necrotizing fasciitis, involves early detection and an aggregate treatment protocol to circumvent the increased morbidity and mortality hazards associated with these presentations. Early treatment and diagnosis minimize mortality and also prevent late complications that gravely affect patients' quality of life. Future efforts will need to focus on bridging knowledge gaps among healthcare providers through targeted educational programs and on developing standardized protocols. Improved communication between primary care and referral units will also enhance clinical outcomes. Ultimately, the integration of multidisciplinary care, evidence-based practice, and ongoing research will further advance the field, improving prognosis and patient safety in these life-threatening dermatologic emergencies (Almoalli & Cheikh, 2021; Alfuraih et al., 2023).

The complex management of dermatologic emergencies, such as Stevens-Johnson Syndrome (SJS), Toxic Epidermal Necrolysis (TEN), erythroderma, and necrotizing fasciitis, demands a profound understanding of their pathophysiology, clinical presentation, and therapeutic modalities. The conditions have superimposable manifestations involving extensive skin involvement and systemic sequelae, which could complicate the process of early diagnosis and cause a delay in life-sustaining therapies. Early diagnosis remains a feature, particularly between SJS and TEN based on body surface area affected, whereby their mortality rates vary significantly. Supportive care tailored to prevent secondary infection, fluid loss, and organ failure is required in all four conditions. Furthermore, coordination of multidisciplinary teams optimizes patient outcomes by addressing dermatological pathology alongside systemic manifestations, thereby making a holistic clinical approach essential. Central to treatment planning is the removal and identification of offending agents, especially drug offensives, which are the most relevant precipitants in SJS and TEN. Adjunctive treatments, although variably supported, are immunomodulatory medicines intravenous immunoglobulin or corticosteroids, whose use continues to be critically evaluated. Treatment in erythroderma is the reversal of the pathologic process, either inflammatory, infectious, or neoplastic, while preserving skin barrier integrity. Necrotizing fasciitis necessitates aggressive debridement surgery in conjunction with broad-spectrum antibiotics to halt fascial necrosis and systemic spread. Understanding these separable yet complementary principles of treatment underscores the imperative of timely intervention, alongside patient-specific variables such as comorbidities and immune status, to optimize prognosis in these dermatologic emergencies. Finally, management of the clinical complexity of SJS, TEN, erythroderma, and necrotizing fasciitis not only includes immediate diagnosis and supportive treatment but also relentless advances in therapeutic modalities to promote survival. The inclusion of organ system assessment, as emphasized in the rheumatology literature, is consistent with the multidisciplinary treatment modality necessary for these conditions (Almoalli & Cheikh, 2021). Even in the presence of evidence-based recommendations, patient-to-patient variability in clinical presentation necessitates individualized care plans that account for each patient's unique pathophysiological state and potential complications. Ultimately, heightened clinical awareness, ongoing research, and interprofessional collaboration remain essential to advancing understanding and management of these critical dermatologic emergencies, reducing mortality, and improving quality of life for affected patients.

KEY TERMS FROM THIS CHAPTER

- Anaerobic bacteria
- Antiepileptics
- Computed tomography (CT)
- Cutaneous T-cell lymphoma
- Dermatologic catastrophe
- Differential diagnosis
- Etiological contributors
- Functional recovery
- Healthcare resources
- Antibiotics
- Chronic kidney disease
- Cutaneous diseases
- Cytotoxic lymphocytes
- Dermatologic emergencies
- Erythroderma
- Exfoliative dermatitis
- Generalized skin inflammation
- HLA alleles

CRITICAL THINKING QUESTIONS

1. **Which of the following is most commonly associated with Stevens-Johnson Syndrome (SJS) and Toxic Epidermal Necrolysis (TEN)?**
   a. Viral infection
   b. Drug reaction
   c. Bacterial infection
   d. Food allergy
2. **Which of the following clinical features is most characteristic of erythroderma?**
   a. Vesicles and bullae
   b. Full-thickness necrosis
   c. Diffuse erythema involving >90% of the body surface area
   d. Localized red patches
3. **Which pathogen is most commonly implicated in necrotizing fasciitis?**
   a. *Pseudomonas aeruginosa*
   b. Group A *Streptococcus* (*Streptococcus pyogenes*)
   c. *Escherichia coli*
   d. *Staphylococcus epidermidis*
4. **What is the most appropriate initial diagnostic test for suspected necrotizing fasciitis?**
   a. MRI or CT scan of the affected area
   b. Skin biopsy
   c. Blood culture
   d. Punch biopsy of the lesion
5. **Which of the following is a key component of effective management of SJS/TEN?**
   a. Systemic corticosteroids only
   b. Empirical antibiotics for all patients
   c. Daily debridement of skin lesions
   d. Immediate cessation of the offending drug and supportive care in an ICU or burn unit

Short Answer Questions

1. What are the key clinical differences between Stevens-Johnson Syndrome (SJS) and Toxic Epidermal Necrolysis (TEN)?
2. What are the most common drug triggers for SJS and TEN, and how can these conditions be prevented?
3. How does erythroderma present clinically, and what underlying conditions are most frequently associated with it?
4. What are the typical signs and symptoms of necrotizing fasciitis, and which pathogens are most commonly responsible?
5. Which diagnostic tools and tests are critical in confirming SJS, TEN, and necrotizing fasciitis?
6. Why is early recognition and differential diagnosis important in dermatologic emergencies like SJS/TEN and necrotizing fasciitis?

Answer to Critical Thinking Questions

1. (b); 2. (c); 3. (b); 4. (a); 5. (d)

REFERENCES

1. Adaskevich, V. P. (2016). *Skin Diseases and Sexually Transmitted Infections.* https://core.ac.uk/download/80150454.pdf (accessed on 21st July 2025).
2. Alsudairy, N. M., Aljuhani, R. a. F., Alhassan, Z. a. J., Alharbi, A. S. A., Alshammari, H. S. A., Alshammari, H. M. F., Almalki, A. S. O., Alasmari, S. A., Alduhailan, Y. A., Alshmri, M. F., Alneami, A. M., Mansur, S. A., Alhuthayli, A. K. A., & Alsahli, H. M. (2023). Dermatological Emergencies in Family Medicine: recognition, management, and referral considerations. *Journal of Advanced Zoology*. https://doi.org/10.53555/jaz.v44i5.3389Alsudairy, N. M., Aljuhani, R. A. F., Alhassan, Z. A. J., Alharbi, A. S. A., Alshammari, H. S. A., Alshammari, H. M. F., Almalki, A. S. O., et al. (2023). Dermatological emergencies in family medicine: Recognition, management, and referral considerations. *Journal of Advanced Zoology, 44*(5). https://doi.org/10.53555/jaz.v44i5.3389 (accessed on 21st July 2025).
3. Ardizzoni, A., De Ponti, F., Gatti, M., Gelsomino, F., Poluzzi, E., & Raschi, E. (2020). Lessons to be learnt from real-world studies on immune-related adverse events with checkpoint inhibitors: A clinical perspective from pharmacovigilance. https://core.ac.uk/download/385957945.pdf (accessed on 21st July 2025).
4. Badia Castello, M., Casanova i Seuma, J. M., Codina, J., Montserrat, et al. (2020). Dermatological manifestations in the intensive care unit: A practical approach. https://core.ac.uk/download/421878579.pdf (accessed on 21st July 2025).
5. Berkeley, R. P., & Parker, J. R. (2010). Toxic epidermal necrolysis from a cigarette burns. https://core.ac.uk/download/pdf/8433926.pdf (accessed on 21st July 2025).
6. Brém, E., Koyfman, A., & Long, B. J. (2020). Oncologic emergencies: Immune-based cancer therapies and complications. https://core.ac.uk/download/305124082.pdf (accessed on 21st July 2025).
7. Chong, S., Jack, A. R., Nichols, B. J., et al. (2011). Cutaneous conditions leading to dermatology consultations in the emergency department. https://core.ac.uk/download/pdf/8656087.pdf (accessed on 21st July 2025).
8. Falodun, O., & Ogunbiyi, A. (2010). Dermatological emergencies: Current trends in management. https://core.ac.uk/download/478397283.pdf (accessed on 21st July 2025).
9. Jose, J. (2018). A pilot study of serum granulysin in drug-induced exanthems and severe cutaneous adverse reactions (SCARs). https://core.ac.uk/download/235668525.pdf (accessed on 21st July 2025).
10. Kellen, R., & Berlin, J. M. (2018). Dermatology emergencies. *Journal of the Dermatology Nurses' Association, 10*, 164–173. https://doi.org/10.1097/jdn.0000000000000394 (accessed on 21st July 2025).
11. Maalik Babu, A. N. M. (2015). A clinical study of non-venereal genital dermatoses. https://core.ac.uk/download/235667095.pdf (accessed on 21st July 2025).
12. Almoallim H, Cheikh M, editors. Skills in Rheumatology [Internet]. Singapore: Springer; 2021. Available from: https://www.ncbi.nlm.nih.gov/books/NBK585743/ doi: 10.1007/978-981-15-8323-0(accessed on 21st July 2025).
13. Pătraşcu, A. I., Vâţă, D., Temelie-Olinici, D., Mocanu, M., Guguluş, D. L., Marinescu, M., Stafie, L., et al. (2024). Skin lesions with loss of tissue and cutaneous-onset sepsis: The skin infection–

sepsis relationship. *Diagnostics, 14*, 659–659. https://doi.org/10.3390/diagnostics14060659 (accessed on 21st July 2025).

14. Skayem, C., Drahy, F., Hirsch, G., Hua, C., & Duong, T. A. (2024). Expertise in dermatologic emergencies: Real-world study on in-person vs. teledermatology emergencies in a reference center. *JDDG Journal der Deutschen Dermatologischen Gesellschaft, 22*, 1272–1274. https://doi.org/10.1111/ddg.15475 (accessed on 21st July 2025).

INDEX

C

D

F

G

H

I

K

L

M

N

O

Z